Channie Hui

ADVANCED
NUTRITION
and
HUMAN
METABOLISM

ADVANCED
NUTRITION
and
HUMAN
METABOLISM

James L. Groff
Georgia State University

Sareen S. Gropper
Auburn University

Sara M. Hunt

WEST PUBLISHING COMPANY
Minneapolis/St. Paul   New York   Los Angeles
San Francisco

Production Management: Michael Bass & Associates
Copyediting: Linda Purrington
Text and Cover Design: Linda Robertson
Composition: BookMasters, Inc.

WEST'S COMMITMENT TO THE ENVIRONMENT

In 1906, West Publishing Company began recycling materials left over from the production of books. This began a tradition of efficient and responsible use of resources. Today, up to 95 percent of our legal books and 70 percent of our college and school texts are printed on recycled, acid-free stock. West also recycles nearly 22 million pounds of scrap paper annually—the equivalent of 181,717 trees. Since the 1960s, West has devised ways to capture and recycle waste inks, solvents, oils, and vapors created in the printing process. We also recycle plastics of all kinds, wood, glass, corrugated cardboard, and batteries, and have eliminated the use of Styrofoam book packaging. We at West are proud of the longevity and the scope of our commitment to the environment.

Production, Prepress, Printing and Binding by West Publication Company.

 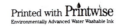

TEXT IS PRINTED ON 10% POST CONSUMER RECYCLED PAPER   Printed with **Printwise** Environmentally Advanced Water Washable Ink

British Library Cataloguing-in-Publication Data. A catalogue record for this book is available from the British Library.

Library of Congress Cataloging-in-Publication Data

Groff, James L.
    Advanced nutrition and human metabolism / James L. Groff, Sareen S.
  Gropper, Sara M. Hunt. — 2nd ed.
        p.   cm.
    Includes bibliographical references and index.
    ISBN 0-314-04467-1
    1. Nutrition.   2. Metabolism.   I. Gropper, Sareen Annora
  Stepnick.   II. Hunt, Sara M.   III. Title.
  QP141.G76   1995
  612.3\9—dc20
                                                    94-24711
                                                       CIP

DEDICATION

To Gerda for a level of spousal support and understanding above and beyond the call during this adventure.

Jim

To Michelle Lauren and Michael James Gropper, the little readers in my house, and to Daniel for his patience and support.

Sareen

BRIEF CONTENTS

CONTENTS

PREFACE

We conceived the first edition of *Advanced Nutrition and Human Metabolism*, published in 1990, to fill the need that teachers expressed for a text on normal metabolism, designed for upper-division nutrition students. The positive response to the first edition has encouraged us to maintain the same general scope, level, and organization of material in this edition. Most of the changes we have made concern new discoveries and reshaped concepts in the field. We have also used more examples, to help students better relate the printed word to current nutritional practice. In addition, helpful suggestions from reviewers and from both student and instructor users of the first edition have helped us revise the sequence of topics to provide a more natural flow of information.

Because this book focuses on normal human nutrition and physiologic function, students majoring in nutrition science and in dietetics can use it with equal effectiveness. As an advanced nutrition text, the book has been written for students at a level that presumes a sound background in the biological sciences. However, we review basic sciences—particularly biochemistry and physiology, which are important for understanding the material—at an appropriate level and scope, to rekindle faded memories. The text broadly applies biochemistry to nutrient use from consumption through digestion, absorption, distribution, and cellular metabolism, and is thus a valuable reference for health care workers. Health practitioners often want to refresh their memory of metabolic and physiologic interrelationships, or they want a concise update on current scientific discoveries or concepts related to human nutrition.

We have represented nutrition as the science that integrates life processes from the cellular level on through the multisystem operation of the whole organism. Our primary goal has been to give a comprehensive picture of cell reactions at the tissue, organ, and system levels. Subject matter was selected for its relevance in meeting this goal. The annotated bibliography familiarizes students with current research on each subtopic. We have also introduced a generous amount of cross-referencing, to strengthen the reader's access to indepth discussions of each topic.

Each of the 17 chapters begins with a topical outline followed by a brief introduction to that chapter's subject. Each chapter has a brief summary that ties together the ideas presented and concludes with an annotated bibliography. Fifteen of the chapters have as their final section one or two *Perspectives*. These relate chapter subject matter to a currently important aspect of human nutrition and health, and have their own annotated bibliographies.

We divided the text into five sections. Section I (Chapters 1, 2, and 3) focuses on the structure, function, and nourishment of the cell, and reviews energy transformation. Section II (Chapters 4 through 8) discusses the metabolism of macronutrients. In this section, we review primary metabolic pathways for carbohydrates, lipids, and proteins, emphasizing reactions that have particular relevance for health. We include a chapter on dietary fiber, and a chapter on the interrelationships among the macronutrient metabolic pathways as well as the metabolic dynamics of the feeding–fasting cycle.

Section III (Chapters 9 through 12) concern nutrients considered regulatory in nature: the vitamins (water- and fat-soluble), and the minerals, both macro and micro. These chapters cover nutrient features such as digestion, absorption, transport, function, metabolism, excretion, deficiency, and toxicity. We also discuss Recommended Dietary Allowances (RDAs) for each.

Section IV, "Homeostatic Maintenance," includes Chapters 13 through 16. We discuss, in order, body fluid and electrolyte balance, body composition, energy balance and weight control, and nutrition and the central nervous system. We singled out the central nervous system for discussion because of the current popular interest in relationships between nutrition and human behavior.

The last chapter (17) constitutes Section V. It is supplementary to the rest of the book. Titled "Experimental Design and Critical Interpretation of Research," this chapter discusses the types of research and the methodologies by which research can be conducted. The chapter is designed to familiarize the student with research organization and implementation, to point out problems and pitfalls inherent in research, and to help him or her critically evaluate scientific literature.

The appendices that round out the book include the following:

• Recommended Dietary Allowances 1989
• Calculation of available dietary iron
• Forms for estimating total energy expenditure
• Food exchange lists

A Glossary of Abbreviations follows.

ACKNOWLEDGMENTS

This textbook could not have been written without the helpful comments, encouragement, and patience of those close to us, both at the workplace and at home.

Our special thanks to our colleagues at Georgia State University and Auburn University for recognizing the size of the task, and showing the interest and understanding that "kept the wind at our backs."

We are indebted to Alexandra Grand, Frank Heredeen, and Lisa Stasco at Auburn University for their invaluable assistance in preparing the manuscript. We also wish to thank Michael Jenkins, at Kent State University, for his assistance in proofing the artwork and text.

Others to whom the authors owe special thanks are the reviewers whose thoughtful comments, criticisms, and suggestions were indispensable in shaping the text: Kathryn Anderson, Florida State University; Barbara Bayard, University of Wisconsin–Stout; Margaret Craig-Schmidt, Auburn University; Peter Horvath, SUNY at Buffalo; Silas Hung, University of California–Davis; Rita Johnson, Indiana University of Pennsylvania; Jay Kandiah, Ball State University; James Kirkland, University of Guelph; Robert D. Lee, Central Michigan University; Michael McIntosh, University of North Carolina–Greensboro; Kris Morey, California Polytechnic State University–San Luis Obispo; Phylis Moser-Veillon, University of Maryland; Amy Olson, College of St. Benedict; Arlette Rasmussen, University of Delaware; Kathryn Silliman, California State University–Chico; Robert Tyzbir, University of Vermont; Simin Bolourchi Vaghefi, University of North Florida; and Marian Wang, University of Georgia.

CELLS AND THEIR NOURISHMENT

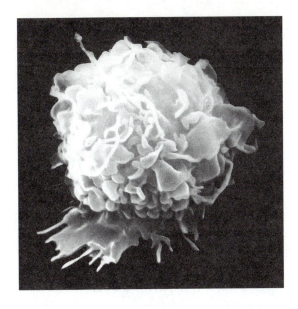

THE CELL: A MICROCOSM OF LIFE

Components of Typical Cells
Plasma Membrane
Cytoplasmic Matrix
Mitochondrion
Nucleus
Endoplasmic Reticulum and Golgi Apparatus
Lysosomes and Peroxisomes

Cellular Proteins
Receptors
Transport Proteins
Catalytic Proteins (enzymes)

Perspective: **The Glucose Transporters**

Photo: A human scavenger cell

Life is impossible without cells. Cells, individual units of life, group together to form a living human body. Cells vary greatly in size, chemical composition, and function, but each one is a remarkable miniaturization of human life. Cells move, grow, ingest food and excrete wastes, react to their environment, and even reproduce.

Cells of all multicellular organisms are called *eukaryotic cells* (from the Greek *eu*, meaning "true," and *karyon*, "nucleus"). By their having a defined nucleus, eukaryotic cells are distinguished from other, more primitive cell types called *prokaryotic cells*, from which they are known to have evolved. Eukaryotic cells are also larger and much more complex structurally and functionally than the prokaryotes. Because this text addresses human metabolism and nutrition, all discussions of cellular structure and function in this and subsequent chapters pertain to eukaryotic cells.

Specialization among cells is a necessity for the living, breathing human, but cells in general have certain basic similarities. All human cells have a plasma membrane and a nucleus (or have had a nucleus), and most of them contain endoplasmic reticulum, Golgi apparatus, and mitochondria. For convenience of discussion, a so-called typical cell is considered so that the various organelles and their functions, which characterize cellular life may be identified. Considering the relationship between the normal functioning of a typical cell and the health of the total organism—the human being—one is reminded of the old rule: "A chain is only as strong as its weakest link."

Figure 1.1a shows the fine structure of a typical animal cell (hepatocyte), while Figure 1.1b gives a schematic view of a typical animal absorptive cell (such as an intestinal epithelial cell), showing its major components or organelles. The discussion begins with consideration of the plasma membrane, which forms the outer boundary of the cell, and then moves inward to examine the organelles held within this membrane.

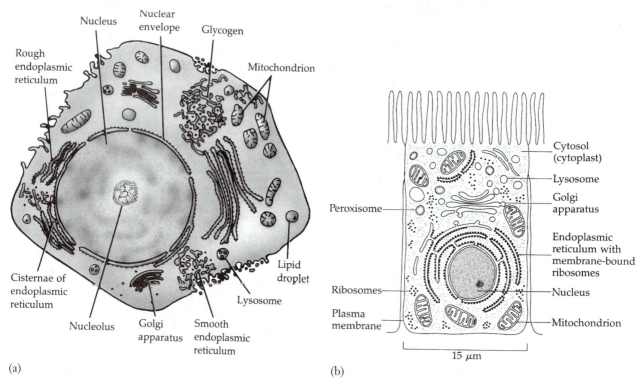

FIGURE 1.1 The fine structure of a typical animal cell (hepatocyte) is shown in (a) while (b) depicts a typical animal absorptive cell.

COMPONENTS OF TYPICAL CELLS

Plasma Membrane

The plasma membrane is the membrane encapsulating the cell. By surrounding the cell, it lets the cell become a unit by itself. The plasma membrane, like other membranes found within the cell, has distinct functions and structural characteristics. Nevertheless, all membranes share some common attributes:

- Membranes are sheetlike structures composed primarily of lipids and proteins held together by non-covalent interactions.

- Membrane lipids consist primarily of phospholipids, which have both a hydrophobic and hydrophilic moiety. This structural property of phospholipids lets them spontaneously form bimolecular sheets in water, called *lipid bilayers*, as shown in Figure 1.2. These bilayer sheets, because of their hydrophobic core, retard the passage of many water-soluble compounds into and out of the cell. Although such an arrangement requires transportation systems across the membrane, it allows retention of essential water-soluble substances within the cell.

- Phosphoglycerides and phosphingolipids (phosphate-containing sphingolipids) compose most of the membrane phospholipids. Of the phosphoglycerides, phosphatidylcholine and phosphatidylethanolamine are particularly abundant in higher animals. Another important membrane lipid is cholesterol, but its amount varies considerably from membrane to membrane. Molecular structures of these lipids are detailed in Chapter 6.

- Membrane proteins confer on biological membranes their functionality: they serve as pumps, gates, receptors, energy transducers, and enzymes. Figure 1.3 schematically illustrates the functions and positioning of some membrane proteins.

- Membranes are asymmetric. The inside and outside faces of the membrane are different.

- Membranes are fluid structures in which lipid and protein molecules can move laterally with ease and rapidity.

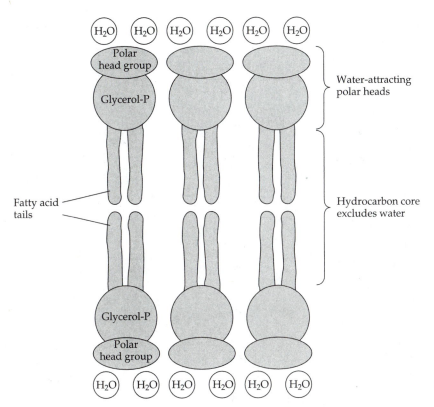

FIGURE 1.2 Lipid bilayer structure of biologic membranes. Structures are schematic representations of phosphoglycerides (glycerophosphatides), which consist of fatty acid tails attached to polar "heads." Contained within the polar heads are glycerol, phosphate (P), and a polar head group, which can be choline, ethanolamine, serine, or inositol.

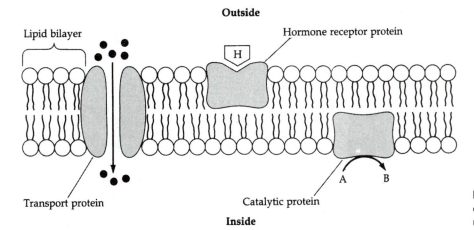

FIGURE 1.3 Schematic representation of various functions performed by cell membrane proteins.

Membranes can no longer be considered entities that are structurally distinct from the aqueous compartments that they surround. For example, the cytoplasm, which is the cell's aqueous ground substance, affords a connection among the various membranes of the cell. It is believed that such an interconnection creates a structure that makes it possible for a signal generated at one part of the cell to be quickly and efficiently transmitted to other regions of the unit [1].

The plasma membrane functions to provide protection to the cellular components while at the same time allowing them sufficient exposure to their environment for stimulation, nourishment, and removal of wastes. Characteristics of the plasma membrane that distinguish it from membranes of cell organelles are (1) its greater carbohydrate content due to the presence of glycolipids and glycoproteins. Although some carbohydrate is found in all membranes, most of the glycolipids and glycoproteins are associated with the plasma membrane. (2) Plasma membrane shows the highest content of cholesterol. Cholesterol enhances the mechanical stability of the membrane and regulates its fluidity.

Figure 1.4 illustrates the positioning of a cholesterol molecule between two phospholipid molecules and its influence on the fatty acid tails of the phospholipids. The cholesterol molecules orient themselves in the bilayer with their hydroxyl groups close to the polar head groups of the phospholipids [2]. Their rigid planar steroid rings are positioned so as to interact with and stabilize those regions of the hydrocarbon chains closest to the polar head groups. The rest of the hydrocarbon chain remains flexible and fluid. Cholesterol, by regulating fluidity of the membrane, regulates membrane permeability, thereby exercising some control over what may pass into and out of the cell. Fluidity of the membrane also appears to affect the structure and function of the proteins embedded in the lipid membrane.

The carbohydrate moiety of the glycoproteins and the glycolipids in membranes helps maintain the asymmetry of the membrane. This is because the oligosaccharide side chains are located exclusively on the membrane layer facing away from the cytoplasmic matrix. In plasma membranes, therefore, the sugar residues are all exposed to the outside of the cell, forming what is called the *glycocalyx*, the layer of carbohydrate on the cell's outer surface. On the membranes of the organelles, however, the oligosaccharides are directed inwardly into the lumen of the membrane-bound compartment [3]. Figure 1.5 schematically illustrates the glycocalyx and the location of oligosaccharide side chains in the plasma membrane.

Although the exact function of the sugar residues is unknown, it is believed that they act as specificity markers for the cell, and as "antennae" to pick up signals for transmission of substances in the cell [1]. The membrane glycoproteins are crucial to the life of the cell, very possibly serving as the receptors for hormones, for certain nutrients, and for various other substances that influence cellular function. Also, glycoproteins may help to regulate the intracellular communication necessary for cell growth and tissue formation. The term *intracellular communication* refers to pathways by which information is conveyed from one part of a cell to another in response to external stimuli. Generally, it involves the passage of chemical messengers from organelle to organelle or within the lipid bilayers of membranes [4].

Whereas the lipid bilayer determines the structure of the plasma membrane, proteins are primarily responsible for the many membrane functions. The membrane proteins are interspersed within the lipid bi-

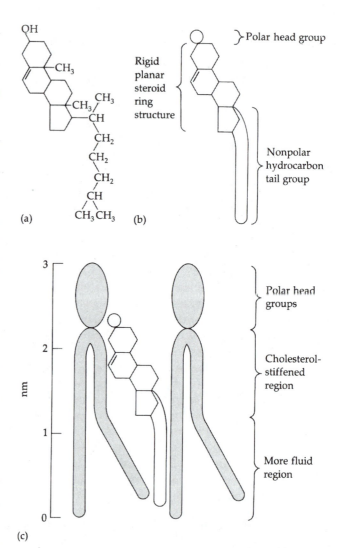

FIGURE 1.4 The structural role of cholesterol in the cell membrane is represented by a formula (a), a schematic drawing (b), and as it interacts with two phospholipid molecules in a monolayer (c).

layers, where they mediate information transfer (e.g., receptors), transport ions and molecules (e.g., pores, carriers, and pumps), and speed up metabolic activities (e.g., enzymes). Figure 1.3 is a schematic representation of the location and functions of these proteins. The importance of proteins for the transport of molecules into and out of the cell is illustrated in Figure 1.6.

Membrane proteins are classified as either integral or peripheral. The integral proteins are attached to the membrane through hydrophobic interactions and are embedded in the membrane. Peripheral proteins, in contrast, are associated with membranes via ionic interactions, and are located on or near the membrane sur-

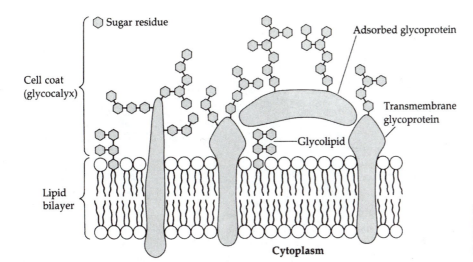

FIGURE 1.5 Diagram of the cell membrane glycocalyx, illustrating that all carbohydrate is located on the outside of the membrane.

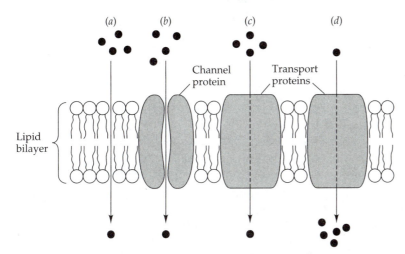

FIGURE 1.6 Schematic illustration of the role of proteins in transport, showing four ways in which molecules (•) may cross cellular membranes: (A) simple diffusion through the lipid bilayer, (B) diffusion through membrane pores created by channel proteins, (C) facilitated diffusion or transport, necessitating a carrier protein specific for the molecule, and (D) active transport, a mechanism that, like facilitated transport, requires a specific transporter, but that also requires the expenditure of energy in the form of ATP hydrolysis. Molecules crossing membranes by simple or facilitated diffusion are moved only from a region of higher concentration on one side of the membrane to a region of lower concentration on the other. Actively transported molecules, in contrast, can be moved against a concentration gradient.

face (Fig. 1.7). Peripheral proteins are believed to be attached to integral membrane proteins either directly or through intermediate proteins [1,2].

Most receptor and carrier proteins are integral proteins, whereas the glycoproteins of the cell recognition complex are peripheral proteins [2]. Functions of membrane proteins, as well as functions of proteins located intracellularly, are discussed later in the chapter.

Cytoplasmic Matrix

A new frontier in the study of cell structure and cell physiology was made possible with the advent of the high-voltage electron microscope. Particularly exciting was the identification of a microtrabecular lattice that supports and controls the movement of cell organelles. The word *trabecula* is from the Latin, meaning a little beam. It describes a fibrous cord of connective tissue that serves as a supporting fiber. It is now believed that the microtrabecular lattice is actually an intercommunication system of proteins and other macromolecules held in some state of aggregation. A model of this lattice, as shown in Figure 1.8, depicts the microtrabeculae as being continuous with the proteins underlying the plasma membrane, the surface of the endoplasmic reticulum, the microtubules, and the filaments of the stress fibers. The lattice also appears to support certain extracellular extensions emanating from the cell surface. For example, the microvilli, which are extensions of intestinal epithelial cells, are associated with the microtrabeculae [5]. Microvilli are designed to present a large surface area for the absorption of dietary nutrients.

The discovery that the ground substance of the cell is actually structured rather than being a homogeneous

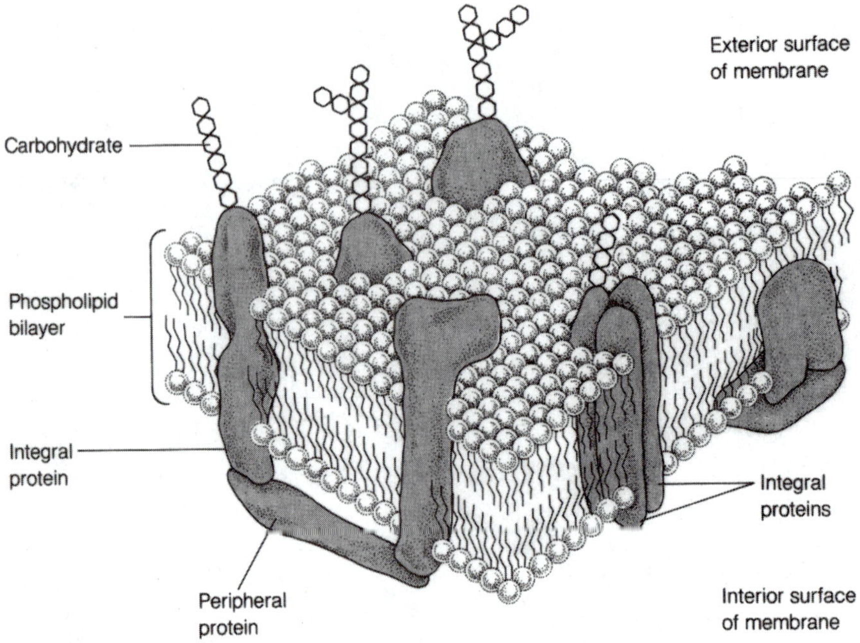

FIGURE 1.7 Positioning of proteins in plasma membrane. Proteins that penetrate into the interior of the lipid bilayer are called *integral proteins*. Proteins that lie on the surface and do not penetrate the lipid bilayer are called *peripheral* or *extrinsic* proteins. Polysaccharides are frequently attached to membrane proteins and membrane lipids on the exterior side of the membrane.

solution necessitates a different nomenclature from the one formerly used (i.e., cytoplasm). Instead of *cytoplasm*, the ground substance is more appropriately named *cytoplast*, thereby connoting a functional unity [5].

Like the microtrabecular lattice, microfilaments and microtubules are apparently complex polymers of many different proteins, including actin, myosin, and tubulin, the latter being a protein necessary for the formation of microtubules. These structures provide mechanical support for the cell, but they also serve as binding surfaces for soluble macromolecules such as proteins and nucleic acids present in the aqueous portion of the cytoplasmic matrix. In fact, there is evidence that the non-filamentous aqueous phase of the cell contains very few macromolecules, and that many proteins in the cytoplasmic matrix are bound to the filaments for a large portion of their lives. Filling the intertrabecular spaces is the fluid phase of the cytoplasmic matrix, containing small molecules such as glucose, amino acids, oxygen, and carbon dioxide. This arrangement of the polymeric and fluid phases apparently gives the cytoplasm (cytoplast) its gel-like consistency [5].

The spatial arrangement of the lattice, or polymeric phase, with the aqueous phase improves the efficiency of the many enzyme-catalyzed reactions that take place in the cytoplast. The aqueous phase contacts the polymeric phase over a very broad surface area. For this reason, enzymes that are associated with the polymeric phase are brought into close proximity to their substrate molecules in the aqueous phase, thereby facilitating the reaction (see discussion of enzymes, p. 18). Furthermore, if enzymes catalyzing the reactions of a metabolic pathway were oriented sequentially so that the product of one reaction was released in very close proximity to the next enzyme for which it is a substrate, the velocity of the overall pathway would be greatly enhanced. There is evidence that such an arrangement of the enzymes participating in glycolysis does in fact exist.

Possibly all metabolic pathways occurring in the cytoplasmic matrix may be influenced by its structural arrangement. Metabolic pathways of particular significance that occur in the cytoplasmic matrix and that might be affected by the structure include *glycolysis, hexose monophosphate shunt (pentose phosphate pathway), glycogenesis* and *glycogenolysis, fatty acid synthesis,* and *production of nonessential, unsaturated fatty acids.*

Normal intracellular communication among all cellular components is vital for cell activation and survival. The importance of the microtrabecular network is therefore evident, considering that its function is to support and interconnect cellular components.

Mitochondrion

The mitochondria are the primary sites of oxygen use in the cell and are responsible for most of the metabolic energy (adenosine triphosphate, or ATP) produced in cells.

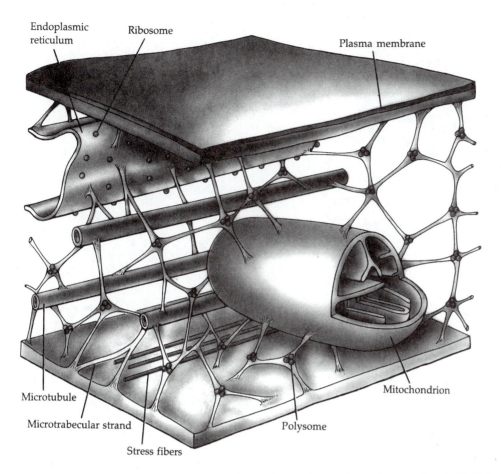

Endoplasmic reticulum

Ribosome

Plasma membrane

Microtubule

Microtrabecular strand

Stress fibers

Polysome

Mitochondrion

FIGURE 1.8 A model of the cytoplast (microtrabecular lattice). The cytoplast is shown at about 300,000 times its actual size, and was derived from hundreds of images of cultured cells viewed in the high-voltage electron microscope. The model illustrates how the microtrabecular filaments are related to other components of the cell cytoplasm: the substance of the cell outside the cell nucleus. In the model the microtrabeculae suspend the elongated structures of the endoplasmic reticulum, the mitochondria, and the microtubules. At junctions of the microtrabecular lattice are polysomes: organized clusters of ribosomes. *(Adapted from "The Grand Substance of the Cell" by Porter and Tucker. Copyright © 1981 by Scientific American, Inc. All rights reserved.)*

The size and shape of the mitochondria in different tissues vary according to the function(s) of the tissue. In the muscle tissue, for example, the mitochondria are held tightly among the fibers of the contractile system. In the liver, however, the mitochondria have fewer restraints, appear spherical in shape, and move freely through the cytoplasmic matrix.

The mitochondrion consists of a matrix or interior space surrounded by a double membrane (Fig. 1.9). The mitochondrial outer membrane is relatively porous, whereas the inner membrane is only selectively permeable, thereby serving as a permeability barrier between the cytoplasmic matrix and the mitochondrial matrix. The inner membrane has many invaginations called the *cristae*. These cristae serve to increase the surface area of

the inner membrane in which are embedded all the components of the electron transport (respiratory) chain.

The electron transport chain is central to the process of oxidative phosphorylation, the mechanism by which most cellular ATP is produced. Its components act as carriers of electrons in the catalytic oxidation of nutrient molecules by enzymes functioning in the mitochondrial matrix. Flow of electrons through the electron transport chain is strongly exothermic, and the energy released is used in part for the synthesis of ATP, an endothermic process. Molecular oxygen is ultimately, but indirectly, the oxidizing agent in these reactions. The purpose of the electron transport chain is to couple the energy released by nutrient oxidation to the formation of ATP. The precise positioning of the chain compo-

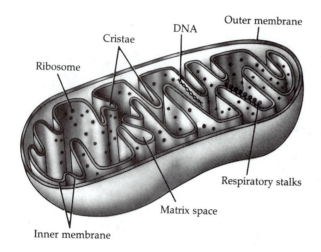

FIGURE 1.9 The mitochondrion.

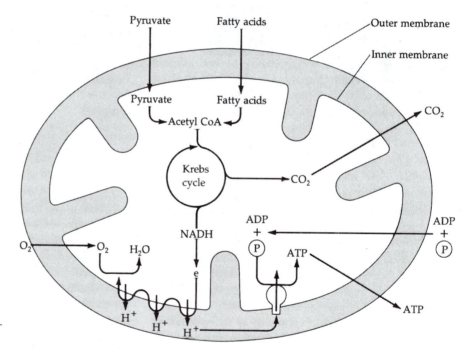

FIGURE 1.10 The flow of major reactants in and out of the mitochondrion.

nents within the inner membrane is fortuitous, because it brings them into close proximity to both the oxidizable products released in the matrix and to molecular oxygen. Figure 1.10 shows the flow of major reactants into and out of the mitochondrion.

Among the metabolic enzyme systems functioning in the mitochondrial matrix are those catalyzing reactions of the Krebs cycle and fatty acid oxidation. Other enzymes are involved in the oxidative decarboxylation

and carboxylation of pyruvate (p. 92, 93), and in certain reactions of amino acid metabolism.

The mitochondrial matrix contains a small amount of DNA and a few ribosomes so that limited protein synthesis within the mitochondrion is possible. It is of interest that the genes contained in mitochondrial DNA, unlike those in the nucleus, are inherited only from the mother. The primary function of mitochondrial genes is to code for proteins vital to the production of ATP [6].

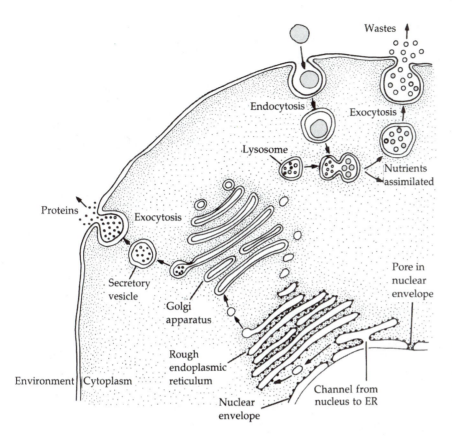

FIGURE 1.11 Communication between nucleus and other cell components. Membrane material in the nuclear envelope, the endoplasmic reticulum, the Golgi apparatus, and the plasma membrane are cycled continuously, as illustrated.

Most of the enzymes operating in the mitochondrion, however, are coded by nuclear DNA (deoxyribonucleic acid), are synthesized on the rough endoplasmic reticulum (RER) in the cytoplasm, and are then incorporated into existing mitochondria.

All cells in the body, with the exception of the erythrocyte, possess mitochondria. The erythrocyte (p. 268), in the process of maturing, disposes of its mitochondria and must depend solely on the energy produced through anaerobic mechanisms, primarily glycolysis (p. 84).

Nucleus

The nucleus of the cell is the largest of the organelles, and because of its DNA content, is the initiator and regulator of most cellular activities. Surrounding the nucleus is the nuclear envelope, composed of two membranes that appear to be dynamic structures. The dynamism of these membranes makes possible communication between the nucleus and the cytoplasmic matrix, and allows a continuous channel between the nucleus and the endoplasmic reticulum. At various intervals the two membranes of the nuclear envelope fuse, thereby creating pores in the envelope (Fig. 1.11).

The matrix held within the nuclear envelope is composed of chromatin plus all the enzymes and minerals necessary for the activity of the nucleus. Condensed regions of the chromatin are called *nucleoli*, in which are found not only DNA and its associated alkaline proteins (histones) but also considerable amounts of RNA (ribonucleic acid). This particular RNA is believed to give rise to the microsomal RNA (i.e., RNA associated with endoplasmic reticulum).

At cell division the chromatin is condensed into chromosomes, each chromosome containing a single molecule of DNA. The DNA exists as two large strands of nucleic acid that are intertwined to form a double helix. During cell division the two unravel at one end, each forming a template for the synthesis of a new strand via pairing of the complementary purines and pyrimidines (adenine with thymine, guanine with cytosine). The end result of the process is two new DNA chains that permit the production of *two* helical DNA molecules from the one parent molecule. The process constitutes *replication*, or the copying of a parent DNA molecule to form two identical daughter molecules. Because of the replication, each new cell of a tissue carries within its nucleus identical information to direct its functioning.

Throughout the entire life cycle of the cell, chromatin DNA is involved in transcription and translation, processes whereby protein synthesis is initiated. In *transcription*, various sections of the DNA molecule unravel, and one strand serves as the template for the synthesis of RNA. The genetic code is transcribed into RNA via base pairing, as in DNA replication, except that the pyrimidine *uracil*, instead of thymine, pairs with the purine adenine. The newly synthesized RNA is then processed in the nucleus to produce messenger RNA (mRNA). Following processing, the mRNA is exported into the cytoplasmic matrix where it is attached to the ribosomes of the RER or to the freestanding polysomes. On the ribosomes, the transcribed genetic code becomes translated so as to bring amino acids into a specific sequence to produce a protein with a clearly delineated function. This process is called *translation*. In the process, the specific amino acids coded for by the mRNA are activated by ATP at their carboxyl end and become attached to a transfer RNA (tRNA), specific for a particular amino acid. The transfer RNA, in turn, brings the code-designated amino acids to the protein synthesis site on the ribosomal mRNA. Peptide bonds are then formed between the aligned amino acids, as the protein chain elongates and simultaneously dissociates from the mRNA. This is the *elongation* phase of the overall process of protein synthesis. The synthesis of cellular proteins, as directed by DNA, determines the fate of the cell. Figure 1.12 briefly outlines the process of protein synthesis.

Endoplasmic Reticulum and Golgi Apparatus

The endoplasmic reticulum is a network of membranous channels pervading the cytoplast and providing continuity between the nuclear envelope, the Golgi apparatus, and the plasma membrane. This structure, therefore, is a mechanism for communication from the innermost part of the cell to its exterior (Fig. 1.11). The endoplasmic reticulum cannot be separated from the cell as an entity by laboratory preparation. During mechanical homogenization, its structure is disrupted and reforms into small spherical particles called *microsomes*.

The endoplasmic reticulum is classified as either rough (granular) or smooth (agranular). The granularity or lack of granularity is determined by the presence or absence of *ribosomes*. Rough endoplasmic reticulum (RER), so named because it is studded with ribosomes, abounds in cells where protein synthesis is a primary function.

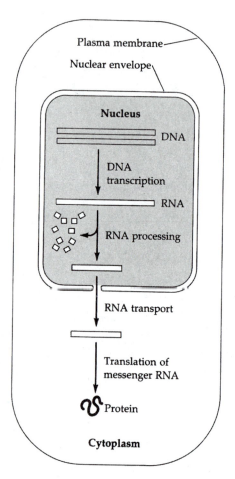

FIGURE 1.12 A schematic representation of protein synthesis (DNA → RNA → protein). RNA processing and subsequent transport through the nuclear envelope are interposed between transcription and translation of mRNA into protein. *(Alberts B, Bray D, Lewis J. Molecular biology of the cell. New York: Garland, 1983:385.)*

Smooth endoplasmic reticulum (SER) is found in most cells. However, since it is the site of synthesis for a variety of lipids, it is more abundant in cells that synthesize steroid hormones (e.g., the adrenal cortex and gonads) and in liver cells, which synthesize fat transport molecules (the lipoproteins). In skeletal muscle, SER is called *sarcoplasmic reticulum*, and is the site of the calcium ion pump, a necessity for the contractile process.

Ribosomes associated with the RER are composed of ribosomal RNA (rRNA) and structural protein. They are the primary site for protein synthesis. All proteins to be secreted (or excreted) from the cell or destined for incorporation within an organelle membrane in the cell more than likely are synthesized on the RER. The clusters of ribosomes (i.e., polyribosomes or polysomes) that are freestanding in the cytoplast are also the synthesis site for some proteins, but all proteins synthesized here are believed to remain within the cytoplasmic matrix.

Located on the SER of liver cells is a system of enzymes that is very important in the detoxification and metabolism of many different drugs. It consists of a family of cytochromes, designated the P450 system, that functions along with other enzymes. The system is particularly active in the oxidation of drugs, but because its action results in the simultaneous oxidation of other compounds as well, the system is collectively referred to as the mixed-function oxidase system. Lipophilic substances—for example, the steroid hormones and numerous drugs—can be made hydrophilic by oxidation, reduction, or hydrolysis. Becoming hydrophilic allows these substances to be excreted easily via the bile or urine.

The Golgi apparatus, thought to be an extension of the endoplasmic reticulum (ER), consists of secretory vesicles and a series of cisternae (Fig. 1.11). The Golgi apparatus is particularly prominent in neurons and secretory cells. It is believed that the membrane of the ER buds off into vesicles that fuse with the Golgi membrane. These vesicles carry in them materials that have been synthesized in the ER. As this membrane flows, the Golgi apparatus becomes the site for membrane differentiation and the development of surface specificity. For example, the polysaccharide moieties of mucopolysaccharides and of the membrane glycoproteins are synthesized and attached to the polypeptide during its passage through the Golgi apparatus. Such an arrangement allows for the continual replacement of cellular membranes, including the plasma membrane.

Proteins synthesized in the RER and destined for secretion from the cell are packaged within the Golgi apparatus and then secreted via secretory vesicles. Secretion of cellular products such as proteins can be either constitutive or regulated. If secretion follows a constitutive course, it means the secretion rate remains relatively constant, uninfluenced by external regulation. Regulated secretion, as the word implies, is affected by regulatory factors, and therefore its rate is changeable. Vesicles destined for the regulatory pathway all contain coats of the protein clathrin. Current research [7] suggests that the different proteins passing through the Golgi apparatus are sorted into different vesicles in the last compartment of the Golgi apparatus called the *trans-Golgi network* (TGN). The model for sorting is shown in Figure 1.13.

Lysosomes and Peroxisomes

Lysosomes and peroxisomes are cell organelles packed with enzymes. Whereas the lysosomes serve as the cell's digestive system, the peroxisomes perform some specific oxidative catabolic reactions.

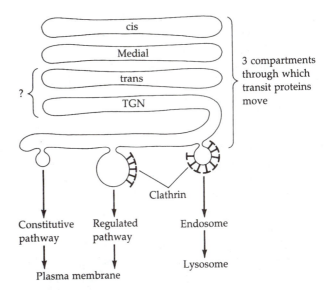

FIGURE 1.13 A model for sorting proteins in the trans-Golgi network (TGN). The model identifies compartments of the Golgi apparatus through which proteins must pass. Distinction between the compartment labeled "trans" and the TGN is a tentative one. *(Griffiths G, Simons K. The trans-Golgi network: sorting at the exit site of the Golgi complex. Sci 1986; 234:439.)*

Lysosomes are particularly large and abundant in those cells that perform digestive functions; for example, the macrophages and leukocytes. Approximately 36 powerful enzymes capable of splitting complex substances such as proteins, polysaccharides, nucleic acids, and phospholipids are held within the confines of a single, thick membrane. The lysosome, just like a protein synthesized for excretion, is believed to develop through the combined activities of the ER and Golgi apparatus, the result of which is a very carefully packaged group of lytic enzymes (Figs. 1.11 and 1.13). The membrane surrounding these catabolic enzymes has the capacity for very selective fusion with other vesicles so that catabolism (or digestion) may occur as necessary. Wastes thereby produced can be removed from the cells by exocytosis, as indicated in Figure 1.11.

Important catabolic activities performed by the lysosomes include participation in *phagocytosis*, in which foreign substances taken up by the cell may be digested or rendered harmless. An example of digestion by lysosomes is their action in the proximal tubules of the kidney. Lysosomes of the proximal tubule cells are believed to digest the albumin absorbed via endocytosis from the glomerular filtrate. Lysosomal phagocytosis serves as protection against invading bacteria and following a wound or infection, it becomes part of the normal repair process.

A second catabolic activity of lysosomes is autolysis (p. 185), in which intracellular components, including organelles, are digested as a result of degeneration or cellular injury [8]. Autolysis also can serve as a survival mechanism for the cell as a whole. Digestion of dispensable intracellular components can provide the nutrients necessary to fuel functions essential to the life of the cell. The mitochondrion is an example of an organelle whose degeneration requires autolysis. It is estimated that the mitochondria of liver cells must be renewed approximately every 10 days.

Another catabolic activity of the lysosomes is bone resorption, an essential process in the normal modeling of bone. Lysosomes of the osteoclasts promote the dissolution of mineral and the digestion of collagen, both of which actions are necessary in bone resorption and for regulation of calcium and phosphorus homeostasis.

Lysosomes, with their special membrane and numerous catabolic enzymes, also function in hormone secretion and regulation. Of particular significance is the role of lysosomes in the secretion of the thyroid hormones (p. 392).

Only recently (early 1960s) have the *peroxisomes* been recognized as separate intracellular organelles. These small bodies are believed to originate via "budding" from the SER. They are similar to the lysosomes in that they are bundles of enzymes surrounded by a single membrane. Rather than having digestive action, however, the enzymes within the peroxisomes are catabolic oxidative enzymes. Although the mitochondrial matrix is the major site of fatty acid oxidation to acetyl coenzyme A (acetyl CoA), the peroxisomes can also carry out a similar series of reactions. Acetyl CoA produced in peroxisomes, however, cannot be further oxidized for energy at that site, and must therefore be transported to the mitochondria for oxidation via the Krebs cycle.

Peroxisomes are also the site for certain reactions of amino acid catabolism. Some of the oxidative enzymes involved in these pathways catalyze the release of hydrogen peroxide (H_2O_2) as an oxidation product. H_2O_2 is a very reactive chemical that could cause cellular damage if not promptly removed or converted, and for this reason H_2O_2-releasing reactions are segregated within these organelles. Present in large quantities in the peroxisomes is the enzyme *catalase*, which degrades the potentially harmful H_2O_2 into water and molecular oxygen. Other enzymes in the peroxisomes are important in detoxifying reactions. Particularly important is the oxidation of ethanol to acetaldehyde.

CELLULAR PROTEINS

Proteins synthesized on the cell's ribosomes may be destined for secretion, or they may remain within the cell to perform their specific structural, digestive, regulatory, or other functions. One of the most interesting areas of biomolecular research during the past few years has been the delineation of how newly synthesized protein that is to remain in the cell finds its way from the ribosomes to its intended destination. Leader sequences are required for (1) proteins destined for secretion from the cell, (2) proteins to be retained in the cell's lysosomes and peroxisomes, and (3) proteins intended for incorporation into various membranes of the cell. Leader, or signaling, sequences are amino acid sequences attached to the amino end of the newly synthesized protein to direct it to its ultimate destination. Interaction between the leader sequences and specific receptors located on the various membranes permits the protein to enter its designated membrane. As the proteins move into their site of localization, the leader sequence is cleaved. Figure 1.14, which depicts the movement of a secretory protein into the ER, illustrates the principle of the leader (or signal) sequences.

There exists a long list of metabolic diseases attributed to a deficiency of, or inactivity of, certain enzymes. Tay-Sachs disease, phenylketonuria, maple syrup urine disease, and the lipid and glycogen storage diseases are a few well-known examples. As a result of research on certain mitochondrial proteins, current thinking is that in at least some cases it is not necessarily the enzymes themselves that are inactive or deficient, but rather, these enzymes fail to reach their correct destination [9,10,11].

Cellular proteins of particular interest to the health science student are (1) *receptors*, proteins that modify the cell's response to its environment; (2) *transport proteins*, those that regulate the flow of nutrients into and out of the cell; and (3) *enzymes*, the catalysts for the hundreds of biochemical reactions taking place in the cell.

Receptors

Receptors are highly specific proteins located in the cellular membrane facing away from the cytoplasmic matrix. Bound to the outer surface of these specific proteins are oligosaccharide chains, which are believed to act as recognition markers. Membrane receptors act as attachment sites for specific external stimuli such as hormones, growth factors, antibodies, lipoproteins, and certain nutrients. Molecular stimuli such as these, which bind specifically to receptors, are called *ligands*. Less is known

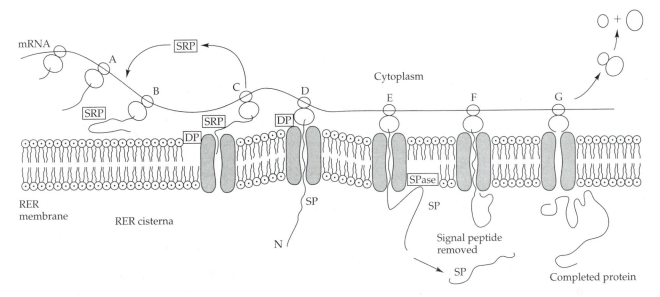

FIGURE 1.14 The signal (leader) peptide hypothesis. A membrane-free ribosome begins the synthesis of protein on a mRNA specific for the particular protein to be secreted. The signal peptide (consisting of approximately 80 amino acids) emerges first from the ribosome (A) and is recognized (B, C) by a complex of several proteins called the *signal recognition particle (SRP)*. Translation stops (C) until the ribosome–SRP complex binds to the rough endoplasmic reticulum (RER) membrane via a specific receptor for the SRP called the *docking protein* (DP). Translation then resumes following the dissociation of the SRP (D). The binding of the SRP to the DP created a channel in the RER membrane through which the signal peptide (SP) travels, emerging in the RER cisterna, where it is eventually removed from the rest of the protein by a proteolytic enzyme, the membrane-bound signal peptidase, SPase (E). Protein synthesis continues, with the completed protein folding within the RER (G).

about the receptors found in the membrane of cell organelles, but they appear to be glycoproteins necessary for the correct positioning of newly synthesized cellular proteins.

Although most receptor proteins are probably integral membrane proteins, some may be peripheral. In addition, receptor proteins can vary widely in their composition and mechanism of action. Although composition and mechanism of action of many receptors have not yet been determined, at least three distinct types of receptors are known to exist: (1) those that bind the ligand stimulus and convert it into an internal signal that alters behavior of the affected cell; (2) those that function as ion channels; and (3) those that internalize their stimulus intact. Following are examples of these three types of receptors.

The internal chemical signal that is most often produced by a stimulus–receptor interaction is 3′-, 5′-cyclic adenosine monophosphate (cyclic AMP, or cAMP). It is formed from adenosine triphosphate (ATP) by the enzyme adenylate cyclase. Cyclic AMP is frequently referred to as the second messenger in the stimulation of target cells by hormones. Figure 1.15 schematically describes one model for the ligand-binding action of receptors, which leads to production of the internal signal cAMP. As shown in the figure, the stimulated receptor reacts with the guanosine triphosphate (GTP)-binding protein (G protein), which is responsible for the activation of adenylate cyclase and the production of cAMP from ATP. The mechanism of action of cAMP signaling within the cell is complex, but it can be viewed briefly as follows: cAMP is an activator of protein kinases. These are enzymes that phosphorylate (add phosphate groups to) other enzymes, and in doing so, convert the enzymes from inactive forms into active forms. Protein kinases that can be activated by cAMP contain two subunits, a catalytic and a regulatory subunit. In the inactive form of the kinase, the two subunits are bound together in such a way that the catalytic portion of the molecule is inhibited sterically by the presence of the regulatory subunit. Phosphorylation of the enzyme by cAMP causes dissociation of the subunits, thereby freeing the catalytic subunit, which regains its full catalytic capacity.

Receptors can also act as ion channels in stimulating a cell. In some cases, the binding of ligand to its receptor causes a voltage change, which then becomes the signal for an appropriate cellular response. Such is the case when the neurotransmitter acetylcholine is the stimulus.

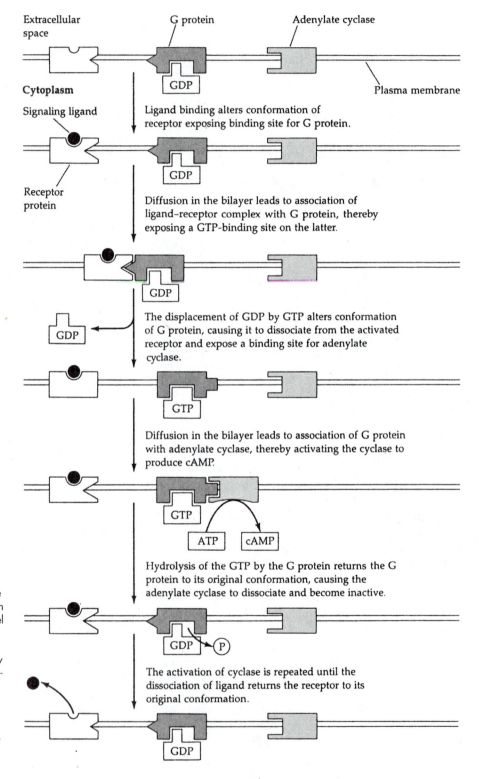

Extracellular space

G protein

Adenylate cyclase

Cytoplasm

Signaling ligand

Plasma membrane

Ligand binding alters conformation of receptor exposing binding site for G protein.

Receptor protein

Diffusion in the bilayer leads to association of ligand–receptor complex with G protein, thereby exposing a GTP-binding site on the latter.

GDP

The displacement of GDP by GTP alters conformation of G protein, causing it to dissociate from the activated receptor and expose a binding site for adenylate cyclase.

Diffusion in the bilayer leads to association of G protein with adenylate cyclase, thereby activating the cyclase to produce cAMP.

ATP   cAMP

Hydrolysis of the GTP by the G protein returns the G protein to its original conformation, causing the adenylate cyclase to dissociate and become inactive.

The activation of cyclase is repeated until the dissociation of ligand returns the receptor to its original conformation.

FIGURE 1.15 A proposed model for production of internal signal, cAMP. The response to an activated receptor protein is much greater than shown in this model because each activated receptor protein activates many molecules of G protein. Also, rather than diffusing independently through the plasma membrane and interacting only after the ligand binds to the receptor protein, the G protein and adenylate cyclase may be permanently associated. (Alberts B, Bray D, Lewis J. Molecular biology of the cell. New York: Garland. 1983, p. 385.)

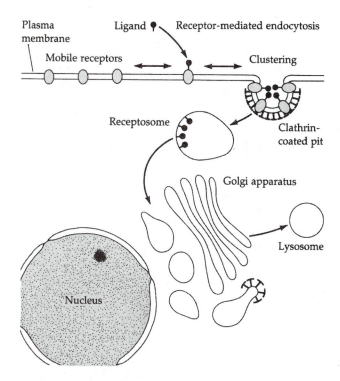

FIGURE 1.16 Receptor-mediated endocytosis, summarizing the steps involved in the binding, clustering, and entry of a typical ligand into a fibroblast.

The receptor for acetylcholine appears to function as an ion channel in response to voltage change. Stimulation by acetylcholine becomes a signal for the channels to open, allowing Na ions to pass through an otherwise impermeable membrane [12].

The internalization of a stimulus into a fibroblast via its receptor is illustrated in Figure 1.16. Receptors performing in such a manner exist for a variety of biologically active molecules, including the hormones *insulin* and *triiodothyronine* [13]. Low-density lipoproteins (LDLs) are internalized in much the same fashion (see "Perspective" section, Chapter 6), except that their receptors, rather than being mobile, are already clustered in coated pits. Coated pits—vesicles formed from the plasma membrane—are coated with several proteins, primary among which is clathrin. A coated pit containing the receptor with its ligand soon loses the protein coating and forms a smooth-walled vesicle. This vesicle delivers the ligand into the depths of the cell, and then along with the receptor is recycled into the plasma membrane.

The reaction of a fibroblast to changes in blood glucose levels is a good example of cellular adjustment to existing environment, made possible through receptor proteins. When blood glucose levels are low, muscular activity leads to release of the hormone epinephrine by the adrenal medulla. Epinephrine becomes attached to its receptor protein on the fibroblast, thereby activating the receptor and causing the receptor to stimulate the G protein and adenylate cyclase, which catalyzes the formation of cAMP from ATP. Then cAMP initiates a series of enzyme phosphorylation modifications, as described earlier in this section, that result in the *phosphorolysis* of glycogen to glucose 1-phosphate for use by the fibroblast (p. 83).

In contrast, when blood glucose is elevated, the hormone insulin, secreted by the β-cells of the pancreas, reacts with its receptors on the fibroblast and is transported into the cell via receptor-mediated endocytosis (Fig. 1.16). The action of insulin is to allow diffusion of glucose into the cell, but the mechanism of action is not fully understood. It is postulated that insulin increases the number of glucose receptors in the cell membrane and that these in turn promote diffusion of glucose via its transport protein (see "Perspective" section at the end of this chapter). The hormone itself is degraded within the cell [2].

Transport Proteins

Transport proteins are responsible for regulating the flow of nutrients and other substances into and out of the cell. They may function by acting as carriers (or pumps) for the substances, or they may provide protein-lined passages (pores) through which water-soluble materials of small molecular weight may diffuse. Figure 1.6 is a schematic diagram of these various transport proteins.

The active transport protein that has been studied most is the sodium (Na^+) pump. Not only is the Na^+ pump essential for the maintenance of ionic and electrical balance, but it also is necessary for the intestinal absorption and renal absorption of certain key nutrients (e.g., glucose and certain amino acids). These nutrients move into the epithelial cell of the small intestine against a concentration gradient, necessitating the need for a carrier and source of energy, both of which are provided by the Na^+ pump.

The proposed mechanism by which glucose is actively absorbed is termed *symport* because it is a simultaneous transport of two compounds (Na^+ and glucose) in the same direction. A transport protein with two binding sites binds both Na^+ and glucose. The attachment of Na^+ to the carrier increases the transport protein's affinity for the glucose. Sodium, because it is moving down a concentration gradient created by energy released through Na^+/K^+ adenosine triphosphatase (ATPase), is able to carry along with it glucose that is moving up a concentration gradient. When Na^+ is released inside

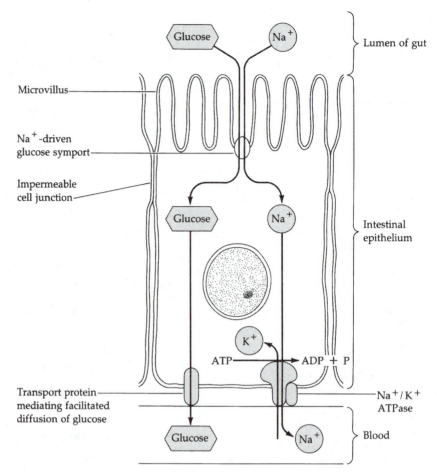

FIGURE 1.17 The active transport of glucose. Glucose is pumped into the cell's apical membrane by a Na+-powered glucose symport, and glucose passes out of the cell by facilitated diffusion. The Na+ gradient driving the glucose symport is maintained by the Na+/K+-ATPase in the basal and lateral plasma membrane, which keeps the internal concentration of Na+ low.

the cell, the carrier's affinity for glucose is decreased, and glucose can be released into the cell also. Na+/K+-ATPase then "pumps" the Na ions back out of the cell (Fig. 1.17).

Na+/K+-ATPase works by first combining with ATP in the presence of Na+ on the inner surface of the cell membrane. The enzyme then is phosphorylated by breakdown of ATP to adenosine diphosphate (ADP) and is consequently able to move three Na+ ions out of the cell. On the outer surface of the cell membrane, ATPase becomes dephosphorylated by hydrolysis in the presence of K ions and is then able to return two K ions into the cell. This pump is responsible for most of the active transport in the body.

Transport of glucose and amino acids into the epithelial cells of the intestinal tract is active in that the carriers needed for their transport are dependent on the concentration gradients achieved by action of Na+/K+-ATPase at the basolateral membrane. The activity of Na+/K+-ATPase is the major energy demand of the body at rest.

The process of facilitated (non–energy-dependent) transport is also a very important mechanism for regulating the flow of nutrients into the cell. It is used broadly across a wide range of cell types. Proteins involved in this function are often called *transporters*, probably the most thoroughly studied of which are the glucose transporters (see "Perspective" section at the end of this chapter).

Catalytic Proteins (enzymes)

Enzymes are distributed throughout all cellular compartments. Those that are components of the cellular membranes usually are found on the inner surface of the membranes. Exceptions are the digestive enzymes: β-galactosidase (lactase), the α-glycosidases (sucrase, glucoamylase), and certain peptidases that are located on the brush border of the epithelial cells lining the small intestine (p. 42).

Membrane-associated enzymes are found distributed throughout the cell organelles, but the greatest concentration is found in the mitochondria. As mentioned earlier, the enzymes of the electron transport chain, where energy transformation occurs, are located within the inner membrane of the mitochondria.

Metabolic processes occurring in the cells are governed by the enzymes that, for the most part, have been synthesized on the cell's RER under the direction of nuclear DNA. The functional activity of most enzymes, however, depends not only on the protein portion of the molecule but also on a nonprotein prosthetic group or coenzyme. If the nonprotein group is an organic compound, it usually contains a chemically modified B-complex vitamin. Very commonly, however, the prosthetic group may be inorganic (that is, metal ions such as Mg, Zn, Cu, Mn, Fe).

Enzymes have an active center that possesses a high specificity. This means that a substrate must fit perfectly into the specific contours of the active center. The K_m, or Michaelis constant, is a useful parameter that aids in establishing how enzymes will react in the living cell. K_m represents the concentration of a substrate that will be found in an occurring reaction when the reaction is at one-half its maximum velocity. If an enzyme has a high K_m value, an abundance of substrate must be present to raise the rate of reaction to half its maximum. In other words, this enzyme has a low affinity for its substrate. An example of an enzyme with a high K_m is *glucokinase*, an enzyme operating in the liver cells. Because glucose can diffuse freely into the liver, the fact that glucokinase has a high K_m is very important in the regulation of blood glucose. This low affinity of glucokinase for glucose prevents too much glucose from being removed from the blood during periods of fasting. Conversely, when the glucose load is high—for example, following a high-carbohydrate meal—the excess glucose will still be able to be converted by glucokinase, which does not function at its maximum velocity when glucose levels are basal. The enzyme can therefore be thought of as a protection against high cellular concentrations of glucose.

The nature of enzyme catalysis can be described by the following reactions:

$$\text{Enzyme (E)} + \text{substrate (S)} \longleftrightarrow \text{E–S complex}$$
$$\text{(reversible reaction)}$$
$$\text{E–S} \longleftrightarrow \text{E–P}$$

The substrate activated by combination with the enzyme is converted into an enzyme–product complex through rearrangement of the substrate's ions and atoms.

$$\text{E–P} \longrightarrow \text{E} + \text{P}$$

The product is released, and the enzyme is free to react with more of the substrate.

Most biochemical reactions are reversible, meaning that the same enzyme can catalyze a reaction in both directions. The extent to which a reaction can proceed in a reverse direction depends on several factors, the most important of which are relative concentrations of substrate (reactant) and product, and the differences in energy content between reactant and product. In those instances when a very large disparity in energy content or concentration exists between reactant and product, the reaction can proceed in only one direction. Such a reaction is *unidirectional* as opposed to reversible. In unidirectional reactions, the same enzyme cannot catalyze in both directions. Instead, a different enzyme is required to catalyze the reverse direction of the reaction (see Chapter 3). Comparing glycolysis with gluconeogenesis allows us to see how unidirectional reactions may be reversed by the introduction of a different enzyme (p. 93).

Simultaneous reactions, catalyzed by various multienzyme systems or pathways, constitute cellular metabolism. Enzymes are compartmentalized within the cell and function in sequential chains. A good example of such a multienzyme system is the Krebs cycle located in the mitochondrial matrix (p. 90). Each sequential reaction is catalyzed by a different enzyme, and some of the reactions are reversible while others are unidirectional. Although some reactions in almost any pathway are reversible, it is important to understand that the removal of one of the products drives the reaction toward formation of more of that product. Removal (or use) of the product, then, becomes the driving force that causes reactions to proceed primarily in the desired direction.

A very important aspect of nutritional biochemistry is the regulation of metabolic pathways. Anabolic and catabolic reactions must be kept in balance appropriate for life (and perhaps growth) of the organism. Regulation involves primarily the adjustment of the catalytic activity of certain participating enzymes, and there are three major mechanisms for doing this: (1) covalent modification of enzymes via hormone stimulation, (2) modulation of allosteric enzymes, and (3) increasing enzyme concentration by induction.

The first of these mechanisms, *covalent modification* of enzymes, is usually achieved by the addition of, or hydrolytic removal of, phosphate groups to and from the enzyme. This is the mechanism involving cAMP and protein kinase activation previously discussed on page 15. An example of covalent modification of enzymes is the regulation of glycogenesis and glycogenolysis (p. 96).

The second important regulatory mechanism is that exerted by certain unique enzymes called *allosteric enzymes*. The term *allosteric* refers to the fact that they possess an allosteric or specific "other" site besides the catalytic site. Specific compounds, called *modulators*, can bind to these allosteric sites and influence profoundly the activity of these regulatory enzymes. Modulators may be positive (i.e., causing an increase in enzyme activity), or they may exert a negative effect and inhibit activity. Modulating substances are believed to alter the activity of the allosteric enzymes by changing the conformation of the polypeptide chain or chains of the enzyme, thereby altering the binding of its catalytic site with the intended substrate. Negative modulators are often the end products of a sequence of reactions. As an end product accumulates above a certain critical concentration, it can inhibit, through an allosteric enzyme, its own further production.

An excellent example of an allosteric enzyme is phosphofructokinase in the glycolytic pathway. Glycolysis gives rise to pyruvate, which is decarboxylated and oxidized to acetyl CoA and which enters the Krebs cycle by combination with oxaloacetate to form citrate. By its regulatory function, *phosphofructokinase* helps prevent an excess production of citrate because increased levels of citrate can act as a negative modulator of the enzyme, thereby inhibiting continuation of glycolysis. In contrast, an accumulation of AMP or ADP—signifying the need of the cell for additional energy in the form of ATP—will act to modulate phosphofructokinase positively. The result is an active glycolytic pathway leading to production of acetyl CoA, which can be oxidized via the Krebs cycle and electron transport chain for release of energy (ATP).

The third mechanism of enzyme regulation, *enzyme induction*, creates changes in the concentration of certain *inducible* enzymes. Inducible enzymes are *adaptive*, meaning that they are synthesized at rates dictated by cellular circumstances. This is in contrast to *constitutive* enzymes, which are synthesized at a relatively constant rate, uninfluenced by external stimuli. Induction usually occurs through the action of certain hormones such as the steroid hormones and thyroid hormones, and is exerted through changes in the expression of genes encoding the enzymes. Dietary changes can elicit the induction of enzymes necessary to cope with the changing nutrient load. This is a relatively slow regulatory mechanism, however, as opposed to the first two mechanisms discussed, which exert effects very quickly; that is, in terms of seconds or minutes.

Specific examples of enzyme regulation will be cited in subsequent chapters dealing with metabolism of the major nutrients. It should be noted at this point, however, that *enzymes targeted for regulation catalyze essentially unidirectional reactions*. In every metabolic pathway, there is at least one reaction that is essentially irreversible, exergonic, and *enzyme-limited*. That is, the rate of the reaction is limited only by the activity of the enzyme catalyzing it. Such enzymes are frequently the regulatory enzymes, capable of being stimulated or suppressed by one of the mechanisms described. It is logical that an enzyme catalyzing a reaction reversibly at near equilibrium in the cell cannot be regulatory. This is because its up or down regulation would affect its forward and reverse activities equally. This, in turn, would not accomplish the purpose of regulation, which is the stimulation of one direction of a metabolic pathway relative to its reverse direction.

Enzymes participating in cellular reactions are located throughout the cell both in the cytoplasmic matrix (cytoplast) and in the various organelles. Location of specific enzymes depends on the site of the metabolic pathways or metabolic reactions in which these enzymes participate. Enzyme classification therefore is based on the type of reaction catalyzed by the various enzymes. Enzymes fall within six general classifications:

1. *Oxidoreductases* (dehydrogenases, reductases, oxidases, peroxidases, hydroxylases, oxygenases), enzymes catalyzing all reactions in which one compound is oxidized and another is reduced. Good examples of oxidoreductases are the enzymes found in the electron transport chain located on the inner membrane of the mitochondria. Other good examples are the cytochrome P450 enzymes located on the ER of the liver.

2. *Transferases*, enzymes catalyzing reactions not involving oxidation and reduction in which a functional group is transferred from one substrate to another. Included in this group of enzymes are *transketolase*, *transaldolase*, *transmethylase* and the *transaminases*. The transaminases (alpha-amino transferases), which figure so prominently in protein metabolism, fall under this classification and are located primarily in the mitochondrial matrix.

3. *Hydroxylases* (esterases, amidases, peptidases, phosphatases, glycosidases), enzymes catalyzing cleavage of bonds between carbon atoms and some other kind of atom by the addition of water. Digestive enzymes fall within this classification, as do those enzymes contained within the lysosome of the cell.

4. *Lyases* (decarboxylases, aldolases, synthetases, cleavage enzymes, deaminases, nucleotide cyclases, hydrases or hydratases, and dehydratases), enzymes that catalyze cleavage of carbon–carbon, carbon–sulfur, and certain carbon–nitrogen bonds (peptide bonds excluded) without hydrolysis or oxidation-reduction. Citrate lyase, which frees acetyl CoA for fatty acid synthesis in the cytoplast, is a good example of an enzyme belonging to this classification.

5. *Isomerases* (isomerases, racemases, epimerases, and mutases), enzymes catalyzing the interconversion of optical or geometric isomers. Phosphohexose isomerase that converts glucose 6-phosphate to fructose 6-phosphate in glycolysis (occurring in the cytoplast) shows the action of this particular class of enzyme.

6. *Ligases*, enzymes that catalyze the formation of bonds between carbon and a variety of other atoms, including oxygen, sulfur, and nitrogen. Formation of bonds catalyzed by ligases require energy that usually is provided by hydrolysis of ATP. A good example of a ligase is acetyl CoA carboxylase, which is necessary to initiate fatty acid synthesis in the cytoplast. Through the action of acetyl CoA carboxylase, a bicarbonate ion (HCO_3^-) is attached to acetyl CoA to form malonyl CoA, the initial compound in *de novo* fatty acid synthesis (p. 139).

Many cells are specific in their function. Among these are hepatocytes, adipocytes, and erythrocytes, which are of particular interest to the student of nutrition. The characteristics and functions of adipocytes and erythrocytes are described in Chapters 6 and 8 respectively. Because of the multifunctional role of the liver in metabolism, the hepatocyte is alluded to throughout the text.

SUMMARY

This brief walk through the cell, beginning with its outer surface, the plasma membrane, and moving into its innermost part, where the nucleus is located, has provided a view of how this living entity functions.

Characteristics of the cell that seem particularly notable are

- The flexibility of the plasma membrane in adjusting or reacting to its environment while protecting the rest of the cell as it monitors what may pass into or out of the cell. Very prominent in the membrane's reaction to its environment are the receptor proteins, which are believed to have been synthesized on the RER and to have moved through the Golgi apparatus to their intended site on the plasma membrane.

- The communication among the various components of the cell made possible through the cytoplast with its microtrabecular network and also through the endoplasmic reticulum and Golgi apparatus. The networking is such that communications flow not only among components within the cell but also between the nucleus and the plasma membrane.

- The efficient division of labor among the cell components (organelles). Each component has its own specific functions to perform, and there is little overlap. Furthermore, much evidence is accumulating to support the concept of an "assembly line" not only in oxidative phosphorylation on the inner membrane of the mitochondrion but also in almost all operations wherever they occur.

- The superb management exercised by the nucleus so that all the proteins needed for a smooth operation are synthesized. Proteins needed as recognition markers, receptors, transport vehicles, and catalysts are available as needed.

Despite all the efficiency of the cell, it is still not a totally self-sufficient unit. Its continued operation is contingent on receiving appropriate and sufficient nutrients. Nutrients needed are not only those that can be used for production of immediate metabolic energy (ATP) or for storage as chemical energy but also those required as building blocks for protein synthesis. In addition, the cell must have an adequate supply of the so-called regulatory nutrients (i.e., vitamins, minerals, and water).

With a view of the structure of the "typical cell," the division of labor among its component parts, and the location within the cell for many of the key metabolic reactions necessary for the continuation of life, consideration can now be given to how the cell receives its nourishment so that life can continue.

References Cited

1. Benga G, Holmes RP. Interactions between components in biological membranes and their implications for membrane function. Prog Biophys Mol Biol 1984;43:195–257.
2. Berdanier CD. Role of membrane lipids in metabolic regulation. Nutr Rev 1988;46:145–149.
3. Alberts B, Bray D, Lewis J, Roff M, Roberts K, Watson J. Molecular biology of the cell. New York: Garland, 1983.
4. Barritt GJ. Networks of extracellular and intracellular signals. In: Communication within animal cells. Oxford, England: Oxford University Press, 1992;1–19.
5. Porter KR, Tucker JB. The ground substance of the living cell. Sci Am 1981;244:57–67.
6. Young, P. Mom's mitochondria may hold mutation. Sci News 1988;134:70.
7. Griffiths G, Simons K. The trans Golgi network: Sorting at the exit site of the Golgi complex. Science, 1986; 234:438–443.
8. Ericcson JLE. Mechanism of cellular autophagy. In: Dingle JT, Fell HB, eds. Lysosomes in biology and pathology. 2nd ed. New York: Wiley Interscience, 1969:345–394.
9. How do proteins find mitochondria? Science 1985;228: 1517–1518.
10. Newly made proteins zip through the cell. Science 1980; 207:164–167.

11. Wickner WT, Lodish JT. Multiple mechanisms of protein insertion into and across membranes. Science 1985; 230:400–407.
12. A potpourri of membrane receptors. Science 1985;230: 649–651.
13. Pastan, IH, Willingham MC. Journey to the center of the cell: Role of the receptosome. Science 1981;214:504–509.

Additional References

Pike RL, Brown ML. Nutrition—an integrated approach. 3rd ed. New York: Wiley, 1984.
McMurray WC. Essentials of human metabolism. 2nd ed. Philadelphia: Harper & Row, 1983.
Vick RL. Contemporary medical physiology. Menlo Park, Calif.: Addison-Wesley, 1984.

Suggested Reading

Barritt GJ. Networks of extracellular and intracellular signals. In: Communication within animal cells. Oxford, England: Oxford University Press, 1992;1–19.
A clearly written, comprehensive review of cell signaling mechanisms and the functions of intracellular chemical messengers.
Benga G, Holmes R. Interaction between components in biological membranes and their implications for membrane function. Prog Biophys Mol Biol 1984;43:195–257.
This is an excellent review of membrane components, their functions and interactions. A great deal of information is condensed into an understandable paper.
Porter KR, Tucker JB. The ground substance of the living cell. Sci Am 1981;244:57–67.
The model for a highly structured cytoplasm (designated as cytoplast) is elucidated. The many implications of this model for cellular communication and metabolism are identified and discussed.
Pastan IH, Willingham MC. Journey to the center of the cell: Role of the receptosome. Science 1981;214:504–509.
An excellent description of the internalization pathway of certain hormones and nutrients as effected by coated pits on the cell's surface is given in this very well written paper.

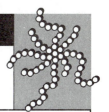

Glucose Transporters, Obesity, and Type 2 Diabetes Mellitus

Glucose transporter proteins, commonly abbreviated GLUT, have been the focus of considerable research, the results of which have led to a better understanding of the means by which glucose enters cells, the mechanism of insulin action, and the cellular defects underlying diabetes mellitus. A discussion of the structure, cellular localization, and function of these transporters was chosen for this Perspective because it will unify some of the information on organelle function and intracellular communication presented in this chapter.

Glucose is our most important nutrient. Its requirement begins at an early stage of fetal development, and continues throughout life. The sugar is effectively used by a wide variety of cell types under normal conditions, and its concentration in the blood must be precisely controlled. The symptoms associated with diabetes mellitus are a graphic example of the consequences of a disturbance in glucose homeostasis. The cellular uptake of glucose requires that it cross the cell's plasma membrane. This cannot occur by simple diffusion because the highly polar glucose molecule cannot be solubilized in the nonpolar matrix of the lipid bilayer. The cellular use of glucose therefore requires an efficient transport system for moving the molecule into and out of cells. In certain absorptive cells, such as epithelial cells of the small intestine and renal tubule, glucose can cross the plasma membrane (actively) against a concentration gradient, pumped by a Na^+/K^+-ATPase symport system (described in the chapter). Nearly all cells in the body, however, admit glucose passively by a carrier-mediated diffusion mechanism that does not require energy. The protein carriers involved in this process are called *glucose transporters.*

Considered collectively, all transporter proteins share a unique structure. They are integral proteins, penetrating and spanning the lipid bilayer of the plasma membrane. Most transporters, in fact, span the membrane several times. They are oriented such that hydrophilic regions of the chain protrude into the extracellular and cytoplasmic media while the hydrophobic regions traverse the membrane, juxtaposed with the membrane's lipid matrix. A model for a glucose transporter, reflecting this spatial arrangement of the molecule, is illustrated in Figure 1 [1]. In its simplest form, a transporter (1) has a specific combining site for the molecule being transported; (2) undergoes a conformational change on binding the molecule, causing the

molecule to be translocated to the other side of the membrane and released; and (3) has the ability to reverse the conformational changes without the molecule's being bound to the transporter, so that the process can be repeated.

Five isoforms of glucose transporters have been described: GLUT1, GLUT2, GLUT3, GLUT4, and GLUT5. All cells express on their plasma membranes at least one of these isoforms. The different isoforms have distinct tissue distribution and biochemical properties, and they contribute to the precise disposal of glucose according to varying physiological conditions. Tissue distribution of the glucose transporters are summarized in Table 1.

The GLUT1 and GLUT3 isoforms are believed to be responsible for basal, or constitutive, glucose uptake. Their number on a given area of cell surface is relatively static and does not increase on insulin stimulation. This is also true for the liver isoform (GLUT2), which is responsible for the bidirectional transport of glucose by the hepatocyte. It may also be involved in the movement of glucose out of absorptive epithelial cells into the circulation following the active transport of the glucose into the cells by symporters. GLUT4, in contrast, is quite sensitive to insulin, its concentration on the plasma membrane increasing dramatically in response to the hormone. It follows that the increase in the membrane transporter population is accompanied by an accelerated increase in the uptake of glucose by the stimulated cells. It is therefore the presence of GLUT4 in skeletal muscle and adipose tissue that makes these tissues responsive to insulin. Liver, brain, and erythrocytes lack the GLUT4 isoform, and are therefore not sensitive to the hormone.

Diabetes mellitus, the disease characterized by the body's inability to metabolize glucose, manifests as one of two types: type 1, or insulin-dependent diabetes mellitus (IDDM), and type 2, non–insulin-dependent diabetes mellitus (NIDDM). The hyperglycemia of type 1 diabetes can be attributed to a primary failure of the β-cells of the pancreas to produce and secrete insulin. The cause of type 2 diabetes has not been completely resolved, but it appears to be associated with insulin resistance in peripheral target tissue. This condition is caused not by a failure of target cells to bind insulin but by a postbinding abnormality, arising somewhere in the sequence of events that follows the binding of insulin to its receptor and leading to the cell's

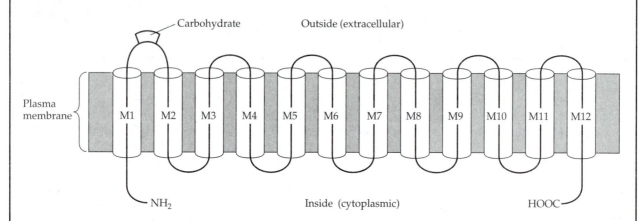

FIGURE 1 A model of a glucose transporter (GLUT1), showing its structural orientation in the plasma membrane. Alpha helical regions of the protein span the membrane 12 times at transmembrane sites designated M1–M12. Transmembrane segments consist largely of hydrophobic amino acids while the loops on the extracellular and cytoplasmic sides of the membrane are primarily hydrophilic. The transporter is a single polypeptide chain comprised of approximately 500 amino acid residues.

normal response to that signal. There is experimental evidence that a primary cause for the interrupted insulin signal is compromised synthesis or mobilization of the cell's glucose transporters. Insulin resistance has also been described in obesity as well as NIDDM. Its link to glucose transporter abnormalities in these conditions is considered next.

Synthesis and storage of the insulin-responsive transporter GLUT4 occurs as described in the chapter for all proteins. Following its synthesis from mRNA on the ribosomes of the rough endoplasmic reticulum, the transporter enters the compartments of the Golgi apparatus, where it is ultimately packaged in tubulovesicular structures in the trans-Golgi network. In the basal, unstimulated state of the adipocyte, GLUT4 resides in these structures and also, to some extent, in small cytoplasmic vesicles [2]. This subcellular distribution of GLUT4 is also found in skeletal muscle cells [3]. On stimulation by insulin, the tubulovesicle-enclosed transporters are translocated to the plasma membrane, where they become expressed on the cell surface. The proposed mechanism is illustrated in Figure 2. In skeletal muscle cells, insulin resistance associated with NIDDM has been shown to be caused by a reduction in glucose transporter activity, specifically the failure of the vesicles to translocate in response to insulin. The error can be thought of as a block or short-circuit in the insulin signal that normally initiates the translocation process. The result is a reduced concentration of transporters at the cell surface, and a consequent re-

duction in the rate of glucose uptake. Although a similar defect was found in adipocytes of NIDDM patients, it is not the major cause of the insulin resistance in these cells. The consequence of NIDDM in adipocytes is a marked depletion of mRNA encoding the GLUT4 transporter, resulting in depleted intracellular stores of the protein. This describes a pretranslational defect, meaning that it interferes with protein synthesis at a level before the translation process, the step that requires mRNA as template. Therefore, even if the vesicle translocation process were not compromised, an inadequate number of surface receptors would still be expressed upon insulation stimulation.

The insulin resistance related to obesity is mechanistically similar to the NIDDM effect on adipocytes. Reduction in GLUT4 mRNA in obese subjects results in a decrease in *de novo* synthesis of the transporter. Furthermore, the extent to which mRNA expression is suppressed appears to relate directly to increasing adiposity [4].

In summary, NIDDM is characterized by insulin resistance in peripheral target tissues, due to a diminished population of functional glucose transporters. In muscle cells, the defect appears to arise from a failure, on insulin stimulation, of vesicle-bound transporters to translocate to the plasma membrane. In adipocytes, translocation is also compromised, but the major mechanism for insulin resistance in these cells, in both NIDDM and obesity, is a pretranslational depletion of GLUT4 mRNA.

PERSPECTIVE   (continued)

TABLE 1 Human Glucose Transporters

Designation	Size (n amino acids)	Major sites of expression
Facilitative glucose transporters		
GLUT1 (erythrocyte)	492	Placenta, brain, kidney, and colon
GLUT2 (liver)	524	Liver, β-cell, kidney, and small intestine
GLUT3 (brain)	496	Many tissues, including brain, placenta, and kidney
GLUT4 (muscle/fat)	509	Skeletal muscle, heart, and brown and white fat
GLUT5 (small intestine)	501	Small intestine (jejunum)

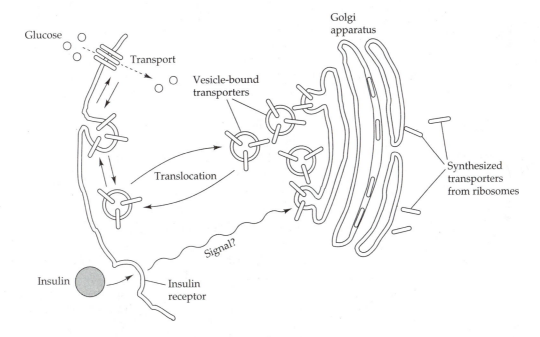

FIGURE 2 Proposed mode of insulin action on glucose transport. Theoretical sequence of events are (1) The binding of insulin to its specific receptor induces a signal of yet unknown nature that stimulates the translocation of vesicles containing the glucose transporters to the plasma membrane. (2) The vesicles fuse with the plasma membrane, releasing the transporters and allowing them to position themselves in the membrane. (3) On removal of insulin from its receptor, membrane-bound transporters are retranslocated back to the intracellular pool by an endocyte-like mechanism.

References Cited

1. Bell GI, Kayano T, Buse JB, et al. Molecular biology of mammalian glucose transporters. Diabetes Care 1990;13:198–208.
2. Bloc J, Gibbs EM, Lienhard GE, Slot JW, and Geuze HJ. Insulin-induced translocation of glucose transporters from post-Golgi compartments to the plasma membrane of 3T3-L1 adipocytes. J Cell Biol 1988;106:69–76.
3. Freidman JE, Dudek RW, Whitehead DS, et al. Immunolocalization of glucose transporter GLUT4 within human skeletal muscle. Diabetes 1991;40:150–154.
4. Garvey WT, Maianu L, Huecksteadt TP, et al. Pre-translational suppression of a glucose transporter protein causes insulin resistance in adipocytes from patients with non–insulin-dependent diabetes mellitus. J Clin Invest 1991;87:1072–1081.

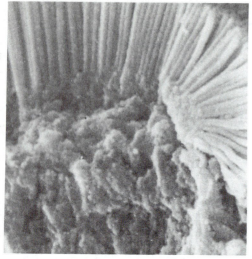

CHAPTER 2

THE DIGESTIVE SYSTEM: MECHANISM FOR NOURISHING THE BODY

Photo: Intestinal microvilli

Nutrition is the science of nourishment. Ingestion of foods and beverages provides the body with at least one, if not more, of the nutrients needed to nourish the body. There are six classes of nutrients that the body needs: carbohydrate, lipid, protein, vitamins, minerals, and water. In order for the body to use carbohydrate, lipid, and protein found in foods, the food must be digested. In other words, the food must be broken down mechanically and chemically. The process of digestion occurs in the digestive tract and on its completion yields nutrients ready for absorption and use by the body.

AN OVERVIEW OF THE STRUCTURE OF THE DIGESTIVE TRACT

The digestive tract includes organs that comprise the alimentary canal, also called the *gastrointestinal tract*, as well as certain accessory organs, primarily the pancreas, liver, and gallbladder. Figure 2.1 illustrates the digestive tract and accessory organs.

The Upper Gastrointestinal Tract

The mouth and pharynx constitute the oral cavity and provide the entryway to the digestive system. Food is passed from the mouth through the pharynx and into the esophagus. Figure 2.2 provides a cross section of the wall of the esophagus. The wall of the alimentary canal consists of the same layers as found in the esophagus (i.e., epithelium, submucosa, muscularis mucosa, and circular and longitudinal muscles). Secretory glands are found distributed throughout the digestive tract, with the exception of the colon. The secretory glands release secretions into a duct (exocrine), or release secretions into the blood (endocrine). Sphincters, which are circular muscles, are also located throughout the digestive tract. For example, an area of the esophagus referred to as the lower esophageal sphincter (LES)

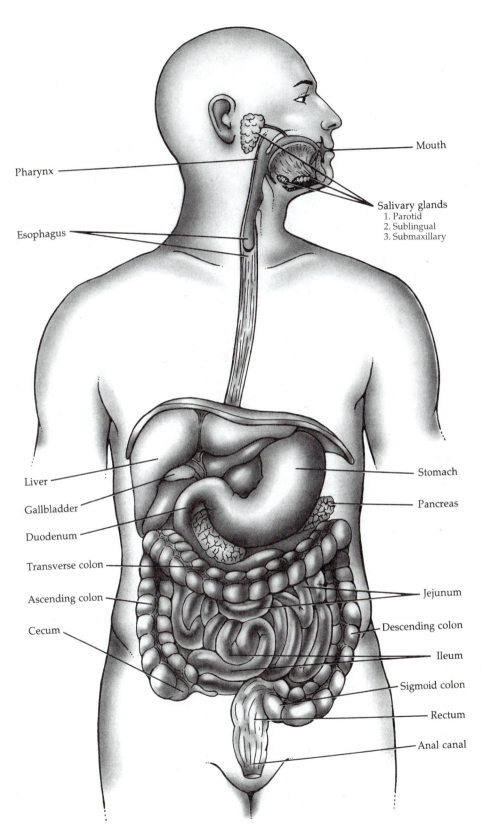

Mouth

Pharynx

Salivary glands
1. Parotid
2. Sublingual
3. Submaxillary

Esophagus

Liver

Gallbladder

Duodenum

Transverse colon

Ascending colon

Cecum

Stomach

Pancreas

Jejunum

Descending colon

Ileum

Sigmoid colon

Rectum

Anal canal

FIGURE 2.1 The digestive system.

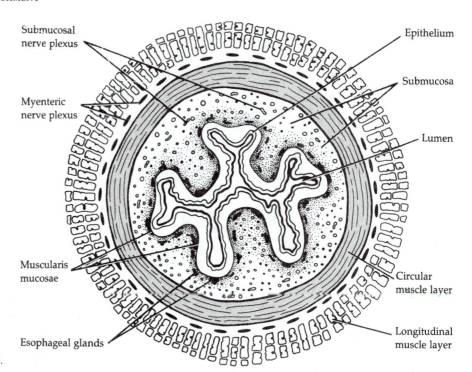

Submucosal
nerve plexus

Myenteric
nerve plexus

Muscularis
mucosae

Esophageal glands

Epithelium

Submucosa

Lumen

Circular
muscle layer

Longitudinal
muscle layer

FIGURE 2.2 A cross section of the esophagus illustrating the basic structure of the wall of the alimentary canal.

lies just above the juncture of the esophagus and stomach. Relaxation of this sphincter permits the passage of food from the esophagus into the stomach. The stomach is a J-shaped organ located under the diaphragm, extending from the LES to the duodenum, the upper or proximal section of the small intestine. The volume of the stomach when empty is about 50 mL (almost 2 oz), but on being filled, as usually shown in diagrams, can expand to accommodate approximately 1 to 1.5 L (about 37 to 52 oz) [1,2]. The pyloric sphincter at the distal end of the stomach controls the release of chyme (partially digested food existing as a semiliquid mass) from the stomach into the duodenum. The functions and additional structural features of the stomach are presented in more detail later in the chapter in the section "The Process of Digestion."

The Lower Gastrointestinal Tract and Accessory Organs

The small intestine is composed of the duodenum (slightly less than 1 ft long), and the jejunum and ileum (which together are about 9 ft long). Microscopy is needed to identify where one of these sections of the small intestine ends and the other begins. The small intestine represents the main site for nutrient digestion and absorption. The duodenum receives secretions from the liver, gallbladder, and pancreas, which are accessory organs. These secretions are necessary for the digestion of nutrients.

The liver, pictured in Figures 2.1 and 2.3, is the largest, single, internal organ of the body. With respect to digestion, specifically fat digestion, liver cells (hepatocytes) synthesize bile. Bile is then released into bile canaliculi, which lie between the hepatocytes in the hepatic plates and drain into bile ducts. As shown in Figure 2.4, right and left hepatic bile ducts join to form the common hepatic duct. The common hepatic duct unites with the cystic duct, which leads into and out of the gallbladder, to form the common hepatic bile duct (Fig. 2.4).

The gallbladder, a small organ with a capacity of approximately 40 to 50 mL (1.4 to 1.8 oz), is located on the visceral surface of the liver. The gallbladder functions to concentrate and store the bile made in the liver until needed in the small intestine for fat digestion. Bile flow into the duodenum is regulated by the intraduodenal segment of the common hepatic bile duct and the sphincter of Oddi, located at the junction of the common hepatic bile duct and the duodenum.

The pancreas, another accessory organ, is a slender, elongated organ ranging in length from about 15 to 23 cm (6 to 9 inches). The pancreas is found behind the greater curvature of the stomach, lying between the stomach and the duodenum (Figs. 2.1 and 2.5). Two types of active tissue are found in the pancreas: the acini or ducted exocrine tissue that produces the digestive enzymes, and the ductless endocrine tissue that secretes hormones, primarily insulin and glucagon. The enzyme-producing cells of the pancreas are arranged into circu-

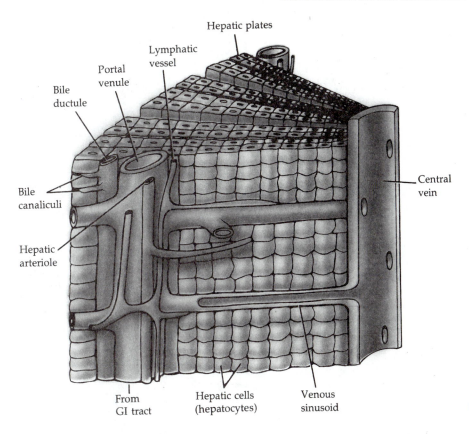

FIGURE 2.3 Structure of a liver lobule.

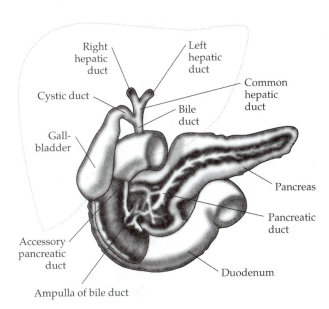

FIGURE 2.4 Connections of the ducts of the gallbladder, liver, and pancreas. (Reproduced, with permission, from Bell GH, Emslie-Smith D, Paterson CR: Textbook of Physiology and Biochemistry, 9th ed. Churchill Livingstone, 1976.)

lar glands that are attached to small ducts. Enzymes are packaged into secretory structures called *zymogen granules*. Stimulation of pancreatic acinar cells by hormones or the parasympathetic nervous system, results in release of the enzymes by exocytosis [3]. Digestive enzymes along with bicarbonate and other anions and cations, are secreted into small ducts within the pancreas. These small ducts coalesce to form a large main pancreatic

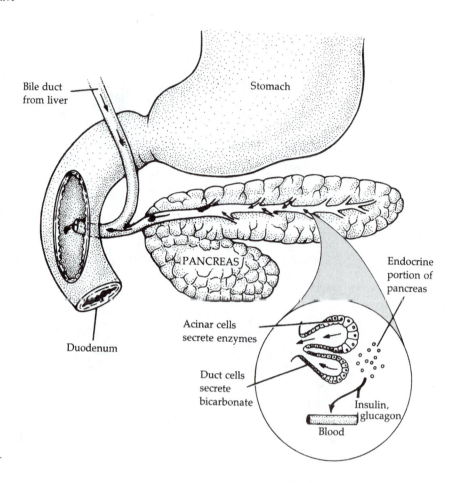

FIGURE 2.5 Structure of the pancreas.

duct, which later joins with the common hepatic bile duct to form the bile pancreatic duct that empties into the duodenum through Oddi's sphincter.

Although the structure of the small intestine contains the same layers as identified in Figure 2.2, the epithelial surface or mucosa of the small intestine is structured to maximize surface area. The small intestine has a surface area of approximately 300 m². This is about equal to a 3-foot-wide sidewalk that is more than three football fields in length. Contributing to this enormous surface area are, first, the large folds of mucosa (folds of Kerckring) that protrude into the lumen of the small intestine. Next are the villi, fingerlike projections lined by hundreds of cells (enterocytes, also called *absorptive epithelial cells*) along with blood capillaries and a central lacteal (lymphatic vessel) for transport of nutrients out of the enterocyte (Fig. 2.6). Finally, there are the microvilli, which are extensions of the plasma membrane of the enterocytes that make up the villi (Fig. 2.7). The microvilli possess a surface coat or glycocalyx, as shown in Figure 2.7, and together these comprise the brush border of the enterocytes. Most of the digestive enzymes produced by the intestinal mu-

cosal cells are found on the brush border, and function to hydrolyze already partially digested nutrients, mainly carbohydrate and protein. Structurally, the digestive enzymes are glycoproteins. The carbohydrate moiety or glyco- portion of these glycoprotein enzymes may in part make up the glycocalyx. The glycocalyx lines the luminal side of the intestine and appears to consist of numerous fine filaments extending in a somewhat perpendicular fashion from the microvillus membrane to which it is attached [4]. Digestion is usually completed on the brush border, but may be completed within the cytoplasm of the enterocytes.

The small intestine also contains small pits called *crypts of Lieberkühn* that lie between the villi. Epithelial cells in these crypts continuously undergo mitosis; the new cells gradually migrate upward and out of the crypts toward the tips of the villi. Shortly after reaching the tip of the villus, the cells will be sloughed off into the intestinal lumen and excreted in the feces. Intestinal cell turnover is rapid, approximately every 3 to 5 days. Cells in the crypts include paneth cells that secrete proteins with unclear functions, goblet cells that secrete mucus, and enterochromaffin cells with endocrine function.

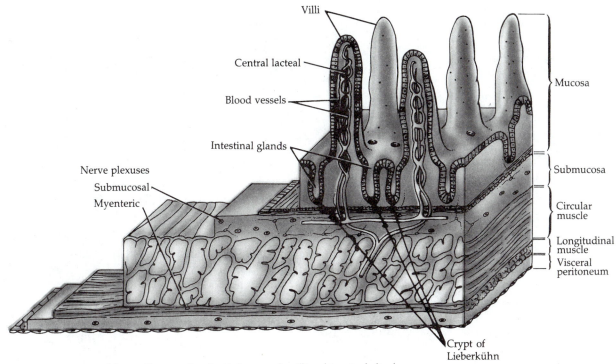

Villi

Central lacteal

Blood vessels

Intestinal glands

Nerve plexuses
Submucosal
Myenteric

Mucosa

Submucosa

Circular
muscle

Longitudinal
muscle

Visceral
peritoneum

Crypt of
Lieberkühn

FIGURE 2.6 Structure of the small intestinal wall with focus on the villi and intestinal glands.

Cells in the crypts of Lieberkühn also secrete fluid and electrolytes into the lumen of the small intestine. This fluid is typically reabsorbed by the villi.

Also present throughout the mucosa and submucosa of the small intestine are lymphoid tissues known as Peyer's patches. Peyer's patches, located underneath epithelial M-cells, contain both T-lymphocytes and B-lymphocytes. Intraepithelial lymphocytes can also be found within the intestinal epithelium between the absorptive cells. The general function of the cells of the Peyer's patches is to provide a defense against bacteria or other foreign substances that may have been ingested with ingested food.

Unabsorbed materials (both endogenous and dietary) leaving the ileum empty via the ileocecal valve into the cecum, the right side of the colon (large intestine). From the cecum, materials move sequentially through the ascending, transverse, descending, and sigmoid sections of the colon (Figs. 2.1 and 2.8). Haustra, or pouches, are characteristic of the colon and are caused by the contraction of the circular muscles and the teniae (also spelled *taenia* or *teneae*) coli, the latter comprising the longitudinal muscle of the colon. Rather than being a part of the entire wall of the alimentary canal as it is in the upper digestive tract, the longitudinal muscle in the colon is gathered into three muscular bands or strips that extend throughout most of the colon. Contraction of a

strip of longitudinal muscle along with contraction of circular muscle, cause the uncontracted portions of the colon to bulge outward, thereby creating pouches or haustra. Contractions typically occur in one area of the colon then move to a different, nearby area. As described by Guyton [5], the fecal material is slowly dug into and rolled over in the colon as one would spade the earth, so that deeper, moister fecal matter is put in contact with the colon's absorptive surface. This process permits dehydration of fecal matter for defecation while increasing fluid and electrolyte absorption.

COORDINATION AND REGULATION OF THE DIGESTIVE PROCESS

Regulatory Peptides

Factors influencing digestion and absorption are thought to be coordinated, in part, by a group of gastrointestinal tract molecules referred to as *regulatory peptides* or more specifically as gastrointestinal hormones and neuropeptides. Together the regulatory peptides affect a variety of digestive functions, including the secretion of digestive enzymes, electrolytes and water, gastrointestinal motility, intestinal absorption,

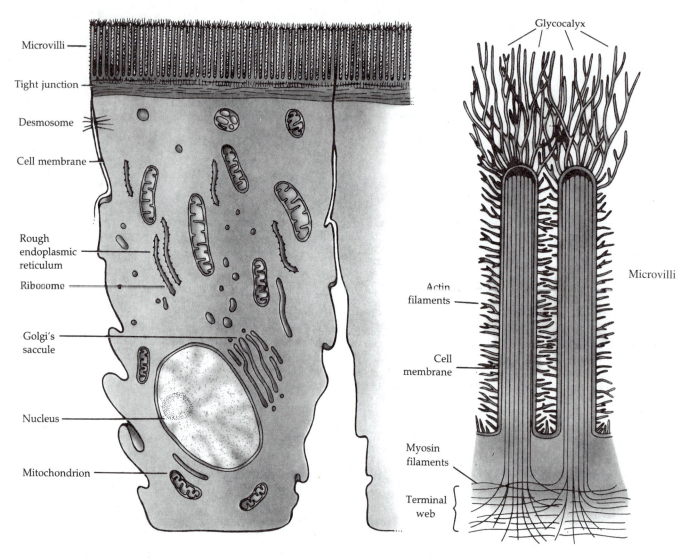

FIGURE 2.7 Structure of the absorptive cell of the small intestine, demonstrating its specialized function in digestion and absorption. The most striking feature of the cell is the brush border on its luminal surface. The brush border is made up of rows of minute projections called *microvilli*.

cell growth, and release of other hormones. Stimuli of peptide release are multiple and varied. For example, gastrin release is affected by vagal stimulation, ingestion of specific substances or nutrients, gastric distention, and hydrochloric acid in contact with gastric mucosa, as well as local and circulating hormones.

Some of the regulatory peptides such as gastrin, cholecystokinin (CCK), secretin, and gastric inhibitory polypeptide (GIP) are considered hormones. Peptides released by endocrine cells but diffusing through the extracellular space to their target tissues rather than being secreted into the blood for transport are termed

paracrines. Somatostatin is thought to act in a paracrine fashion by entering the gastric juice. Somatostatin then mediates the inhibition of gastrin secretion, which occurs in response to acid in contact with gastric mucosa [6]. Neurocrines are peptides that originate from nerves of the gut and include vasoactive intestinal peptide (VIP), gastrin-releasing peptide (GRP, also called *bombesin*), neurotensin, and substance P.

The functions of regulatory peptides with respect to the gastrointestinal tract and the digestive process are numerous. Gastrin, synthesized primarily by cells in the stomach, but also in the proximal small intestine, acts

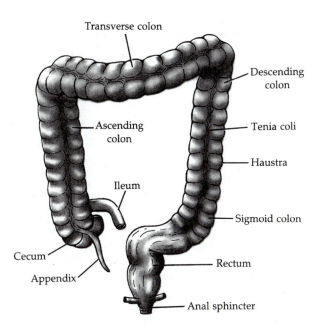

Transverse colon

Descending colon

Ascending colon

Tenia coli

Haustra

Ileum

Sigmoid colon

Cecum

Rectum

Appendix

Anal sphincter

FIGURE 2.8 The human colon.

TABLE 2.1 Actions of Selected GI Hormones

Action	Hormones			
	Gastrin	CCK	Secretin	GIP
Acid secretion	S[a]	S	I[a]	I[a]
Gastric emptying	I	I[a]	I	I
Pancreatic HCO$_3^-$ secretion	S	S[a]	S[a]	O
Pancreatic enzyme secretion	S	S[a]	S	O
Bile HCO$_3^-$ secretion	S	S	S[a]	O
Gallbladder contraction	S	S[a]	S	?
Gastric motility	S	I	I	I
Intestinal motility	S	S	I	?
Insulin release	S	S	S	S[a]
Mucosal growth	S[a]	S	I	?
Pancreatic growth	S	S[a]	S[a]	?

Abbreviations: S, stimulates; I, inhibits; O, no effect; ?, information unavailable.

[a]Particularly important action.

Source: Adapted from Johnson LR. Gastrointestinal physiology 3rd ed. St. Louis: Mosby, 1985:8.

mainly in the stomach. Principally, gastrin stimulates the release of hydrochloric acid, but it also stimulates gastric and intestinal motility and pepsinogen release. Gastrin stimulates the cellular growth of (has trophic action on) the stomach, and both the small and large intestine. CCK, secreted by cells of the proximal small intestine, principally stimulates the secretion of pancreatic juices (water and bicarbonate) and enzymes into the duodenum. It also stimulates the contraction of the gallbladder to facilitate the release of bile into the duodenum. Gastric motility may be slightly inhibited by CCK, whereas intestinal motility is enhanced by CCK. Secretin, secreted by the proximal small intestine in response to the release of acid chyme into the duodenum, acts primarily to stimulate the release of pancreatic juice (water and bicarbonate) into the intestine. Secretin is thought to inhibit motility of most of the gastrointestinal tract, especially the stomach and proximal small intestine [7]. GIP, also produced by cells of the small intestine, inhibits gastric secretions and motility. GIP also stimulates intestinal secretions and, like the other three hormones, stimulates insulin secretion from the pancreas as well. Table 2.1 lists additional actions of gastrin, CCK, secretin, and GIP.

Information on many of the other regulatory peptides is emerging rapidly. Motilin, secreted by the cells of the small intestine, causes contraction of intestinal smooth muscle and may be involved in regulating different phases of the migrating motility complex (MMC), important in maintaining gastrointestinal motility and

described in more detail on page 37 [7,8]. Somatostatin, synthesized by pancreatic and intestinal cells, appears to inhibit gastrin release as well as the release of GIP, secretin, VIP, and motilin. Gastric acid, gastric motility, pancreatic exocrine secretions and gallbladder contraction are also inhibited by somatostatin. VIP is present in neurons within the gut; it is not thought to be present in intestinal endocrine cells [9]. VIP stimulates intestinal secretions, relaxes most gastrointestinal sphincters, inhibits gastric acid secretion, and stimulates pancreatic bicarbonate release into the small intestine [9]. Gastrin-releasing peptide (GRP), released from nerves, stimulates the release of hydrochloric acid, gastrin, and CCK. Neurotensin, produced by small intestine mucosa, has no physiologic role at normal circulating concentrations; however, it may serve to mediate gastric emptying, intestinal motility, and gastric acid secretion after fat ingestion [7]. Substance P, another neuropeptide, increases blood flow to the gastrointestinal tract, inhibits acid secretion and motility of the small intestine, and binds to pancreatic acinar cells associated with enzyme secretion [6,9,10].

Neural Regulation

The nervous system of the gastrointestinal tract is referred to as the enteric (relating to the intestine) nervous system, and lies in the wall of the gastrointestinal tract beginning in the esophagus and extending to the anus. Neural regulation of the gastrointestinal tract involves a combination of neural plexuses and reflexes. The enteric

TABLE 2.2 Digestive Enzymes and Their Actions

Enzyme or Zymogen/Enzyme	Site of Secretion	Preferred Substrate(s)	Primary Site of Action
Salivary α amylase	Mouth	α 1-4 bonds in starch, dextrins	Mouth
Lingual lipase	Mouth	Triacylglycerol	Stomach, small intestine
Pepsinogen/pepsin	Stomach	Carboxyl end of phe, tyr, trp, met, leu, glu, asp	Stomach
Trypsinogen/trypsin	Pancreas	Carboxyl end of lys, arg	Small intestine
Chymotrypsinogen/chymotrypsin	Pancreas	Carboxyl end of phe, tyr, trp, met, asn, his	Small intestine
Procarboxypeptidase/			
carboxypeptidase A	Pancreas	C-terminal neutral amino acids	Small intestine
carboxypeptidase B	Pancreas	C-terminal basic amino acids	Small intestine
Proelastase	Pancreas	Fibrous proteins	Small intestine
Collagenase	Pancreas	Collagen	Small intestine
Ribonuclease	Pancreas	Ribonucleic acids	Small intestine
Deoxyribonuclease	Pancreas	Deoxyribonucleic acids	Small intestine
Pancreatic α amylase	Pancreas	α 1-4 bonds, in starch, maltotriose	Small intestine
Lipase and colipase	Pancreas	Triacylglycerol	Small intestine
Phospholipase A and B	Pancreas	Lecithin and other phospholipids	Small intestine
Cholesterol esterase	Pancreas	Cholesterol esters	Small intestine
Retinyl ester hydrolase	Pancreas	Retinyl esters	Small intestine
Amino peptidases	Small intestine	N-terminal amino acids	Small intestine
Dipeptidases	Small intestine	Dipeptides	Small intestine
Nucleotidase	Small intestine	Nucleotides	Small intestine
Nucleosidase	Small intestine	Nucleosides	Small intestine
Alkaline phosphatase	Small intestine	Organic phosphates	Small intestine
Monoglyceride lipase	Small intestine	Monoglycerides	Small intestine
Alpha dextrinase or isomaltase[a]	Small intestine	α 1-6 bonds in dextrins, oligosaccharides	Small intestine
Glucoamylase, glucosidase, and sucrase	Small intestine	α 1-4 bonds in maltose, maltotriose	Small intestine
Trehalase	Small intestine	Trehalose	Small intestine
Disaccharidases	Small intestine		Small intestine
Sucrase[a]		Sucrose	
Maltase		Maltose	
Lactase		Lactose	

[a]Part of an enzyme complex.

nervous system can be divided into two neuronal networks or plexuses. One plexus lies between the longitudinal and circular muscles and is called the *myenteric plexus*. The myenteric plexus controls primarily peristaltic activity or gastrointestinal motility and is innervated by parasympathetic and sympathetic nervous systems. Acetylcholine most often excites gastrointestinal motility. Norepinephrine and epinephrine, in contrast, typically inhibit gastrointestinal activity. The myenteric plexus also possesses its own neuronal network. The second plexus lies in the submucosa and is called the *submucosal plexus* or the *Meissner's plexus*. This plexus controls mainly gastrointestinal secretions and local blood flow.

Gastrointestinal reflexes involving the enteric nervous system also control gastrointestinal secretions and peristalsis, as well as other processes involved in digestion. For example, reflexes originating from the intestines inhibit gastric motility and secretions, and are called *enterogastric reflexes*. The colonoileal reflex from the colon inhibits the emptying of the contents of the ileum into the colon.

THE PROCESS OF DIGESTION: SECRETIONS AND ENZYMES REQUIRED FOR NUTRIENT DIGESTION

Table 2.2 provides a partial list of enzymes that participate in the digestion of nutrients in foods. Each of these are briefly discussed later as nutrient digestion is traced from the oral cavity throughout the rest of the gastrointestinal tract.

Oral Cavity and Salivary Glands

On entering the mouth, food is chewed by the action of the jaw muscles and is made ready for swallowing by mixing with the secretions released from the salivary glands. Small saliva-secreting salivary glands are found throughout the lining of the oral cavity. Three pairs of bilateral glands—the parotid, the submandibular, and the sublingual—are located along the jaw from the base of the ear to the chin (Figure 2.1). The parotid glands secrete water, electrolytes, and enzymes; the submandibular and sublingual glands secrete water, electrolytes, enzymes, and mucus. Mucus secretions contain glycoproteins, known as *mucins*, that lubricate food and protect the oral mucosa. Antibacterial and antiviral compounds, one example being the antibody IgA (immunoglobin A), are also found in saliva. The principal enzyme of saliva is α amylase (also called *ptyalin*) (Table 2.2). This enzyme hydrolyzes internal alpha 1-4 bonds within starch. A second digestive enzyme that is produced by lingual serous glands in the mouth is lingual lipase. This enzyme, which hydrolyzes dietary triacylglycerols in the stomach and small intestine, is mostly of importance to infants.

The passage of food from the mouth through the pharynx into the esophagus constitutes swallowing. Swallowing can be divided into several stages, voluntary, pharyngeal, and esophageal. Swallowing is a reflex response initiated by a voluntary action and regulated by the swallowing center in the medulla of the brain. As food passes through the pharynx, this swallowing center acts to inhibit the respiratory center, thereby preventing food from being aspirated into the larynx and lungs.

Esophagus

When food moves into the esophagus, both the striated muscle of the upper portion of the esophagus and the smooth muscle of the distal portion are stimulated by cholinergic (parasympathetic) nerves. The result is peristalsis, a progressive wavelike motion [1] that moves the food through the esophagus into the stomach.

At the lower (distal) end of the esophagus, just above the upper end of the stomach, lies the lower esophageal sphincter (LES). The area referred to as the LES may be a misnomer, since there is no consensus about this particular muscle area being sufficiently hypertrophied to constitute a true sphincter.

Normally LES pressure is higher than intragastric pressure. On swallowing, the LES pressure drops, relaxing the sphincter so that food may pass from the esophagus into the stomach. The musculature of the LES possesses increased tonic pressure that functions between meals to prevent gastroesophageal reflux. Multiple mechanisms, including neural and hormonal, regulate LES pressure. Moreover, certain foods and/or food-related substances appear to increase, probably indirectly, the re-

laxation of the LES. LES incompetence, manifested as heartburn, occurs when LES pressure is decreased or the LES is relaxed. Examples of substances that promote LES relaxation include smoking [11], chocolate [12], high-fat foods [12], alcohol [13], and carminatives such as peppermint [14].

Stomach

Additional Structural Information After passage through the LES, food enters the upper section of the stomach known as the *fundus.* The body and the antrum make up the two major parts of the stomach, shown in Figure 2.9. The body makes up approximately the first three-quarters of the stomach; it includes the fundus and extends from the LES to the angular notch. The body of the stomach serves primarily as the reservoir for swallowed food and is the production site for much of the gastric juice. The antrum extends from the angular notch to the duodenum, and functions to grind and mix food with the digestive juices to form chyme. The antrum also provides strong peristalsis for gastric emptying.

Gastric Juices Mixing of food with gastric juices begins primarily in the body of the stomach. Gastric juice is produced by three functionally different gastric glands found deep within the gastric mucosa. Gastric glands penetrate into the entire epithelium of the stomach and include (1) cardiac glands, found in a narrow rim at the juncture of the esophagus and stomach; (2) oxyntic glands, found in the body of the stomach; and (3) pyloric glands, located primarily in the antrum [15]. Several cell types secreting different substances may be found within a gland. For example, oxyntic glands, depicted in Figure 2.10, contain neck (mucus) cells, located close to the surface mucosa, as well as endocrine cells, parietal (oxyntic) cells, and chief (peptic or zymogenic) cells. Neck cells secrete bicarbonate and mucus. Parietal or oxyntic cells secrete hydrochloric acid and intrinsic factor. Chief, peptic, or zymogenic cells secrete pepsinogens. The cardiac glands contain no parietal cells, but produce mucus (mucus cells) and possess endocrine cells. The pyloric glands contain both mucus and parietal cells as well as endocrine G cells that produce the hormone gastrin. Gastrin is released from the G cells into the circulatory system and is carried to its target tissues.

In review, the main constituents of gastric juice produced by the different cells of the gastric glands include water, electrolytes, hydrochloric acid, enzymes, mucus, and intrinsic factor. Some of the functions of these constituents are discussed hereafter. Hydrochloric acid functions to activate the inactive proenzyme or zymogen

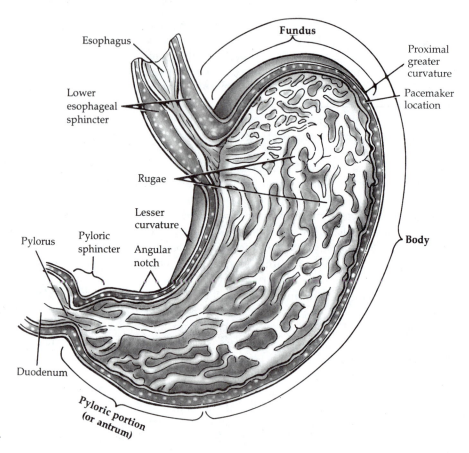

FIGURE 2.9 *Structure of the stomach.*

pepsinogen to active pepsin, as well as to denature proteins. Denaturation results in the destruction of tertiary and secondary protein structure and thereby opens interior bonds to the proteolytic effect of pepsin. Hydrochloric acid also releases various nutrients from organic complexes and serves as a bactericide, killing many of the bacteria ingested along with food. The principal active enzyme in the stomach is pepsin, which is derived from pepsinogen. Pepsinogen can be classified into one of two groups. Pepsinogen I is found primarily in areas of the stomach where hydrochloric acid is secreted. Maximal acid secretion correlates positively with pepsinogen I levels. Pepsinogen II is found both in the acid-secreting area of the stomach and in the antrum. The distinction between the two groups of pepsinogens has no known implications with respect to digestion; however, higher concentrations of pepsinogen I have been associated with an increased incidence of peptic ulcers [2]. On stimulation by acetylcholine and/or by acid, chief cells secrete zymogen granules containing pepsinogens. Pepsinogens are proenzymes, or zymogens, and are inactive. Pepsinogen is converted to pepsin, an active enzyme, in an environment with a low

pH or in the presence of previously formed pepsin. Optimal pepsin activity occurs at a pH < 3.5. Pepsin (Table 2.2) functions as an endopeptidase, meaning that it hydrolyzes interior peptide bonds within proteins. Specifically, pepsin appears to have an affinity for peptide bonds adjacent to the carboxyl end of methionine, leucine, the dicarboxylic amino acids (glutamate and aspartate), and the aromatic amino acids (phenylalanine, tyrosine, and tryptophan). Another enzyme present in the gastric juice is α-amylase that originated from the salivary glands in the mouth. This enzyme retains some activity in the stomach until it is inactivated by the low pH of gastric juice. Mucus, also present within the stomach, serves as a lubricant for ingested gastrointestinal contents and to coat the gastric mucosa and protect it from mechanical and chemical damage. Intrinsic factor, secreted by parietal cells, is necessary for the absorption of vitamin B_{12}, and will be discussed in more detail in Chapter 9, "Water-Soluble Vitamins."

In summary, very little chemical digestion of nutrients occurs in the stomach except for the initiation of protein hydrolysis by the protease pepsin. The only absorption that occurs is that of water and a few fat-

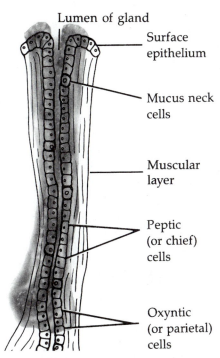

Lumen of gland

Surface epithelium

Mucus neck cells

Muscular layer

Peptic (or chief) cells

Oxyntic (or parietal) cells

FIGURE 2.10 The oxyntic gland from the body of the stomach.

soluble drugs such as ethyl alcohol and aspirin and a few minerals. Nourishment and survival, therefore, are possible without the stomach. Nevertheless, a healthy stomach makes adequate nourishment much easier.

Regulation of Gastric Secretions Gastric secretion and motility are regulated by multiple mechanisms as described in a general fashion in this chapter in the section "Coordination and Regulation of the Digestive Process," page 31. Some additional information regarding regulation of gastric secretions and motility will be presented here.

Release of acetylcholine from the vagus nerve stimulates both the parietal cells to secrete hydrochloric acid, and other gastric cells to secrete pepsinogen and mucus. In addition, on stimulation by acetylcholine, some nerves release GRP, which in turn stimulates the release of gastrin. Gastrin, an endocrine secretion, enters the blood and is transported to the oxyntic glands where it stimulates hydrochloric acid release from parietal cells. Gastrin secretion is also stimulated by elevated blood epinephrine concentrations and by amino acids and peptides in the gastric lumen. Acidification of the contents of the lumen of the antrum stimulates somatostatin release from the pancreas. Somatostatin and acidification of the gastric luminal contents inhibit gastrin release; somatostatin also directly inhibits hydrochloric acid secre-

tion [10,16]. In addition to gastrin and acetylcholine, another potent secretogogue (a compound that stimulates secretion) of hydrochloric acid is histamine, which is secreted from mast cells throughout the gastrointestinal tract. Histamine, a paracrine, binds to H_2 receptors on parietal cells to stimulate hydrochloric acid release. Together, acetylcholine, gastrin, and histamine prompt the release of substantial amounts of hydrochloric acid necessary for digestion. An understanding of how these three substances promote acid secretion facilitates an understanding of how drug therapies for peptic ulcers decrease acid production. For example, several drugs—cimetidine (Tagamet), ranitidine (Zantac), famotidine (Pepcid), and nizatidine (Axid)—used to treat ulcers act to prevent histamine from binding to H_2 receptors, and thereby, decrease acid release. Nutrients, foods, or substances in foods can also promote acid secretion. For example, alcohol is a potent stimulant of gastric acid secretion [17]. In contrast to caffeine, coffee, both decaffeinated and caffeinated, increases acid secretion [18,19]. Oral intake of calcium also stimulates gastrin and acid secretion [20].

Gastric Emptying and Motility When food is swallowed, the proximal portion of the stomach relaxes to accommodate the ingested food. Two processes mediated by the vagus nerve (receptive relaxation and gastric accommodation) influence this relaxation process, considered to be a reflex [1,15]. Signals for antral contraction, which occur at regular intervals, begin in the proximal stomach at a point along the greater curvature and migrate distally toward the pylorus [1]. Response of the antrum to signals by the pacemaker, located between the fundus and body of stomach, is thought to be affected by gastrointestinal hormones and neuropeptides [1]. The pacemaker determines the frequency of the contractions that occur [1,2]. As the food moves into the antrum, the rate of contractions increases so that in the distal portion of the stomach, food is liquefied into chyme.

The migrating motility complex (MMC), a series of contractions with several phases, moves distally like a wave down the gut. The migrating motility complex occurs in both the stomach and intestine. The waves or migrating motility complex occur approximately every 80 to 120 minutes during interdigestive periods. The migrating motility complex functions to sweep gastrointestinal contents and prevent bacterial overgrowth in the intestine; changes in migrating motility complex occur with eating [1,2,6,8]. The timing and site of initiation of the migrating motility complex are not constant [8].

Although contractions within the stomach promote physical disintegration of solid foods into a liquid form, complete liquefaction is not necessary for the emptying of the stomach contents through the pyloric sphincter into the duodenum. Particles as large as 3 mm in diameter (about 1/8 inch) can be emptied from the stomach, but solid particles are usually emptied with fluids when they have been degraded to a diameter of about 2 mm or less [1,2]. Approximately 1 to 5 mL (5 mL = 1 teaspoon) of chyme are allowed to enter the duodenum about twice per minute [2,21]. Contraction of the pylorus and proximal duodenum is thought to be coordinated with antral contraction of the gastric peristaltic wave [22]. Receptors of the duodenal bulb (proximal duodenum) are sensitive to osmolarity of chyme, volume of chyme present in the duodenum, and presence of acid and/or irritants in the small intestine. Gastric emptying is also partially affected by the macronutrient composition of the food. Carbohydrate and protein appear to empty at approximately the same rate from the stomach; fat, however, slows gastric emptying into the duodenum. Salts and monosaccharides inhibit gastric emptying, as do many free amino acids like tryptophan and phenylalanine. Complex carbohydrates, especially soluble fiber, decrease the rate of gastric emptying. Neural gastrointestinal reflexes, along with the release of regulatory peptides such as secretin by the duodenal bulb, also influence gastric emptying.

Small Intestine

Chyme, once in the small intestine, is mixed and moved through the small intestine by various contractions under nervous system influence. Contractions of longitudinal muscle may be referred to as *sleeve contractions* and function to mix the intestinal contents with the digestive juices [1]. Segmentation, or standing contractions of circular muscles, produces bidirectional flow [1], occurs many times per minute, and serves to mix and churn the chyme with digestive secretions in the small intestine. Peristaltic waves, or progressive contractions, also accomplished primarily through action of the circular muscles, move the chyme along the intestinal mucosa toward the ileocecal valve.

Chyme, moving from the stomach into the duodenum, initially has a low pH due to its gastric acid content. The duodenum is protected from this gastric acidity by pancreatic secretions with buffering capacity released into the duodenum and by secretions from the Brunner's glands. The Brunner's glands are located in the mucosa and submucosa of the first few centimeters of the duodenum or duodenal bulb. The mucus-containing secretions are viscous and alkaline with a pH approximately 8.2 to 9.3. Other secretions by intestinal cells include those from glands within the crypts of Lieberkühn. These glands secrete large volumes of intestinal juices, which facilitate digestion of nutrients throughout the small intestine. Distal to the duodenal bulb is a small projection termed the *duodenal papillae* or *papillae of Vater*. The bile pancreatic duct carrying secretions from the pancreas and gallbladder empties into this duct. These secretions are discussed next.

The Interrelationship Between the Small Intestine and Pancreas in the Digestive Process   The pancreas produces secretions containing fluid, electrolytes, bicarbonate, and enzymes that are released into the duodenum. The enzymes are responsible for the digestion of approximately 50% of all carbohydrates, 50% of all proteins, and 90% of all fat [23]. Bicarbonate released into the duodenum is important for neutralizing the acid chyme passing into the duodenum from the stomach and for maximizing enzyme activity within the duodenum.

Hormones such as secretin and CCK play important roles in the digestive process occurring in the small intestine. Secretin release is triggered by duodenal acidification with gastric hydrochloric acid. Secretin's major action is to increase the pH of the small intestine by stimulating secretion of water and bicarbonate by the pancreas. This hormone further promotes alkalization of intestinal contents by inhibiting gastric acid secretion and gastric emptying. CCK stimulates the secretion of pancreatic juices and enzymes into the duodenum. CCK is also thought to slightly inhibit gastric motility but to stimulate intestinal motility.

Enzymes produced by the pancreas and necessary for nutrient digestion are listed in Table 2.2 (p. 34). Pancreatic enzymes responsible for the digestion of protein, carbohydrate, and lipid are discussed in the following text, and are discussed in detail in Chapters 4, 6, and 7. Proteases—enzymes that digest proteins—found in pancreatic juice and secreted into the duodenum include trypsinogen, chymotrypsinogen, procarboxypeptidases, proelastase, and collagenase. Trypsinogen, a zymogen or proenzyme, is converted to its active form, trypsin, by the enzyme enteropeptidase (formerly called *enterokinase*) and by free trypsin. Enteropeptidase is stimulated by CCK. Trypsin is an endopeptidase specific for peptide bonds at the carboxyl end of basic amino acids (lysine and arginine). Chymotrypsinogen is activated to chymotrypsin by trypsin as well as by enteropeptidase. Chymotrypsin, also an endopeptidase, hydrolyzes interior peptide bonds adjacent to the carboxyl end of aromatic amino acids as well as methionine, asparagine, and histidine. Procarboxypeptidases are converted to active carboxypeptidases by trypsin. Carboxypeptidase A, an exopeptidase, cleaves carboxyterminal neutral (including aromatic) amino acids, whereas carboxypeptidase B, also an exopeptidase, cleaves carboxyterminal basic amino acids. Elastase hydrolyzes fibrous proteins, and collagenase hydrolyzes collagen.

As a group, proteases hydrolyze peptide bonds, either internally or from the ends, and the net result of their collective actions is the production of polypeptides shorter in length than the original polypeptide, oligopeptides (typically 4 to 10 amino acids in length), tripeptides, dipeptides, and free amino acids. The latter three may be absorbed into the enterocyte. Oligopeptides and some tripeptides may be further hydrolyzed by brush border aminopeptidases prior to absorption.

Pancreatic alpha (α) amylase secreted by the pancreas into the duodenum is a principal enzyme necessary for starch digestion. Like the α-amylase secreted by salivary glands, pancreatic α-amylase hydrolyzes alpha 1-4 bonds within starch to yield oligosaccharides, dextrins, maltotriose, and maltose. The oligosaccharides and dextrins produced may possess α 1-6 branches, which will require further hydrolysis by alpha dextrinase or isomaltase. The maltotrioses and maltoses also will need further hydrolysis by intestinal brush border enzymes prior to absorption.

Enzymes necessary for lipid digestion are also produced by the pancreas. Pancreatic lipase, the major fat-digesting enzyme, hydrolyzes triacylglycerols to yield monoacylglycerols, free fatty acids, and glycerol. In the presence of bile, phospholipase A_1 and A_2 hydrolyze fatty acids from phospholipids. Cholesterol esterase hydrolyzes fatty acids from cholesterol as well as from triacylglycerols. Bile is also needed for cholesterol esterase activity. The role of bile in fat digestion is discussed later.

The Interrelationships Among the Small Intestine, Liver, and Gallbladder in the Digestive Process
Bile Synthesis Bile acids are synthesized in the hepatocytes from cholesterol. Cholesterol, in a series of reactions, is oxidized to chenodeoxycholic acid and cholic acid, which are then conjugated principally with the amino acid glycine, and to a lesser extent with the amino acid taurine to form conjugated bile acids. For example, cholic acid conjugates with glycine and taurine to form glycocholic acid and taurocholic acid respectively. Chenodeoxycholic acid conjugates with glycine and taurine to form glycochenodeoxycholic acid and taurochenodeoxycholic acid, respectively. Conjugation occurs between the carboxy carbon of the acid and the amino group of the amino acid. Conjugation of the bile acids with these amino acids results in better ionization, and thus improved ability to form micelles. The role of micelles is described in the section "The Function of Bile," below. Hepatocytes also secrete cholesterol and phospholipids, especially lecithin, into the bile. These bile components make up the *bile acid-dependent* fraction of bile, and it is of importance that these bile components remain in proper ratio to prevent cholesterol precipitation and gallstone formation [24]. Immunoglobulin A (IgA), synthesized by plasma cells adjacent to biliary ducts and derived from plasma, is also found in bile. IgA, being an antibody, acts as a first line of defense against infectious microorganisms. Water, electrolytes, and bilirubin (a waste end product of hemoglobin degradation) conjugated with glucuronic acid, are secreted into bile by hepatocytes. This fraction of the bile is referred to as *bile acid independent*.

During the interdigestive periods, bile is sent from the liver to the gallbladder, where it is concentrated and stored. The gallbladder concentrates the bile such that as much as 90% of the water, and some of the electrolytes are reabsorbed by the gallbladder mucosa. The fluid reabsorption thus leaves the remaining bile constituents (i.e., bile acids and salts, cholesterol, lecithin, and bilirubin) in a less dilute form. Concentration of the bile permits greater storage of bile produced by the liver between periods of food ingestion. Contraction of the gallbladder is stimulated by CCK released in response to products of protein digestion (primarily tryptophan and phenylalanine) and of fat digestion (especially long-chain fatty acids). Bile is secreted into the duodenum through Oddi's sphincter.

The Function of Bile The general bile acid structure is given in Figure 2.11a. Bile acids are present in bile mostly in the conjugated form (i.e., conjugated with glycine or taurine). Furthermore, at bile's pH range, most bile acids are present as bile salts. Sodium is the predominant biliary cation, although potassium and calcium are also present.

Bile acids and bile salts act as detergents. In other words, the bile functions to decrease the surface tension of the fat, thus permitting emulsification (i.e., dispersion or increase in the exposed surface area of the lipids, and stabilization in a watery medium such as the intestinal lumen). Bile acids and salts are effective as a detergent because they contain both polar (hydrophilic) and nonpolar (hydrophobic) areas (i.e., they are amphipathic).

In addition to emulsification of lipids, bile acids and salts help in the absorption of lipids by forming spherical complexes called *micelles*. As bile salt concentrations increase, bile salt monomers aggregate to form simple micelles. As fatty acids and monoacylglycerols enter the micelles, mixed micelles are formed. The hy-

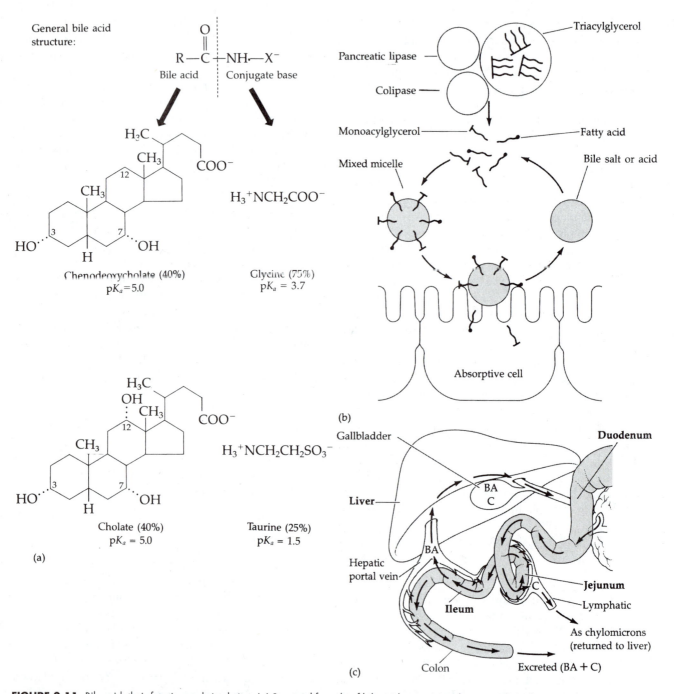

FIGURE 2.11 Bile acid, their function and circulation: (a) Structural formula of bile acid occurring in humans. Chenodeoxycholate and cholate each make up approximately 40% of the total bile acids. The remaining 20% of bile acids are secondary products, the result of bacterial action on chenodeoxycholate and cholate. (b) Schematic representation of the role of bile acids (micelle formation) in digestion and absorption of triacylglycerol. (c) Enterohepatic circulation of bile acids (BA) and cholesterol (C).

drophobic fat portion of the micelle is positioned in the interior of the sphere. Polar portions project outward from the surface of the micelle, thus permitting solubility in the watery digestive fluids, and transport to the brush border for absorption. Figure 2.11b shows the

action of the bile acids in forming micelles and delivering the lipids to the enterocytes for absorption. Other lipids in the intestinal lumen, such as fat-soluble vitamins and cholesterol, may also be incorporated into the micelle for delivery to the intestinal brush border. Once

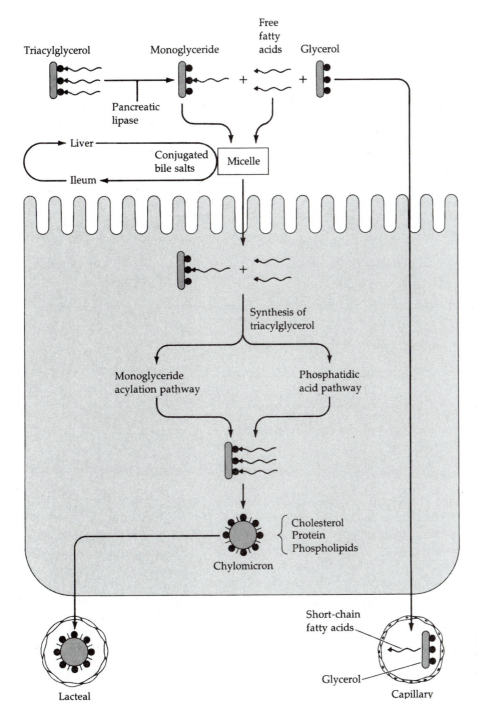

FIGURE 2.12 Summary of digestion and absorption of triacylglycerol. *(Reproduced by permission of Johnson LR. Gastrointestinal physiology, 3rd ed. St. Louis: Mosby, 1985.)*

at the brush border, the monoacylglycerols and fatty acids diffuse through the unstirred or stagnant water layer lying above the glycocalyx of the microvilli and into the enterocytes; the bile acids are released for reuse. Figure 2.12 summarizes the digestion and absorption of triacylglycerol.

The Recirculation and Excretion of Bile Greater than 90% of the bile acids secreted into the duodenum are reabsorbed by active transport in the ileum. Small amounts of the bile may be passively reabsorbed in the jejunum and the colon [25]. Of the cholesterol contained within the bile, about one half is taken up by the jejunum and is

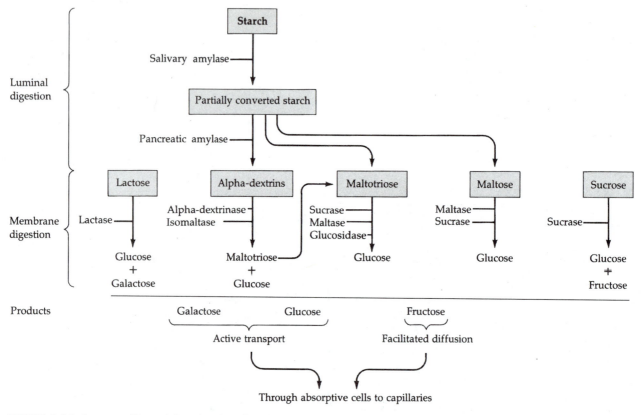

FIGURE 2.13 Summary of luminal digestion of starch and membrane digestion of disaccharides and oligosaccharides. Also indicated is the mechanism(s) for absorption of digestive products.

used in the formation of chylomicrons. The remainder of the cholesterol is excreted (Fig. 2.11c). The human body contains a total bile acid pool of about 2.5 to 4.0 g [25]. Only small amounts of bile acids, about 15 to 35% of the total pool, are not reabsorbed. Bile that is absorbed in the ileum enters the portal vein for transport in the blood (attached to albumin) back to the liver. Once in the liver, the reabsorbed bile acids are reconjugated if necessary and secreted into bile along with the newly synthesized bile acids. New bile acids are typically synthesized in amounts about equal to those which are lost in the feces. New bile mixed with recirculated bile is sent via the cystic duct for storage in the gallbladder. The circulation of bile, termed *enterohepatic circulation*, is pictured in Figure 2.11c. The pool of bile is thought to recycle as often as twice per meal [25].

Of the bile acids that are not reabsorbed in the ileum, some may be deconjugated by bacteria in the colon and possibly terminal ileum. Deconjugated bile acids form secondary bile acids. For example, cholic acid is converted to deoxycholic acid, which can be reabsorbed. Chenodeoxycholic acid is converted to lithocholic acid,

which is then primarily excreted in the feces. About 0.5 g of bile salts are lost daily in the feces. [25].

Knowledge of the recirculation and excretion of bile helps in the understanding of various drug therapies used for some people with high blood cholesterol concentrations. Drugs—powdered resins such as cholestyramine (Questran)—have been manufactured with the purpose of binding bile to enhance its excretion from the body. The increased excretion of the bile necessitates the use of body cholesterol for the synthesis of new bile acids. The goal from the use of such drugs is the lowering of blood cholesterol concentrations, and a reduced risk of cardiovascular disease.

The Role of the Intestinal Brush Border in the Digestive Process Several enzymes necessary for digestion are found on the brush border of the small intestine (Table 2.2, p. 34). Enzymes are present in the small intestine that are responsible for carbohydrate digestion (Fig. 2.13). Isomaltase is an oligosaccharidase found on the brush border. The enzyme functions as part of a complex with sucrase. Isomaltase hydrolyzes

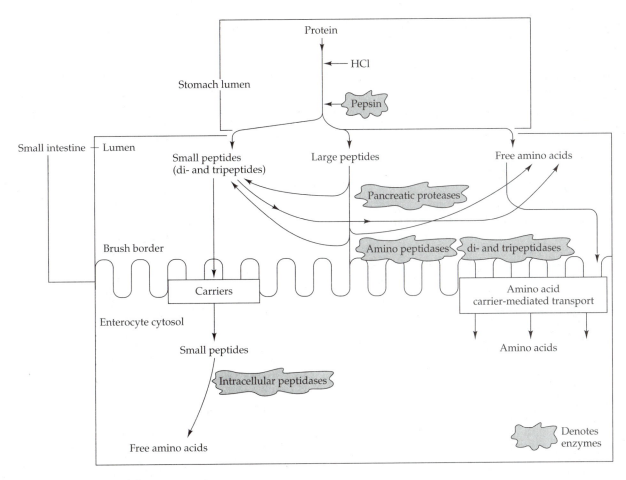

FIGURE 2.14 Summary of dietary protein digestion.

alpha 1-6 bonds in oligosaccharides and dextrins. Sucrase (invertase) hydrolyzes sucrose to yield glucose and fructose; however, it is also active against maltose and maltotriose. Maltose and maltotriose are generated from the action of pancreatic amylase. Glucoamylase, glucosidase, and maltase also hydrolyze α-1-4 bonds in oligosaccharides, maltotriose, and maltose. Three disaccharidases hydrolyze the three disaccharides into monosaccharides. Maltase hydrolyzes maltose into two glucose molecules. Lactase hydrolyzes lactose into glucose and galactose. Sucrase hydrolyzes sucrose to yield glucose and fructose. Further and more detailed information on carbohydrate digestion is provided in Chapter 4.

The brush border also contains enzymes for protein digestion (Fig. 2.14). These protein-digesting enzymes include (1) several aminopeptidases (with different specificities) that hydrolyze N-terminal amino acids from oligopeptides, tripeptides, and dipeptides; (2) tripeptidases that hydrolyze tripeptides into free amino acids and a dipeptide; and (3) dipeptidases that hydrolyze dipep-

tides into two free amino acids. Further information on protein digestion can be found in Chapter 7.

The Interrelationship Between the Digestive and Absorptive Processes in the Small Intestine
Most nutrients must be digested, that is, broken down into smaller pieces, prior to absorption. Digestion of nutrients occurs both in the lumen of the gastrointestinal tract and on the brush border. Although some absorption of some nutrients may occur in the stomach, absorption of most nutrients begins in the duodenum and continues throughout the jejunum and ileum. Generally, most absorption occurs in the proximal portion of the small intestine.

For absorption to occur, nutrients typically move through an unstirred or stagnant layer of water lying above the glycocalyx of the microvilli. Digestion and absorption of nutrients within the small intestine are rapid, with most of the carbohydrate, protein, and fat being absorbed within 30 minutes after chyme has reached the

Diffusion. Some substances such as water and small lipid molecules cross membranes freely. The concentration of substances that can diffuse across cell membranes tends to equalize on the two sides of the membrane, so that the substance moves from the higher concentration to the lower; that is, it moves down a concentration gradient.

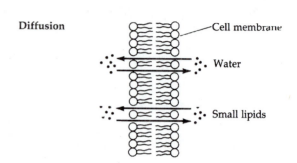

Facilitated diffusion. Other compounds cannot cross cell membranes without a specific carrier. The carrier may affect the permeability of the membrane in such a way that the substance is admitted or it may shuttle the compound from one side of the membrane to the other. Facilitated diffusion, like simple diffusion, allows an equalization of the substance on both sides of the membrane. The figure illustrates the shuttle process:
1. Carrier loads particle on outside of cell
2. Carrier releases particle on inside of cell
3. Reversal of (1) and (2)

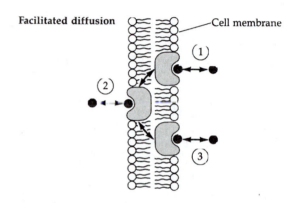

Active transport. Substances that need to be concentrated on one side of the cell membrane or the other require active transport, which involves energy expenditure. The energy is supplied by ATP and Na^+ is usually involved in the active transport mechanism. The figure illustrates the unidirectional movement of a substance requiring active transport:
1. Carrier loads particle on outside of cell
2. Carrier releases particle on inside of cell
3. Carrier returns to outside to pick up another particle.

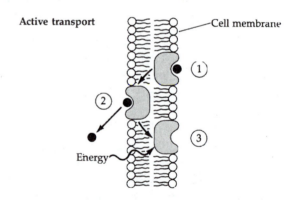

Pinocytosis. Some large molecules are moved into the cell via engulfment by the cell membrane. The figure illustrates the process:
1. Substance contacts cell membrane
2. Membrane wraps around or engulfs the substance
3. The sac formed separates from membrane and moves into the cell.

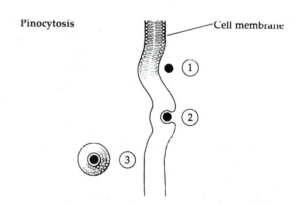

FIGURE 2.15 Primary mechanisms for nutrient absorption.

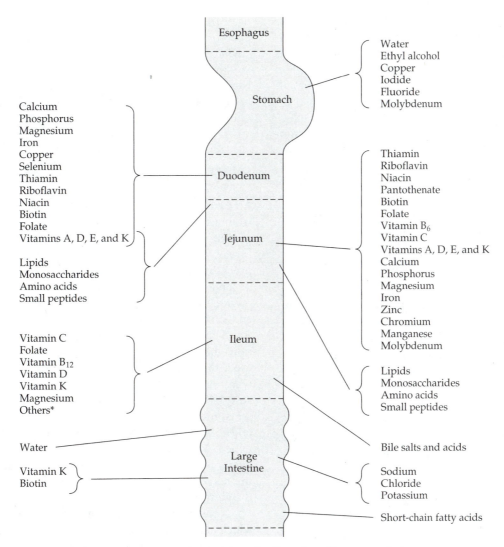

*Many additional nutrients may be absorbed from the ileum depending on transit time.

FIGURE 2.16 Sites of nutrient absorption in the gastrointestinal tract.

small intestine. The presence of unabsorbed food in the ileum may increase the time period in which material remains in the small intestine, and may therefore increase nutrient absorption [26].

Absorption of nutrients into enterocytes may be accomplished by diffusion, facilitated diffusion, active transport, or, occasionally, by pinocytosis or endocytosis (Fig. 2.15). In addition, a few nutrients may be absorbed by a paracellular (between cells) route. The mechanism of absorption depends on the solubility (fat versus water) of the nutrient, the concentration or electrical gradient, and the size of the molecule to be absorbed. The absorption and transport of amino acids,

peptides, monosaccharides, and lipid, the end products of macronutrient digestion, are considered in depth in Chapters 4, 6, and 7. The sites of absorption for each of the vitamins and minerals are shown in Figure 2.16, and are discussed in detail in Chapters 9–12. Following intestinal fluid and electrolyte exchange, unabsorbed intestinal contents are passed through the ileocecal valve into the colon.

Colon or Large Intestine

Intestinal material leaving the ileum empties via the ileocecal valve into the cecum, the right side of the large intestine. Figure 2.8 (p. 33) depicts the anatomy of the human colon. Initially on entering the colon, the intestinal material is still quite fluid. Colonic movements are coordinated so as to mix contents gently and to keep material in the proximal (ascending) colon for sufficient time to allow nutrient absorption to occur [27]. The proximal colonic epithelia absorb sodium, chloride, and water more effectively than does the small intestinal mucosa [28]. Of the water and sodium entering the colon daily, about 90 to 95% is absorbed with little back flux into the lumen of the colon unless the colon becomes irritated or inflamed [28,29]. Colonic absorption of sodium is influenced by a number of factors including hormones. Antidiuretic hormone (ADH), for example, decreases absorption of sodium, while glucocorticoids and mineralocorticoids increase sodium absorption in the colon [29].

Secretions into the lumen of the colon are few. Cells in the crypts of Lieberkühn secrete mucus. Mucus protects the colonic mucosa and acts as a lubricant for fecal matter. Potassium is secreted, as is bicarbonate, in exchange for chloride absorption. Bicarbonate provides an alkaline environment that helps to neutralize acids produced by colonic anaerobic bacteria. Both gram-negative and gram-positive bacteria strains representing over 400 species, of at least 40 genera have been isolated from human feces [30,31]. Acids produced in the colon include principally short-chain fatty acids, acetate, butyrate, and propionate, from bacterial action on carbohydrate. These fatty acids, and especially butyrate, may be absorbed by the colon. Butyrate is thought to represent a preferred energy source for use by colonic epithelial cells [30]. Other products generated by colonic bacteria include gases and ammonia. Bacterial fermentation of carbohydrates may generate gas (methane, hydrogen, and/or carbon dioxide) in some people. Ammonia generated by bacterial urease action on urea (secreted into the gastrointestinal tract from the blood) can be reabsorbed by the colon and recirculated to the liver, where it is reused to synthesize urea or amino acids [29]. About 25%, or about 8 g, of the body's urea may be handled in this fashion [29,32], and must be controlled in people with liver disease to prevent hepatic encephalopathy. Uric acid and creatinine may also be released into the digestive tract and may be metabolized by colonic bacteria [33,34].

As intestinal matter passes through the sections of the colon, contractions by longitudinal and circular muscles promote absorption of water and electrolytes. Fluids from the moist fecal matter are absorbed into the cells of the colon as the fecal matter moves through the colon. The end result is a progressive dehydration of the unabsorbed materials such that the liter or more of chyme that enters the large intestine daily is reduced to less than 200 g of defecated material containing dead bacteria, inorganic matter, water, small amounts of undigested and unabsorbed nutrients, and constituents of digestive juices [2].

SUMMARY

An examination of the various mechanisms in the gastrointestinal tract that allow food to be ingested, digested, absorbed, and then its residue to be excreted reveals the complexity of the digestive and absorption processes. Normal digestion and absorption of nutrients depends not only on a healthy alimentary canal but also on integration of the digestive system with the nervous, endocrine, and circulatory systems.

The many factors influencing digestion and absorption, including the dispersion and mixing of ingested food, the quantity and composition of gastrointestinal secretions, enterocyte integrity, the expanse of intestinal absorptive area, and the transit time of intestinal contents, must be coordinated so that nourishment of the body can occur while homeostasis of body fluids is maintained. Much of the coordination required is provided by regulatory peptides, some of which are provided by the nervous system as well as by the endocrine cells of the gastrointestinal tract.

Although the basic structure of the alimentary canal, which consists of the epithelium, submucosa, muscularis mucosa, and circular and longitudinal muscles, remains the same throughout, structural modifications allow for more specific functions by various segments of the gastrointestinal tract. Gastric glands that underlie the gastric mucosa secrete fluids and compounds necessary for digestive functions of the stomach. Also, particularly noteworthy is the presence of the folds of Kerckring, the villi, and the microvilli, all of which serve to increase dramatically the surface area exposed to the contents of the intestinal lumen. This enlarged surface area helps to maximize absorption, not only of ingested nutrients but also of endogenous secretions released into the gastrointestinal tract.

Study of the digestive system makes abundantly clear the fact that adequate nourishment of an individual, and therefore his or her health, depends in large measure on a normal functioning gastrointestinal tract. Particularly crucial to nourishment and health is a normally functioning small intestine, where the greatest amount of digestion and absorption occurs. Later chapters expand on the digestion and absorption of the various individual nutrients.

References Cited

1. Christensen J. Gastrointestinal motility: The regulation of nutrient delivery. In: Green M, Greene HL, eds. The role of the gastrointestinal tract in nutrient delivery. New York: Academic Press, 1984;3:83–106.
2. Vick RL. Contemporary medical physiology. Menlo Park: Addison-Wesley, 1984.
3. Grossman A. An overview of pancreatic exocrine secretion. Comp Biochem Physiol 1984;78B:1–13.
4. Madara JL, Trier JS. Functional morphology of the mucosa of the small intestine. In Johnson LR et al., eds. Physiology of the gastrointestinal tract. New York: Raven Press, 1987;1209–1249.
5. Guyton AC. Textbook of medical physiology. 8th ed. Philadelphia: Saunders, 1991.
6. Ganong WF. Review of medical physiology. 16th ed. Norwalk: Appleton and Lange, 1993.
7. Walsh JH. Gastrointestinal hormones. In: Johnson LR et al., eds. Physiology of the gastrointestinal tract. New York: Raven Press, 1987;181–253.
8. Weisbrodt NW. Motility of the small intestine. In: Johnson LR et al., eds. Physiology of the gastrointestinal tract. New York: Raven Press, 1987;631–663.
9. Dockray GJ. Physiology of enteric neuropeptides. In: Johnson LR et al., eds. Physiology of the gastrointestinal tract. New York: Raven Press, 1987;41–66.
10. Debas HT, Mulvihill SJ. Neuroendocrine design of the gut. Am J Surg 1991;161:243–249.
11. Dennish GW, Castell DO. Inhibitory effect of smoking on the lower esophageal sphincter. N Engl J Med 1971;284:1136–1137.
12. Babka JC, Castell DO. On the genesis of heartburn: The effects of specific foods on the lower esophageal sphincter. Am J Dig Dis 1973;18:391–397.
13. Hogan WJ, Andrade SRV, Winship DH. Ethanol-induced acute esophageal motor dysfunction. J Appl Physiol 1972;32:755–760.
14. Sigmund CJ, McNally EF. The action of a carminative on the lower esophageal sphincter. Gastroenterology 1969;56:13–18.
15. Meyer JH. Motility of the stomach and gastroduodenal junction. In: Johnson LR et al., eds. Physiology of the gastrointestinal tract. New York: Raven Press, 1987;613–629.
16. Walsh JH. Gastric secretion. In: Green M, Greene HL, eds. The role of the gastrointestinal tract in nutrient delivery. New York: Academic Press, 1984;3:107–118.
17. Lenz HJ, Rerrari-Taylor J, Isenberg JI. Wine and five percent alcohol are potent stimulants of gastric acid secretion in humans. Gastroenterology 1983;85:1082–1087.
18. Cohen S, Booth GH. Gastric acid secretion and lower esophageal sphincter pressure in response to coffee and caffeine. N Engl J Med 1975; 293:897–899.
19. Feldman EJ, Isenberg JI, Grossman MI. Gastric acid and gastrin response to decaffeinated coffee and a peptone meal. JAMA 1981;246:248–250.
20. Levant JA, Walsh JH, Isenberg JI. Stimulation of gastric secretion and gastrin release by single oral doses of calcium carbonate in man. N Engl J Med 1973;289:555–558.
21. Van Itallie TB, Kissileff HR. Physiology of energy intake: An inventory control model. Am J Clin Nutr 1985; 42:914–923.
22. Heading RC. Role of motility in the upper digestive tract. Scand J Gastroenterol 1984;19(suppl 96):39–44.
23. Guyton AC. Anatomy and physiology. Philadelphia: Saunders, 1985.
24. Greenberger NJ, Isselbacher KJ. Diseases of the gallbladder and bile ducts. In: Wilson JD, Braunwald E, Isselbacher KJ, Petersdorf RG, Martin JB, Fauci AS, Root RK. Harrison's principles of internal medicine. 12th ed. New York: McGraw-Hill, 1991;1358–1368.
25. Makhlouf GM. Function of the gallbladder. Nutr Today 1982;17:10–15.
26. Read NW. Small bowel transit time of food in man: Measurement, regulation and possible importance. Scand J Gastroenterol 1984;19(suppl 96):77–85.
27. Read NW. The relationship between colonic motility and transport. Scand J Gastroenterol 1984;19(suppl 93):35–42.
28. Phillips SF, Stephen AM. The structure and function of the large intestine. Nutr Today 1981;16:4–12.
29. Phillips SF. Functions of the large bowel: An overview. Scand J Gastroenterol 1984;19(suppl 93):1–12.
30. Savage DC. Gastrointestinal microflora in mammalian nutrition. Ann Rev Nutr 1986;6:155–178.
31. Simon GL, Gorbach SL. Intestinal flora in health and disease. Gastroenterology 1984;86:174–193.
32. Walser M, Bodenlos LJ. Urea metabolism in man. J Clin Invest 1959;38:1617–1626.
33. Sorensen LB. Degradation of uric acid in man. Metabolism 1959;8:687–703.
34. Jones JD, Burnett PC. Creatinine metabolism in humans with decreased renal function: Creatinine deficit. Clin Chem 1974;20:1204–1212.

Suggested Reading

Makhlouf GM. Function of the gallbladder. Nutr Today 1982; 17:10–15.
Moog F. The lining of the small intestine. Sci Am 1981;245: 164–176.
Phillips SF, Stephen AM. The structure and function of the large intestine. Nutr Today 1981;16:4–12.
These three well-written articles provide a good overview of the anatomy and physiology of the gallbladder, small intestine, and large intestine, respectively.
Grossman A. An overview of pancreatic exocrine secretion. Comp Biochem Physiol 1984;78B:1–13.

This paper is an excellent review of synthesis, translocation and secretion of proteins by exocrine glands.

Johnson LR, et al., eds. Physiology of the gastrointestinal tract. 2d ed. Vols. 1 and 2. New York: Raven Press, 1987.

These two books provide an outstanding review of the physiology of the gastrointestinal tract.

Langkamp-Henken B, Glezer JA, Kudsk KA. Immunologic structure and function of the gastrointestinal tract. Nutr Clin Prac 1992;7:100–108.

This article provides an excellent overview of the immune system and immunologic processes with respect to the gastrointestinal tract.

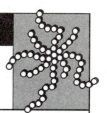

An Overview of Selected Disorders of the Digestive System with Implications for Nourishing the Body

In Chapter 2, digestion is defined as a process by which food is broken down mechanically and chemically in the gastrointestinal (GI) tract. Digestion ultimately provides nutrients ready for absorption into the body through the cells of the GI tract, principally the cells of the small intestine (enterocytes). Secretions required for digestion of nutrients are produced by multiple organs of the GI tract. These secretions include principally enzymes, but also hydrochloric acid for gastric digestion and bicarbonate and bile for digestion in the intestine. Malfunction of one or more of the organs due to pathology (the causes, nature, and effects of disease) can in turn diminish the production and/or release of secretions into the GI tract. Without secretions or with less than normal amounts of secretions, digestion of nutrients may be impaired and result in nutrient malabsorption.

Some GI tract diseases may cause decreased synthesis and release of secretions needed for nutrient digestion; other conditions or diseases affecting the GI tract can alter motility or clearing of the GI contents through the organs of the GI tract. Malfunction of sphincters can alter clearing or passage of the GI contents through the various organs of the GI tract. Clearing problems may cause back fluxes (refluxes) of secretions from, for example, the stomach into the esophagus; normally the contents of the GI tract move from the esophagus to the stomach and not vice versa. Conditions in which the GI mucosa is inflamed or damaged as well as conditions that increase transit time or speed up the movement of GI contents (food and nutrients) through the GI tract typically result in nutrient malabsorption due to diminished time for digestion and absorption of nutrients.

Understanding both the physiology of the GI tract and its accessory organs and the pathology affecting the GI tract are primary in understanding how an individual's diet will need to deviate from standard dietary recommendations for healthy populations of the United States. Standard dietary recommendations are based on the Recommended Dietary Allowances (RDA) [1], the Food Guide Pyramid, the Dietary and Health Recommendations [2], the Dietary Guidelines for Americans [3], and the Dietary Goals for the United States [4].

This Perspective addresses, in a general fashion, three disorders affecting the digestive tract and what

implications these conditions have with respect to nourishing the body.

Disorder 1. Reflux (backward flow) Esophagitis (inflammation of the esophagus)
After chewing and swallowing food, food enters the esophagus then passes through the lower esophageal sphincter (LES) into the stomach. Decreases in pressure at the LES, sometimes called *LES incompetence*, can result in reflux esophagitis in which gastric contents including hydrochloric acid flow backward into the esophagus from the stomach. Recurring reflux of hydrochloric acid into the esophagus can damage the esophageal mucosa. The individual experiencing reflux esophagitis typically complains of heartburn.

To address nutrition implications of this condition, we first need to re-examine some of the foods, nutrients, or substances in foods that influence LES pressure and that may promote increased acid production. High-fat meals and chocolate decrease LES pressure [5,6]. Carminatives (loosely and broadly defined as agents that may produce a warm sensation and also relieve symptoms of gas in the GI tract) or more specifically volatile oil extracts of plants, most often oils of spearmint and peppermint, decrease LES pressure [7]. Smoking [8] (nicotine) decreases LES pressure. Alcohol decreases LES pressure [9] and stimulates acid production [10]. Decaffeinated and caffeinated coffee increase acid secretion [11–13], and methylxanthine stimulates gastric secretion [14]. Ingestion of these substances or foods is likely to promote gastroesophageal reflux or aggravate irritated esophageal mucosa.

With this knowledge, the recommendations for the patient with reflux esophagitis or LES incompetence will make sense to you. Recommendations are aimed at (1) avoiding substances that can further lower LES pressure, which is already low due to the condition, and to a lesser extent (2) avoiding substances that may promote the secretion of acid, which would then be present in higher concentrations than normal if refluxed. Some of the recommendations are as follows: avoiding high-fat foods or meals, and avoiding chocolate, coffee, alcohol, and carminatives such as peppermint. Higher protein intake is encouraged, because protein increases LES pressure [14]. To some extent, however, excessive protein intakes, especially from foods high in calcium, such as dairy products, are not recommended. The reason behind this latter recommendation relates to the fact that amino acids and peptides (generated from digestion of the protein in the dairy products) and calcium in dairy products are both known to stimulate gastrin release [15]. Although gastrin increases LES pressure, it is also a potent stimulator of hydrochloric acid secretion.

In addition, in making nutrition recommendations for individuals with gastric reflux, it is important to remember that reflux is more likely to occur with increased gastric volume (i.e., eating large meals), with increased gastric pressure (obesity), and with placement of gastric contents near the sphincter (bending and lying down or recumbent positions). Thus, ingestion of smaller meals is recommended versus consumption of larger meals, and fluids should primarily be drunk between meals instead of with a meal to help minimize gastric volume. If an individual is overweight or obese, weight loss may help to diminish reflux. Avoidance of tight-fitting clothes is also suggested. Lastly, one should avoid lying down as well as lifting and bending for at least two hours after eating.

Disorder 2. Inflammatory Bowel Diseases

IBDs (inflammatory bowel diseases) include ulcerative colitis and Crohn's disease or regional enteritis. IBDs cause chronic inflammation of various segments of the GI tract, especially the intestines. Although the causes of IBDs are unknown, nutrient malabsorption is a significant problem. Because of the inflammation of the mucosa, nutrient hydrolysis by brush border disaccharidases and peptidases is diminished. Nutrient transit time is typically decreased (shortened). Absorption of many nutrients is impaired due to diminished digestion and enterocyte damage. People who have IBD generally experience diminished bowel function, both digestive and absorptive processes. Diarrhea and/or steatorrhea (excessive fat in the feces) are common. Blood may also be found in the feces with severe inflammation or ulceration of deeper areas of the GI mucosa. Moreover, food intake is usually decreased, especially during acute attacks.

The nutritional problems of individuals with IBD are multiple. The discussion that follows addresses a few of these problems along with nutrition recommendations. Blood lost in diarrhea results in the loss of iron and protein from the blood into the feces; potassium, other electrolytes, and fluids pulled from the blood are also typically lost with diarrhea. When these losses are coupled with poor nutrient intake, the individual becomes dehydrated, has poor protein and iron status, and usually has electrolyte imbalances. If IBD has affected the ileum, the absorption of vitamin B_{12}

may be impaired (absorption of this vitamin occurs in the ileum), reabsorption of bile salts from the ileum may be diminished, and fat malabsorption may occur. Although pancreatic lipase is available to hydrolyze dietary triacylglycerols, the lack of sufficient bile or diminished bile function due to bacterial alteration of bile can decrease micelle formation and thus decrease absorption of fatty acids and fat-soluble vitamins into the enterocyte. Unabsorbed fatty acids bind to calcium and magnesium in the lumen of the intestine; the resulting insoluble complex, sometimes called a *soap*, is excreted in the feces.

Some dietary recommendations for people with IBD include (1) increased intakes above the RDA for iron due to increased losses with the bloody diarrhea and decreased absorption; (2) a low-fat diet, due to impaired fat absorption; (3) increased intakes of calcium and magnesium due to diminished absorption secondary to soap formation and overall malabsorption with diarrhea; (4) a high-protein diet to improve protein status diminished by protein loss from the blood into the feces with bloody diarrhea and malabsorption of amino acids; (5) fat-soluble vitamin supplements, possibly given in a water-miscible form to improve absorption; (6) increased fluids for rehydration; and (7) increased nutrient intake to meet energy needs. Easily digestible carbohydrates that are low in fiber, high protein, low fat foods with minimal residue, and lactose-free foods will need to provide the bulk of the individual's energy needs if oral intake is deemed appropriate. Medium-chain triacylglycerol (MCT) oil, which is absorbed directly into portal blood and does not need bile for absorption, may be added in small amounts to different foods throughout the day to increase energy intake.

Disorder 3. Pancreatitis (inflammation of the pancreas)

Pancreatitis provides an excellent example of the nutritional ramifications of a condition affecting an accessory organ of the GI tract. Remember, the pancreas produces several enzymes needed for the digestion of all nutrients. People with pancreatitis experience malabsorption, especially of fat and fat-soluble vitamins. Diminished secretion of pancreatic lipase into the duodenum results in malabsorption of fat and fat-soluble vitamins. Thus, a low-fat diet is needed for people with pancreatitis. Bicarbonate secretion into the duodenum is also diminished with pancreatitis. Bicarbonate, in part, functions to increase the pH of the small intestine. Intestinal enzymes function best at an alkaline pH, which is provided by the release of bicarbonate into the intestine. Oral supplements of pancreatic enzymes may be needed to replace the diminished output of these enzymes by the malfunctioning, inflamed pan-

PERSPECTIVE   (continued)

creas. In addition, antacids may need to be taken with the oral pancreatic replacement enzymes. The antacids are taken to replace the role of the bicarbonate, and thus, to help maintain an appropriate pH for enzyme function. Administration of exogenous insulin may also be needed to replace the insulin no longer produced by damaged pancreatic endocrine cells.

These conditions have been presented to exemplify malfunction of a sphincter (LES incompetence), destruction of enterocyte function (IBD), and malfunction of an accessory organ (pancreatitis) of the gastrointestinal tract that provides secretions needed for nutrient digestion. The conditions exemplify the need to alter nutrient intakes to less than recommended levels for some nutrients and to greater than recommended levels, according to the Recommended Dietary Allowances (RDA). Bidirectional dietary modifications are typical of many conditions affecting not only the gastrointestinal tract, but other organ systems as well.

References Cited

1. Food and Nutrition Board, Commission on Life Sciences, National Research Council. Recommended dietary allowances, 10th ed. Washington DC: National Academy Press, 1989.
2. Committee on Diet and Health, Food and Nutrition Board, Commission on Life Sciences, National Research Council. Diet and health: Implications for reducing chronic disease risk. Washington DC: National Academy Press, 1989.
3. U.S. Department of Agriculture, U.S. Department of Health and Human Services. Dietary Guidelines for Americans, 3rd ed. Washington DC: U.S. Government Printing Office, 1990.
4. U.S. Senate, Select Committee on Nutrition and Human Needs. Dietary goals for the United States, 2nd ed. Washington DC: Government Printing Office, 1977.
5. Babka JC, Castell DO. On the genesis of heartburn: The effects of specific foods on the lower esophageal sphincter. Am J Dig Dis 1973;18: 391–397.
6. Wright LE, Castell DO. The adverse effect of chocolate on lower esophageal sphincter pressure. Digest Dis 1975;20:703–707.
7. Sigmund CJ, McNally EF. The action of a carminative on the lower esophageal sphincter. Gastroenterology 1969;56:13–18.
8. Dennish GW, Castell DO. Inhibitory effect of smoking on the lower esophageal sphincter. N Engl J Med 1971;284:1136–1137.
9. Hogan WJ, Andrade SRV, Winship DH. Ethanol-induced acute esophageal motor dysfunction. J Appl Physiol 1972;32:755–760.
10. Lenz HJ, Rerrari-Taylor J, Isenberg JI. Wine and five percent alcohol are potent stimulants of gastric acid secretion in humans. Gastroenterology 1983;85:1082–1087.
11. Cohen S, Booth GH. Gastric acid secretion and lower esophageal sphincter pressure in response to coffee and caffeine. N Engl J Med 1975;293: 897–899.
12. Feldman EJ, Isenberg JI, Grossman MI. Gastric acid and gastrin response to decaffeinated coffee and a peptone meal. JAMA 1981;246:248–250.
13. Thomas FB, Steinbaugh JT, Fromkes JJ, Mekhjian HS, Caldwell JH. Inhibitory effect of coffee on lower esophageal sphincter pressure. Gastroenterology 1980;79:1262–1266.
14. Harris JB, Nigon K, Alonso D. Adenosine-3′,5′-monophosphate: Intracellular mediator for methylxanthine stimulation of gastric secretion. Gastroenterology 1969;57:377–384.
15. Levant JA, Walsh JH, Isenberg JI. Stimulation of gastric secretion and gastrin release by single oral doses of calcium carbonate in man. N Engl J Med 1973;289:555–558.

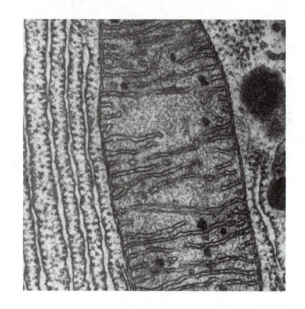

CHAPTER 3

·······································

ENERGY TRANSFORMATION

Photo: A mitochondrion

Many of the processes that sustain life require energy. In its most obvious connotation, "energy" implies physical verve and vitality, defining one's capacity for physical feats and endurance. Indeed, this view of energy does have biochemical foundation because the contraction of muscle fibers associated with mechanical work is an energy-demanding process. The process is accomplished at the expense of adenosine triphosphate (ATP), the major supplier of molecular energy. But there are other equally important, although perhaps more subtle, bodily requirements for energy. These include (1) the biosynthetic (anabolic) systems by which substances can be formed from simpler precursors, (2) active transport systems by which compounds or metal ions can be moved across membranes against a concentration gradient (p. 17), and (3) the transfer of genetic information.

Energy is derived from the energy-containing nutrients—carbohydrate, fat, and protein. If the covalent bonds contained within these molecules are cleaved, the bonding forces "relax," and their energy is released. Release of energy may simply be expressed as heat, such as would occur in the combustion of flammable substances. In the case of cellular metabolism, however, energy may be salvaged in the form of new, high-energy bonds that represent a usable source of energy for driving energy-requiring processes. Such stored energy is generally contained in phosphate anhydride bonds, chiefly those of ATP (Fig. 3.1). The analogy between the combustion and the metabolic oxidation of a typical nutrient (palmitic acid) is illustrated in Figure 3.2.

The unit of energy used throughout this text is the *calorie*, abbreviated *cal.* In the expression of the higher caloric values encountered in nutrition, the unit of kilocalories (kcal) is often used: 1 kcal = 1,000 cal. The reader should be aware of another unit of energy called the *joule* (J), and its higher-value counterpart, the kilojoule (kJ), which has become widely used in bio-

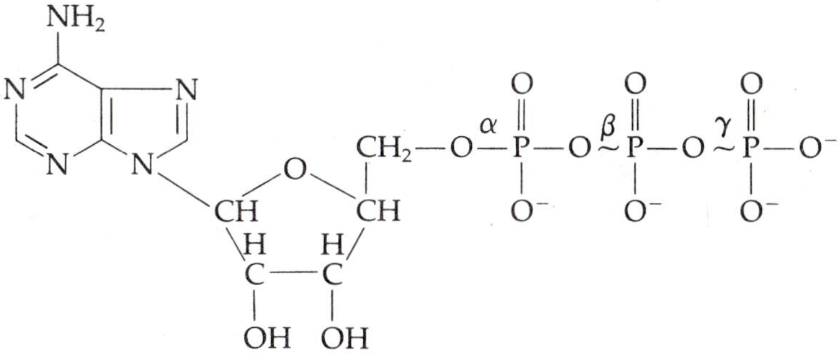

FIGURE 3.1 Adenosine triphosphate (ATP). The bonds connecting the α- and the β-phosphates and the β- and γ-phosphates are anhydride bonds, which release a large amount of energy when hydrolyzed. The bonds are shown as wavy lines, which are customarily used to denote a high-energy source.

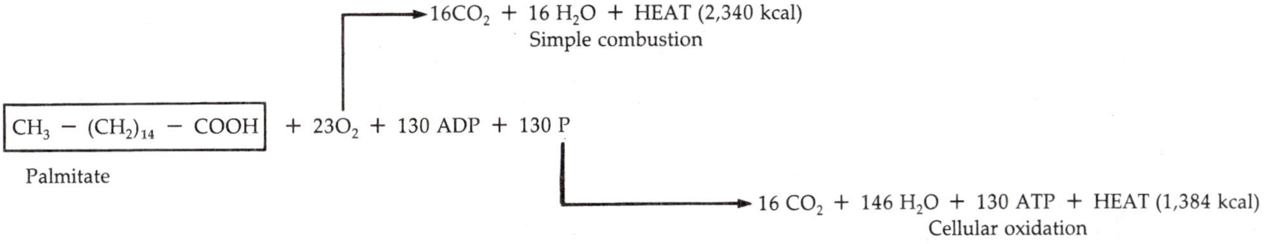

$$16CO_2 + 16\ H_2O + HEAT\ (2{,}340\ kcal)$$
Simple combustion

$$CH_3 - (CH_2)_{14} - COOH\ + 23O_2 + 130\ ADP + 130\ P$$

Palmitate

$$16\ CO_2 + 146\ H_2O + 130\ ATP + HEAT\ (1{,}384\ kcal)$$
Cellular oxidation

FIGURE 3.2 A comparison of the simple combustion and the metabolic oxidation of the fatty acid palmitate. The energy liberated from combustion assumes the form of heat only, while approximately 40% of the energy released by metabolic oxidation is salvaged as ATP, with the remainder released in the form of heat.

chemistry. Calories can be easily converted to joules by the factor 4.18:

$$1\ cal = 4.18\ J, \text{ or } 1\ kcal = 4.18\ kJ$$

Nutrition and the calorie have been so closely linked over the years, however, that the authors feel that students of nutrition may be more comfortable with the kilocalorie unit, and that digression from this unit may not be appropriate at this time.

ENERGY RELEASE OR CONSUMPTION IN CHEMICAL REACTIONS

The potential energy inherent in the chemical bonds of nutrients is released if the molecules undergo oxidation either through combustion or through the controlled oxidation within the cell. This energy is defined as *free energy* (G) if, on its release, it is capable of doing work at constant temperature and pressure. Since the cell does function under conditions of constant temperature and pressure, the energy it uses to drive energy-requiring reactions or processes is therefore free energy.

The products of the complete oxidation of organic molecules containing only carbon, hydrogen, and oxygen are CO_2 and H_2O, and they too have an inherent

free energy. However, since energy was released in the course of the oxidation of the organic molecules, the reactants in this case, the free energy of the products would necessarily be lower than that of the reactants. The difference in the free energy between the products and the reactants in a given chemical reaction is a very useful parameter for estimating the tendency for that reaction to occur. This difference is symbolized as:

$$G_{products} - G_{reactants} = \Delta G \text{ of the reaction}$$

If the G value of the reactants is greater than the G value of the products, as in the case of the oxidation reaction, the reaction is said to be *exothermic*, or energy releasing, and the sign of the ΔG is negative. In contrast, a positive ΔG indicates that the G of the products is greater than that of the reactants, indicating that energy would have to be supplied to the system to convert the reactants into the higher-energy products. Such a reaction is called *endothermic*, or energy requiring. Exothermic and endothermic reactions are sometimes referred to as *downhill* and *uphill* reactions respectively, a view that may help to clarify the concept of energy input and release. The free-energy levels of reactants and products in a typical exothermic or downhill reaction can be likened to a boulder on a hillside that can occupy the two positions A and B as illustrated in Figure 3.3. As the boulder descends to level B from level A, energy capable of doing

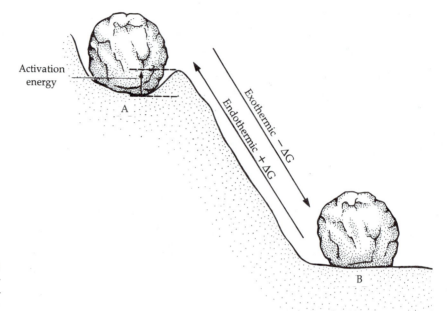

Activation
energy

Exothermic −ΔG
Endothermic +ΔG

A

B

FIGURE 3.3 The uphill–downhill concept illustrating energy-releasing and energy-demanding processes. Also indicated is the activation energy, which is the amount required to activate the reactant (the boulder, when occupying position A in this case) to its transition state.

work is clearly liberated, and the change in free energy is a negative value. The reverse reaction, moving the boulder uphill to level A from level B, necessitates the input of energy, an endothermic process, and a positive ΔG. It is important to understand that *the quantity of energy released in the downhill reaction is precisely the same as the quantity required for the reverse (uphill) reaction*. Only the sign of the ΔG changes.

Although exothermic reactions are favored over endothermic reactions in that they require no external energy input, they do not occur spontaneously. Otherwise, no energy-producing nutrients or fuels would exist throughout the universe, since they would have transformed spontaneously to their lower energy level. A certain amount of energy must be introduced into reactant molecules in order to activate them to what is referred to as their *transition state*, a higher energy level or barrier at which the exothermic conversion to products can indeed take place. This energy that must be imposed on the system to promote the reactants to their transition state is called the *activation energy*. Referring again to the boulder-and-hillside analogy of Figure 3.3, the boulder does not spontaneously descend until the required activation energy can dislodge it from its resting place to the brink of the slope.

The cell derives its energy from chemical reactions, each one of which exhibits a free-energy change. The reactions occur sequentially as the nutrients are systematically oxidized through a pathway of intermediates, ultimately to CO_2 and H_2O. All the reactions are enzyme-catalyzed. Within a given catabolic pathway, for example, the oxidation of glucose to CO_2 and H_2O, some reactions may be energy consuming ($+\Delta G$). However, energy-releasing ($-\Delta G$) reactions will prevail, so that the *net* energy transformation for the entire pathway is highly exothermic.

Most cellular reactions are reversible, meaning that an enzyme (E) that can catalyze the conversion of hypothetical substance A into substance B can also catalyze the reverse reaction, as shown:

$$A \underset{\longleftarrow}{\overset{\longrightarrow}{\quad E \quad}} B$$

To review briefly the concept of reversibility in a chemical reaction using the A, B interconversion as an example, in the presence of the specific enzyme E, substance A will be converted to substance B. Initially, the reaction is unidirectional, because only A is present. However, because the enzyme is also capable of converting B to A, this reaction becomes significant as B increases in concentration. Therefore, from the moment the reaction is initiated, the amount of A will decrease, while that of B will increase to the point that the *rate* of the two reactions becomes equal and the concentration of A and B will consequently no longer change. At this point the system is said to be in equilibrium, and whether the A $\longrightarrow$ B reaction or the B $\longrightarrow$ A reaction is energetically favored is indicated by the equilibrium constant, K_{eq}, of the reaction, which in this case is simply the ratio of the equilibrium concentration of product B to that of reactant A:

$$K_{eq} = [B]/[A]$$

Obviously, the K_{eq} increases in value to the extent that the $A \longrightarrow B$ conversion is favored over the $B \longrightarrow A$. If the K_{eq} has a value greater than 1, the formation of B from A is favored, whereas a value less than 1 indicates that the equilibrium favors the formation of A from B. It follows that if no bias exists for either reaction, the equilibrium constant becomes unity. The K_{eq} of a reaction can be used to calculate its standard free-energy change, which is discussed next.

The standard free-energy change (ΔG^0) for a chemical reaction is a constant for that particular reaction. It is defined as the difference between the free-energy content of the reactants and the free energy of the products under standard conditions. Standard conditions are defined precisely: a temperature of 25°C (298°K), a pressure of 1.0 atm (atmospheres), and the reactants and products must be present at their standard concentrations, namely 1.0 mol/L. Under such conditions, the ΔG^0 is mathematically related to the K_{eq} by the equation

$$\Delta G^0 = -2.3 \ RT \log K_{eq}$$

in which R is the gas constant (1.987 cal/mol × degrees K), and T is the absolute temperature, 298°K in this case. The relationship clearly shows that the equilibrium constant of a reaction determines the sign and magnitude of the standard free-energy change. Referring once again to the $A \longrightarrow B$ reaction as an example, the log of a K_{eq} value greater than 1.0 will be a positive integer, and the sign of the ΔG^0 will consequently be negative, therefore establishing that the reaction $A \longrightarrow B$ is energetically favored. Conversely, a K_{eq} of less than 1.0 would have a negative log value and therefore a positive ΔG^0 *for the reaction* $A \longrightarrow B$. The $+\Delta G$ in this case indicates that the formation of A from B is favored in the equilibrium. A pH of 7 is, by convention, designated the *standard pH in biochemical reactions.* In this special case, the free-energy change of reactions is designated $\Delta G^{0\prime}$ and will be used henceforth in this discussion.

There is an important difference between the free-energy change, ΔG, and the standard free-energy change, $\Delta G^{0\prime}$, of a chemical reaction. The difference in the two values can explain why a reaction having a positive $\Delta G^{0\prime}$ can proceed exothermically ($-\Delta G$) in the cell, where standard conditions do not exist. As an example, consider the reaction catalyzed by the enzyme triosephosphate isomerase shown in Figure 3.4. This particular reaction occurs in the glycolytic pathway through which glucose is converted to pyruvate. The pathway is discussed in detail in Chapter 4. The reaction catalyzed by the enzyme aldolase produces 1 mol each of

dihydroxyacetone phosphate (DHAP) and glyceraldehyde 3-phosphate (G-3-P) from 1 mol of fructose 1,6-bisphosphate. However, of the two products, only the G-3-P is directly degraded in the subsequent reactions of glycolysis, resulting in a significantly lower concentration of this metabolite compared to the DHAP. Therefore there are two important conditions within the cell that deviate from standard conditions, namely, the temperature (approximately 37°C, or 310°K) and the fact that the reactants and products are *not* at equal, 1.0 mol/L concentrations. The actual ΔG of the triosephosphate isomerase reaction for the conditions existing in the cell can be calculated from the $\Delta G^{0\prime}$ of the reaction and the cellular, steady-state equilibrium concentrations of reactant and product.

$$\Delta G = \Delta G^{0\prime} + 2.3 \ RT \log [\text{product}]/[\text{reactant}]$$

The $\Delta G^{0\prime}$ for the reaction DHAP (reactant) $\longrightarrow$ G-3-P (product) is +1,830 calorie/mol, indicating that under standard conditions the formation of DHAP is preferred over the formation of G-3-P. For the sake of illustration, however, let us assume that the cellular concentration of DHAP is 50 times that of G-3-P for the reason already explained. Substituting these values in the equation:

$$
\begin{aligned}
\Delta G &= +1,830 + 2.3(1.987)(310°K) \log 1/50 \\
&= +1,830 + 1,416 \log 0.02 \\
&= +1,830 + 1,416 \ (-1.7) \\
&= +1,830 - 2,407 \\
&= -577 \ \text{cal/mol}
\end{aligned}
$$

The negative ΔG therefore shows that the reaction is indeed proceeding to the right, as shown, despite the positive $\Delta G^{0\prime}$ for this reaction.

THE ROLE OF HIGH-ENERGY PHOSPHATE IN ENERGY STORAGE

The preceding section addressed the fundamental principle of free-energy changes in chemical reactions, and the fact that the cell obtains this free energy through the catabolism of nutrient molecules. Furthermore, it was pointed out that this energy must somehow be used to drive the various energy-requiring processes and anabolic reactions so important in normal cell function. Liberated energy can be used to form the phosphate anhydride bonds of ATP, and these bonds can in turn be hydrolyzed to release the energy when needed. Therefore, ATP can be thought of as an energy reservoir, serving as the major linking intermediate between energy-yielding and energy-demanding chemical reac-

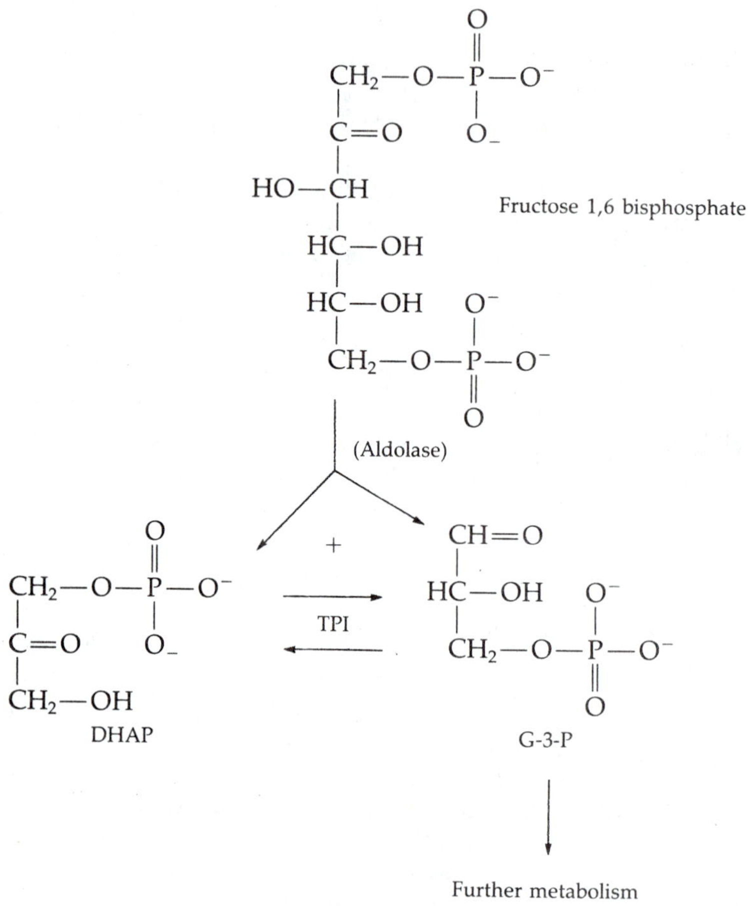

$$CH_2-O-P-O^-$$
... (Fructose 1,6 bisphosphate structure)

FIGURE 3.4 A segment of the glycolytic pathway of glucose metabolism, illustrating the interconversion by the enzyme triosephosphate isomerase (TPI) of dihydroxyacetone phosphate (DHAP) and glyceraldehyde 3-phosphate (G-3-P). The two triose phosphates are formed from the splitting of fructose 1,6 bisphosphate by aldolase. Under standard conditions, the TPI equilibrium is shifted toward the formation of DHAP, but in cellular metabolism the further conversion of G-3-P to other metabolites depletes its equilibrium concentration, and causes the rate of the DHAP $\longrightarrow$ G-3-P reaction to increase.

Fructose 1,6 bisphosphate

(Aldolase)

+

TPI

DHAP

G-3-P

Further metabolism

tions in the cell. In nearly all cases, the energy release from the molecule is effected by the enzymatic hydrolysis of the anhydride bond connecting the β- and γ-phosphates. The products of this hydrolysis are adenosine diphosphate (ADP) and a free phosphate group that in certain instances is transferred to various phosphate acceptors, a reaction that activates the acceptors to higher energy levels. The involvement of ATP as a link between the energy-releasing and energy-requiring cellular reactions and processes is summarized in Figure 3.5.

THE HIGH-ENERGY PHOSPHATE BOND

Hydrolysis of the anhydride bond connecting the β- and γ-phosphates of ATP is a highly exothermic reaction. The reaction, which releases ADP and inorganic phosphate (P_i), has a $\Delta G^{0\prime}$ of $-7{,}300$ cal/mol. The hydrolysis of the anhydride bond connecting the α- and β-phosphates also has a $\Delta G^{0\prime}$ of $-7{,}300$ cal/mol. How-

ever, the bond linking the α-phosphate to the adenosine is a phosphate ester, a bond that characteristically possesses considerably less free energy than a phosphate anhydride bond. The hydrolysis of adenosine monophosphate (AMP) to yield adenosine and phosphate liberates 3,400 cal/mol, typical of phosphate ester hydrolysis, the range for which is generally 2,000 to 5,000 cal/mol. As a family, therefore, phosphate esters rank below ATP and other nucleoside triphosphates on the scale of hydrolytic energy production.

Based on the preceding discussion of phosphate bond energies, it is tempting to think in terms of high-energy and low-energy phosphate bonds, with ATP and other nucleoside triphosphates being high energy, and phosphate esters representing low energy. However, the wide range of ester energy and the fact that there are phosphorylated compounds having even higher energy than ATP complicates the high-energy–low-energy concept. Phosphoenolpyruvate and 1,3 diphosphoglycerate, which occur as intermediates in the metabolic pathway of glycolysis (p. 84) are examples of compounds having phosphate bond energies significantly

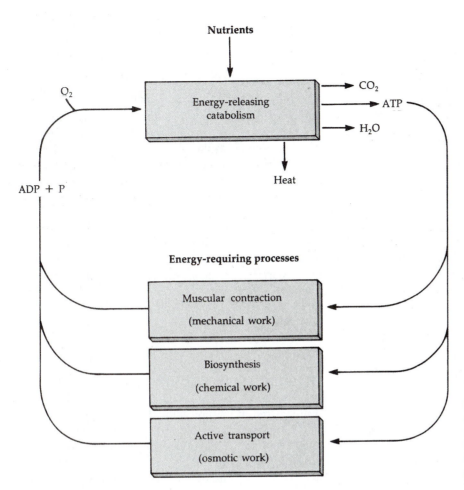

FIGURE 3.5 An illustration of how ATP is generated from the coupling of ADP and phosphate through the oxidative catabolism of nutrients, and how it is in turn used for energy-requiring processes.

higher than ATP. These structures are shown in Figure 3.6. Note that "high energy" bonds are depicted as a wavy line (~), referred to as a *tilde*, indicating that the free energy of hydrolysis is higher than for the more stable phosphate esters. Table 3.1 lists the standard free energy of hydrolysis of selected phosphate-containing compounds.

COUPLED REACTIONS IN THE TRANSFER OF ENERGY

It has been pointed out that the $\Delta G^{0\prime}$ value for the phosphate bond hydrolysis of ATP is intermediate between certain particularly high energy phosphate compounds and those compounds possessing relatively low energy phosphate esters. Its central position on the energy scale lets ATP serve as an intermediate carrier of phosphate groups. ADP can accept the phosphate groups from high-energy phosphate donor molecules, and then, as ATP, transfer them to lower-energy receptor molecules.

By receiving the phosphate groups, the acceptor molecules become activated to a higher energy level from which they can undergo subsequent reactions. The end result, therefore, is the transfer of chemical energy from donor molecule through ATP to receptor molecule.

If a given quantity of energy is released in an exothermic reaction, it is important to understand that the same amount of energy must be added to the system if the reaction is to be driven in the reverse direction. For example, the hydrolysis of the phosphate ester bond of glucose 6-phosphate liberates 3,300 cal/mol of energy, whereas the reverse reaction, the addition of the phosphate to glucose to form the ester, necessitates the input of 3,300 cal/mol. These reactions can be expressed in terms of their standard free-energy changes.

1. Glucose 6-phosphate $\longrightarrow$ Glucose + phosphate

$$\Delta G^{0\prime} = -3,300 \text{ cal/mol}$$

2. Phosphate + glucose $\longrightarrow$ Glucose 6-phosphate

$$\Delta G^{0\prime} = +3,300 \text{ calorie/mol}$$

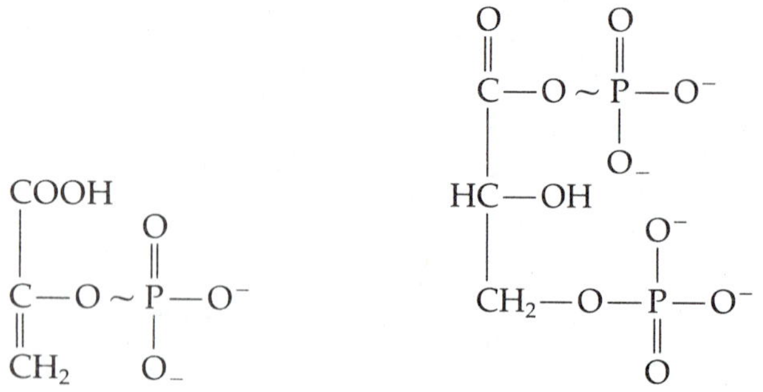

FIGURE 3.6 Examples of very high energy phosphate compounds. The hydrolysis of the phosphate bonds represented by the wavy line liberates more energy than the terminal phosphate of ATP, making it energetically possible to transfer these phosphate groups to ADP.

TABLE 3.1 Free Energy of Hydrolysis of Some Phosphorylated Compounds

	$\Delta G^{0\prime}$ (calories)
Phosphoenolpyruvate	−14,800
1,3-bisphosphoglycerate	−11,800
Creatine phosphate	−10,300
ATP	− 7,300
Glucose 1-phosphate	− 5,000
Adenosine monophosphate (AMP)	− 3,400
Glucose 6-phosphate	− 3,300

The addition of phosphate to a molecule is called a phosphorylation reaction and generally is accomplished by the enzymatic transfer of the terminal phosphate group of ATP to the compound, rather than by the addition of free phosphate, as suggested by reaction 2. Reaction 2 is hypothetical, designed only to illustrate the energy requirement for phosphorylation of the glucose molecule. In fact, the enzymatic phosphorylation of glucose by ATP is the important initial reaction that glucose undergoes on entering the cell. This reaction promotes glucose to a higher energy level, from which it may be indirectly incorporated into glycogen as stored carbohydrate or systematically oxidized for energy (p. 82). Phosphorylation can therefore be viewed as occurring in two reaction steps: (1) the hydrolysis of ATP to ADP and phosphate, and (2) addition of the phosphate to the substrate (glucose) molecule. *A net energy change for the two reactions coupled together* can be expressed.

$$(\text{Hydrolysis}) \text{ ATP} \longrightarrow \text{ADP} + \text{P}_i$$
$$\Delta G^{0\prime} = -7,300 \text{ cal/mol}$$
$$(\text{P-addition}) \text{ Glucose} + \text{P}_i \longrightarrow \text{glucose 6-P}$$
$$\Delta G^{0\prime} = +3,300 \text{ cal/mol}$$

Therefore

$$\text{ATP} + \text{glucose} \longrightarrow \text{ADP} + \text{glucose 6-P}$$
$$\Delta G^{0\prime} = -4,000 \text{ cal/mol}$$
(the coupled reaction)

The important implication of these reactions is that even though energy is consumed in the endothermic formation of glucose 6-phosphate from glucose and phosphate, the energy released by the ATP hydrolysis is of sufficient magnitude to drive the endothermic reaction, with 4,000 cal/mol left over. The reaction is catalyzed by the enzymes hexokinase or glucokinase, both of which hydrolyze the ATP and transfer the phosphate group to glucose. The enzyme brings the ATP and the glucose into close proximity to each other, reducing the activation energy of the reactants and facilitating the phosphate group transfer. The overall reaction, which depicts the activation of glucose at the expense of ATP, is energetically favorable, as evidenced by its high, negative standard free-energy change.

FORMATION OF ATP

Emphasized in the preceding discussion is that ATP is capable of activating molecules by phosphorylation. The phosphorylation itself is an endothermic reaction but is made possible by the highly exothermic hydrolysis of the terminal phosphate of ATP. From this, it can be seen that the ADP produced by the reaction must be reconverted by phosphorylation back to ATP to maintain the concentration of the ATP pool. But how is this accomplished, considering the large amount of energy ($\Delta G^{0\prime} = +7,300$ cal/mol) required for the reaction? Obviously there must be outside sources of considerable energy that can be linked to the phosphorylation of ADP. Actually, two such mechanisms function: *substrate-level phosphorylation* and *oxidative phosphorylation*, the latter being the more important of the two, from the standpoint of the amount of ATP generated.

Substrate-Level Phosphorylation

As discussed previously, phosphorylated molecules have a wide range of free energies of hydrolysis of their phosphate groups. Many of them release less energy than ATP, but some release more. The $\Delta G^{0\prime}$ of hydrolysis of the compounds listed in Table 3.1 is termed the *phosphate group transfer potential*, which is a measure of the compounds' capacities to donate phosphate groups to other substances. The more negative the transfer potential, the more potent the phosphate-donating power. Therefore, a compound that releases more energy on hydrolysis of its phosphate can transfer that phosphate to an acceptor molecule having a relatively more positive transfer potential. For this to occur in actuality, however, there must be a specific enzyme to catalyze the transfer. Therefore, just as ATP is capable of phosphorylating glucose to form glucose 6-phosphate, it can be predicted from Table 3.1 that those compounds having a more negative phosphate group transfer potential than ATP can phosphorylate ADP to ATP. This does, in fact, occur in metabolism. The phosphorylation of ADP by creatine phosphate, for example, represents an important mode for ATP formation in muscle, and the reaction exemplifies a substrate-level phosphorylation.

$$\text{Creatine-P} + \text{ADP} \longrightarrow \text{creatine} + \text{ATP}$$
$$\Delta G^{0\prime} = -3,000 \text{ cal/mol}$$

Oxidative Phosphorylation

This mechanism is the major means by which ATP is formed from ADP. The necessary energy is tapped from a pool of energy generated by the flow of electrons from a substrate molecule undergoing oxidation. The electrons are then passed through a series of intermediate compounds, ultimately to molecular oxygen, which becomes reduced to H_2O in the process. The compounds participating in this sequential reduction–oxidation constitute the *respiratory chain*, so named because the electron transfer is linked to the uptake of O_2, which is made available to the tissues by respiration. The *electron transport chain* is a more commonly used alternate term and is used throughout this text. The chain functions within the cell mitochondria, and reference to these organelles as the power plants of the cell is founded on the large amount of energy liberated by electron transport (p. 9). Although most of this energy assumes the form of heat to maintain body temperature, much of it is used to form ATP from ADP and phosphate. Therefore the term oxidative phosphorylation is a descriptive blend of two processes operating simultaneously, the oxidation of a metabolite by O_2 via electron transport, and the phosphorylation of ADP. Cellular oxidation, electron transport, and oxidative phosphorylation therefore are unified in function and are considered next in more detail.

BIOLOGICAL OXIDATION AND THE ELECTRON TRANSPORT CHAIN

The production of energy is intimately associated with the oxidation of the energy nutrients, as exemplified by the oxidation of the fatty acid palmitate shown in Fig-

(3A)

ure 3.2. Cellular oxidation of a compound can occur by different reactions: the addition of oxygen, the removal of electrons, and the removal of hydrogens. All these reactions are catalyzed by enzymes collectively termed *oxidoreductases* (p. 20). Among these, the *dehydrogenases*, which remove hydrogens and electrons from nutrient metabolites, are particularly important in energy transformation. This is because the hydrogens and electrons removed from metabolites by dehydrogenase reactions pass along the components of the electron transport chain and cause the release of large amounts of energy. In reactions in which oxygen is incorporated into a compound, or hydrogens are removed by other than dehydrogenases, the electron transport chain is not called into play and no energy is released. Such reactions are catalyzed by oxidoreductase enzymes generally referred to as *oxidases* and are not considered further in this section.

The hydrogens removed from a substrate molecule by a dehydrogenase enzyme are transferred to a cosubstrate, such as the vitamin-derived nicotinamide adenine dinucleotide (NAD^+) or flavin adenine dinucleotide (FAD). As a result of this transfer, the metabolite molecule, in its reduced form, which will be designated MH_2, becomes oxidized to M, while the oxidized forms of the cosubstrates (either NAD^+ or FAD) become reduced to NADH and $FADH_2$, respectively. Hydrogens and electrons are then enzymatically transferred through the electron transport chain components and eventually to molecular oxygen, which becomes reduced to H_2O. Using the example of NAD^+ as hydrogen acceptor, the overall reaction can be summarized as in 3A.

The energy given off is used in part to synthesize ATP from ADP and phosphate. It originates from the sequence of individual reduction–oxidation (redox) reactions along the electron transport chain, each component having a characteristic ability to donate or accept electrons. The tendency of a compound to give and to receive electrons is expressed in terms of its standard reduction potential, $E_0\prime$. More negative values of $E_0\prime$ reflect a greater ability of the compound to donate electrons to another, while increasingly positive values signify an increasing tendency to accept electrons. The reducing capacity of a compound can be expressed by the E_0' value of its half reaction, which indicates the compound's electromotive potential of electron donation.

Free-energy changes accompany the transfer of electrons between conjugate redox pairs of compounds, and are related to the measurable electromotive force of the electron flow from donor to acceptor. The quantity of energy released is directly proportional to the difference in the standard reduction potentials, $\Delta E_0'$, between the partners of the redox pair. The free energy of a redox reaction and the $\Delta E_0'$ of the interacting compounds are related by the expression

$$\Delta G^{0'} = -n\text{F} \ \Delta E_0'$$

where $\Delta G^{0'}$ is the standard free-energy change in calories, n is the number of electrons transferred (in cellular oxidation, assumed to be two) and F is a constant called the *faraday* (23,062 calories absolute volt equivalent). An example of a reduction–oxidation reaction that occurs within the electron transport system is the transfer of hydrogen atoms and electrons from NADH through the flavin mononucleotide (FMN)-linked enzyme called NADH dehydrogenase to oxidized coenzyme Q (CoQ). The half-reactions and E_0' values for each of these reactions are

$$\text{NADH} + \text{H}^+ \longrightarrow \text{NAD}^+ + 2\text{H}^+ + 2e^-$$
$$E_0' = -0.32 \text{ volts}$$
$$\text{CoQH}_2 \longrightarrow \text{CoQ} + 2\text{H}^+ + 2e^-$$
$$E_0' = +0.04 \text{ volts}$$

Since the NAD$^+$ system has a relatively more negative E_0' value than the CoQ system, it follows from the preceding discussion that it has a greater reducing potential than the CoQ system, since electrons tend to flow toward the more positive system. The reduction of CoQ by NADH is therefore predictable, and the coupled reaction, linked by the FMN of NADH dehydrogenase, can be written

$$\begin{array}{ccc} \text{NADH} + \text{H}^+ & \text{FMN} & \text{CoQH2} \\ E_0' = -0.32 \text{ volts} & & E_0' = +0.04 \text{ volts} \\ \text{NAD}^+ & \text{FMNH}_2 & \text{CoQ} \end{array}$$

$$\Delta E_0' = 0.36 \text{ volts}$$

Inserting this value for $\Delta E_0'$ into the energy equation:

$$\Delta G^{0'} = -2(23,062)(0.36) = -16,604 \text{ cal/mol}$$

The amount of energy liberated from this single reduction–oxidation reaction within the electron transport chain is therefore more than enough to phosphorylate ADP to ATP, which, it will be recalled, requires approximately 7,300 cal/mol. Before considering the electron transport components themselves, it is worthwhile to review the importance of the dehydrogenase reactions that deliver hydrogens to NAD$^+$ and FAD from various substrates undergoing oxidation. Such reactions are common within the pathways of intermediary metabolism, particularly the energy-rich citric acid (Krebs) cycle, which is detailed in Chapter 4. Two dehydrogenase reactions occurring in the Krebs cycle are offered here as examples of cosubstrate reduction linked to substrate (metabolite) oxidation. The reactions are catalyzed by the enzymes malate dehydrogenase (MDH) and succinate dehydrogenase (SDH) (see 3B).

The first three components of the electron transport chain are involved in the transfer of both hydrogens and electrons. In order of their functioning position in the chain, they are NAD$^+$, FMN, and coenzyme Q (CoQ), also referred to as *ubiquinone*. Precisely where, within their molecular structure, these substances accept and release hydrogens and electrons is shown by their reduced and oxidized forms in Figures 3.7, 3.8, and 3.9. The components functioning after CoQ are called *cytochromes*, which are iron-containing, electron-transferring proteins acting sequentially to carry electrons (only) from CoQ to molecular oxygen. No hydrogen transfer takes place within this segment of the chain. The hydrogen atoms collected by CoQ are released into the mitochondrial matrix, and ultimately combine with O_2 to form H_2O, as shown later. Specifically, the cytochromes are heme proteins in which the iron is bound to porphyrin, forming the heme moiety such as is found in hemoglobin (p. 360). The heme group is a red-brown pigment, and because of the high concentration of cytochromes in the mitochondrion, this coloration is imparted to that organelle. Cytochromes designated as cyt a–a_3, cyt b, cyt c_1, and cyt c function as electron carriers, and although subtle structural differences differentiate them, they share the heme moiety. Among them, the structure of cyt c was the first to be defined, and is shown in Figure 3.10. The reduction–oxidation of the cytochromes occurs at the iron atom, which alternates between the ferric (Fe^{+3}) and ferrous (Fe^{+2}) forms as it releases and acquires electrons.

$$Fe^{+2} \longrightarrow Fe^{+3} + e^-$$

Other iron-containing compounds called *iron-sulfur proteins* also function as electron carriers in the electron transport chain. The iron in these compounds is not in the form of heme, as it is in the cytochromes, but is associated with inorganic sulfur atoms and/or the sulfur atoms in the cysteine amino acid residues of the protein (Table 7.1). Two arrangements in which these iron-sulfur centers exist are shown in Figure 3.11.

(3B)

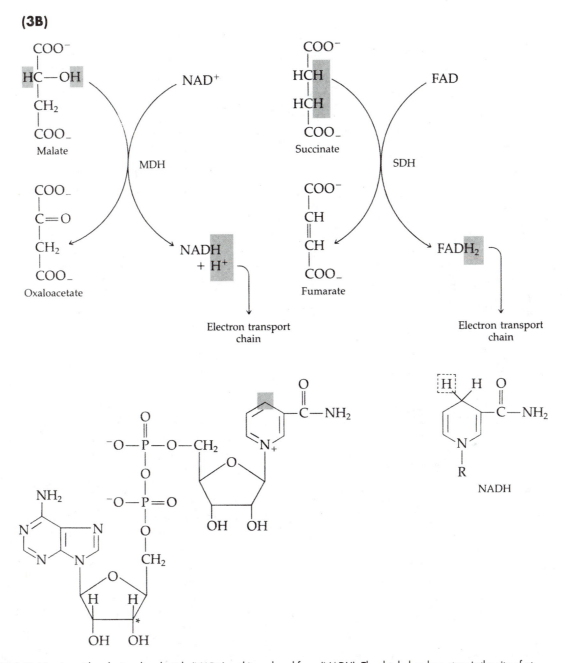

FIGURE 3.7 Nicotinamide adenine dinucleotide (NAD⁺) and its reduced form (NADH). The shaded carbon atom is the site of attachment of one of the two hydrogen atoms transferred from a metabolite undergoing dehydrogenation. The hydrogen is actually acquired as a hydride ion (:H⁻) that attaches to the nicotinamide ring as shown and neutralizes the positive charge on the ring nitrogen. The remainder of the structure, indicated by the symbol R, is unchanged from that of NAD⁺. The second hydrogen transferred from the metabolite is released as a proton. Another dehydrogenase cosubstrate, NADP, differs from NAD⁺ only in the attachment of a phosphate group at the position shown by the asterisk.

In the overall reaction catalyzed by the mitochondrial electron transport chain, electrons move from NADH or FADH₂, as these are formed from dehydrogenation reactions, through the FMN, CoQ, and cytochrome systems, and finally to O₂. These components exist in the form of four different complexes, each of which represents a portion of the electron transport chain. Each complex has its own unique composition, and catalyzes the transfer of electrons through that portion of the chain. Complexes I and II catalyze electron

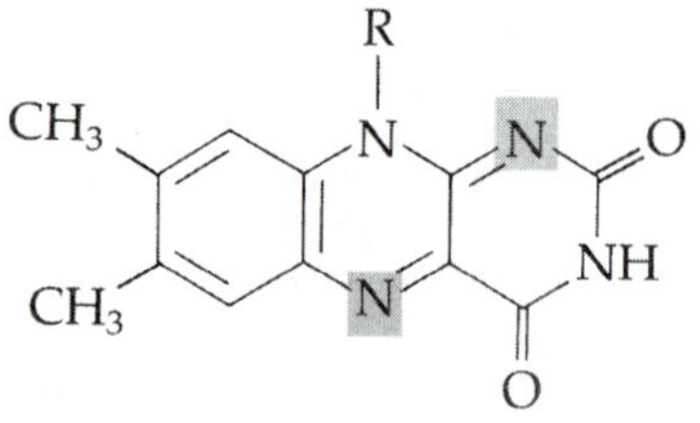

$$R = -CH_2-(CHOH)_3-CH_2-O-PO_3^{-2}$$
Ribitol phosphate

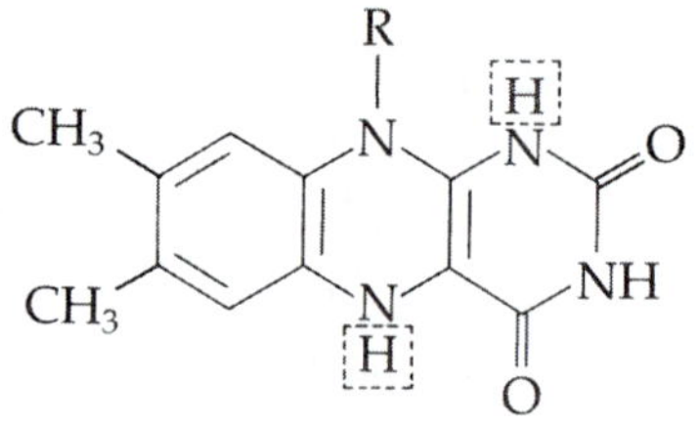

FMN

FMNH_2

FIGURE 3.8 Flavin mononucleotide (FMN) and its reduced form (FMNH_2). Hydrogens transferred from NADH and H^+ attach to the nitrogen atoms shaded in the structures. FMN is the phosphorylated derivative of the vitamin riboflavin (B_2). The cosubstrate FAD differs from FMN in that the ribitol phosphate side chain is linked to adenosine monophosphate (AMP) via a pyrophosphate bond. The site of hydrogen atom attachment to FAD is the same as with FMN.

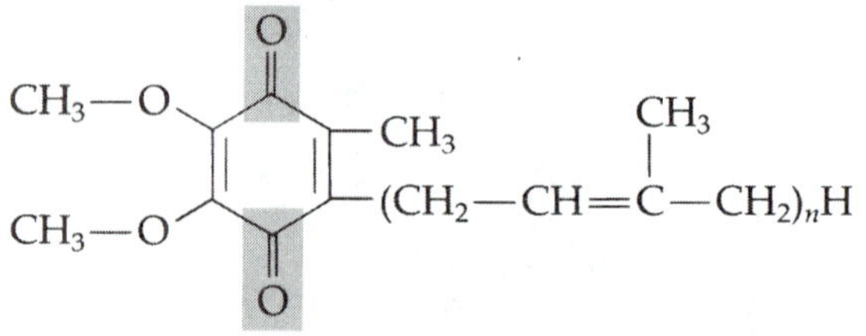

CoQ (**ubiquinone**) (**oxidized**)

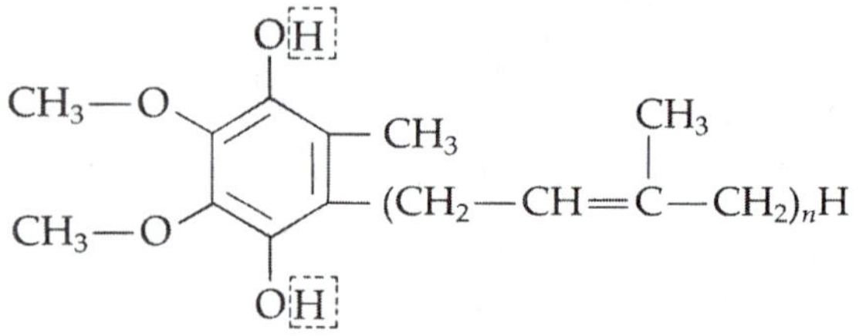

CoQH_2 (**ubiquinol**) (**reduced**)

FIGURE 3.9 Oxidized and reduced forms of coenzyme Q, or ubiquinone. The shaded groups function in the transfer of hydrogen atoms. The subscript n indicates the number of isoprenoid units in the side chain.

transfer to CoQ from two different electron donors: NADH (Complex I) and succinate, through FADH_2 (Complex II). Complex III carries electrons from CoQ to cytochrome c, and Complex IV completes the sequence by transferring electrons from cytochrome c to O_2. Figure 3.12 shows the sequential order of the electron transport intermediates and their division into the four component complexes. The flow of electrons from

NADH to O_2 is "downhill," meaning that each component has a more negative E_0' than its partner on the O_2 side and that energy is therefore released at each step in the sequence. However, the $\Delta E_0'$ between the redox pairs varies considerably, and, accordingly, so does the quantity of energy released. The $\Delta G^{0'}$ for each reaction site, calculated from the corresponding $\Delta E_0'$ values is shown in Table 3.2.

There are three sites at which the release of energy is sufficient to effect the phosphorylation of ADP, meaning that *for each molecule of NADH reoxidized to NAD^+ by O_2, via the electron transport chain, three ATPs are generated.* These sites of oxidative phosphorylation are indicated in Table 3.2 and also Figure 3.12. It is important to point out that the number of ATPs produced by oxidative phosphorylation is less if the dehydrogenase reaction uses the flavin cosubstrate FAD rather than NAD^+. This is because CoQ collects electrons directly from FADH_2 through an iron-sulfur center, thereby bypassing the NAD^+ ⟶ FMN ⟶ CoQ phosphorylation site. Therefore the FAD-requiring succinate dehydrogenase reaction generates only two ATPs rather than three.

The electron carriers are situated precisely, and most opportunistically, within the inner membrane of the mitochondrion. Complex I, for example, is oriented so that it can easily interact with the NADH produced by any of the dehydrogenases active in the matrix. The positioning of Complex IV (also called *cytochrome oxidase*) facilitates its picking up of electrons from Complex III and transferring them on to O_2 on the matrix side

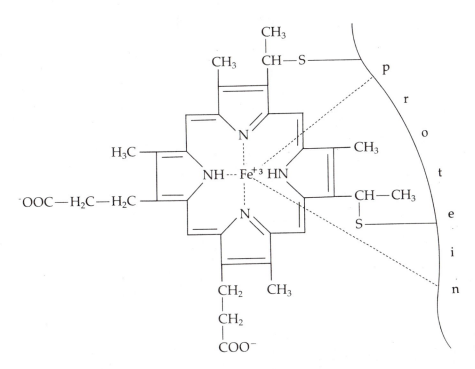

FIGURE 3.10 Oxidized cytochrome c. In its reduced form, the iron exists as Fe^{+2}.

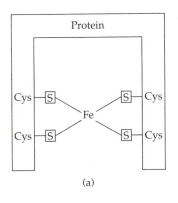

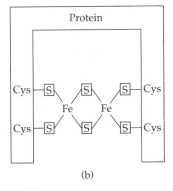

FIGURE 3.11 A schematic represen- tation of the binding of iron ions in the iron-sulfur centers of the mitochondrial electron transport system. Sulfur atoms can be covalently attached to the protein via cysteine amino acid residues (a), or they can, in addition, be free, as shown in structure (b).

of the membrane. Cytochrome c, in the intermembrane space, shuttles the electrons from Complex III to Complex IV. The spatial arrangement of the electron transport chain is illustrated schematically in Figure 3.13. Notice that electron flow through Complexes I, III, and IV is accompanied by the flow of protons from the matrix into the intermembrane space.

The difference in the E_0' values between the NAD^+–NADH and the one-half O_2–H_2O systems makes it possible to calculate the overall change in free energy across the entire electron transport chain:

$$\Delta E_0' = E_0'(O_2) - E_0'(NAD^+)$$
$$= 0.82 - (-0.32) = 1.14 \text{ volts}$$

then

$$\Delta G^{0'} = -2(23,062)(1.14) = -52,581 \text{ cal/mol}$$

Under the standard conditions, 21,900 cal/mol (3 × 7,300) of this total energy is conserved for future use as ATP, while the remaining 30,681 calories, representing 60% of the total, is in the form of heat that is necessary to help maintain a normal body temperature.

The precise mechanism by which the energy from electron transport is used to synthesize ATP is not entirely understood, but the preferred explanation is the *chemiosmotic theory*, a brief overview of which follows:

Energy released by the downhill (lower to higher E_0' values) flow of electrons in Complexes I, III, and IV is used to pump protons against a concentration gradient, from the matrix into the intermembrane space. This produces a marked disparity of both proton concentra-

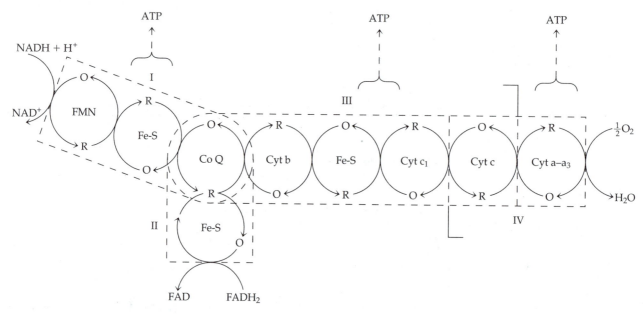

FIGURE 3.12 The sequential arrangement of the components of the electron transport chain, showing its division into four complexes, I, II, III, and IV. Coenzyme Q (ubiquinone) is shared by complexes I, II, and III. Cyt c is shared by complexes III and IV. Reduced cosubstrates, NADH and $FADH_2$, released in the matrix by dehydrogenase enzymes, are ultimately reoxidized by molecular oxygen as the intermediates undergo reversible reduction (R) and oxidation (O). Also indicated are the sites in complexes I, III, and IV where electron transfers between reduction–oxidation pairs furnish enough energy for the synthesis of ATP from ADP.

TABLE 3.2 Free-Energy Changes at Various Sites Within the Electron Transport Chain Showing Phosphorylation Sites

Reaction	$\Delta G^{0'}$	ADP Phosphorylation
NAD $\longrightarrow$ FMN	$-$ 922	
FMN $\longrightarrow$ CoQ	$-15,682$	ADP + P $\longrightarrow$ ATP
CoQ $\longrightarrow$ cyt b	$-$ 1,380	
cyt b $\longrightarrow$ cyt c_1	$-$ 7,380	ADP + P $\longrightarrow$ ATP
cyt c_1 $\longrightarrow$ cyt c	$-$ 922	
cyt c $\longrightarrow$ cyt a	$-$ 1,845	
cyt a $\longrightarrow$ ½ O_2	$-24,450$	ADP + P $\longrightarrow$ ATP

tion and electrical charge on either side of the membrane. Permeating the membrane are proton channels, through which protons passively diffuse back into the matrix from the intermembrane space. The driving force for the diffusion is the large difference in proton concentration in the two compartments. The channels are constructed from protein aggregates, and exist as two distinct sectors designated F_1 and F_0. F_1 is the catalytic sector, residing on the matrix side of the membrane, while F_0 is the membrane sector, involved primarily with proton translocation. Together, these components comprise what is called the *F_1F_0 ATPase aggregate*, also referred to as *Complex V*.

The return flow of protons furnishes the energy necessary for the synthesis of ATP from ADP and P_i. The proton flow is directed by the F_0 sector to the F_1 headpiece, which has binding sites for ADP and P_i. One oxygen atom of the inorganic phosphate is believed to react with two of the energetic protons, eliminating H_2O from the molecule. The precise mechanism of phosphorylation is complicated and not fully understood. It is believed, however, that the energy of oxidative phosphorylation is needed not for the actual coupling of ADP and P_i, but for the binding of the substrates (ADP and P_i) to the enzymatic binding sites of the F_1 sector, and the subsequent release of the ATP formed. A schematic representation of the chemiosmotic theory of oxidative phosphorylation is shown in Figure 3.14. Comprehensive reviews of electron transport, oxidative phosphorylation, and chemiosmotic coupling are available to the interested reader [1,2,3].

SUMMARY

This chapter has dealt with a subject of vital importance in nutrition, namely the conversion of the energy contained within nutrient molecules into energy usable by the body. The major portion of this energy is needed to

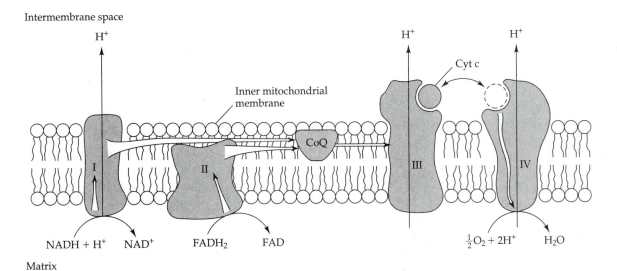

FIGURE 3.13 The spatial orientation of the complexes of the electron transport chain in the inner membrane of the mitochondrion. The energy of electron flow from reduced cosubstrates (NADH and FADH$_2$) to oxygen, within complexes I, III, and IV, pumps protons from the matrix to the intermembrane space against a concentration gradient.

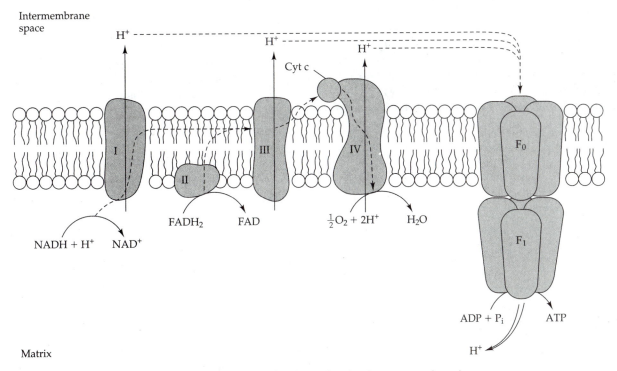

FIGURE 3.14 An illustration of the chemiosmotic theory of oxidative phosphorylation. Energy from electron transport pumps protons into the intermembrane space from the matrix against a concentration gradient. The passive diffusion of protons back into the matrix through the F$_0$F$_1$ ATP-synthase aggregate furnishes the energy to synthesize ATP from ADP and inorganic phosphate. For more details, see text.

maintain normal body temperature, but much of it is also conserved in the form of high-energy phosphate bonds, principally ATP. The ATP can, in turn, activate various substrates by phosphorylation to higher-energy levels from which they can undergo metabolism by specific enzymes. The exothermic hydrolysis of the ATP phosphate is sufficient to drive the endothermic phosphorylation, thereby completing the energy transfer from nutrient to metabolite.

ATP can be generated by two distinct mechanisms: (1) the transfer of a phosphate group from a very high energy phosphate donor to ADP, a process called substrate-level phosphorylation; and (2) oxidative phosphorylation, by which the energy derived from mitochondrial electron transport is used to unite ADP with an active phosphate. Oxidative phosphorylation is the major route for ATP production. Electron flow in the electron transport chain is from reduced cosubstrates to molecular oxygen, which therefore becomes the ultimate oxidizing agent and which becomes reduced to H_2O in the process. The downhill flow of electrons generates sufficient energy to effect oxidative phosphorylation at multiple sites along the chain.

Chapter 4 focuses on carbohydrate metabolism, including the energy-producing, systematic oxidation of glucose to CO_2 and H_2O. Within this pathway, reactions exemplifying both substrate level and oxidative phosphorylation are encountered. The reader is encouraged to thoughtfully consolidate the principles of energy transformation learned in the present chapter with the design and purpose of the metabolic pathways of the energy nutrients in following chapters. It is important to understand the link between the controlled oxidation of the energy nutrients and how released energy is ultimately used. Reference to this chapter will be made frequently in order to strengthen this unification of cellular processes.

References Cited

1. Racker E. Mechanisms of energy transformations. Ann Rev Biochem 1977;46:1006–1014.
2. Mitchell P. Vectorial chemiosmotic processes. Ann Rev Biochem 1977;46:996–1005.
3. Hatefi Y. The mitochondrial electron transport and oxidative phosphorylation system. Ann Rev Biochem 1985; 54:1015–1069.

Suggested Reading

Jequier E, Acheson K, Schutz Y. Assessment of energy expenditure and fuel utilization in man. Ann Rev Nutr 1987;7: 187–208.
The assessment of nutrient energy use is emphasized in this review of energy expenditure.
Lehninger AL, Nelson DL, Cox MM. Oxidative Phosphorylation and Photophosphorylation. In: Principles of Biochemistry, 2nd ed. New York: Worth, 1993: chap. 18.
This is a clearly written and graphically illustrated survey of energy transduction in the mitochondrion.

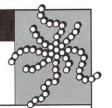

PERSPECTIVE

Energy Transformation in Brown Fat—Its Possible Implication in Weight Control

Among the nutritional curiosities that have invited extensive research for many years, perhaps none is more perplexing than the obesity problem. Particularly interesting is the fact that certain individuals remain lean with no effort to control caloric intake while others become obese despite conscientious efforts to control their consumption of food. Recently there has been a revival of interest in brown adipose tissue as possibly being implicated in this inconsistency. Brown fat is known to be an energy "buffer" capable of dissipating energy derived from ingested food as heat, a process called *thermogenesis*. Two types of external stimuli trigger thermogenesis: the ingestion of food and prolonged exposure to cold temperature, both of which stimulate the tissue via sympathetic innervation. The end result of this stimulation is that the phosphorylation of ADP by electron transport in the mitochondria of the brown fat cells becomes "uncoupled," resulting in less ATP formation but considerably more heat production. As ATP production diminishes, the dynamics of the catabolic breakdown and biosynthesis of stored nutrients would shift to catabolism in an effort to replenish the ATP. Theoretically, therefore, weight reduction should accompany a higher activity of brown fat. It is interesting to note that the percentage of brown fat relative to white fat is higher in hibernating animals, in animals adapted to living in a cold environment, and in early postnatal life, in which case thermogenesis is of obvious benefit.

Brown adipose tissue obtains its name from its high degree of vascularity and the abundant mitochondria present. The mitochondria, it will be recalled, are pigmented, due to the cytochromes and perhaps other oxidative pigments associated with electron transport. Not only are there larger numbers of mitochondria in brown fat compared with white fat, but they are also structurally different so as to promote thermogenesis at the expense of phosphorylation. Brown fat mitochondria have special H^+ pores in their inner membrane, formed by an integral protein called *thermogenin*, or the *uncoupling protein (UCP)*. It had previously been referred to as the *GDP-binding protein* because of its ability to bind guanosine diphosphate. UCP is a translocator of protons, allowing the external H^+ pumped out by electron transport to flow back into the mitochondria, rather than through the F_0F_1 ATP-synthase site of phosphorylation. Figure 13.15 illustrates how the proposed mechanism of brown fat thermogenesis relates to the chemiosmotic theory of oxidative phosphorylation. Protons within the mitochondrial matrix are pumped outside the inner membrane by the electron transport energy. Then the downhill flow of protons through the F_0F_1 aggregate channels provides the energy for ADP phosphorylation. Membrane pores of brown fat, which allow the futile cycling of protons, appear to be regulated by the 32,000-dalton uncoupling protein. A sympathetic signal, created by cold or dietary stimuli, and mediated by the hormone norepinephrine, has a stimulatory and hypertrophic effect on brown adipose tissue. This results in enhanced expression of the UCP in the inner membrane of the mitochondrion as shown in Figure 13.15, as well as accelerated synthesis of lipoprotein lipase and glucose transporters. The higher UCP concentration allows a greater proton flux into the matrix, which in turn encourages greater electron transport activity in answer to the reduced proton pressure in the intermembrane space. Enhancement of lipoprotein lipase and glucose transporters provide fuel (fatty acids and glucose, respectively) to meet the higher metabolic demand. The result is a shift toward thermogenesis, and away from ATP synthesis.

In mammals, brown adipose tissue is located in small depots principally in the interscapular, subscapular, and axillary regions; the nape of the neck; and in small patches between the ribs. It contributes about 1 to 5% of body weight. In older animals, including humans, a quantity of brown fat involutes, but it can be increased by exposure to the cold or during hibernation. Although there is considerable evidence that thermogenesis is defective in instances of obesity, direct evidence that the defect is in brown adipose tissue is tenuous. Studies using thermographic skin measurements have shown defective thermogenesis in the brown fat depots of obese subjects who had received catecholamine hormone. Such measurements are imprecise, however, due to the insulation provided by the thick, subcutaneous adipose tissue of obese people. In fact, some researchers are of the opinion that a simple, single test to assess appropriate brown fat function in obese subjects is lacking. Despite this shortcoming, the demonstration of the catecholamine stimulation of brown fat thermogenesis deserves further investigation, and it raises the tempting possibility that this tissue may relate to human obesity both in a causal way and as a focus for therapy. The following references

P E R S P E C T I V E   (continued)

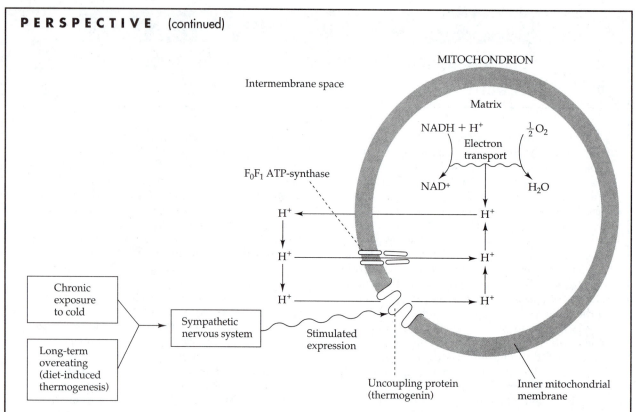

FIGURE 1   The stimulatory effect of cold and diet on brown adipocyte thermogenesis. Enhanced activity of the uncoupling protein, which translocates protons from the intermembrane space to the matrix, shifts the energy released from the proton flow toward thermogenesis and away from ATP synthesis.

are representative of review articles that have been published on the brown fat–thermogenesis connection, and are recommended as supplemental reading.

References Cited
1. Bray GA. Brown tissue and metabolic activity. Nutr Today 1982;17(1):23–27.
2. Himms-Hagan J. Brown adipose tissue thermogenesis in obese animals. Nutr Rev 1983:41(9): 261–267.
3. Himms-Hagan J. Thermogenesis in brown adipose tissue as an energy buffer. N Engl J Med 1984; 311(24):1549–1558.
4. Himms-Hagan J. Brown adipose thermogenesis: interdisciplinary studies. FASEB J 1990;4: 2890–2898.

MACRO-NUTRIENTS AND THEIR METABOLISM

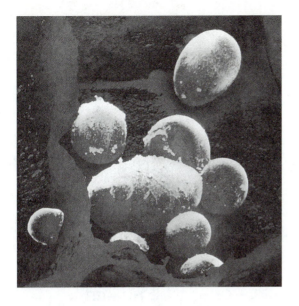

CARBOHYDRATES

Photo: Starch granules in a potato cell

The major source of energy fuel in the average human diet is carbohydrate, supplying nearly half of the total caloric intake. Roughly half of dietary carbohydrate is in the form of polysaccharides such as starches and dextrins, derived largely from cereal grains and vegetables. The remaining half is supplied as simple sugars, the most important of which include sucrose, lactose, and to a lesser extent, maltose, glucose, and fructose.

Carbohydrates are polyhydroxy aldehydes, or ketones, or substances that produce such compounds when hydrolyzed. They are constructed from the atoms of carbon, oxygen, and hydrogen, occurring in proportion that approximates that of a "hydrate of carbon," CH_2O, therefore accounting for the term *carbohydrate*. They exist in three major classes: the monosaccharides, the oligosaccharides, and the polysaccharides.

Monosaccharides are structurally the simplest form of carbohydrate, in that they cannot be hydrolyzed to smaller units by hydrolysis. For this reason they are sometimes referred to as *simple sugars*. The most abundant monosaccharide in nature and certainly the most important nutritionally is the 6-carbon sugar glucose.

Oligosaccharides consist of short chains of monosaccharide units joined by covalent bonds. The number of units is designated by the prefixes *di-*, *tri-*, *tetra-*, and so on, followed by the word *saccharide*. Among the oligosaccharides, the disaccharides, having just two monosaccharide units, are the most abundant. Within this group, sucrose, which consists of a glucose and a fructose residue, is nutritionally most significant, furnishing approximately one-third of total dietary carbohydrate in an average diet.

Polysaccharides are long chains of monosaccharide units that may number from several into the hundreds or even thousands. The major polysaccharides of interest in nutrition are glycogen, found in certain animal, including human, tissues, and starch and cellulose, which are both of plant origin. All these polysaccharides consist of repeating units of glucose only.

STRUCTURAL FEATURES

Monosaccharides and Stereoisomerism

As they occur in nature, or arise as intermediate products in digestion, these simple sugars contain from three to seven carbon atoms, and are accordingly termed *trioses, tetroses, pentoses, hexoses,* and *heptoses.* In addition to hydroxyl groups, these compounds possess a functional carbonyl group that can be either an aldehyde or a ketone, therefore necessitating the additional classification of aldoses, those sugars having an aldehyde group, and ketoses, those possessing a ketone. These two classifications are used together with the number of carbon atoms in describing a particular monosaccharide. For example, a five-carbon sugar having a ketone group is called a ketopentose; a six-carbon, aldehyde-possessing compound is an aldohexose, and so forth.

Many organic substances, including the carbohydrates, are optically active, which means that if plane-polarized light is passed through a solution of the substances, the plane of light will be rotated to the left (such substances are called levorotatory) or to the right (dextrorotatory). The direction and extent of the rotation is characteristic of a particular compound and is measurable by an instrument called a polarimeter.

The right or left direction of rotation is expressed as dextrorotatory (+) or levorotatory (−), and the number of angular degrees indicates the extent of rotation. As an example, a solution of glucose is known to have a rotation of +52.7°.

Optical activity is attributed to the presence of one or more asymmetric or chiral carbon atoms in the molecule. Chiral carbon atoms have four different atoms or groups covalently attached to them. Shown in 4A is a chiral carbon atom with its bonds directed toward the hypothetical atoms or groups W, X, Y, and Z. It can be thought of as being situated in the geometric center of a tetrahedron, with its four bonds directed toward the corners of that tetrahedron. Because the molecule is asymmetric, it is possible to construct a similar but not identical figure simply by exchanging the relative positions of any two of the groups. The two models shown bear the same groups and therefore the same molecular formula, but they are not identical, as evidenced by the reader's inability to superimpose them by mental manipulation. They are, in fact, mirror images of each other and are said to be *enantiomers,* a special class within

(4A)

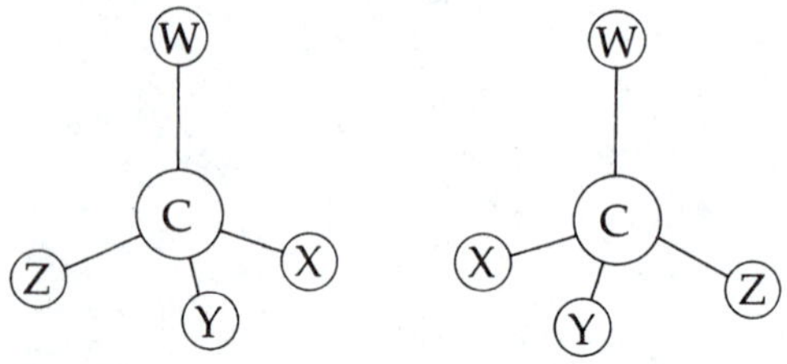

(4B)

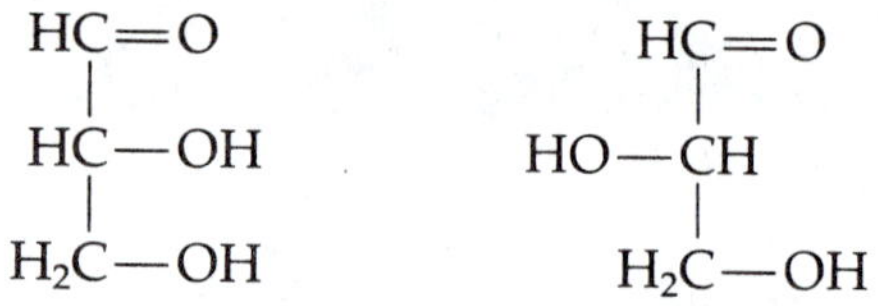

D-glyceraldehyde   L-glyceraldehyde

a broader family of compounds called *stereoisomers.* Stereoisomers are compounds having two or more chiral carbon atoms, which have the same four groups attached to those carbon atoms but which are not mirror images of each other. If an asymmetric substance rotates the plane of polarized light a certain number of degrees to the right, its enantiomer will rotate the light the same number of degrees to the left. Enantiomers exist in D or L orientation, and if a compound is structurally D, its enantiomer will be L. The D–L designation does not predict the direction of rotation of plane-polarized light. Instead, the designation simply refers to structural analogy to the reference compound glyceraldehyde, whose D and L forms are by convention drawn as shown in 4B. The distinction between D and L configurations of stereoisomers therefore rests with the direction of the −OH bond on the single, chiral carbon of the molecule. Notice that in the D form it points to the right, and in the L configuration to the left. Remember, these forms are not superimposable. Monosaccharides having more than three carbons will have more than one chiral center, but only the highest-numbered chiral carbon is the indicator as to whether the molecule is of the D or L configuration. The configuration is determined by the right or left direction of the hydroxyl group attached to that carbon atom. Carbon atom numbering and the D versus L designation are illustrated in the following structures for the aldohexose glucose and the ketohexose fructose. Since the highest numbered asymmetric carbon atom in these structures is number 5, this becomes the designator atom for either the D or L stereoisomer. Notice, however, that in going from the D

(4C)

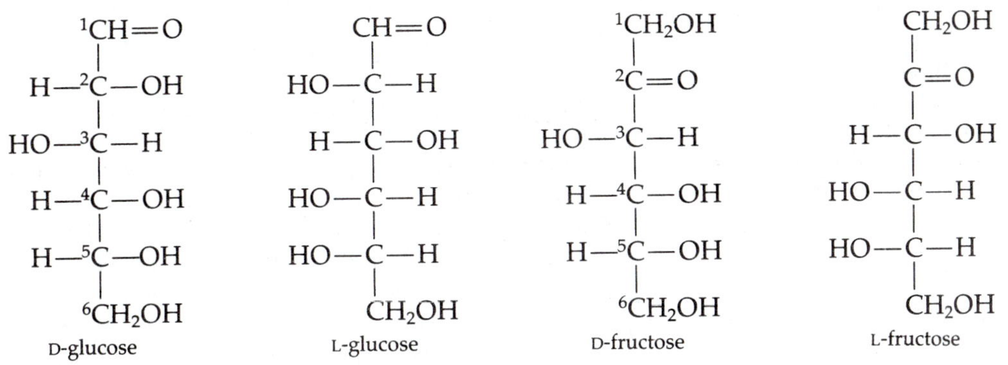

| D-glucose | L-glucose | D-fructose | L-fructose |

(4D)

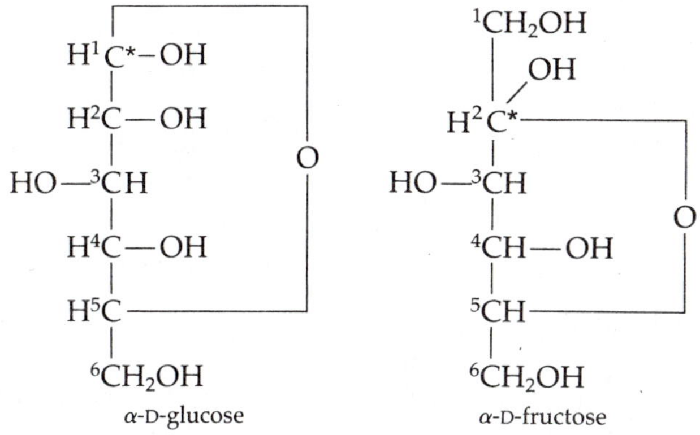

α-D-glucose   α-D-fructose

to L isomer, the direction of the hydroxyl groups on all asymmetric carbons is reversed, not only that on the number 5 carbon (see 4C). Monosaccharides of the D configuration are much more important nutritionally than their L isomers because they exist as such in dietary carbohydrate, and are specifically metabolized in that form. This is because the enzymes involved in carbohydrate digestion and metabolism are stereospecific for D sugars, meaning that they convert D sugars only, and are inactive toward the L forms.

The structures in 4C are shown as open-chain, or Fischer projection models, in which the carbonyl (aldehyde or ketone) functions are free. The monosaccharides do not generally exist in open-chain form, as explained later, but are shown that way here to clarify the D–L concept and to illustrate the so-called anomeric carbon, which is the carbon atom comprising the carbonyl function. Notice that the anomeric carbon is number 1 in the aldose (glucose) and number 2 in the ketose (fructose).

The fact that the monosaccharides do not exist in open-chain form while in solution is evidenced by the fact that they do not undergo reactions characteristic of true aldehydes and ketones. Actually the molecules cyclize, producing forms called *hemiacetals*, if the sugar is an aldose, and *hemiketals*, if the sugar is a ketose. The hemiacetal or hemiketal bonds are formed by the reaction of an alcohol group with an aldehyde or ketone group respectively. Therefore, the participating groups within a monosaccharide are the aldehyde or ketone of the anomeric carbon atom, and the alcohol group attached to the highest-numbered chiral carbon atom. This is illustrated using the examples of D-glucose and D-fructose (see 4D). The formation of the hemiacetal or hemiketal produces a new chiral center at the anomeric carbon, designated by an asterisk in the structures, and therefore the bond direction of the newly formed hydroxyl becomes significant. In the cyclized structures shown, the anomeric hydroxyls at position 1 for D-glucose and position 2 for D-fructose are arbitrarily directed to the right, resulting in an alpha (α) configuration. Should the anomeric hydroxyl be directed to the left, the structure would be in a beta (β) configuration. Cyclization to the hemiacetal or hemiketal can produce either the α- or β-isomer; however, in aqueous solution, an equilibrium mixture of the isomers exists, with the concentration of the β-form being roughly twice that of the α-form. If a pure solution of either isomer is prepared, the optical rotation of the solution will change as the equilibrium concentrations of the two forms are approached. This change in optical rotation is called *mutarotation*, and it results from the interconversion of the α- and β-isomers.

Stereoisomerism among the monosaccharides and also other nutrients such as amino acids has important metabolic implications due to the stereospecificity of certain metabolic enzymes. An interesting example of stereospecificity is the action of the digestive enzyme α-amylase, which hydrolyzes polyglucose molecules such as the starches, in which the glucose units are connected through an α-linkage (p. 76). Cellulose, also a polymer of glucose but one in which the monomeric glucose residues are connected via β-bonds, is resistant to amylase hydrolysis.

The structures of the cyclized monosaccharides are more conveniently and accurately represented by Haworth models, which will be used throughout the remainder of this text. In such models the carbons and oxygen comprising the five- or six-membered ring are depicted as lying in a horizontal plane, with the hydroxyl groups pointing down or up from the plane. Those that are directed to the right in the open-chain structure point down in the Haworth model, and those directed to the left point up. Table 4.1 shows the structural relationship among simple projection and Haworth formulas for the major, naturally occurring hexoses—glucose, galactose, and fructose.

Compared to the hexoses shown in Table 4.1, pentose sugars furnish very little dietary energy because of their low content in the diet. However, they are readily synthesized in the cell from hexose precursors and are incorporated into metabolically important compounds. The aldopentose ribose, for example, is a constituent of key nucleotides such as the adenosine phosphates—adenosine triphosphate (ATP), adenosine diphosphate (ADP), adenosine monophosphate (AMP), cyclic adenosine monophosphate (cAMP)—and the nicotinamide adenine dinucleotides (NAD$^+$, NADP$^+$) (p. 61). Ribose and its deoxygenated form, deoxyribose, are also part of the structures of ribonucleic acid (RNA) and deoxyribonucleic acid (DNA), respectively. Ribitol, a reduction product of ribose, is a constituent of the vitamin riboflavin and of the flavin coenzymes, flavin adenine dinucleotide (FAD) and flavin mononucleotide (FMN) (see 4E) (p. 62).

Oligosaccharides

Oligosaccharides are short-chain polymers of monosaccharide units covalently attached to one another through acetal bonds. Acetal bonds, as they occur in the special case of carbohydrate structures, are also called *glycosidic bonds*, and are formed between a hydroxyl group of one monosaccharide unit and a hydroxyl group of the next unit in the polymer, with the elimination of one molecule of water. Generally oligosaccharides are considered to have from two to ten monomeric units, but the two-unit structures, the disaccharides, are the most common and are major energy-supplying nutrients. The glycosidic bonds generally involve the hydroxyl group on the anomeric carbon of one member of the monosaccharide pair and the hydroxyl group on carbon 4 or 6 of the second. Furthermore, the glycosidic bond can be alpha or beta in orientation, depending on whether the anomeric hydroxyl group was alpha or beta before the glycosidic bond was formed. Specific glycosidic bonds may therefore be designated α-1,4, β-1,4, α-1,6, and so on.

The most common disaccharides are maltose, lactose, and sucrose (see 4F, 4G, and 4H). Maltose is formed primarily from the partial hydrolysis of starch, and therefore is found in malt beverages such as beer and malt liquors. It consists of two glucose units linked through an α-1,4 glycosidic bond, as illustrated. The residue on the right is shown in the β-form, although it also may exist in α-form (see 4F). Lactose is found naturally only in milk and milk products. It is composed of galactose, linked by a β-1,4 glycosidic bond to glucose, which can exist in either α- or β-form (see 4G). Sucrose (cane sugar, beet sugar) is the most widely distributed of the disaccharides and is the most commonly used natural sweetener. It is composed of glucose and fructose, and it is structurally unique in that its glycosidic bond involves the anomeric hydroxyl of both the residues. The linkage is α- with respect to the glucose and β- with respect to the fructose residue (see 4H).

Polysaccharides

The glycosidic bonding of monosaccharide residues may be repeated many times to form high molecular weight polymers called *polysaccharides*. If the structure is comprised of a single type of monomeric unit, it is re-

TABLE 4.1 Various Structural Representations Among the Hexoses—Glucose, Fructose, and Galactose

Hexose	Fischer projection	Cyclized Fischer projection	Haworth	Simplified Haworth
α-D-glucose	$^1CH{=}O$ $H^2C{-}OH$ $HO{-}^3CH$ $H^4C{-}OH$ $H^5C{-}OH$ $^6CH_2OH$	OH H^1C $H^2C{-}OH$ $HO{-}^3C{-}H$ $H^4C{-}OH$ H^5C $^6CH_2OH$	$^6CH_2OH$ ... ^5O ... ^4OH ... $HO\,^3$ ... $^2\,OH$ ... OH	(simplified Haworth ring, positions 6,5,4,3,2,1,O)
β-D-galactose	$^1CH{=}O$ $H^2C{-}OH$ $HO{-}^3C{-}H$ $HO{-}^4C{-}H$ $H^5C{-}OH$ $^6CH_2OH$	HO ^1CH $H^2C{-}OH$ $HO{-}^3C{-}H$ $HO{-}^4C{-}H$ H^5C $^6CH_2OH$	$^6CH_2OH$ ... $HO\,^5$ ... ^4OH ... ^{3} ... ^{2} ... $O\,OH$ ... OH	(simplified Haworth ring, positions 6,5,4,3,2,1,O)
β-D-fructose	$^1CH_2OH$ $^2C{=}O$ $HO{-}^3CH$ $H^4C{-}OH$ $H^5C{-}OH$ $^6CH_2OH$	$^1CH_2OH$ $HO{-}^2C$ $HO{-}^3CH$ $H^4C{-}OH$ H^5C $^6CH_2OH$	$^6CH_2OH$ ... ^{5} ... ^{4} ... ^{3} ... ^{1} ... $HO\,^2$ ... $O\,OH$ ... CH_2OH ... OH	(simplified Haworth ring, positions 6,5,4,3,2,1,O)

ferred to as a *homopolysaccharide*. If two or more different types of monosaccharides make up its structure, it is called a *heteropolysaccharide*. Both types exist in nature; however, the homopolysaccharide is of far greater importance in nutrition because of the abundance of the substance in many natural foods. The polyglucoses, starch and glycogen, for example, are the major storage forms of carbohydrate in plant and animal tissues respectively. They range in molecular weight from a few thousand to 500,000.

Monosaccharides that are cyclized into hemiacetals or hemiketals are sometimes referred to as *reducing sugars* because they are capable of reducing other substances, such as the copper ion from Cu^{++} to Cu^+. In describing polysaccharide structure, this property is useful in distinguishing one end of a linear polysaccharide from the other end. In a polyglucose chain, for example, the glucose residue at one end of the chain has a hemiacetal group because its anomeric carbon atom is not involved in acetal bonding to another glucose residue. The

(4E)

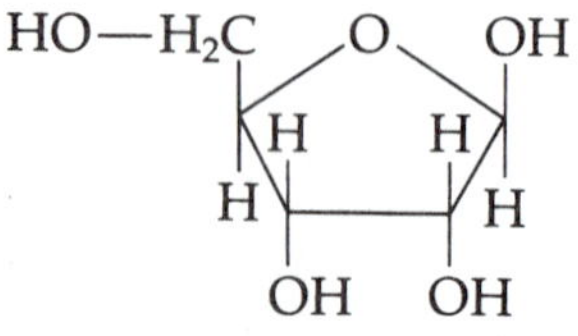

β-D-ribose

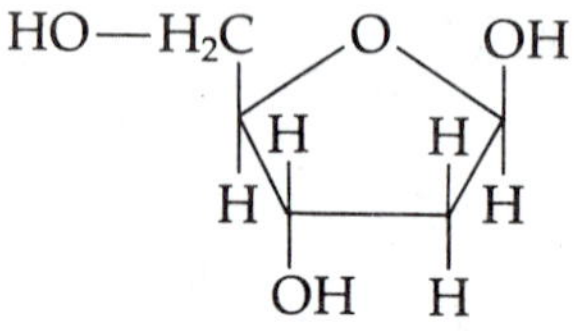

β-D-2-deoxyribose

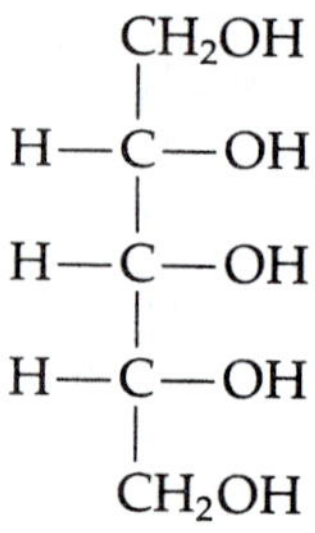

Ribitol

(4F)

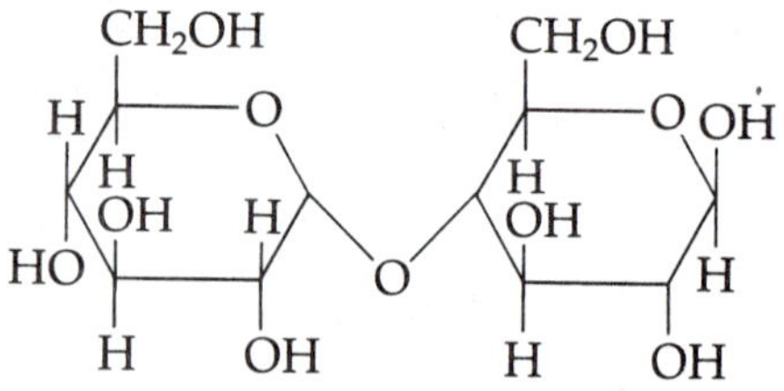

Maltose (β-form)

(4G)

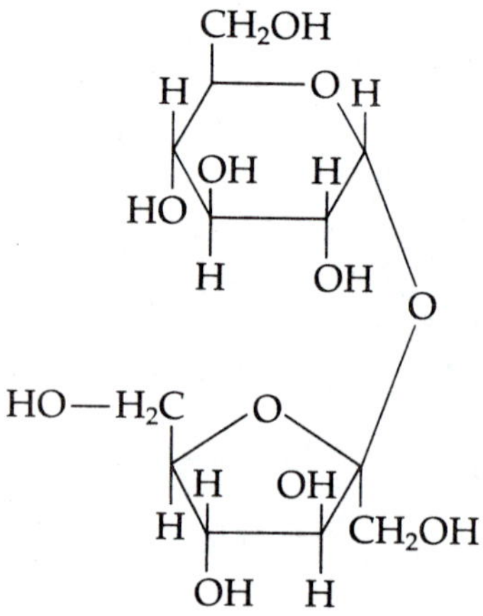

(Lactose)

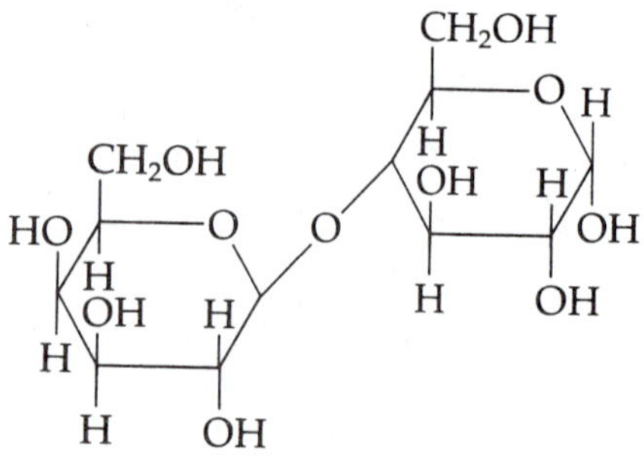

Lactose (α-form)

(4H)

Sucrose

residue at the other end of the chain, in contrast, is not in hemiacetal form because it is attached by acetal bonding to the next residue in the chain. A linear polyglucose molecule therefore has a reducing end (the hemiacetal end) and a non-reducing end, at which no hemiacetal exists. This notation is of use in designating at which end of a polysaccharide certain enzymatic reactions occur.

Starch   The most common digestible polysaccharide in plants is starch, and it can exist in two forms, *amylose* and *amylopectin*, both of which are polymers of D-glucose. The amylose molecule is a linear, unbranched structure in which the glucose residues are attached solely through α-1,4 glycosidic bonds.

Amylopectin, however, is a branched-chain polymer, the branch points occurring through α-1,6 glycosidic bonds, as illustrated in Figure 4.1. Both forms occur in cereals, potatoes, legumes, and other vegetables, with amylose contributing about 15–20%, and amylopectin 80–85% of the total starch content.

Glycogen   The major form of stored carbohydrate in animal tissues is glycogen, which is localized primarily in liver and skeletal muscle. Like amylopectin, it is a highly branched polyglucose molecule, and differs from the starch only in the fact that it is more highly branched (see Fig. 4.1b). The glucose residues within glycogen serve as a rich source of energy. When dictated by the

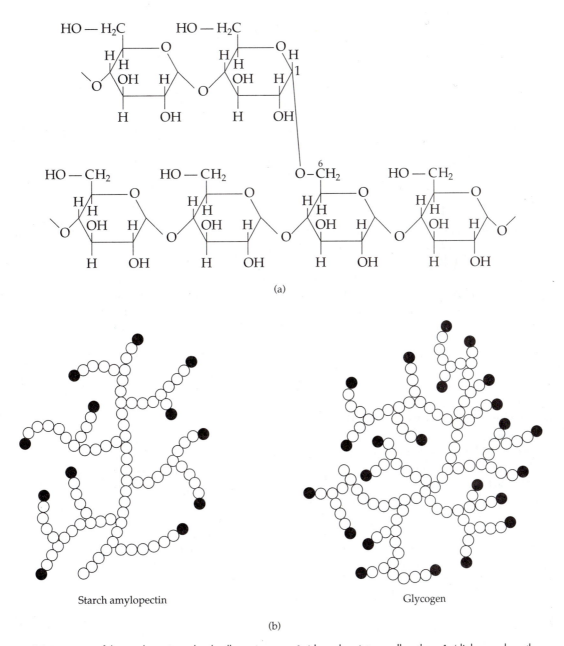

FIGURE 4.1 (a) A segment of the amylopectin molecule, illustrating an α-1,6 branch point as well as the α-1,4 linkages along the linear segments. Branch points may occur as frequently as every 25 to 30 residues. (b) Comparison of the gross structures of starch amylopectin and glycogen, showing the difference in the degree of branching. Circles represent glucose residues. Solid circles are those residues located at nonreducing ends of chains. Only one reducing end is present in each molecule.

body's energy demands, they are sequentially hydrolyzed enzymatically from the nonreducing ends of the glycogen chains and enter energy-releasing pathways of metabolism. This process (glycogenolysis) is discussed later in this chapter. The high degree of branching in glycogen and amylopectin is a distinct metabolic advantage, because it presents a large number

of nonreducing ends from which glucose residues can be cleaved.

Cellulose Cellulose is the major component of cell walls in plants. Like the starches, it is a homopolysaccharide of glucose but is different in that the glycosidic bonds connecting the residues are β-1,4. This renders

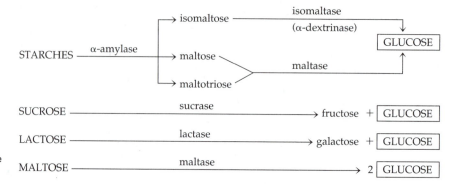

FIGURE 4.2 The enzymatic hydrolysis of carbohydrates, illustrating the importance of glucose as a component of these major nutrients.

the molecule resistant to the digestive enzyme amylase, the specificity of which favors α-1,4 linkages. Since cellulose is not digestible by mammalian degradative enzymes, it is defined as a dietary fiber and is considered not to provide energy. However, as a source of fiber, cellulose assumes importance as a bulking agent and potential energy source for intestinal bacteria (p. 103).

DIGESTION

The dietary carbohydrates that are most important nutritionally are polysaccharides and disaccharides, because free monosaccharides are not commonly present in the diet in significant quantities. There is, however, some free glucose and fructose in honey, in certain fruits, and in the carbohydrates that are added to processed foods. The cellular use of carbohydrates depends on their absorption from the gastrointestinal (GI) tract into the bloodstream, a process normally restricted to monosaccharides. Therefore polysaccharides and disaccharides must be hydrolyzed to their constituent monosaccharide units. The hydrolytic enzymes involved are collectively called *glycosidases*, or, alternatively, *carbohydrases*.

Polysaccharides

The key enzyme in the digestion of dietary polysaccharides is α-amylase, a glycosidase that specifically hydrolyzes α-1,4 glycosidic linkages. Resistant to the action of this enzyme, therefore, are the β-1,4 bonds of cellulose and the α-1,6 linkages that form branch points in starch amylopectin.

Digestion of starches actually begins in the mouth, because α-amylase activity is found in saliva. But considering the short period of time that food is in the mouth prior to being swallowed, this phase of digestion is of little consequence. However, the salivary amylase action continues in the stomach until the gastric acid penetrates the food bolus and lowers the pH sufficiently

to inactivate the activity of the enzyme. At this point, partial hydrolysis of the starches has occurred, the major products being dextrins, which are short-chain polysaccharides, and maltose. Further digestion of the dextrins is resumed in the small intestine by the α-amylase of pancreatic origin, which is secreted into the duodenal contents. Here, the presence of bile and pancreatic bicarbonate elevate the pH to a level favorable for enzymatic function. If the dietary starch form is amylose, which is unbranched, the products of α-amylase hydrolysis are maltose and the trisaccharide maltotriose, which undergoes slower hydrolysis to maltose and glucose. The hydrolytic action of α-amylase on amylopectin, a branched starch, produces glucose and maltose, as it did with amylose. However, the α-1,6 bonds linking the glucose residues at the branch points of the molecule cannot be hydrolyzed by α-amylase. This results in the release of disaccharide units called *isomaltose*, the glycosidic bond of which is α-1,6.

The action of α-amylase on dietary starch, therefore, releases maltose, isomaltose, and glucose as principal hydrolytic products, as illustrated in Figure 4.2. The further breakdown of the disaccharide products to glucose is brought about by specific glycosidases described in the next section.

Disaccharides

Virtually no digestion of disaccharides or small oligosaccharides occurs in the mouth or stomach. In the human, it takes place entirely in the upper small intestine. Unlike α-amylase, disaccharidase activity is associated with the microvilli of the intestinal mucosal cells (the brush border) rather than with the intestinal lumen (p. 42). Among the enzymes located on the mucosal cells are lactase, sucrase, maltase, and isomaltase. Lactase catalyzes the cleavage of lactose to equimolar amounts of galactose and glucose, and sucrase hydrolyzes sucrose to yield one glucose and one fructose residue. Isomaltase (also called an α-dextrinase) hydrolyzes the α-1,6 bond of isomaltose, the branch point disaccharide remaining from the incomplete breakdown of branched starches. The products are two molecules of glucose.

In summary, nearly all dietary starches and disaccharides are ultimately hydrolyzed completely by specific glycosidases to their constituent monosaccharide units. Monosaccharides, together with small amounts of remaining disaccharides can then be absorbed by the intestinal mucosal cells. The reactions involved in the digestion of starches and disaccharides are summarized in Figure 4.2.

ABSORPTION AND TRANSPORT

The wall of the small intestine is comprised of absorptive mucosal cells and mucus-secreting goblet cells that line projections, called *villi*, that extend into the lumen. The absorptive cells have hairlike projections on the surface on the lumen side called *microvilli* (the *brush border*). A square millimeter of cell surface is believed to have as many as 2×10^5 microvilli projections. The microstructure of the small intestinal wall is illustrated in Figures 2.6 and 2.7. The anatomic advantage of the villi–microvilli structure is that it presents an enormous surface area to the intestinal contents, thereby facilitating absorption. It has been estimated that the absorptive capacity of the human intestine amounts to about 5,400 g/d for glucose and 4,800 g/d for fructose—a capability that is, of course, never challenged in a normal diet.

Glucose and galactose are absorbed into the mucosal cells by active transport, whereas fructose enters by facilitated diffusion [1,2]. Active transport implies that the process requires energy and that a specific receptor is involved. The exact nature of the glucose–galactose carrier is unclear, but is known to be a protein complex dependent on the Na^+/K^+-ATPase pump (p. 17), which, at the expense of ATP, furnishes energy for the transport of sugar through the mucosal cell. Glucose or galactose cannot attach to the carrier until it has been preloaded with Na^+.

Glucose appears to leave the mucosal cell at the basolateral surface by three routes: approximately 15% leaks back across the brush border into the intestinal lumen, about 25% diffuses through the basolateral membrane into the circulation; but the major portion (approximately 60%) is transported from the cell into the circulation via a carrier in the serosal membrane [3].

Facilitated diffusion, the process by which fructose crosses the mucosal cells, is not energy requiring and can only proceed down a concentration gradient. There is a carrier involved, however, and so the system is saturable

and can be competitively inhibited. Because fructose is very efficiently trapped and phosphorylated by the liver, there is virtually no circulating fructose in the bloodstream. Therefore, the downhill concentration gradient for fructose across the intestinal mucosa is ensured. Although it is known that facilitated diffusion is the mechanism involved in fructose absorption, the process is still not completely understood. Its absorption takes place more slowly than glucose or galactose, which are actively absorbed, but faster than sugars such as sorbitol and xylitol, which are absorbed by purely passive transfer. Increased interest in fructose absorption has followed the finding that its absorption is limited in nearly 60% of normal adults, and that intestinal distress, symptomatic of malabsorption, frequently appears following ingestion of 50 g of pure fructose [4]. This observation raises the interesting speculation that malabsorption of fructose, to at least some degree, may be common in humans. Symptoms diminish if glucose is co-consumed with the fructose.

Following transport across the gut wall, the monosaccharides enter the portal circulation, wherein they are carried directly to the liver. The liver is the major site of metabolism of galactose and fructose, which are readily taken up by the liver cells via specific hepatocyte receptors. They then enter the cells by facilitated diffusion, and are subsequently metabolized. Both fructose and galactose can be converted to glucose derivatives through pathways that will be discussed later, and then stored as liver glycogen, or they may be catabolized for energy according to the body's energy demand. The blood levels of galactose and fructose are not directly subject to the strict hormonal regulation that is such an important part of glucose homeostasis. However, if their dietary intake is a significantly higher than normal percentage of total carbohydrate intake, they may be regulated indirectly as glucose, due to their metabolic conversion to that sugar.

Glucose is nutritionally the most important monosaccharide, since it is the exclusive constituent of the starches, and since it also occurs in each of three major disaccharides (Fig. 4.2). Like fructose and galactose, glucose is extensively metabolized in the liver, but its uptake by that organ is not as complete as in the case of fructose and galactose. The remainder of the glucose passes on into the systemic blood supply and is then distributed among other tissues such as muscle, kidney, and adipose tissue. It enters these cells by facilitated diffusion. In skeletal muscle and adipose tissue the process is insulin dependent, while in the liver it is insulin independent.

The maintenance of normal blood glucose concentration is a major function of the liver. Regulation is the

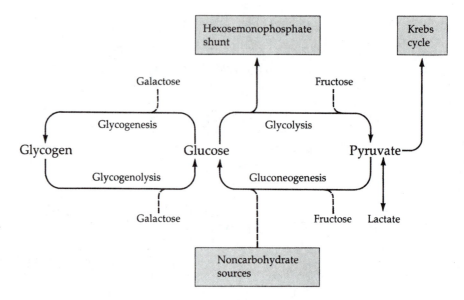

FIGURE 4.3 An overview of the major pathways of carbohydrate metabolism, emphasizing the fate of glucose but also indicating the sites of entry of galactose and fructose into the pathways.

net effect of the organ's metabolic processes that remove glucose from the blood for either glycogen synthesis or for energy production, and of processes that return glucose to the blood, such as glycogenolysis and gluconeogenesis. These pathways, which are examined in detail in the next section, are hormonally influenced, primarily by the antagonistic pancreatic hormones insulin and glucagon, and by the glucocorticoid hormones of the adrenal cortex. The rise in blood glucose following the ingestion of carbohydrate, for example, triggers the release of insulin while reducing the secretion of glucagon. This increases uptake of glucose by muscle and adipose tissue, returning blood glucose to homeostatic levels. A fall in blood glucose concentration, conversely, signals the reversal of the pancreatic hormonal secretions; that is, decreased insulin and increased glucagon release. In addition, an increase in glucocorticoid hormone secretion occurs in answer to, and to offset, a falling blood glucose level. The result is an increased activity of hepatic gluconeogenesis, a process described in the following sections.

INTEGRATED METABOLISM IN TISSUES

The metabolic fate of the monosaccharides depends to a great extent on the energy demands of the body. According to these demands, the activity of certain metabolic pathways are regulated in such a way that some may be stimulated, while others may be suppressed. The major regulatory mechanisms are hormonal (involving the action of hormones such as insulin, glucagon, epinephrine, and the corticosteroid hormones), and allosteric enzyme activation or suppression (p. 94). Allosteric enzymes are regulatory enzymes, the activities of which can be altered by compounds called *modulators*. A negative modulator of an allosteric enzyme reduces the activity of the enzyme and slows its velocity, while a positive modulator increases the activity of an allosteric enzyme, increasing its velocity. The effect of a modulator, negative or positive, is exerted on its allosteric enzyme as a result of increasing concentrations of the modulator. Each of these mechanisms of regulation is discussed in detail in the section dealing with regulation of metabolism.

The metabolic pathways of carbohydrate use and storage consist of glycogenesis, glycogenolysis, glycolysis and hexose monophosphate shunt, the Krebs cycle, and gluconeogenesis. An integrated overview of these pathways is given in Figure 4.3, and a detailed review of their intermediary metabolites, sites of regulation, and, most importantly, their function in the overall scheme of things are now considered. Reactions within the pathways are numbered to allow elaboration on those that are particularly significant from a nutritional standpoint. Because of the central role of glucose in carbohydrate nutrition, its metabolic fate is featured. The entry of fructose and galactose into the metabolic pathways is introduced later in the discussion.

Glycogenesis

The term *glycogenesis* refers to the pathway by which glucose is ultimately converted into glycogen. This

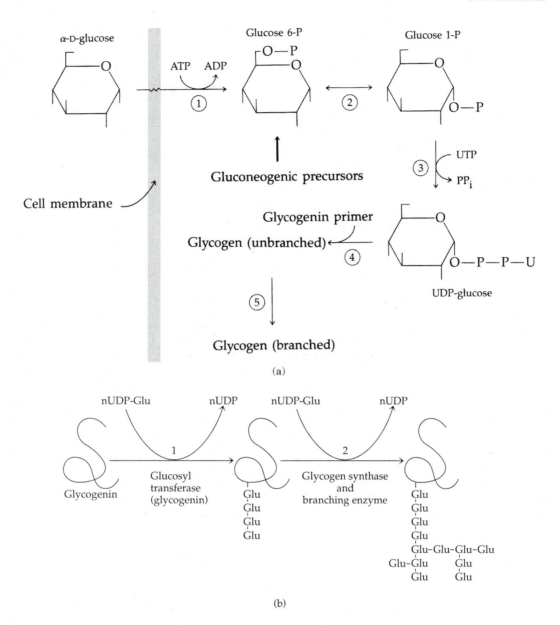

FIGURE 4.4 (a) Reactions of glycogenesis, by which the formation of glycogen from glucose occurs. Glycogen appears to be formed principally from gluconeogenic precursor substances rather than from glucose directly [8]. (b) The primer function of glycogenin. The glucosyl transferase activity of glycogenin catalyzes the attachment to itself of from two to seven glucose residues transferred from UDP-glucose (reaction 1). Remaining glucose units of the glycogen molecule are incorporated into the molecule by glycogen synthase, and linked together by glycogen synthase and the branching enzyme (reaction 2). The letter n represents an unspecified number of UDP-glucose molecules.

pathway is particularly important in hepatocytes because the liver is the major site of glycogen synthesis and storage. Glycogen accounts for as much as 7% of the wet weight of this organ. The other major site of glycogen storage is skeletal muscle and, to a lesser extent, adipose tissue. In human skeletal muscle, glycogen generally accounts for a little less than 1% of the wet weight of the tissue. The glycogen stores in muscle are used first when the body is confronted by an energy demand such as physical exertion or emotional stress, so the glycogenic pathway is of vital importance in ensuring a reserve of instant energy. The pathway is illustrated in Figure 4.4a. The following are comments on selected reactions:

1. On entering the cell, glucose is first phosphorylated by ATP, producing a phosphate ester at the number 6 carbon of the glucose. In muscle cells, the enzyme catalyzing this phosphate transfer is hexokinase, an allosteric enzyme that is negatively modulated by the reaction product, glucose 6-phosphate. Glucose phosphorylation in the liver is catalyzed primarily by glucokinase (sometimes referred to as hexokinase D). Although the reaction product, glucose 6-phosphate, is the same, interesting differences distinguish it from hexokinase. For example, hexokinase is negatively modulated by glucose 6-phosphate, while glucokinase is not. Also, glucokinase has a much higher K_m than hexokinase, meaning that it can convert glucose to its phosphate form at a higher velocity should the cellular concentration of glucose rise significantly (e.g., after a carbohydrate-rich meal). The much lower K_m of hexokinase indicates that it is catalyzing at maximum velocity even at average glucose concentrations. Therefore, the liver has the capacity to reduce blood glucose concentration when it becomes high. Furthermore, glucokinase is inducible by the hormone insulin, the activity of which is stimulated by elevated blood glucose levels. In diabetes mellitus, type 1 (see "Perspective" section in Chapter 8), glucokinase activity is therefore below normal values, since such patients are deficient in insulin. This contributes to the cell's inability to take up and metabolize glucose. The concept of K_m and its significance, as it applies to this reaction, has been discussed in Chapter 1. The hexokinase–glucokinase reaction is energy consuming, because the glucose was activated (phosphorylated) at the expense of ATP.

2. The phosphate is transferred from the number 6 carbon of the glucose to the number 1 carbon in a complex reaction catalyzed by the enzyme phosphoglucomutase.

3. Nucleoside triphosphates sometimes function as activating substances in intermediary metabolism. In this reaction, energy derived from the hydrolysis of the α–β–phosphate anhydride bond of uridine triphosphate allows the coupling of the resulting uridine monophosphate to the glucose 1-phosphate to form uridine diphosphate glucose (UDP-glucose).

4. Glucose is incorporated directly into glycogen as UDP glucose. The reaction is catalyzed by glycogen synthase, and it requires some preformed glycogen (primer) to which the incoming glucose units can be attached. The nature of the glycogen primer has become understood during only recent years. Before then, the unanswered question was that if glycogen synthase requires a primer, how is a new glycogen molecule initiated? The answer lies in an intriguing protein called *glycogenin*. Glycogenin itself acts as the primer to which the first glucose residue is covalently attached, and it also catalzyes (is the enzyme for) the reaction by which the attachment occurs. It also catalyzes the attachment of additional glucose residues to form chains of up to eight units. At that point, glycogen synthase takes over, extending the glycogen chains further. The role of glycogenin in glycogenesis has been reviewed [5], and a simplified view of the process is shown schematically in Figure 4.4b.

Glycogen synthase exists in an active (dephosphorylated) form and a less active (phosphorylated) form. The relative amount of each form is regulated by the cellular level of cAMP, which is in turn regulated by insulin. The glycogen synthase reaction is the primary target of insulin's stimulatory effect on glycogenesis.

5. Branching within the glycogen molecule is very important because it increases its solubility and compactness. It also makes available many nonreducing ends of chains from which glucose residues can be cleaved and used for energy, the process known as *glycogenolysis*, which is described in the following section. Glycogen synthase cannot form the α-1,6 bonds of the branch points. This is left to the action of the branching enzyme, which transfers small oligosaccharide segments from the end of the main glycogen chain to carbon number 6 hydroxyl groups throughout the chain. The overall pathway of glycogenesis, like most synthetic pathways, consumes energy, because an ATP (reaction 1) and a uridine triphosphate (UTP) (reaction 3) are consumed for each molecule of glucose introduced.

Glycogenolysis

The potential energy of glycogen is contained within the glucose residues that comprise its structure. As the body's energy demand dictates, the residues can be systematically cleaved one at a time from the ends of the glycogen branches and routed through energy-producing pathways. The breakdown of glycogen into individual glucose units, in the form of glucose 1-phosphate, is called *glycogenolysis*. Like its counterpart, glycogenesis, it is regulated by hormones, most importantly by glucagon, of pancreatic origin, and the catecholamine hormone epinephrine, produced in the adrenal medulla. Both of these hormones stimulate glycogenolysis, and are directed at the initial reaction, glycogen phosphorylase. Therefore, they function antagonistically to insulin in regulating the balance between free and stored glucose. The steps involved in glycogenolysis are shown in Figure 4.5. The following are comments on selected reactions:

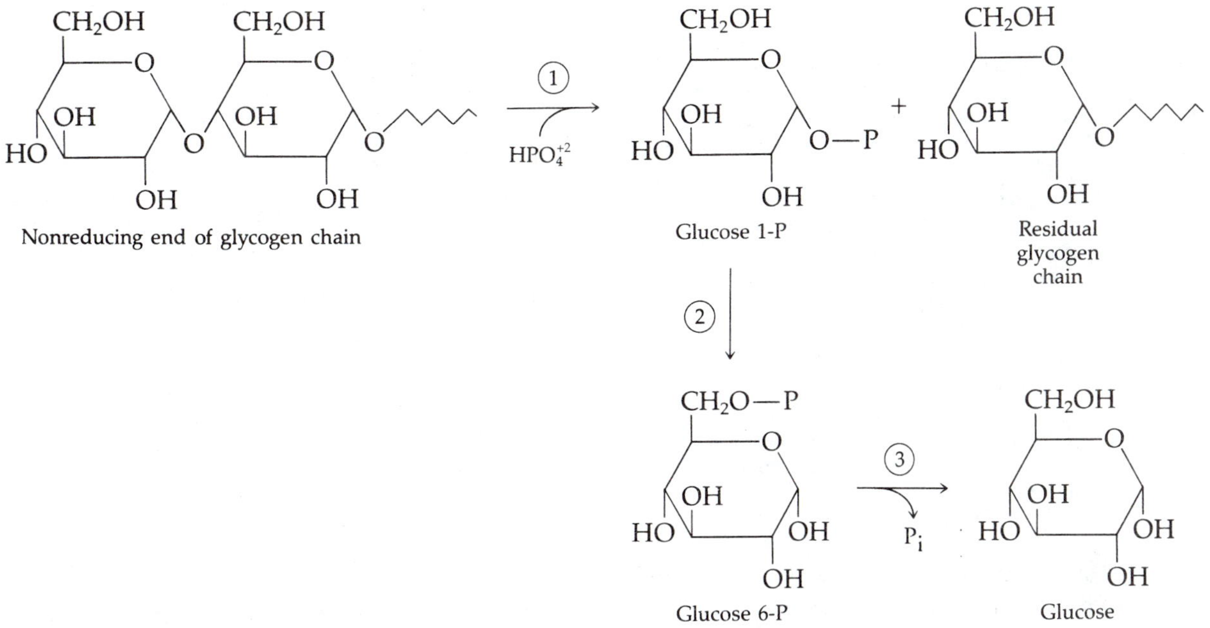

FIGURE 4.5 The reactions of glycogenolysis, by which glucose residues are sequentially removed from the non-reducing ends of glycogen segments. Reactions 1 and 2 are shared by both liver and muscle cells. In liver cells, glucose 6-phosphate can be converted to free glucose (reaction 3) by glucose 6-phosphatase. Muscle cells lack glucose 6-phosphatase, and therefore cannot carry out reaction 3.

1. The sequential release of individual glucose units from glycogen is a *phosphorolysis* process by which the glycosidic bonds are cleaved by phosphate addition. The products of one such cleavage reaction are glucose 1-phosphate and the remainder of the intact glycogen chain minus the one glucose residue. The reaction is catalyzed by glycogen phosphorylase, an important site of metabolic regulation by both hormonal and allosteric enzyme modulation. Different forms of glycogen phosphorylase exist, including phosphorylase a, a phosphorylated active form, and phosphorylase b, a dephosphorylated, inactive form. The two forms are interconverted by other enzymes, which can either attach phosphate groups to the phosphorylase enzyme or remove phosphate groups from it. The enzyme catalyzing the phosphorylation of phosphorylase b to its active "a" form is called *phosphorylase b kinase*. The enzyme that removes phosphate groups from the active (a) form of phosphorylase, producing the inactive "b" form, is called *phosphorylase a phosphatase*. The rate of glycogen breakdown to glucose 1-phosphate therefore depends on the relative activity of these enzymes.

The regulation of phosphorylase activity in the breakdown of liver and muscle glycogen is complex. It can involve *covalent regulation*, which is the phosphorylation–dephosphorylation regulation just described, and

it may also involve *allosteric regulation* by modulators. These, and other mechanisms of regulation are broadly reviewed in the section "Regulation of Metabolism." Covalent regulation is strongly influenced by the hormones epinephrine, which stimulates glycogenolysis in muscle, and glucagon, which stimulates glycogenolysis in liver. Both of these hormones exert their effect by stimulating phosphorylase b kinase, thereby promoting the formation of the more active ("a") form of the enzyme. This hormonal activation of phosphorylase b kinase is mediated through cAMP, the cellular concentration of which is increased by the action of the hormones. The allosteric regulation of phosphorylase generally involves the positive modulator AMP, which induces a conformational change in the inactive "b" form, resulting in a fully active "b" form. ATP competes with AMP for the allosteric site of the enzyme, therefore preventing the shift to its active form, and tending to keep it in its inactive form. There is no covalent (phosphorylation) regulation involved in allosteric modulations. The interconversion of phosphorylases a and b, and the active and inactive forms of phosphorylase b by covalent and allosteric regulation, respectively, is shown in Figure 4.6. For the interested reader, the textbook by Lehninger [6] includes a more indepth account of the regulation of the phosphorylase reaction.

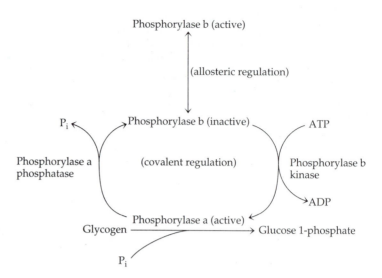

FIGURE 4.6 An overview of the regulation of glycogen phosphorylase. The enzyme is regulated covalently by phosphorylation to an active "a" form, and dephosphorylation to an inactive "b" form, reactions mediated through cAMP by hormones such as epinephrine and glucagon. It is also regulated allosterically by AMP and ATP, which cause shifts in the equilibrium between inactive and active "b" forms. AMP positively modulates the enzyme by shifting the equilibrium toward its active "b" form. ATP inhibits the effect of AMP, thereby favoring the formation of the inactive "b" form. For more details, see text under reaction 1.

2. At times of heightened glycogenolytic activity, the formation of increased amounts of glucose 1-phosphate shifts the equilibrium of the glucose phosphate isomerase reaction toward production of the 6-phosphate isomer.

3. The conversion of glucose 6-phosphate to free glucose requires the action of glucose 6-phosphatase. This enzyme functions in liver and kidney cells but not muscle cells or adipocytes. Therefore free glucose can be formed from liver glycogen and transported via the bloodstream to other tissues for oxidation. In this manner, the liver, but not muscle, can control the concentration of glucose in the blood. It follows that although muscle and, to some extent, adipose tissue have stores of glycogen, these stores can only be broken down for use in these locations.

Glycolysis

Glycolysis is the pathway by which glucose is degraded into two units of pyruvate, a triose. From pyruvate, the metabolic course of the glucose depends largely on the availability of oxygen, and therefore the course is said to be either aerobic or anaerobic. Under anaerobic conditions—that is, in a situation of oxygen debt—pyruvate is converted to lactate. Under otherwise normal conditions, this would occur mainly in times of strenuous exercise when the demand for oxygen by the working muscles, to satisfy their energy needs, exceeds that which is available. In such a case, lactate can accumulate in the muscle cells, contributing in part to the aches and pains associated with overexertion. Under anaerobic conditions glycolysis does, however, release a small amount of usable energy, which can sustain the muscles even in a state of oxygen debt. This is the major function of the anaerobic pathway to lactate.

Pyruvate can also follow an aerobic course of reactions, the Krebs cycle, wherein it becomes completely oxidized to CO_2 and H_2O. Complete oxidation is accompanied by the release of relatively large amounts of energy. Since the glycolytic enzymes function within the cytoplasmic matrix of the cell, while the enzymes catalyzing the Krebs cycle reactions are located within the mitochondrion (p. 8), pyruvate must enter the mitochondrion for oxidation. Glycolysis followed by Krebs cycle activity (aerobic catabolism of glucose) demands an ample supply of oxygen, a condition that is generally met in normal, resting mammalian cells. In a normal, aerobic situation, complete oxidation of the pyruvate generally occurs, with only a small amount of lactate being formed. The primary importance of glycolysis in energy metabolism, therefore, is that it provides the initial sequence of reactions (to pyruvate) necessary for glucose to be oxidized completely via the Krebs cycle.

In cells that lack mitochondria, such as the erythrocyte, the pathway of glycolysis is the sole provider of ATP by the mechanism of substrate-level phosphorylation of ADP, as discussed in Chapter 3. Nearly all cell types conduct glycolysis, but most of the energy derived from carbohydrates originates in liver, muscle, and adipose tissue.

The pathway of glycolysis, under both aerobic and anaerobic conditions, is summarized in Figure 4.7. Also indicated in the figure is the mode of entry of dietary fructose and galactose into the pathway for metabolism. The following are comments on selected reactions:

1. The hexokinase–glucokinase reaction consumes 1 mol ATP/mol glucose. Hexokinase (not glucokinase) is negatively regulated by the product of the reaction, glucose 6-phosphate.

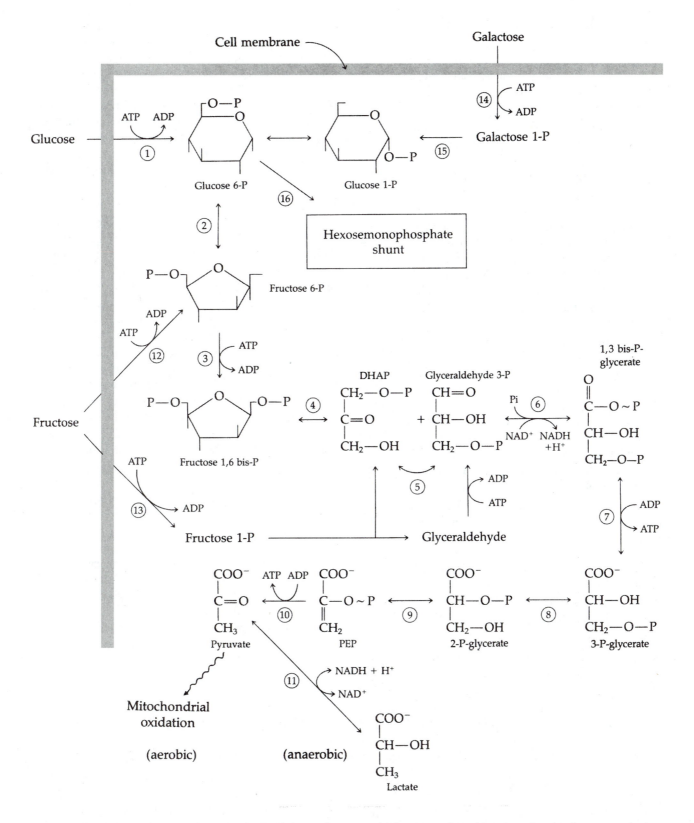

FIGURE 4.7 Glycolysis, indicating the mode of entry of glucose, fructose, and galactose into the pathway, as well as the alternative entry of glucose 6-phosphate into the hexosemonophosphate shunt. Under conditions of oxygen debt (anaerobic), pyruvate is converted to lactate. If the supply of oxygen is adequate, pyruvate can be oxidized completely in the mitochondrion to carbon dioxide and water.

2. Glucose phosphate isomerase catalyzes this interconversion of isomers.

3. The phosphofructokinase reaction, an important regulatory site, is modulated negatively by ATP and citrate and positively by AMP and ADP. Another ATP is consumed in the reaction.

4. The aldolase reaction results in the splitting of a hexose bisphosphate into two triose phosphates.

5. The isomers glyceraldehyde 3-phosphate and dihydroxyacetone phosphate (DHAP) are interconverted by the enzyme triosephosphate isomerase. In an isolated system, the equilibrium favors DHAP formation. But in the cellular environment it is shifted completely toward the production of glyceraldehyde 3-phosphate, since this metabolite is continuously removed from the equilibrium by the subsequent reaction catalyzed by glyceraldehyde 3-phosphate dehydrogenase.

6. In this reaction, glyceraldehyde 3-phosphate is oxidized to a carboxylic acid, while inorganic phosphate is incorporated as a high-energy anhydride bond. The enzyme is glyceraldehyde 3-phosphate dehydrogenase, which uses NAD^+ as its hydrogen-accepting cosubstrate. Under aerobic conditions, the NADH formed is reoxidized to NAD^+ by O_2 via the electron transport chain in the mitochondria as explained in the following section. The reason why O_2 is not necessary to sustain this reaction under anaerobic conditions is that the NAD^+ consumed is restored by a subsequent reaction (see reaction 11, following).

7. This reaction, catalyzed by phosphoglycerate kinase, exemplifies a substrate-level phosphorylation of ADP. Refer to Chapter 3 for a more detailed review of this mechanism by which ATP can be formed from ADP by the transfer of a phosphate from a high-energy donor molecule (p. 58).

8. Phosphoglyceromutase catalyzes the transfer of the phosphate group from the carbon-3 to the carbon-2 of the glyceric acid.

9. Dehydration of 2-phosphoglycerate by the enzyme enolase introduces a double bond that imparts high energy to the phosphate bond.

10. The product of reaction 9, phosphoenolpyruvate (PEP), donates its phosphate group to ADP in a reaction catalyzed by pyruvate kinase. This is the second site of substrate-level phosphorylation of ADP in the glycolytic pathway.

11. The lactate dehydrogenase reaction transfers two hydrogens from NADH and H^+ to pyruvate, reducing it to lactate. NAD^+ is formed in the reaction and can replace the NAD^+ consumed in reaction 6 under anaerobic conditions. It must be emphasized that this reaction is most active in situations of oxygen debt, as in prolonged muscular activity. Under normal, aerobic conditions, pyruvate enters the mitochondrion for complete oxidation. A third important option available to pyruvate is its conversion to the amino acid alanine by transamination with the amino group donor glutamate (p. 000). This, together with the fact that pyruvate is also the product of the catabolism of various amino acids, makes it an important link between protein and carbohydrate metabolism.

12 and 13. These two reactions provide the means by which dietary fructose enters the glycolytic pathway. Fructose is an important factor in the average American diet, since nearly half of the carbohydrate consumed is sucrose, and high-fructose corn syrup is becoming more popular as a food sweetener. Reaction 12 functions in extrahepatic tissues and involves the direct phosphorylation by hexokinase to form fructose 6-phosphate. This is a relatively unimportant reaction. It is slow and occurs only in the presence of high levels of fructose. Reaction 13 is the major means by which fructose is converted to glycolysis metabolites. The phosphorylation occurs at carbon-1 and is catalyzed by fructokinase, an enzyme found only in liver cells. The fructose 1-phosphate is subsequently split by aldolase (designated aldolase B to distinguish it from the enzyme acting on fructose 1,6-bisphosphate), forming DHAP and glyceraldehyde. The latter can then be phosphorylated by glyceraldehyde kinase (or triokinase) at the expense of a second ATP to produce glyceraldehyde 3-phosphate. Fructose is therefore converted to glycolytic intermediates, and as such can follow the pathway to pyruvate formation and Krebs cycle oxidation. Alternatively, they can be used in the liver to produce free glucose by a reversal of the first part of the pathway through the action of gluconeogenic enzymes. Glucose formation from fructose is particularly important if fructose provides the major source of carbohydrate in the diet.

Since the phosphorylation of fructose is essentially the responsibility of the liver, eating large amounts of the ketose can deplete hepatocyte ATP, reducing the rate of various biosynthetic processes such as protein synthesis.

14. Like glucose and fructose, galactose is first phosphorylated. The transfer of the phosphate from ATP is catalyzed by galactokinase, and the resulting phosphate ester is at carbon 1 of the sugar. The major dietary source of galactose is lactose, from which the monosaccharide is released hydrolytically by lactase.

15. Galactose 1-phosphate can be converted to glucose 1-phosphate through the intermediates uridine diphosphate (UDP)-galactose and uridine diphosphate (UDP)-glucose. The enzyme galactose 1-phosphate uridyl transferase transfers a uridyl phosphate residue from UDP-glucose to the galactose 1-phosphate, yielding glucose 1-phosphate and UDP-galactose. In a reaction catalyzed by epimerase, UDP-galactose can then be converted to UDP-glucose in which form it can be converted to glucose 1-phosphate by the uridyl transferase reaction already referred to, or it can be incorporated into glycogen by glycogen synthase, as described in the Glycogenesis section. It can also enter the glycolytic pathway as glucose 6-phosphate, made possible by the reaction series: UDP-glucose $\longrightarrow$ glucose 1-phosphate $\longrightarrow$ glucose 6-phosphate. As glucose 6-phosphate, it can also be hydrolyzed to free glucose in liver cells.

16. This indicates the entry of glucose 6-phosphate into another pathway called the *hexose monophosphate shunt* (pentose phosphate pathway), which will be considered next.

NADH in Anaerobic and Aerobic Glycolysis: The Shuttle Systems

Under *anaerobic* conditions, the one NADH produced in the pathway of glycolysis (the glyceraldehyde 3-phosphate dehydrogenase reaction) cannot undergo reoxidation by mitochondrial electron transport because molecular oxygen is the ultimate oxidizing agent in that system. Instead, it is used in the lactate dehydrogenase reduction of pyruvate to lactate, thereby becoming reoxidized to NAD$^+$ without the involvement of oxygen. In this manner, NAD$^+$ is restored to sustain the glyceraldehyde 3-phosphate dehydrogenase reaction, and allow the pathway to continue in the absence of oxygen.

When the system is operating *aerobically*, and the supply of oxygen is ample to allow total oxidation of incoming glucose, lactic acid is not formed. Instead, pyruvate enters the mitochondrion, as does a carrier molecule of hydrogen atoms that were transferred to it from NADH. NADH cannot enter the mitochondrion directly. Instead, reducing equivalents in the form of carriers of hydrogen atoms removed from the NADH in the cytoplast are shuttled across the mitochondrial membrane. Once in the mitochondrial matrix, the carriers are enzymatically dehydrogenated, and NAD$^+$ becomes reduced to NADH. The latter can then become oxidized by electron transport, and consequently generate three ATPs/mol NADH by oxidative phosphorylation (p. 64). In this manner, six moles of ATP are consequently formed per mole of glucose. The result of the shuttle system is therefore equivalent to a transfer of NADH from the cytoplasm into the mitochondrion, although it does not occur directly. Shuttle substances that transport the hydrogens removed from cytoplasmic NADH into the mitochondrion are malate or glycerol 3-phosphate.

The most active shuttle compound, malate, is reoxidized by malate dehydrogenase in the mitochondrion as NAD$^+$ becomes reduced to NADH, therefore generating the three ATPs/mol. This shuttle system is called the *malate–aspartate shuttle system* because the intramitochondrial malate is eventually converted to aspartate, in which form it returns to the cytoplasm. The glycerol 3-phosphate shuttle, in contrast, leads to only two ATPs/mol NADH because the intramitochondrial reoxidation of glycerol 3-phosphate is catalyzed by glycerol phosphate dehydrogenase, which uses FAD instead of NAD$^+$ as hydrogen acceptor. If the glycerol 3-phosphate shuttle is in effect, therefore, only four ATPs will be formed per mole of glucose by oxidative phosphorylation. Figure 4.8 illustrates how these shuttle systems function in the reoxidation of cytoplastic NADH. The shuttle systems are specific to certain tissues. The more active malate–aspartate shuttle functions in the liver, kidney, and heart, while the glycerol 3-phosphate shuttle occurs in the brain and skeletal muscle.

To summarize energy release from glycolysis in terms of ATP produced, a net of two ATPs are formed as a result of substrate-level phosphorylation reactions. If the starting point of glycolysis is glycogen rather than free glucose, the hexokinase reaction is bypassed. The result is that the energy yield is therefore increased by one ATP for glycolysis of glycogen glucose under either aerobic or anaerobic conditions.

If the cell is functioning anaerobically, the two ATPs formed by substrate-level phosphorylation are the total produced. Under aerobic conditions, in contrast, additional ATPs are formed by oxidative phosphorylation. This is because the cytoplasmic NADH produced is not used in the (anaerobic) lactate dehydrogenase reaction, but is reoxidized to NAD$^+$ by electron transport and oxygen. The number of additional ATPs formed depends on which shuttle system is used to move the NADH hydrogens into the mitochondrion. If the malate–aspartate shuttle is in effect, six ATPs are produced, bringing the total to eight. In tissues using the glycerol 3-phosphate shuttle, just four ATPs are formed by oxidative phosphorylation, or a glycolytic total of six.

The Hexosemonophosphate Shunt

The purpose of a shunt is to generate biochemically important intermediates not produced in other path-

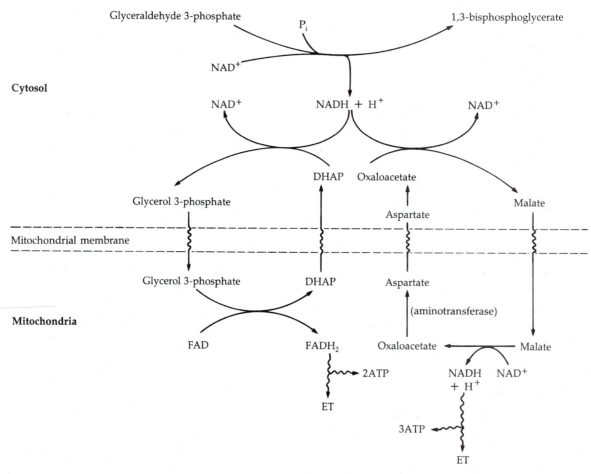

FIGURE 4.8 The glycerol 3-phosphate and malate–aspartate shuttle systems by which cytosolic NADH can be indirectly reoxidized by mitochondrial electron transport. Reducing equivalents of NADH are reoxidized by either FAD- or NAD+-requiring enzymes leading to the production of either two or three ATPs respectively per mole of cosubstrate. DHAP, dihydroxyacetone phosphate; ET, electron transport.

ways. Two very important products of the hexose-monophosphate shunt are pentose phosphates and the reduced cosubstrate NADPH. Two consecutive dehydrogenase reactions, glucose 6-phosphate dehydrogenase (G-6-PD) and 6-phosphogluconate dehydrogenase, initiate the sequence of reactions of the shunt. Both reactions require NADP+ as cosubstrate. Consequently a large amount of NADPH is formed, and this reduced cosubstrate is used for other important metabolic functions, such as the biosynthesis of fatty acids (p. 139) and the maintenance of reducing substrates in red blood cells necessary to ensure the functional integrity of the cells.

Production of pentose sugars in the shunt is necessary for the synthesis of DNA and RNA. This is achieved by the decarboxylation of 6-phosphogluconate to form the pentose phosphate, ribulose 5-phosphate, which in turn is isomerized to its aldose isomer, ribose

5-phosphate. The reactions leading to the production of ribose 5-phosphate and the formation of NADPH from NADP+ are referred to as the oxidative reactions of the pathway. In tissues that require mainly pentose phosphates for nucleic acid synthesis, the pathway ends at this point, as is summarized in Figure 4.9. But in those tissues that are particularly active in fatty acid synthesis, such as the mammary gland, adipose tissue, the adrenal cortex, and the liver, NADPH is the most important pathway product. In these tissues, the pathway continues through a non-oxidative series of reactions by which the pentose phosphates are recycled back into glucose 6-phosphate, thereby repeating the NADPH-producing dehydrogenations. Included among the non-oxidative reactions are those catalyzed by transaldolase and transketolase, enzymes that interconvert three-, four-, and seven-carbon phosphate sugars. The eventual prod-

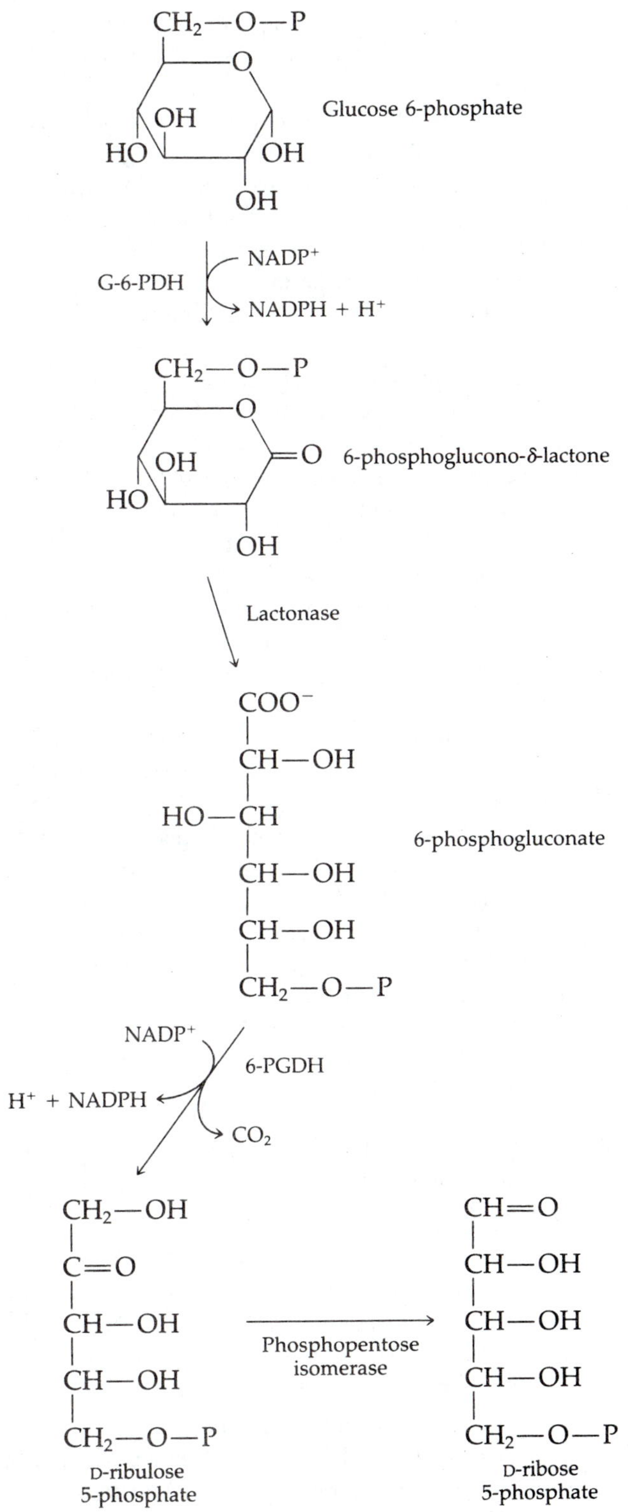

Glucose 6-phosphate

G-6-PDH
- NADP$^+$
→ NADPH + H$^+$

6-phosphoglucono-δ-lactone

Lactonase

COO$^-$
|
CH—OH
|
HO—CH
|
CH—OH
|
CH—OH
|
CH$_2$—O—P

6-phosphogluconate

NADP$^+$
6-PGDH
H$^+$ + NADPH
CO$_2$

CH$_2$—OH
|
C=O
|
CH—OH
|
CH—OH
|
CH$_2$—O—P
D-ribulose
5-phosphate

Phosphopentose
isomerase

CH=O
|
CH—OH
|
CH—OH
|
CH—OH
|
CH$_2$—O—P
D-ribose
5-phosphate

FIGURE 4.9 The portion of the hexosemonophosphate shunt showing the generation of NADPH by the G 6-PDH (glucose 6-phosphate dehydrogenase) and 6-PGDH (6-phosphogluconate dehydrogenase) reactions. Adding to the importance of the latter reaction is that it also forms pentose phosphates by the decarboxylation of 6-phosphogluconate. The series of reactions shown represents the oxidative portion of the shunt.

uct resulting from these interconversions is glucose 6-phosphate, representing a return to the glycolytic pathway.

The shunt is active in liver, adipose tissue, adrenal cortex, thyroid gland, testis, and lactating mammary gland. Its activity is low in skeletal muscle because of the limited demand for NADPH (fatty acid synthesis) in this tissue, and also due to muscle's reliance on glucose for energy rather than biosynthesis.

The Krebs Cycle

Also referred to as the *tricarboxylic acid cycle* or the *citric acid cycle*, the Krebs cycle represents the forefront of energy metabolism in the body. It can be thought of as the common and final catabolic pathway because products of carbohydrate, fat, and amino acids feed into the cycle where they can be completely oxidized to CO_2 and H_2O, with the accompanying generation of large amounts of ATP. Not all entrant substances are totally oxidized. Some Krebs cycle intermediates are used to form glucose by the process of gluconeogenesis, which is discussed in the next section, and some can be converted to certain amino acids by transamination (p. 170). However, the importance of the cycle as the nucleus of energy production is evidenced by the estimation that over 90% of energy released from food occurs here.

The high energy output of the Krebs cycle is attributed to mitochondrial electron transport, with oxidative phosphorylation providing the means for ATP formation, as discussed in Chapter 3. The oxidation reactions occurring in the cycle are actually dehydrogenations in which an enzyme catalyzes the removal of two hydrogens to an acceptor cosubstrate such as NAD^+ or FAD. Since the enzymes of the cycle and the enzymes and electron carriers of electron transport are both compartmentalized within the mitochondria, the reduced cosubstrates, NADH and $FADH_2$ are readily reoxidized by O_2 via the electron transport chain.

In addition to its production of the reduced cosubstrates NADH and $FADH_2$, which furnish the energy through their oxidation via electron transport, the Krebs cycle produces most of the carbon dioxide through decarboxylation reactions. In terms of glucose metabolism, it must be recalled that two pyruvates are produced from one glucose during cytoplasmic glycolysis. These pyruvates are in turn transferred into the mitochondria, where decarboxylation leads to the formation of two acetyl CoA units and two molecules of CO_2. The two carbons represented by the acetyl CoA are additionally lost as CO_2 through Krebs cycle decarboxylations. Most of the CO_2 produced is exhaled through the lungs, although some is used in certain synthetic reactions called *carboxylations*.

The Krebs cycle is shown in Figure 4.10. The acetyl CoA, which couples with oxaloacetate to begin the pathway, is formed from numerous sources, including the breakdown of fatty acids, glucose (through pyruvate), and certain amino acids. Its formation from pyruvate is considered now, because pyruvate links cytoplasmic glycolysis to the Krebs cycle, which takes place in the mitochondrion.

The reaction shown in 4I is referred to as the pyruvate dehydrogenase reaction. Actually, however, the reaction is a complex one requiring a multienzyme system and various cofactors. The enzymes and cofactors are contained within an isolable unit called the *pyruvate dehydrogenase complex*. The cofactors include coenzyme A (CoA), thiamine pyrophosphate (TPP), Mg^{+2}, NAD^+, FAD, and lipoic acid. Four vitamins are therefore necessary for the activity of the complex: pantothenic acid (a component of CoA), thiamine, niacin, and riboflavin. The role of these vitamins and others as precursors of coenzymes is discussed in Chapter 9. The enzymes include pyruvate decarboxylase, dihydrolipoyl dehydrogenase, and dihydrolipoyl transacetylase. The net effect of the complex results in decarboxylation and dehydrogenation of pyruvate, with NAD^+ serving as the terminal hydrogen acceptor. This reaction therefore yields energy, because the reoxidation by electron transport of the NADH produces 3 mol of ATP by oxidative phosphorylation. The reaction is regulated negatively by ATP and by NADH.

The condensation of acetyl CoA with oxaloacetate initiates the Krebs cycle reactions. The following are comments on reactions:

1. The formation of citrate from oxaloacetate and acetyl CoA is catalyzed by citrate synthase. The reaction is regulated negatively by ATP.

2. The isomerization of citrate to isocitrate involves cis aconitate as an intermediate. The isomerization, catalyzed by aconitase, involves dehydration followed by sterically reversed hydration, resulting in the repositioning of the —OH group onto an adjacent carbon.

3. The first of four dehydrogenation reactions within the cycle, the isocitrate dehydrogenase reaction supplies energy through the respiratory chain reoxidation of the NADH. Note that the first loss of CO_2 in the cycle occurs at this site. It arises from the spontaneous decarboxylation of an intermediate compound, oxalosuccinate. The reaction is positively modulated by ADP and negatively modulated by ATP and NADH.

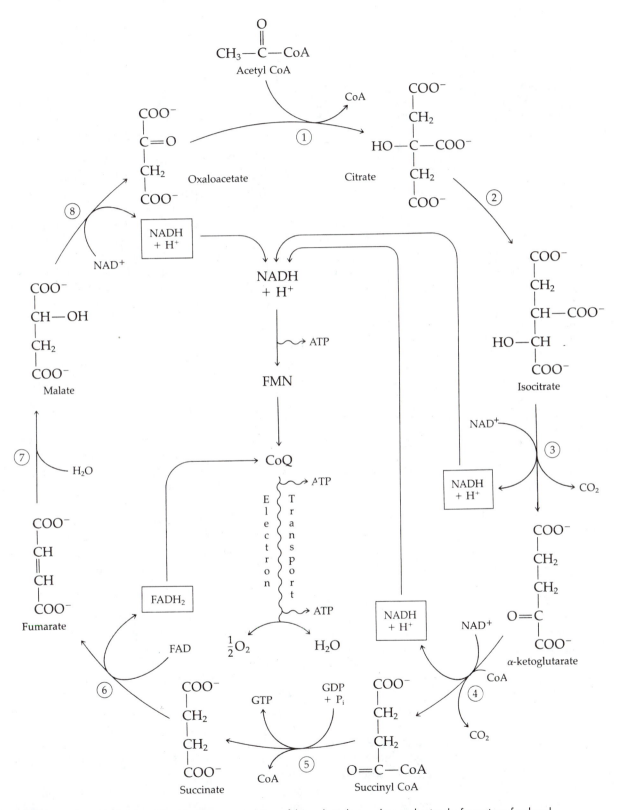

FIGURE 4.10 The Krebs (citric acid) cycle. This representation of the cycle is designed to emphasize the formation of reduced coenzymes and how their reoxidation by electron transport contributes to the synthesis of ATP.

(41)

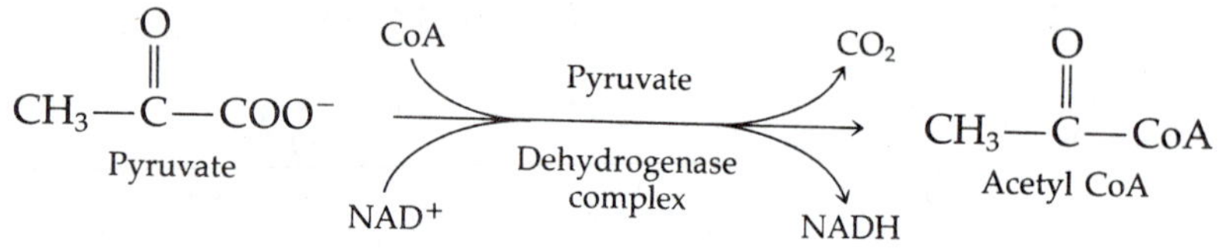

4. The decarboxylation–dehydrogenation of α-ketoglutarate is mechanistically identical to the pyruvate dehydrogenase complex reaction in its multienzyme–cofactor requirement. In the reaction, referred to as the α-*ketoglutarate dehydrogenase reaction*, NAD$^+$ serves as hydrogen acceptor, and a second carbon is lost as CO_2. The pyruvate dehydrogenase, isocitrate dehydrogenase, and α-ketoglutarate dehydrogenase reactions account for the loss of the three-carbon equivalent of pyruvate as CO_2.

5. Energy is conserved in the thioester bond of succinyl CoA. The hydrolysis of that bond by succinyl thiokinase releases sufficient energy to drive the phosphorylation of guanosine diphosphate (GDP) by inorganic phosphate. The resulting GTP is a high-energy phosphate anhydride compound like ATP; as such, GTP can serve as phosphate donor in certain phosphorylation reactions. One such reaction occurs in the gluconeogenesis pathway (p. 93).

6. The succinate dehydrogenase reaction uses FAD instead of NAD$^+$ as hydrogen acceptor. The FADH$_2$ is reoxidized by electron transport to O_2, but only two ATPs are formed by oxidative phosphorylation instead of three.

7. Fumarase incorporates the elements of H_2O across the double bond of fumarate to form malate.

8. The conversion of malate to oxaloacetate completes the cycle. NAD$^+$ acts as a hydrogen acceptor in this dehydrogenation reaction catalyzed by malate dehydrogenase. It is the fourth site of reduced cosubstrate formation and therefore of energy release in the cycle.

In summary, the complete oxidation of glucose to CO_2 and H_2O can be shown by the equation

$$C_6H_{12}O_6 + 6\,O_2 \longrightarrow 6\,CO_2 + 6\,H_2O + \text{energy}$$

This is achieved by the combined reaction sequences of the glycolytic and Krebs cycle pathways. Under aerobic conditions, the amount of released energy conserved as ATP is therefore as follows.

The glycolytic sequence, glucose $\longrightarrow$ two pyruvates, produces two ATPs by substrate-level phosphorylation and either four or six by oxidative phosphorylation, depending on the shuttle system for NADH-reducing equivalents. Generally six will be formed, due to the overall greater activity of the malate shuttle system. The intramitochondrial pyruvate dehydrogenase reaction yields 2 mol of NADH, one for each pyruvate oxidized, and therefore six additional ATPs by oxidative phosphorylation.

The oxidation of 1 mol of acetyl CoA in the Krebs cycle yields a total of 12 ATPs. The sites of formation, indicated by reaction number, follow:

3. 3 ATPs

4. 3 ATPs

5. 1 ATP (as GTP)

6. 2 ATPs

8. 3 ATPs
_____

Total 12 ATPs

Since 2 mol acetyl CoA derive from one glucose, however, the actual total is 24 ATPs. The total number of ATPs produced for the complete oxidation of 1 mol of glucose is therefore 38, equivalent to 262.8 kcal. Recall from Chapter 3 that this figure represents only about 40% of the total energy released by mitochondrial electron transport. The remaining 60%, or approximately 394 kcal, is released as heat to maintain body temperature.

As already mentioned, acetyl CoA is produced by fatty acid oxidation and amino acid catabolism as well as from the pyruvate derived from glycolysis, a fact that is readdressed in Chapters 6 and 7. This clearly leads to an imbalance between the amount of acetyl CoA and oxaloacetate, which condense one to one stoichiometrically in the citrate synthase reaction. It is therefore important that oxaloacetate and/or Krebs cycle intermediates, which can form oxaloacetate, be replenished in the cycle. Such a mechanism does exist. Oxaloacetate, fumarate, succinyl CoA, and α-ketoglutarate can all be formed from certain amino acids, but the single most important mechanism for ensuring an ample supply of oxaloacetate is the reaction by which it is formed directly from pyruvate. This reaction, shown here, is catalyzed by pyruvate carboxylase. The "uphill" in-

(4J)

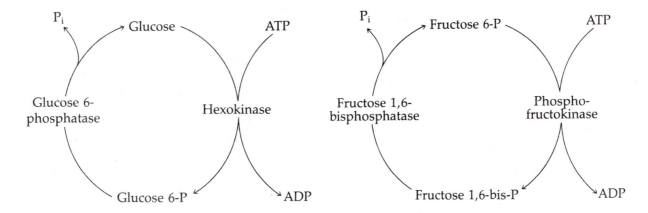

(4K)

corporation of CO_2 is accomplished at the expense of ATP, and the reaction requires the participation of biotin—see 4J. The conversion of pyruvate into oxaloacetate is called an *anaplerotic* (filling up) process because of its role in restoring oxaloacetate to the cycle. It is of interest that pyruvate carboxylase is regulated positively by acetyl CoA, thereby accelerating oxaloacetate formation in response to increasing levels of acetyl CoA.

Gluconeogenesis

D-glucose is an essential nutrient for the proper function of most cells. Particularly dependent on glucose as a nutrient are the brain and other tissues of the central nervous system (CNS), and red blood cells. When dietary intake of carbohydrate is reduced, and blood glucose concentration declines, a hormonal triggering of accelerated glucose synthesis from noncarbohydrate sources occurs. Lactate, pyruvate, glycerol (a catabolic product of triacylglycerols), and certain amino acids represent the important noncarbohydrate sources. The process of producing glucose from such compounds is termed *gluconeogenesis*. The liver is the major site of this activity, although under certain circumstances, such as starvation, the kidneys become increasingly important in gluconeogenesis.

Gluconeogenesis is essentially a reversal of the glycolytic pathway. Most of the cytoplasmic enzymes involved in the conversion of glucose to pyruvate catalyze their reactions reversibly and therefore provide the means for also converting pyruvate to glucose. There are three reactions in the glycolytic sequence that are *not reversible*—the hexokinase, phosphofructokinase, and pyruvate kinase reactions (sites 1, 3, and 10, Fig. 4.7). They are unidirectional by virtue of the high, negative-free energy change of the reactions. Therefore the process of gluconeogenesis requires that these reactions be bypassed or circumvented by other enzyme systems. The presence or absence of these enzymes determines if a certain organ or tissue is capable or incapable of conducting gluconeogenesis. As shown in 4K, the hexokinase and phosphofructokinase reactions are bypassed by specific phosphatases (glucose 6-phosphatase and fructose 1,6-bisphosphatase, respectively) that remove phosphate groups by hydrolysis.

The bypass of the pyruvate kinase reaction involves the formation of oxaloacetate as an intermediate. Mitochondrial pyruvate can be converted to oxaloacetate by pyruvate carboxylase, a reaction that has been discussed as an anaplerotic process. Oxaloacetate can, in turn, be decarboxylated and phosphorylated to phosphoenolpyruvate by PEP carboxykinase, thereby completing the bypass of the pyruvate kinase reaction. The PEP carboxykinase reaction is a cytoplasmic reaction, however, and oxaloacetate must therefore leave the mitochondrion to be acted on by the enzyme. The mitochondrial membrane is, however, impermeable to oxaloacetate, which therefore must first be converted to either malate (by malate dehydrogenase) or aspartate (by transamination with glutamate; see Chapter 7), either of which freely traverse the mitochondrial membrane. In the cytoplasm, the malate or aspartate can be converted to oxaloacetate by malate dehydrogenase or aspartate aminotransferase (glutamate oxaloacetate transaminase) respectively. This mechanism allows the carbon skeletons of various amino acids to enter the gluconeogenic pathway and lead to a net synthesis of glucose. Such amino acids are accordingly called *glucogenic.* They can be metabolically converted to pyruvate and to Krebs cycle intermediates. As such, they can ultimately leave the mitochondrion in the form of malate or aspartate, as discussed. Reactions showing the entry of noncarbohydrate substances into the gluconeogenic system are shown in Figure 4.11, along with the bypass of the pyruvate kinase reaction.

Liver gluconeogenesis accounts for that organ's ability to control the high levels of blood lactate that may accompany strenuous physical exertion. Muscle and adipose tissue, for example, are unable to form free glucose from noncarbohydrate precursors because they lack glucose 6-phosphatase. This suggests that muscle and adipose lactate cannot serve as a precursor of free glucose. Also, muscle cells convert lactate into glycogen only very slowly, especially in the presence of glucose [7]. How, then, is the high level of muscle lactate that can be encountered in situations of oxygen debt, dealt with? Recovery is accomplished by the gluconeogenic capability of the liver. The lactate leaves the muscle cells, and is transported via the general circulation to the liver, where it is able to be converted to glucose. The glucose can then be returned to the muscle cells to re-establish homeostatic concentrations there. This circulatory transport of muscle-derived lactate to the liver and the return of glucose to the muscle is referred to as the *Cori cycle.*

During the past decade, evidence has emerged from *in vitro* studies that glucose, as the sole substrate at physiologic concentrations, has limited use by the liver and is, in fact, a poor precursor of liver glycogen. However, use is greatly enhanced if gluconeogenic substances such as fructose, glycerol, or lactate are available along with the glucose. The simple incorporation of glucose into glycogen *in vivo*, but its limited conversion *in vitro*, in the absence of other gluconeogenic compounds, has been referred to as the glucose paradox [8]. It is now believed that glucose ingested during a meal takes a somewhat roundabout path to glycogen. It is first taken up by red blood cells in the bloodstream and converted to lactate by glycolysis. The lactate is then taken up by the liver and converted to glucose 6-phosphate (and thence to glycogen) by gluconeogenesis.

REGULATION OF METABOLISM

The purpose of regulation is to both maintain homeostasis and to alter the reactions of metabolism in such a way as to meet the nutritional and biochemical demands of the body. An excellent example is the reciprocal regulation of the glycolysis and Krebs cycle (catabolic) pathways, and the gluconeogenic (anabolic) pathways. Because the glycolytic conversion of glucose to pyruvate liberates energy, the reversal of the process, gluconeogenesis, must therefore be energy consuming. The pyruvate kinase bypass in itself is energetically expensive, considering that 1 mol of ATP and 1 mol of GTP must be expended in converting intramitochondrial pyruvate to extramitochondrial PEP. It follows that among the factors that regulate the glycolysis–gluconeogenesis activity ratio is the body's need for energy. Our discussion focuses on the body's requirements for energy and on how regulation can speed up or slow down the activity of the metabolic pathways contributing to release or consumption of energy.

In a broad sense, regulation is achieved by three mechanisms:

- Negative or positive modulation of allosteric enzymes by effector compounds
- Hormonal activation or induction of specific enzymes
- Shifts in reaction equilibria by changes in reactant or product concentrations.

Allosteric Enzyme Modulation

Allosteric enzymes can be stimulated or suppressed by certain compounds, usually formed within the pathway in which the enzymes function. An allosteric, or regulatory, enzyme is said to be positively or negatively modulated by a substance (modulator) according to whether the effect is stimulation or suppression, respectively. Modulators generally act by altering the conformational structure of their allosteric enzymes, causing a shift in the equilibrium between so-called tight and relaxed conformations of the enzyme. The enzyme is functionally more active in its relaxed form than when it is in its tight form. A positive modulator causes a shift toward the re-

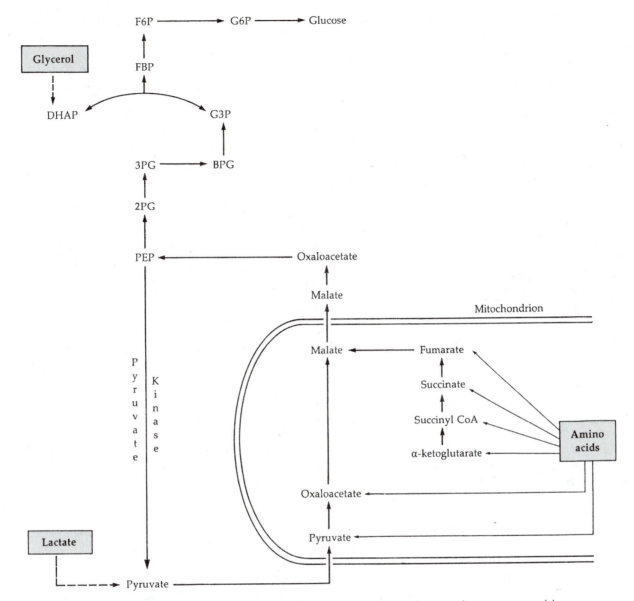

FIGURE 4.11 The reactions of gluconeogenesis, showing the bypass of the unidirectional pyruvate kinase reaction and the entry into the pathway of noncarbohydrate substances such as glycerol, lactate, and amino acids. Abbreviations: G6P, glucose 6-phosphate; F6P, fructose 6-phosphate; FBP, fructose 1,6-bisphosphate; DHAP, dihydroxyacetone phosphate; G3P, glyceraldehyde 3-phosphate; BPG, 1,3-bisphosphoglycerate; 3PG, 3-phosphoglycerate; 2PG, 2-phosphoglycerate; PEP, phosphoenolpyruvate.

laxed configuration, while a negative modulator shifts the equilibrium toward the tight form.

An important regulatory system in energy metabolism is the cellular concentration ratio of ADP (or AMP) to ATP. The usual breakdown product of ATP is ADP, but as ADP increases in concentration, some becomes enzymatically converted to AMP. Therefore, both ADP and/or AMP accumulation can signify an excessive breakdown of ATP, and therefore a depletion of ATP.

AMP, ADP, and ATP all act as modulators of certain allosteric enzymes, but the effect of AMP or ADP will oppose that of ATP. For example, if ATP accumulates, which might occur during a period of muscular relaxation, it can negatively modulate certain regulatory enzymes in energy-releasing (ATP-producing) pathways, so as to reduce the production of additional ATP. An increase in AMP (or ADP) concentration conversely signifies a depletion of ATP and the need to produce more of this energy source. In such a case, AMP or ADP, as their concentration increases, can positively modulate allosteric enzymes functioning in energy-releasing pathways. Two examples of positive modulation by AMP are (1) its ability to bring about a shift from the inactive form of phosphorylase b to an active form of phosphorylase b (see Fig. 4.6), and (2) its stimulation, by a similar mechanism, of the enzyme phosphofructokinase, which catalyzes a reaction in the glycolytic pathway. It can be reasoned that an enhanced activity of either of these reactions encourages glucose catabolism. The resulting shift in metabolic direction, as signaled by the AMP buildup, therefore releases energy and helps restore depleted stores of ATP.

In addition to being positively modulated by AMP, phosphofructokinase is also modulated positively by ADP, and negatively by ATP. So as the store of ATP increases, and further energy release is not called for, ATP can signal the slowing of the glycolytic pathway at that reaction. Phosphofructokinase is an extremely important rate-controlling allosteric enzyme, and is modulated by a variety of substances. Its regulatory function has already been described in Chapter 1.

There are other regulatory enzymes in carbohydrate metabolism that are modulated by ATP, ADP, or AMP. Pyruvate dehydrogenase complex, citrate synthase, and isocitrate dehydrogenase are negatively modulated by ATP. Pyruvate dehydrogenase complex is positively modulated by AMP, and citrate synthase and isocitrate dehydrogenase are positively regulated by ADP.

The ratio of NADH to NAD^+ also has an important regulatory effect. Certain allosteric enzymes are responsive to an increased level of NADH or NAD^+, which therefore regulate their own formation through negative modulation of those enzymes. Since NADH is a product of the oxidative catabolism of carbohydrate, its accumulation would signal for a decrease in catabolic pathway activity. Conversely, higher proportions of NAD^+ signify that a system is in an elevated state of oxidation readiness, and would send a modulating signal to accelerate catabolism. Stated in a different way, the level of NADH in the fasting state is markedly lower because the rate of its reoxidation by electron transport would exceed its formation from substrate oxidation. Fasting, therefore, logically encourages glycolysis and Krebs cycle oxidation of carbohydrates. Dehydrogenase reactions, which involve the interconversion of the reduced and oxidized forms of the cosubstrate, are reversible. If metabolic conditions lead to the accumulation of one form or the other, the equilibrium is shifted so as to consume more of the predominant form. Pyruvate dehydrogenase complex is positively modulated by

NAD^+, and pyruvate kinase, citrate synthase and α-ketoglutarate dehydrogenase are negatively modulated by NADH.

As discussed previously in Chapter 1 (section on enzymes), allosteric enzymes catalyze unidirectional, or nonreversible, reactions. This is because modulators of those enzymes must either stimulate or suppress a reaction in one direction only. The stimulation or suppression of an enzyme that catalyzes both the forward and reverse direction of a reaction would have little value.

Hormonal Regulation

Hormones can regulate specific enzymes by either *covalent regulation* or by *enzyme induction*. The term *covalent regulation* refers to the phosphorylation and dephosphorylation of the enzymes being regulated, which converts them into active or inactive forms. In some instances, phosphorylation activates and dephosphorylation inactivates the enzyme. In other cases, the reverse may be true. Examples are found in the covalent regulation of glycogen synthase and glycogen phosphorylase, enzymes that have been discussed under the glycogenesis and glycogenolysis sections, respectively. Phosphorylation inactivates glycogen synthase, while dephosphorylation activates it. In contrast, phosphorylation activates glycogen phosphorylase, and dephosphorylation inactivates it.

Another very important example of covalent regulation by a hormone is glucagon's control of the relative rates of liver glycolysis and gluconeogenesis. The control is directed at the opposing reactions of the phosphofructokinase (PFK) and fructose bisphosphatase (FBPase) site, and is mediated through a compound called fructose 2-6-bisphosphate. Unlike fructose 1-6-bisphosphate, fructose 2-6-bisphosphate is not a normal glycolysis intermediate, but serves solely as a regulator of pathway activity. *Fructose 2-6-bisphosphate stimulates PFK activity and suppresses FBPase activity, therefore stimulating glycolysis and reducing gluconeogenesis.* Cellular concentration of fructose 2-6-bisphosphate is set by the relative rates of its formation and breakdown. It is formed by phosphorylation of fructose 6-phosphate by phosphofructokinase 2 (PFK-2), and is broken down by fructose bisphosphatase 2 (FBPase-2). The designation 2 distinguishes these enzymes from PFK and FBPase which catalyze the formation and breakdown, respectively, of fructose 1-6-bisphosphate. PFK-2 and FBPase-2 activities are expressed by a single (bifunctional) enzyme, and the relative activity of each is controlled by glucagon. Glucagon stimulates the phosphorylation of the bifunctional enzyme, resulting in a sharply increased activity of FBPase-2 activity and suppression of PFK-2 activity. *Glucagon there-*

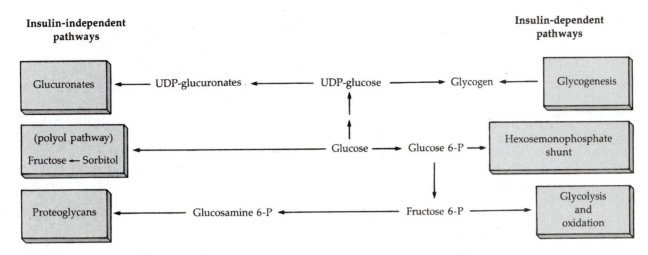

FIGURE 4.12 Insulin-independent and insulin-dependent pathways of glucose metabolism.

fore stimulates hepatic gluconeogenesis and suppresses glycolysis by reducing the concentration of fructose 2-6-bisphosphate, a positive modulator of the glycolytic enzyme PFK. The end result, therefore, is that in response to falling blood glucose levels, the release of glucagon encourages hepatic gluconeogenesis to restore glucose levels.

Covalent regulation is usually mediated through cAMP, which acts as a second messenger in the hormones' action on the cell. It will be recalled that insulin strongly affects the glycogen synthase reaction positively, and that epinephrine and glucagon positively regulate glycogen phosphorylase in muscle and liver, respectively. Each of these hormonal effects are mediated through covalent regulation.

The control of enzyme activity by hormone induction represents another mechanism of regulation. Enzymes functioning in the glycolytic and gluconeogenic pathways can be divided into the three following groups:

Group 1. *Glycolytic enzymes*
  Glucokinase
  Phosphofructokinase
  Pyruvate kinase

Group 2. *Bifunctional enzymes*
  Phosphoglucoisomerase
  Aldolase
  Triosephosphate isomerase
  Glyceraldehyde 3-phosphate dehydrogenase
  Phosphoglycerate kinase
  Phosphoglyceromutase
  Enolase
  Lactate dehydrogenase

Group 3. *Gluconeogenic enzymes*
  Glucose 6-phosphatase
  Fructose biphosphatase
  PEP carboxykinase
  Pyruvate carboxylase

Groups 1 and 3 are inducible enzymes, meaning that their concentrations can rise and fall in response to molecular signals such as a sustained change in the concentration of a certain metabolite. Such a change might arise through a prolonged shift in the dietary intake of certain nutrients. Induction results in the stimulated transcription of new messenger RNA programmed to produce the hormone. Glucocorticoid hormones are known to stimulate gluconeogenesis by inducing the formation of the key gluconeogenic enzymes, and insulin may stimulate glycolysis by inducing an increased synthesis of key glycolytic enzymes. Group 2 enzymes are not inducible, and are produced at a steady rate under the control of constitutive, or basal, gene systems. Non-inducible enzymes are required all the time at a relatively constant level of activity, and their genes are expressed at a more or less constant level in virtually all cells. Genes for enzymes that are not inducible are sometimes called *housekeeping genes*.

The interrelationship among pathways of carbohydrate metabolism is exemplified by the regulation of blood glucose concentration. Largely through the opposing effects of insulin and glucagon, fasting serum glucose level is normally maintained within the approximate range of 60 to 90 mg/dL. Whenever hyperglycemia is excessive or sustained due to an insufficiency of insulin, other insulin-independent pathways of carbohydrate metabolism for lowering blood glucose become increasingly active. Such insulin-independent pathways are indicated in Figure 4.12. The overactivity of these pathways is believed to be partly responsible for the clinical manifestations of diabetes mellitus, type 1 (see "Perspective" section, Chapter 8).

Shifts in Reaction Equilibria

Most enzymes catalyze reactions reversibly, and the preferred direction that a reversible reaction is undergoing at a particular moment is largely dependent on the relative concentration of each reactant. A buildup in concentration of one of the reactants will drive or force the reaction toward formation of the other. For example, consider the hypothetical pathway intermediates A and B, which are interconverted reversibly. Reaction 1 (see following diagrams) may represent the reaction in a metabolic resting state. It shows a net formation of A from B as indicated by the size of the directional arrows. Reaction 2 shows that the "equilibrium" shifts toward the formation of B from A if some metabolic event or demand causes the concentration of A to rise above its homeostatic levels.

$$\textit{Reaction 1.} \quad \overset{\longleftarrow}{\underset{\rightarrow}{} } A \overset{\longleftarrow}{} B \longleftarrow$$

$$\textit{Reaction 2.} \quad \longrightarrow A \overset{\longrightarrow}{\underset{\longleftarrow}{}} B \longrightarrow$$

This concept is exemplified by the phosphoglucomutase reaction, which interconverts glucose 6-phosphate and glucose 1-phosphate, and which functions in the pathways of glycogenesis and glycogenolysis (see Figs. 4.4 and 4.5). At times of heightened glycogenolytic activity (rapid breakdown of glycogen), glucose 1-phosphate concentration rises sharply, driving the reaction toward the formation of glucose 6-phosphate. With the body at rest, glycogenesis and gluconeogenesis is accelerated, increasing the concentration of glucose 6-phosphate. This in turn shifts the phosphoglucomutase reaction toward the formation of glucose 1-phosphate, and ultimately glycogen.

SUMMARY

The major sources of dietary carbohydrates are the starches and the disaccharides. In the course of digestion, these are hydrolyzed by specific glycosidases to their component monosaccharides, which are absorbed into the circulation from the intestine. The monosaccharides are transported to the cells of various tissues, wherein they are first phosphorylated at the expense of

ATP, and can then follow any of several integrated pathways of metabolism. The uptake of glucose occurs in cells of many tissues. It is phosphorylated in most cells by hexokinase, but in the liver, by glucokinase. Phosphorylation of fructose can also be catalyzed by hexokinase, but it is phosphorylated mainly by the liver enzyme fructokinase. Galactose is phosphorylated by galactokinase, also a liver enzyme.

Cellular glucose can be converted into glycogen, primarily in liver and skeletal muscle, or it can be routed through the energy-releasing pathways of glycolysis and the Krebs cycle in these and other tissues for ATP production. Glycolytic reactions convert glucose (or glucose residues from glycogen) to pyruvate. From pyruvate, either an aerobic course (complete oxidation in the Krebs cycle) or anaerobic course (to lactate) can be followed. Nearly all the energy released by the oxidation of carbohydrates to CO_2 and H_2O occurs in the Krebs cycle, as reduced coenzymes are oxidized via mitochondrial electron transport. Approximately 40% of this energy is retained in the high-energy phosphate bonds of ATP. The remaining energy supplies heat to the body.

Noncarbohydrate substances derived from the other major nutrients, fats and proteins, can be converted to glucose or glycogen by the pathways of gluconeogenesis. Basically, the reactions are the reversible reactions of glycolysis, shifted toward glucose synthesis in accordance with reduced energy demand by the body. Three kinase reactions occurring in glycolysis are not reversible, however, requiring the involvement of different enzymes and pathways to circumvent those reactions in the process of gluconeogenesis. Muscle glycogen provides a source of glucose for energy for that tissue only, because muscle lacks the enzyme glucose 6-phosphatase, which forms free glucose from glucose 6-phosphate. The enzyme is active in liver, however, meaning that the liver can release free glucose from its glycogen stores into the circulation for use by other tissues. The Cori cycle describes the liver's uptake and gluconeogenic conversion of working muscle lactate to glucose.

A metabolic pathway is regulated according to the body's need for energy or for maintaining homeostatic cellular concentrations of certain metabolites. Regulation is mainly exerted through hormones, through substrate concentrations (which can affect the velocity of enzyme reactions), and through allosteric enzymes that can be modulated negatively or positively by certain pathway products.

In Chapters 6 and 7, we will see that fatty acids and the carbon skeleton of various amino acids also are ultimately oxidized through the Krebs cycle. The amino acids that do become Krebs cycle intermediates may not, however, be completely oxidized to CO_2 and H_2O but instead may leave the cycle to be converted to glucose or glycogen (by gluconeogenesis), should dietary intake of carbohydrate be low. The glycerol portion of triacylglycerols enters the glycolytic pathway at the level of dihydroxyacetone phosphate, from which point it can be oxidized for energy or used to synthesize glucose or glycogen. The fatty acids of triacylglycerols enter the Krebs cycle as acetyl CoA, which is oxidized to CO_2 and H_2O but which cannot contribute carbon for the net synthesis of glucose. This is considered further in Chapter 6.

These examples of the entrance of noncarbohydrate substances into the pathways discussed in this chapter are cited here to remind the reader that these pathways are not singularly committed to carbohydrate metabolism. Rather, they must be thought of as common ground for the interconversion and oxidation of fats and proteins as well. It is essential to maintain this broadened perspective as we move on into Chapters 6 and 7, in which the metabolism of lipids and proteins, respectively, are examined.

References Cited

1. Crane RK. Hypothesis for mechanism of intestinal active transport of sugars. Fed Proc 1962;21:891–895.
2. Crane RK. Handbook of physiology. Washington DC: American Physiological Society, 1968;3(6):1323–1351.
3. Gray GM, Johnson LR, ed. Physiology of the gastrointestinal tract. New York: Raven Press. 1981;2:1069.
4. Truswell AS, Seach JM, Thorburn AW. Incomplete absorption of pure fructose in healthy subjects and the facilitating effect of glucose. Am J Clin Nutr 1988;48:1424–1430.
5. Smythe C, Cohen P. The discovery of glycogenin and the priming mechanism for glycogen biosynthesis. Eur J Biochem 1991;200:625–631.
6. Lehninger AL, Nelson DL, Cox MM. Principles of Biochemistry, 2nd ed. New York: Worth, 1993;428–430.
7. McLane JA, Holloszy JO. Glycogen synthesis from lactate in three types of skeletal muscle. J Biol Chem 1979;254:6548–6553.
8. Katz J, McGarry JD. The glucose paradox: Is glucose a substrate for liver metabolism? J Clin Invest 1984;74:1901–1909.

Suggested Reading

McGarry JD, Kuwajima M, Newgard CB, Foster DW. From dietary glucose to liver glycogen: The full circle round. Ann Rev Nutr 1987;7:51–73.

The glucose paradox is emphasized, from the standpoint of its emergence, as are the attempts to resolve it.

Pilkis SJ, El-Maghrabi MR, Claus TH. Hormonal regulation of hepatic gluconeogenesis and glycolysis. Ann Rev Biochem 1988;57:755–783.

This is a brief, clearly presented summary of the effect of certain hormones on the important regulatory enzymes in these major pathways of carbohydrate metabolism.

Simpson IA, Cushman SW. Hormonal regulation of mammalian glucose transport. Ann Rev Biochem 1986;55:1059–1089.

This is an excellent review of what is known about the mechanism of insulin action and how it relates to the cellular transport of glucose.

Glycogen Loading in the Athlete

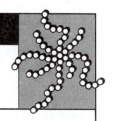

In today's society, emphasis is on the improvement of health and physical performance, a trend that has led to the emergence of sports nutrition as an important science. Nutrition, as a means of positive impact on physical performance, has become a topic of great interest to all those involved in human performance—the scientist as well as the athlete and the trainer of the athlete. To understand how nutrition relates to physical performance at the cellular level, determining various biochemical parameters is necessary. The respiratory quotient (RQ), the ratio of the volume of CO_2 expired to the volume of O_2 consumed, has served for nearly a century as the basis for determining the relative participation of carbohydrates and fats in exercise [1]. During the past 20 years, however, such knowledge has been advanced by invasive techniques such as arteriovenous measurements and the use of needle biopsies to quantify tissue stores.

Despite pronounced involvement of the cardiovascular and respiratory systems during periods of prolonged, strenuous exercise, the limiting factor is the supply and use of intramuscular and extramuscular fuel reserves. The single, most consistently observed factor contributing to fatigue is the depletion of muscle glycogen [2]. Blood glucose levels, the concentrations of muscle and liver glycogen, hepatic glucose output, and working muscle uptake of glucose are among the parameters studied in connection with prolonged exercise. Such measurements are meaningful only when the *quantity* of work is defined, because the extent of deviation from homeostatic reaction rates parallels the extent of exertion. Exercise intensity is most commonly expressed in terms of the percentage of the maximal oxygen consumption ($VO_{2\ max}$), which is the workload that places the highest possible demand on the working muscle of that subject. Studies of the parameters mentioned are generally carried out within the exercise intensity range of 70 to 85% of the $VO_{2\ max}$.

Biopsy of muscle during exercise at 70 to 85% $VO_{2\ max}$ shows an exponential pattern of glycogen depletion. In the latter phase of this curve, the rate of degradation slows, indicative of complete depletion in most of the working muscle fibers. This phase correlates with subject exhaustion, and any required energy at that point is compensated for by increased gluconeogenesis by the liver and by increased fat oxidation [1,3].

Like muscle glycogen, the concentration of blood glucose also falls progressively during prolonged, strenuous exercise. This is due to the fact that glucose uptake by working muscle may increase to as much as 20-fold or more above resting levels, while hepatic glucose output decreases with exercise duration. Interestingly, however, hypoglycemia is not always observed at exhaustion, particularly at exercise intensities above 70% $VO_{2\ max}$ [1]. Hypoglycemia following liver glycogen depletion can apparently be postponed by an inhibition of glucose uptake and by accelerated gluconeogenesis in the liver, using the glycerol produced in lipolysis, and by lactate and pyruvate produced by the glycolytic activity of the working muscles. Furthermore, elevated ketone levels, which are an alternative substrate for the CNS, could diminish the symptoms of hypoglycemia.

Since muscle glycogen was identified as the limiting factor for the capacity to exercise at intensities requiring 70 to 85% $VO_{2\ max}$, dietary manipulation to maximize glycogen stores followed naturally. The most popular subject for research of this nature has been the marathon runner, because of the prolonged physical taxation of the event and the fact that the athlete's performance is readily measurable by the time required to complete the course. There emerged the major dietary concern in the endurance training of marathon runners as to how to elevate muscle glycogen to above-normal levels (i.e., *supercompensated* levels).

The so-called classical regimen resulted from investigations in the late 1960s by Scandinavian scientists [3]. This involved two sessions of intense exercise to exhaustion separated by two days of low-carbohydrate diet (less than 10%), to "starve" the muscle of carbohydrate. This was followed by three days of a high-carbohydrate diet (greater than 90%) and rest. The event would be performed on day 7 of the regimen. After this regimen, muscle glycogen levels approached 220 mmol/kg wet weight (expressed as glucose residues), more than double the athlete's resting level. However, various undesirable side effects of the classical regimen, such as irritability, dizziness, and a diminished exercise capacity, has led to the recent revelation of a less-stringent regimen of diet and exercise that produces comparably high muscle glycogen levels [4]. In this modified regimen, runners perform "tapered-down" exercise periods over the course of five days, followed by one day of rest. During this time, three days of a

PERSPECTIVE (continued)

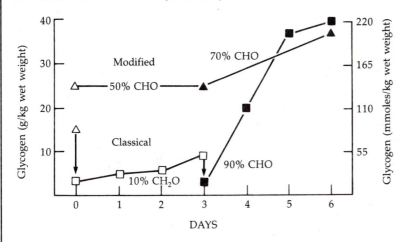

Classical (arrows indicate exhaustive exercise)

□—□ 10% CHO

■—■ 90% CHO

Modified (tapering exercise, 90, 40, 40, 20, 20 min, rest)

△—△ 50% CHO } 73% $\dot{V}O_2$ max
▲—▲ 70% CHO

FIGURE 1 Schematic representation of the "classical" regime of muscle glycogen supercompensation described by Scandinavian investigators and the "modified" regime of muscle glycogen supercompensation, which has been shown to elevate muscle glycogen stores to comparably high levels with "normal" diets and a "tapering-down" sequence of exercise. (From "Carbohydrates, Muscle Glycogen, and Muscle Glycogen Supercompensation" by W. M. Sherman. In Ergogenic Aids in Sport (p. 14) by M. H. Williams (ed.), 1983, Champaign, IL: Human Kinetics Publishers. Reprinted by permission.)

50% carbohydrate diet are followed by three days of a 70% carbohydrate diet. Figure 4.13 illustrates graphically the amount of muscle glycogen formed as a result of each regimen. Predictably, the supercompensation of muscle glycogen by whatever approach has been shown to improve performance in trained runners during races of 30 km and longer. It did not improve performance in shorter races (<21 km) owing to the fact that glycogen depletion is not the limiting factor in such an event.

The timing of the final meal before intense exercise is crucial because fasting results in a reduction of the labile glycogen stores of liver, while carbohydrate meals consumed too close in time to the event may cause hyperinsulinemia. In the latter situation, a rapid reduction in plasma glucose ensues, and work capacity is significantly impaired. In addition, elevated plasma insulin inhibits liver glucose output and the normal rise of plasma-free fatty acid. Under such conditions, excessive muscle glycogen degradation occurs, resulting in early fatigue [5]. The form of carbohydrate (i.e., glucose, fructose, or sucrose) ingested may produce different blood glucose and insulin responses, but the rate of muscle glycogen resynthesis is about the same regardless of the structure [5].

We hope this "Perspective" will make the reader more aware of the importance of nutritional control in maximizing physical performance. Careful attention to the finer details of intermediary metabolism, particularly that of carbohydrate, has helped to promote sports nutrition to the scientific status it enjoys today.

References Cited
1. Hermansen L, Hultman E, Saltin B. Muscle glycogen during prolonged severe exercise. Acta Physiol Scand 1967;71:129–139.
2. Sherman WM, Costill DL. The marathon: Dietary manipulation to optimize performance. Am J Sports Med 1984;12:44–51.
3. Bergstrom J, Hultman E. A study of the glycogen metabolism during exercise in man. Scand J Clin Lab Invest 1967;19:218–228.
4. Sherman WM. Carbohydrates, muscle glycogen, and muscle glycogen supercompensation. In Williams MH, ed. Ergogenic aids in sports. Champaign, IL: Human Kinetics Publishers, 1983; 1–250.
5. Costill DL. Carbohydrate nutrition before, during, and after exercise. Fed Proc 1985;44:364–368.

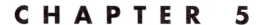
DIETARY FIBER

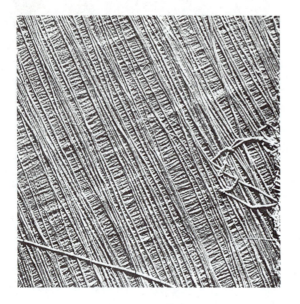

Photo: Cellulose fibrils of plant cell wall

Recognition of dietary fiber as an important food component was reawakened in the mid 1970s [1]. Results from extensive research devoted to dietary fiber during the last 20 or so years have implicated fiber as important in various aspects of gastrointestinal function and in the prevention and/or management of a variety of disease states.

The varying effects of fiber observed by researchers are related to the fact that dietary fiber is made up of different components, each with its own distinctive characteristics. Examining these many components plus their various, distinctive characteristics emphasizes the fact that dietary fiber cannot be considered a single entity.

Fractionation of dietary fiber rather than extraction of plant roughage, or crude fiber, began around 1955 and is continuing to be refined and improved [1–3]. The concept of crude fiber, or indigestible material, and its extraction from animal feed and forages were introduced in Germany during the 1850s. Owing to the lack of simple alternative methods, the crude fiber extraction method has continued to be used, even for human food, until quite recently. Food composition figures of fiber traditionally have referred to *crude fiber*, primarily cellulose, rather than being inclusive for the various components making up dietary fiber. This crude fiber figure, based on food sample residues after treatment with 1.25% sulfuric acid and sodium hydroxide, is believed to underestimate total dietary fiber by at least 40% [2,3]. Nevertheless, no correction factors can be used because the relationship between the crude fiber and dietary fiber varies among foods.

DEFINITION OF DIETARY FIBER

Because dietary fiber is not a constant entity, no universally accepted definition for this food component has yet evolved. Probably the most widely accepted definition for dietary fiber is that proposed by Trowell et al. [4]: "plant polysaccharides and lignin which are resistant to hydrolysis by the digestive enzymes of man." Dissatisfaction with this definition exists because (1) it fails to include all the indigestible residue from food that may reach the colon, and (2) it uses ability to be digested as the basis for identifying fiber [5]. Heaton [5] points out that all undigested food reaching the colon does not necessarily lack the ability to be digested, nor is it necessarily unavailable to the body. Starch in varying amounts reaches the colon in an unaltered state along with nonstarch polysaccharides (NSP). Starch and much of the nonstarch polysaccharides undergo fermentation by colonic bacteria, thereby producing short-chain fatty acids that may be used for energy by the host.

Despite their presence in colonic residue, some researchers do not consider starch and lignin to be true components of dietary fiber [6]; starch because it is digestible by mammalian enzymes, and lignin because it is a noncarbohydrate polymer. It is generally agreed that all the nonstarch polysaccharides should be regarded as fiber components.

Dietary fiber, in spite of the controversy about its exact composition, is derived from plant cells. The plant cell wall is of particular importance in providing the nonstarch polysaccharides; also the plant cell wall is the source of lignin. Table 5.1 demonstrates the relationship between the plant cell wall and the plant components generally accepted as comprising dietary fiber. Identifying the chemical characteristics and various intraplant functions of those substances found in the plant cell wall itself (and/or in contact with the wall) promotes conceptualization of how fiber components may affect physiologic functions in human beings.

CHEMISTRY AND INTRAPLANT FUNCTIONS OF FIBER COMPONENTS

The general chemical structure of various dietary fiber components is shown in Figure 5.1.

TABLE 5.1 Relationship Between Plant Cell Wall and Dietary Fiber

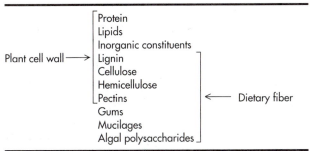

Cellulose

Cellulose, shown in Figure 5.1a, is a long, linear polymer of 1,4 beta-linked glucose units. Hydrogen bonding between sugar residues in adjacent chains imparts a microfibril structure. Cellulose has a truly fibrous structure. Being a large, linear, neutrally charged molecule, cellulose is insoluble. Degradation of cellulose by colonic bacteria varies. In plants, cellulose provides structure to the cell wall. Some examples of foods high in cellulose relative to other fibers include bran, legumes, peas, root vegetables, vegetables of the cabbage family, outer covering of seeds, and apples [1].

Hemicellulose

Hemicellulose is a heterogenous group of substances containing a number of sugars in its backbone and side chains. The sugars found most prominently in hemicellulose are shown in Figure 5.1b. The hemicelluloses may be classified based on their principal sugar. Hemicelluloses with acid molecules are slightly charged and are soluble in water. Other hemicelluloses are insoluble. The hexose and uronic acid components of hemicellulose are somewhat accessible to bacterial enzymes. In plants, hemicelluloses function as part of the cell wall. Some examples of high-hemicellulose foods are bran and whole grains [1].

Pectic Substances

Pectic substances (commonly called *pectin*) are a complex group of polysaccharides in which galacturonic acid is a primary constituent. The backbone structure of pectin is usually an unbranched chain of 1,4-linked D-galacturonic acid units, as shown in Figure 5.1c. Other carbohydrate moieties may be linked to the galacturonic acid chain. Additional sugars sometimes found attached as side chains include rhamnose, arabinose, xylose, and fucose. Pectins form part of the primary cell wall of plants and part of the middle lamella. Pectins are soluble and gel forming, and can be almost completely metabolized by colonic bacteria. Apples, strawberries, and citrus fruits are high in pectins [1]. Pectins are also added to commercial products and to some enteral nutrition formulas administered to tube-fed hospitalized patients.

Lignin

Lignin is the main noncarbohydrate component of fiber. It is a three-dimensional polymer composed of phenol units with strong intramolecular bonding. The primary phenols composing lignin are shown in Figure 5.1d. Lignin forms the structural components of plants. Ma-

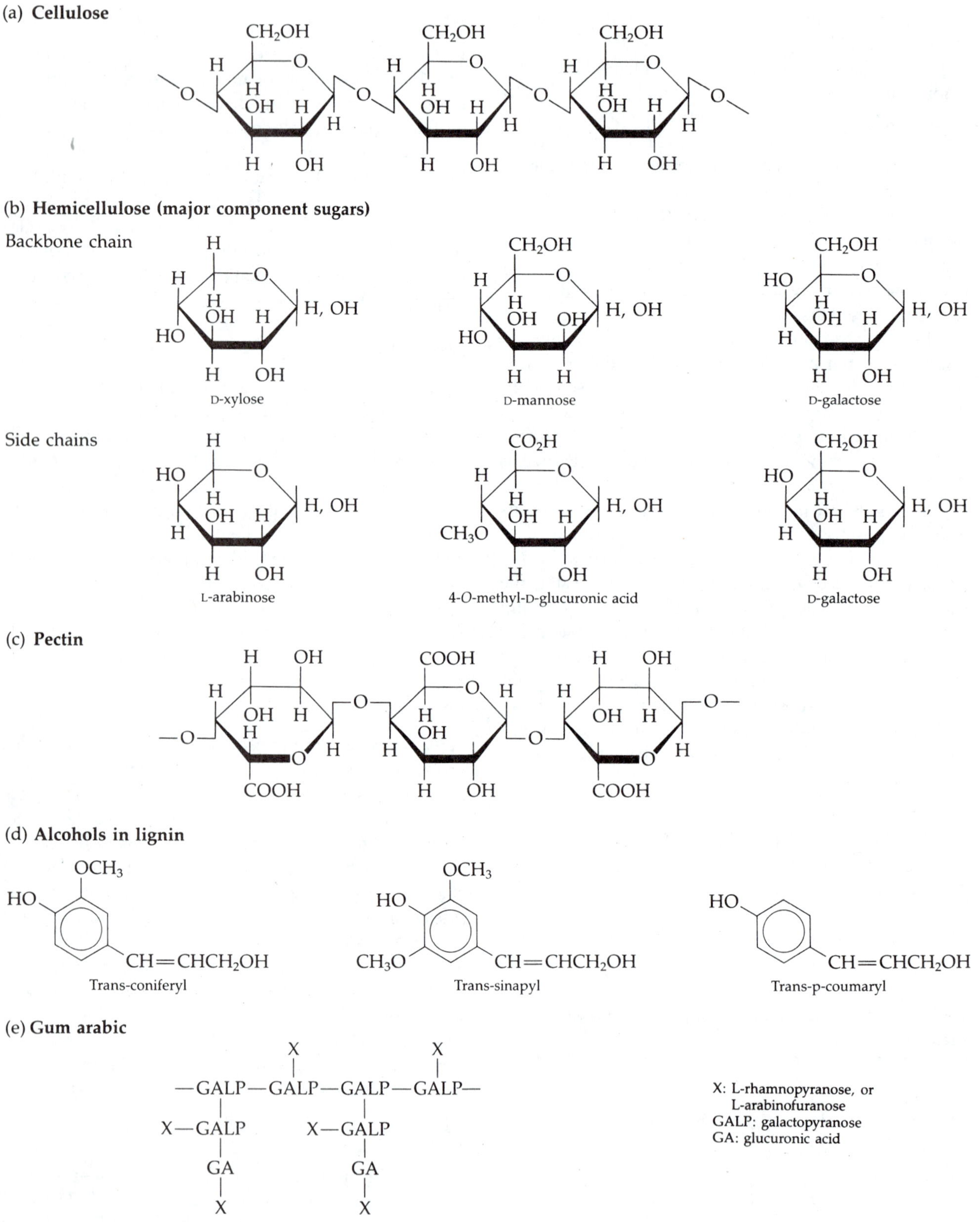

(a) Cellulose

(b) Hemicellulose (major component sugars)

Backbone chain

D-xylose   D-mannose   D-galactose

Side chains

L-arabinose   4-O-methyl-D-glucuronic acid   D-galactose

(c) Pectin

(d) Alcohols in lignin

$CH=CHCH_2OH$ $CH=CHCH_2OH$ $CH=CHCH_2OH$

Trans-coniferyl   Trans-sinapyl   Trans-p-coumaryl

(e) Gum arabic

```
        X                    X
        |                    |
 —GALP—GALP—GALP—GALP—
   X—GALP        X—GALP
        |                    |
       GA                  GA
        |                    |
        X                    X
```

X: L-rhamnopyranose, or
   L-arabinofuranose
GALP: galactopyranose
GA: glucuronic acid

FIGURE 5.1 Chemical structures of dietary fibers.

ture root vegetables such as carrots, wheat, and fruits with edible seeds such as strawberries are high in lignin [1]. Lignin is insoluble in water and has hydrophobic binding capacity. Lignin is not digested by colonic bacterial microflora.

Gums

Gums are one of a group of substances that may be referred to as *hydrocolloids*. They are secreted at the site of plant injury by specialized secretory cells. Gums are composed of a variety of sugars and sugar derivatives. Occurring prominently in the gums are galactose and glucuronic acid as well as uronic acids, arabinose, rhamnose, and mannose, among others. The structure of the gum arabic is given in Figure 5.1e. Gum arabic is the plant hydrocolloid most commonly used as a food additive. Its popularity is due to its physical properties, including high solubility, pH stability, and gelling characteristics [7]. Gums are also found naturally in foods such as oatmeal, barley, and legumes [1,8].

Mucilages and Algal Polysaccharides

Mucilages and algal polysaccharides are both hydrocolloids and similar to gums in chemical structure, although not shown in Figure 5.1. Because of their hydrophilic property, these substances are excellent stabilizers. Mucilages—the best known of which is guar—are synthesized by plant secretory cells to protect the seed endosperm from desiccation. The algal polysaccharides—for example, carrageenan and agar—are derived from algae and seaweed and are commonly added to food.

In addition to the polysaccharides and lignin, a variety of other substances that are plant derived or result from food processing are considered dietary fiber. These substances, usually recovered in the lignin fraction of fiber analysis, include the Maillard product, cutin, and suberin. The Maillard product consists of enzyme-resistant linkages between the amino group of amino acids, especially lysine, and the carboxyl groups of reducing sugars. Maillard products are formed during heat treatment, particularly in the baking and frying of foods [9,10]. Cutin and suberin are both polymeric esters of fatty acids that are both enzyme resistant and acid resistant.

The plant cell wall contributes the greatest percentage of the dietary fiber (Table 5.1). The cell wall consists of both a primary and secondary wall. The primary wall is a thin envelope surrounding the contents of the growing cell; the secondary wall develops as the cell matures. The secondary wall of a mature plant contains many strands of cellulose arranged in an orderly fashion within a matrix of noncellulosic polysaccharides. The primary

wall also contains cellulose, but it occurs in smaller amounts and is less well organized.

Lignin deposits (phenolics) form in specialized cells whose function is to provide structural support to the plant. As the plant matures, lignin spreads through the intracellular spaces, penetrating the pectic substances. Pectic substances function as intercellular cement and are located between and around the cell walls. Lignification begins by permeating the primary wall and then spreads into the developing secondary wall. Suberin is deposited in the cell wall during later stages of plant development [9]. Starch, the energy storage product of the cell, is found within the cell walls. Cutin is a water-impermeable substance secreted onto the plant surface [9].

SELECTED PHYSIOLOGIC ROLES OF DIETARY FIBER

Important characteristics of dietary fiber that affect its physiologic roles include hydration or water-holding capacity, viscosity, adsorptive attraction for organic molecules, cation exchange capacity, and fermentability.

Response of the Upper Gastrointestinal Tract to Fiber

Food sources of fiber vary in the relative amounts of the different fiber components. Dietary fiber composition of a plant depends on the plant species, the part of the plant consumed (leaf, root, stem) and its maturity [1]. For example, wheat bran is primarily hemicellulose, while most fruits and vegetables contain almost equal quantities of cellulose and pectin [10]. The cellulose content of cereals is about 17%, while in raw vegetables it averages approximately 31% [1]. These different types of fibers and the relative amounts of the different types of fibers in food influence the upper gastrointestinal tract.

Fiber may first exert its effect in the mouth. Fiber components that cannot be solubilized (lignin, cellulose, and some hemicelluloses) require increased chewing, thereby stimulating saliva secretion and serving somewhat as a tooth cleanser [5].

Water-Holding Capacity, Hydration, and Viscosity Different types of fibers produce different physiologic effects. Pectins, gums, and some hemicelluloses have a high water-holding capacity. Pectins, gums, mucilages, and algal polysaccharides can also form viscous solutions within the gastrointestinal tract. Overall effects of ingestion of these substances include delayed emptying of food from the stomach; interference with the mixing of the intestinal contents with digestive enzymes, thus disrupting digestion; and delayed nutrient absorption in the proximal intestine. In general, soluble fibers (Fig. 5.2) typically delay small intestine transit time versus insoluble fibers (Fig. 5.2), which increase transit time within the small intestine [11].

The size of the particles and/or degree of processing of the foods providing fiber also influence the gastrointestinal response to ingested fiber. For example, coarsely ground bran has a higher hydration capacity than that which is finely ground. Consequently, coarse bran increases fecal volume. Coarse bran also speeds up the rate of fecal passage through the colon. Maintaining the integrity of cells in grains and legumes rather than subjecting them to traditional milling processes also appears to increase the effect of these fiber sources in the delay of gastric emptying and in nutrient absorption [12].

Various mechanisms have been proposed for the observed gastrointestinal effects of fibers with high water-holding capacity and those which form viscous gels. These mechanisms include blunting of villi in the small intestine, decreased secretion of gastrointestinal and pancreatic hormones, and direct reduction in the activity of pancreatic enzymes [8,13]. Other mechanisms suggested for the delayed absorption of nutrients observed when pectins, gums, mucilages, and algal polysaccharides are ingested include the slowed emptying of the stomach and/or a decreased diffusion rate of nutrients in the proximal intestine. The decreased diffusion rate is probably due to an increased thickness of the unstirred water layer. The primary effect of gums in slowing glucose absorption appears to be due to their decreasing the convective solute movement within the lumen of the intestine [8]. Convective currents induced by peristaltic movements are responsible for bringing nutrients from the lumen to the epithelial surface for absorption. Decreasing the convective solute movement may also help explain the decreased absorption of amino acids and fatty acids caused by viscous fiber [8]. The hydrocolloids may further reduce the availability of amino acids to the

body through inhibition of intestinal peptidases [8,14]. It is unclear whether fiber directly decreases the activity of these digestive enzymes or acts by reducing the rate of enzyme penetration into the food.

Adsorption and Cation Exchange Adsorption (binding) to organic substances such as bile is also a property of some fiber components, especially lignin, gums, and pectins. Adsorption depends on pH, and is influenced by particle size, food processing, and fermentability [15]. Lipid digestion, absorption, and metabolism are affected by fiber. This occurs by mechanisms such as delayed gastric emptying, reduced mixing of gastrointestinal contents with digestive enzymes, and delayed nutrient absorption, but also by adsorption of key compounds involved in lipid digestion. Soluble fibers (such as pectin, guar gum, and oat bran), but also lignin, an insoluble fiber, may affect lipid absorption by adsorbing cholesterol or bile acids. Adsorption to bile acids by fibers results in a lowering of the amount of free bile acids available in the gastrointestinal lumen for micelle formation. In addition, the complexing of bile acids by fiber removes the bile from enterohepatic circulation. A decrease in the bile acids returned to the liver necessitates the use of cholesterol for synthesis of new bile acids. The net effect of the process is a lowering of serum cholesterol. A second proposed mechanism for the hypocholesterolemic (lower blood cholesterol) effect of fiber is the shift of bile acid pools toward chenodeoxycholic acid, and away from cholic acid, which has no inhibitory quality [8]. The increased concentrations of chenodeoxycholic acid inhibit 3-hydroxy-3-methylglutaryl CoA reductase (HMG-CoA reductase), a regulatory enzyme of cholesterol biosynthesis. This shift would reduce the amount of cholesterol synthesized in the liver and theoretically result in lower blood cholesterol concentrations. Neither mechanism, however, can explain the extent to which fiber has been able to lower serum cholesterol in various human studies [8].

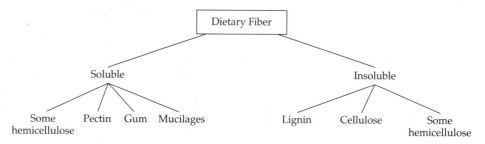

FIGURE 5.2 Soluble and insoluble dietary fiber.

Cation adsorption, particularly adsorption of calcium, zinc, and iron, is another property of fiber in the upper digestive system. The formation of cationic bridges by fiber—especially those with uronic acid such as hemicellulose, pectins, and gums—appears to serve as a mechanism for the adsorption of bile acid, fatty acids, and minerals [16]. Lignin, which has both carboxyl and hydroxyl groups, is also thought to play a role in mineral adsorption [16]. Hydration capacity correlates positively with cation exchange capacity, suggesting a relationship [16]. Cation-binding capacity of fiber is lost when or if a fiber is fermented by colonic bacteria [15]. Thus, the effect (positive or negative) that fiber has on mineral balance depends to some extent on its degree of fermentability or its accessibility to bacterial enzymes [13].

Response of Lower Gastrointestinal Tract to Fiber

By conventional definition, dietary fiber is that portion of the food that enters the cecum unchanged. Therefore it follows that the colon is the organ most profoundly affected by fiber [5,12,15].

Fermentability Fibers, such as pectins, gums, mucilages, algal polysaccharides, and some hemicelluloses, are fermented by the various anaerobic bacteria residing in the colon. Some cellulose and hemicelluloses are also fermentable, but their fermentation is much slower than that of the other fibers. The principal metabolites of fermentable fibers (including any starch that has passed into the cecum) are volatile fatty acids (VFA)—also called *short-chain fatty acids (SCFA)*—primarily acetic, butyric, and propionic acids. By-products of this fiber fermentation are hydrogen, carbon dioxide, and methane gases that are excreted as flatus or are expired by the lungs.

Different fibers are fermented to different short-chain fatty acids in different amounts [17]. For example, ingestion of pectin resulted in higher propionate concentrations in the colon of rats versus wheat bran, which resulted in higher butyrate concentrations [17].

Fatty acids produced by fermentation are rapidly absorbed, and their absorption in turn stimulates water and sodium absorption in the colon [15]. In addition, certain fatty acids such as butyrate appear to promote cell proliferation in the distal colon of rats [17]. Moreover, the colonic epithelial cells metabolize for energy the short-chain fatty acids, particularly butyric acid, produced from fiber fermentation. Butyric acid acts as an important fuel source for these cells, promotes cell proliferation, and performs specific regulatory functions within the cell nucleus [18]. Those fatty acids not used by the colonic cells, primarily the propionic and acetic acids, are carried by the portal vein to the liver, where the propionate and some of the acetate are taken up and metabolized. Most of the acetate, however, passes to the peripheral tissues, where it is metabolized by muscle [18].

The propionic acid generated from fiber fermentation may produce, in part, the hypocholesterolemic effect observed with ingestion of some fibers. Propionic acid, fed to rats, has been shown to inhibit HMG-CoA reductase, the rate-limiting enzyme in hepatic cholesterol biosynthesis. Inhibition of this enzyme, as with increased chenodeoxycholate concentrations, could lower serum cholesterol [8].

Fermentation of carbohydrates by colonic anaerobes makes available to the body much of the energy contained in undigested food reaching the cecum. How much energy is actually realized principally depends on the amount and type of dietary fiber that is ingested [18]. It is estimated that in developed countries as much as 10 to 15% of ingested carbohydrate may be fermented in the colon; in the Third World (developing) countries, this percentage may be considerably higher [19].

Microbe Proliferation and Water Absorption The fiber components that are nonfermentable—principally cellulose and lignin—or that are more slowly fermentable, such as some hemicelluloses, increase fecal bulk through water absorption and/or promotion of microbe proliferation. The fermentation occurring from that portion of fiber that is slowly fermentable is particularly valuable in causing proliferation of microbes.

Microbial proliferation and excretion may be important as a detoxification mechanism as well as a means of increasing fecal volume. The synthesis of increased microbial cells could result in the increased scavenging of and sequestering of degradable nitrogenous substances, which eventually are excreted [16]. The effect of microbial proliferation on mineral balance may not be favorable, however. Microbial proliferation from slowly fermentable fibers may result in increased binding of minerals within the new microbial cells and result in the loss of minerals from the body, assuming colonic mineral absorption. In contrast, the more rapidly fermentable fiber components (such as pectins) appear to have a favorable effect on mineral balance. Calcium, zinc, and iron bound to these fiber components are released as fermentation occurs and may possibly be absorbed in the colon [8,13].

Fecal bulk is formed from unfermented fiber, bacterial mass, salts, and water. In general, fecal bulk increases with decreased fermentation of the fiber. The rapidly fermentable fiber appears to have little or no effect on fecal bulk. Therefore, choosing the appropriate food source(s) of fiber depends on the specific fiber effect(s) being sought and whether the food contains the fiber components producing this effect(s). Wheat bran is one of the most effective fiber laxatives because it can absorb three times its weight of water, thereby producing a much softer, bulky stool. Gastrointestinal responses to wheat bran include (1) increased fecal bulk, (2) greater frequency of defecation, (3) reduced intestinal transit time, and (4) decreased intraluminal pressure. Rice bran has been found to be even more effective than wheat bran in eliciting an increased fecal bulk and a reduced intestinal transit time [20].

Fruits and vegetables, in contrast to wheat bran, contain considerable amounts of pectin, which can delay gastric emptying and reduce glucose absorption because of its gelation quality. It is obvious that knowing only the total fiber content of various foods may not be particularly useful in defining physiologic effects. For this reason, when an effort is being made to increase the amount of fiber ingested, sources of fiber should be somewhat varied so that all the various fiber components are being supplied.

Physiologic effects elicited by fibers are summarized in Table 5.2. Figure 5.3 diagrams the relationship between fibers and the observed physiologic effects.

RECOMMENDED INTAKE OF FIBER: IMPLICATIONS IN DISEASE PREVENTION AND/OR MANAGEMENT

Recommendations for increasing the amount of dietary fiber in the U.S. diet have come from several governmental and private organizations, each with a concern for improving the health of the U.S. public. The recommended intake of fiber for the general population ranges from 20 to 40 g/day but may reach as much as 50 g/day for some individuals [21–25].

The importance of an adequate intake of fiber to the improvement of health is demonstrated by some of the physiologic effects exerted by its various components. Particularly noteworthy are the hypoglycemic and hy-polipidemic effects of soluble fiber. Slowing the absorption rate of carbohydrate can be very helpful to the diabetic in regulating blood glucose levels. Lowering serum cholesterol levels has significant benefits in the prevention of atherosclerosis.

Adequate fiber intake has been implicated in control of various gastrointestinal disorders, including diverticular disease, gallstones, irritable bowel syndrome, and constipation. The nonfermentable fibers, especially cellulose and lignin, and fibers that are more slowly fermentable, such as some hemicelluloses, have been shown to be helpful in overcoming constipation, particularly constipation associated with symptomatic diverticular disease and/or irritable bowel syndrome [13,15]. Sources of such fibers include wheat and rice bran; both are effective in the treatment of constipation. Evidence for the effectiveness of fiber in the control of the other diseases appears equivocal [13,26]; however, populations with high fiber intakes have a lower incidence of these gastrointestinal disorders [11].

A generous fiber intake appears to be beneficial to some people in their efforts at weight control. The bulk provided by fiber may have some satiety value. High-fiber foods may reduce the hunger associated with caloric restriction while simultaneously somewhat reducing nutrient utilization [26]. The effectiveness of a high-fiber diet as a treatment for obesity is not clear [27].

The antitoxic effect of fiber is a physiologic role often overlooked. Results of studies on experimental animals, particularly growing rats, have shown the protective effects of selected fiber supplements against a variety of toxic agents [26]. Burkitt and Trowell [27,28], among others, suggested that a high-fiber diet appears to have a protective effect against the development of colon cancer. Some of the proposed mechanisms of action of fiber in preventing colon cancer include [8,11,29–32]:

- Increase in fecal bulk decreases intraluminal concentrations of carcinogens [8,11].

- Provision of a fermentable substrate to colonic bacteria alters species and numbers of bacteria, and/or their metabolism.

- A shortened fecal transit time decreases the time during which toxins can be synthesized and in which they are in contact with the colon [8].

- Fermentation to short-chain fatty acids decreases the interluminal pH, thereby decreasing synthesis of secondary bile acids, which have been shown to promote the generation of tumors [8,32].

- Degradation of fiber by fermentation may release fiber-bound calcium. The increased calcium in the

TABLE 5.2 Physiologic Effects of Dietary Fiber Ingestion on the Gastrointestinal Tract

- Increased fecal bulk
- Decreased intraluminal pressure
- Greater frequency of defecation
- Reduced intestinal transit time
- Delayed gastric emptying
- Increased postprandial satiety
- Reduced glucose absorption
- Changes in pancreatic and intestinal enzyme activity
- Increased bile acid excretion
- Possible alterations in mineral balances

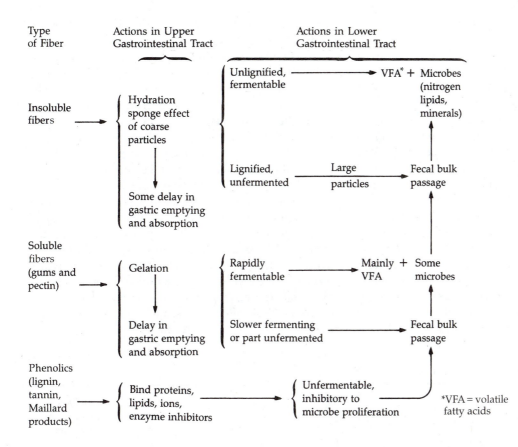

FIGURE 5.3 Diagram showing a model relating type of fiber with gastro-intestinal responses in humans. *(Modified from Peter J. Van Soest, "Some physical characteristics of dietary fibres and their influence on the microbial ecology of the human colon," Proc. Nutr. Soc. 1984; 43:25–33. Reprinted with permission.)*

colon may help eliminate the mitogenic advantage that cancer cells have over normal cells in a low-calcium environment [8].

- Butyric acid produced by fermentation may have antineoplastic properties; however, data are conflicting [31].

On the negative side, wheat bran has been shown in rats to increase proliferation of colonic cells in the right colon [33]. Should carcinogens be present in the right colon at the time of the proliferation, the chances of developing neoplastic change might increase [33]. Harris and associates [34] have proposed three possible mechanisms by which soluble fibers may enhance the development of colorectal cancers. These theories include (1) soluble fibers reduce the ability of insoluble fibers to adsorb hydrophobic carcinogens, thus more carcinogens may enter the colon maintained in solution than adsorbed onto insoluble fibers; (2) on degradation of soluble fibers, carcinogens are released and deposited on the colonic mucosal surface; (3) soluble fibers may cross the intestinal epithelium and transport with them carcinogens maintained in solution [34].

There is little agreement among the numerous studies (in experimental animals) designed to determine the effect of fiber in the development of colon cancer [30]. Most of the evidence for the positive role of fiber in the colon cancer prevention has come from epidemiologic observations. Unfortunately, in these epidemiologic studies, variation in many dietary factors other than fiber intake has been noted. The dietary factors most often identified as being involved in variations in the incidence of colorectal cancer between different population groups are too many total calories, high fat, too much protein, low fiber, low intake of vitamin D and calcium, and a low intake of antioxidants [30,33]. Consequently, evidence for a protective effect of fiber in colon carcinogenesis is inconclusive [30,35].

Recommendations that fiber intake be increased should be interpreted in terms of dietary change rather than addition of fiber supplements, which, more than likely, are devoid of other nutrients. Because much fiber is nonfermentable, an excessive intake may pose the hazard of negative mineral balance, particularly among infants, children, adolescents, and pregnant women whose mineral needs are greater than those for adult men and nonpregnant women [36]. Excessive fiber intake could be particularly detrimental for calcium, zinc, and iron balance when the intake of these minerals is marginal. A fiber intake of 30 to 40 g/day when accompanied by an adequate intake of minerals appears to have no detrimental effects, only possible benefits.

Guidelines suggest increasing complex carbohydrates to 55 to 65% of total calories and increasing fiber using a combination of fibers in food. A minimum of about 20 g/day is recommended by the American Dietetic Association [25] and by the Federation of American Societies for Experimental Biology (FASEB) [21], which suggests 10 g/1000 kcal. Intake of 25 g fiber/day minimum is recommended by others [36] including the National Cancer Institute [23]. The upper level of fiber consumption should be about 40 g/day as recommended by the American Diabetes Association [24]. Both FASEB [21] and the American Dietetic Association [25] suggest an upper limit of 35 g/day. For clients with a family his-

tory of diet-implicated cancers, daily fiber consumption should regularly be about 35 to 40 g/day [38]. Intakes of up to 50 g/day are recommended for diabetics and people with hypercholesterolemia [24,38]. Intakes of fiber beyond the upper range of 40 to 50 g/day may produce intestinal obstruction in susceptible individuals and/or cause a fluid imbalance when the fiber consumed is particularly high in water-binding components [36].

Dietary changes encouraged for accomplishing an increased and balanced fiber intake include (1) a greater consumption of fiber-rich legumes, which may serve as the primary source of protein in a meal; (2) increased consumption of fruits and vegetables; and (3) replacement of refined cereals and flour products by ones made from whole grain. As the percentage of complex carbohydrates increases in relation to the amount of fat and protein in the diet, an increase in fiber becomes almost inevitable. It remains important, however, to eat a variety of cereals, legumes, fruits, and vegetables so that variety in dietary fibers is maximized.

TABLE 5.3 Dietary Fiber Content of Some Common Foods

	Total Dietary Fiber (g/100 g)	Cellulose (g/100 g)	Noncellulose Polysaccharides (g/100 g)	Lignin (g/100 g)	Serving Size	Serving Weight (g)	Total Dietary Fiber per Serving (g)
Breads							
White	2.72	0.71	2.01	Trace	1 slice	23	0.63
Whole meal	8.50	1.31	5.95	1.24	1 slice	23	1.96
Vegetables							
Broccoli	4.10	0.85	2.92	0.03	½ cup	73	2.99
Beans, baked	7.27	1.41	5.67	0.19	⅓ cup	85	6.18
Cabbage (boiled)	2.83	0.69	1.76	0.38	½ cup	73	2.07
Corn (canned)	5.69	0.64	4.97	0.08	½ cup	83	4.72
Lettuce (raw)	1.53	1.06	0.47	Trace	½ cup	55	0.84
Onions (raw)	2.10	0.55	1.55	Trace	1 2¼" onion	100	2.10
Peas (frozen, raw)	7.75	2.09	5.48	0.18	½ cup	73	5.66
Carrots (boiled)	3.70	1.48	2.22	Trace	½ cup	75	2.78
Tomato (fresh)	1.40	0.45	0.65	0.30	1 small tomato	100	1.40
Fruits							
Apple, flesh	1.42	0.48	0.94	0.01	1 medium apple	141	2.00
Apple, peels	3.71	1.01	2.21	0.49	1 medium apple	11	0.41
Banana	1.75	0.37	1.12	0.26	1 6" banana	100	1.75
Peach, flesh and skin	2.28	0.20	1.46	0.62	1 medium peach	100	2.28
Pear, flesh	2.44	0.67	1.32	0.45	½ medium pear	87	1.12
Pear, peels	8.59	2.18	3.72	2.67	½ medium pear	11	0.95
Strawberries	2.12	0.33	0.98	0.81	10 large strawberries	100	2.12
Preserves							
Strawberry jam	1.12	0.11	0.85	0.15	1 tbsp	20	0.22
Peanuts	9.30	1.69	6.40	1.21	1 tbsp	9	0.84
Peanut butter	7.55	1.91	5.64	Trace	1 tbsp	15	1.13

Source: Adapted from Southgate DAT, Bailey B, Collinson E. et al. A guide to calculating intakes of dietary fiber. J Hum Nutr 1976; 30:303–313.

Table 5.3 provides the fiber content of some commonly consumed foods. The contribution of cellulose and lignin (both insoluble components) to the amount of total fiber is listed, but the other fiber components are grouped together as "noncellulose polysaccharides." Within the group of fibers labeled as noncellulose polysaccharides are insoluble and only slowly fermentable fibers as well as the soluble and rapidly fermentable pectic substances and hydrocolloids.

SUMMARY

No definition for *dietary fiber* has evolved that is entirely satisfactory to the scientific community. Some investigators believe the term should include all food components that reach the cecum unaltered. Others maintain that fiber should refer only to the nonstarch polysaccharides. Nevertheless, there is agreement that dietary fiber is not an entity but is a complex made up of several distinctive components. The physiologic roles of fiber in the gastrointestinal tract are as varied as the number of dietary fiber components and are determined by the types and amounts present.

The fact that some fiber components ingested by humans can be fermented by colonic microbes into usable short-chain fatty acids is of tremendous interest. No longer can the potential energy in fiber be considered totally unavailable to the human body.

The proportion of a fiber component to the other components varies according to the food source. To obtain all fiber components via the diet, food sources of fiber need to be complementary. Assurance of a good intake of all dietary fiber components requires consumption of a variety of high-fiber foods: whole-grain cereals and breads, legumes, fruits, and vegetables.

References Cited

1. Slavin JL. Dietary fiber: Classification, chemical analyses, and food sources. J Am Diet Assoc 1987;87:1164–1171.
2. Asp NG, Johansson CG. Dietary fiber analysis. Nutr Abstr Rev 1984;54:736–752.
3. Bing FC. Dietary fiber—a historical perspective. J Am Diet Assoc 1976;69:498–505.
4. Trowell HC, Southgate DAT, Wolever TMS, et al. Dietary fiber redefined. Lancet 1976;1:967.
5. Heaton KW. Dietary fibre in perspective. Hum Nutr Clin Nutr 1983:37C:151–170.
6. Bingham S. Definitions and intakes of dietary fiber. Am J Clin Nutr 1987;45:1226–1231.
7. Sharma SC. Gums and hydrocolloids in oil-water emulsions. Food Tech 1981;35:59–67.
8. Ink SL, Hurt HD. Nutritional implications of gums. Food Tech 1987;41:77–82.
9. McPherson R. Classification of fiber types. In: The clinical role of fibre (proceedings of symposium held in Toronto, February 1985), Medical Educational Services, 1985.
10. Friedman M. Dietary impact of food processing. Ann Rev Nutr 1992;12:119–137.
11. Anderson JW. Physiological and metabolic effects of dietary fiber. Fed Proc 1985;44:2902–2906.
12. Golay A, Coulston AM, Hollenbeck CB, et al. Comparison of metabolic effects of white beans processed into two different physical forms. Diabetes Care 1986;9:260–266.
13. Jenkins DJ, Jenkins AL, Wolever TMS, Rao AV, Thompson LU. Fiber and starchy foods: Gut function and implications in disease. Am J Gastroenterol 1986;81:920–930.
14. Anon. The effect of fiber on protein digestibility. Nutr Rev 1984;42:23–24.
15. Eastwood MA, Passmore R. A new look at dietary fiber. Nutr Today 1984;19:6–11.
16. Van Soest PJ. Some physical characteristics of dietary fibres and their influence on the microbial ecology of the human colon. Proc Nutr Soc 1984;43:25–33.
17. Lupton JR, Kurtz PP. Relationship of colonic luminal short chain fatty acids and pH to in vivo cell proliferation in rats. J Nutr 1993;123:1522–1530.
18. Cummings JH, Englyst HN. Fermentation in the human large intestine and the available substrates. Am J Clin Nutr 1987; 45:1243–1255.
19. McNeil NI. The contribution of the large intestine to energy supplies in man. Am J Clin Nutr 1984;39:338–342.
20. Tomlin T, Read NW. Comparison of effects on colonic function caused by feeding rice bran and wheat bran. Eur J Clin Nutr 1988;42:857–861.
21. Ad Hoc Expert Panel on Dietary Fiber, Federation of American Societies for Experimental Biology. Physiologic and health consequences of dietary fiber. Rockville, MD: FASEB, 1987.
22. American Cancer Society. Nutrition and cancer: Cause and prevention. New York: Am Cancer Soc, 1984.
23. National Cancer Institute. Diet, nutrition and cancer prevention. A guide to food choices. NIH Pub. No. 85-2711. Washington, DC: U.S. Government Printing Office, 1987.
24. American Diabetes Association. Nutritional recommendations and principles for individuals with diabetes mellitus: 1986. Diab Care 1987;10:126–132.
25. American Dietetic Association. Position of the American Dietetic Association: Health implications of dietary fiber. J Am Diet Assoc. 1988;88:216.
26. Kritchevsky D. Dietary fiber. Ann Rev Nutr 1988;8:301–328.

27. Burkitt DP, Trowell ARP, eds. Refined carbohydrates and disease. New York: Academic Press, 1975.

28. Burkitt DP, Walker ARP, Painter NS. Dietary fiber and disease. JAMA 1974;229:1068–1074.

29. Jenkins DJA, Jenkins AL, Rao AV, et al. Cancer Risk: Possible role of high carbohydrate, high fiber diets. Am J Gastroenterol 1986;81:931–935.

30. Ausman LM. Fiber and colon cancer: Does the current evidence justify a preventive policy? Nutr Rev 1993; 51:57–63.

31. Klurfeld DM. Dietary fiber-mediated mechanisms in carcinogenesis. Cancer Res (suppl) 1992;52:2055s–2059s.

32. Potter JD. Colon cancer—do the nutritional epidemiology, the gut physiology and the molecular biology tell the same story? J Nutr 1993;123:418–423.

33. Mendeloff AI. Dietary fiber and gastrointestinal disease. Am J Clin Nutr 1987;45:1267–1270.

34. Harris PJ, Roberton AM, Watson ME, Triggs CM, Ferguson LR. The effects of soluble fiber polysaccharides on the adsorption of a hydrophobic carcinogen to an insoluble dietary fiber. Nutr Cancer 1993;19:43–54.

35. Klurfeld DM. The role of dietary fiber in gastrointestinal disease. J Am Diet Assoc. 1987;87:1172–1177.

36. Southgate DAT. Minerals, trace elements, and potential hazards. Am J Clin Nutr 1987;45:1256–1266.

37. Wynder EL, Weisburger JH, Ng SK. Nutrition: The need to define "optimal" intake as a basis for public policy decisions. Am J Pub Hlth 1992;82:346–349.

38. Floch MH, Maryniuk MD, Bryant C, Franz MJ, Tietyen-Clark J, Marrota RB, Wolever T, Maillet JO, Jenkins AL. Practical aspects of implementing increased dietary fiber intake. Nutr Today 1986;21:27–30.

Suggested Reading

Anderson JW, Smith BM, Gustafson NJ. Health benefits and practical aspects of high-fiber diets. Am J Clin Nutr 1994; 59(suppl):1242S–1247S.

This article reviews the roles of dietary fiber and serum lipids, coronary heart disease, cancer, blood pressure, obesity, diabetes, and gastrointestinal disorders. The article also discusses implementation of a high-fiber diet.

Trowell H, Burkitt D. Physiological role of dietary fiber: A ten year review. J Dent Child 1986;33:444–447.

This article reviews the definitions and constituents of fiber as well as its relationship with colon cancer, diabetes, and coronary heart disease.

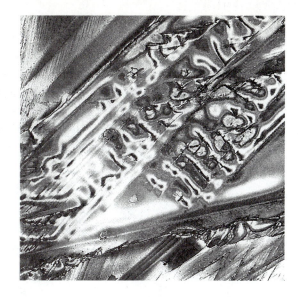

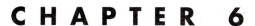
LIPIDS

Photo: Photomicrograph of crystallized
docosahexaenoic acid

The property that sets lipids apart from other major nutrients is their solubility in organic solvents such as ether, chloroform, and acetone. If lipids are defined according to this property, which is generally the case, the scope of their function becomes quite broad. It encompasses the fat-soluble vitamins, corticosteroid hormones, certain mediators of electron transport such as coenzyme Q, as well as those substances required as an energy source or as lipid constituents of cell and organelle membranes.

Among the many compounds classified as lipids, only a small number are important as dietary energy sources or as functional or structural constituents within the cell. The following classification is limited to those lipids germaine to this section of the text dealing with energy-releasing nutrients. Fat-soluble vitamins are discussed in Chapter 10.

1. Simple lipids
   a. Fatty acids
   b. Triacylglycerols, diacylglycerols, and monoacylglycerols.
   c. Waxes (esters of fatty acids with higher alcohols)
      (1) Sterol esters (cholesterol-fatty acid esters)
      (2) Nonsterol esters (vitamin A esters, and so on)

2. Compound lipids
   a. Phospholipids
      (1) Phosphatidic acids (i.e., lecithin, cephalins)
      (2) Plasmalogens
      (3) Sphingomyelins
   b. Glycolipids (carbohydrate-containing)
   c. Lipoproteins (lipids in association with proteins)

3. Derived lipids: derivatives such as sterols and straight-chain alcohols obtained by hydrolysis of those lipids in groups 1 and 2 that still possess general properties of lipids

A discussion of the structure and physiologic function of lipids follows. For this purpose they have been arbitrarily

(6A)

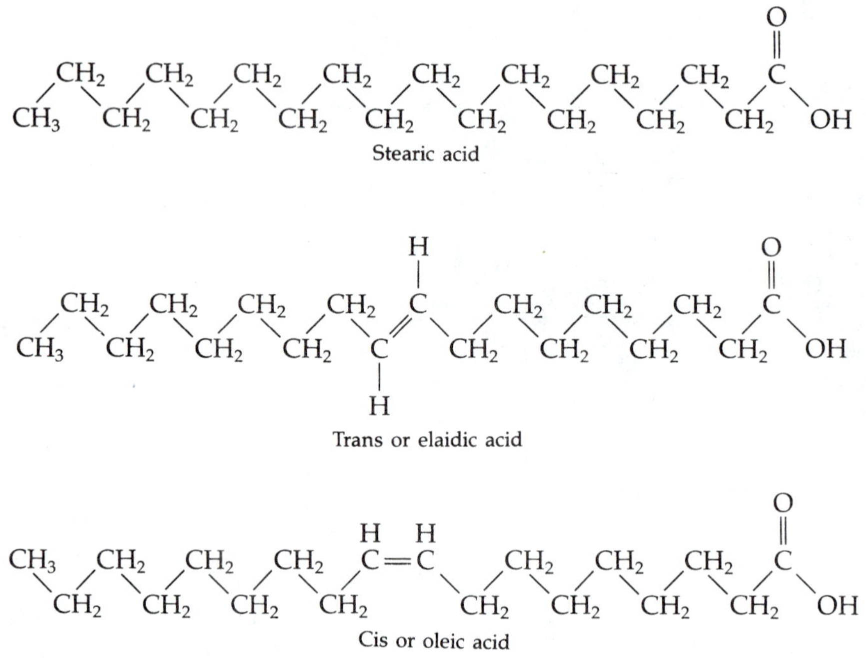

Stearic acid

Trans or elaidic acid

Cis or oleic acid

grouped according to fatty acids, triacylglycerols (triglycerides), sterols and steroids, phospholipids, and glycolipids.

STRUCTURE AND FUNCTION

Fatty Acids

As a class, the fatty acids are the simplest of the lipids. They are comprised of a straight hydrocarbon chain terminating with a carboxylic acid group, therefore endowing the molecules with a polar, hydrophilic end, and a nonpolar, hydrophobic end that is insoluble in water. Fatty acids are components of the more complex lipids, which are discussed in this section. They are of vital importance as an energy nutrient, furnishing most of the calories from dietary fat.

The length of the chains of fatty acids found in foods and body tissues ranges from 4 to about 24 carbon atoms. They may be saturated (SFA), monounsaturated (MUFA, possessing one carbon-carbon double bond), or polyunsaturated (PUFA, having two or more carbon-carbon double bonds). PUFAs of nutritional interest may have as many as six double bonds. Where a carbon-carbon double bond exists, there is an opportunity for either cis or trans geometric isomerism, which significantly affects the molecular configuration of the molecule. Cis isomerism results in a folding back and kinking

of the molecule into a U-like orientation, whereas the trans form has the effect of extending the molecule into a linear form similar to that of saturated fatty acids. The following structures illustrate saturation and unsaturation in an 18-carbon fatty acid and show how cis or trans isomerization affects the molecular configuration (see 6A).

The more carbon-carbon double bonds occurring within a chain, the more pronounced is the bending effect that, in turn, plays an important role in the structure and function of cell membranes. Most naturally occurring unsaturated fatty acids are of the cis configuration, although the trans form does exist in some natural and partially hydrogenated fats and oils. Partial hydrogenation, a process commonly used in making margarine, is designed to solidify vegetable oils. Double bonds of cis orientation, not reduced by hydrogen in the process, undergo an electronic rearrangement to the trans form. The availability of trans fatty acids in the typical U.S. diet has been estimated to be approximately 8.1 g/person/d, the major source of which is margarines and spreads [1].

There has been concern about the possible adverse nutritional effects of dietary trans fatty acids, particularly their reputed role in the etiology of cardiovascular disease. This topic is discussed in this chapter's section dealing with lipoproteins and cardiovascular disease risk.

A notation has been established to denote the chain length of the fatty acids and the number and position of any double bonds that may be present. For example, the notation 18:2 $\Delta^{9,12}$ describes linoleic acid. The first number—18, in this case—represents the number of carbon atoms; the number following the colon refers to the number of double bonds; and the superscripted numbers following the delta symbol designate the carbon atoms, *numbered from the carboxyl end*, at which the double bond(s) begins. Another commonly used system of notation locates the position of double bond(s) on carbon atoms *counted from the methyl, or omega (ω) end of the chain*. The system identifies the total number of carbon atoms in the chain, the number of double bonds, and the location (carbon atom number) of the first double bond. Implied in this system of notation is that multiple double bonds are separated by three carbon atoms; that is, $-CH=CH-CH_2-CH=CH-$. Therefore, the location of multiple double bonds is unambiguous, given their total number and the location of the one closest to the methyl end of the chain. The omega symbol replaces the delta symbol in this manner of notation. For example, the designation of linoleic acid by each of the two systems is 18:2 $\Delta^{9,12}$ or 18:2 ω-6. The fatty acid α-linolenic acid, which contains three double bonds, is identified as 18:3 $\Delta^{9,12,15}$, or 18:3 ω-3. Substitution of the omega symbol with the letter "n" has been popularized. Using this designation, α-linolenic acid would be expressed as 18:3 n-3.

Table 6.1 lists some naturally occurring fatty acids and their dietary sources. The list includes only those fatty acids having chain lengths of 14 or more carbon atoms, because these are most important nutritionally and functionally. For example, palmitic acid (16:0), stearic acid (18:0), oleic acid (18:1), and linoleic acid (18:2) together account for over 90% of the fatty acids in the average U.S. diet. However, it should be understood that shorter-chain fatty acids do occur in nature. Butyric acid (4:0) and lauric acid (12:0) occur in large amounts in milk fat and coconut oil, respectively.

If fat is entirely excluded from the diet of vertebrates, there develops a condition characterized by retarded growth, dermatitis, kidney lesions, and early death. Studies have shown that the feeding of certain unsaturated fatty acids such as linoleic, linolenic, and arachidonic acids is effective in curing the condition. It is therefore evident that certain unsaturated fatty acids cannot be synthesized in animal cells, and that they have to be acquired in the diet from plant foods. These are the essential fatty acids, of which there are two, linoleic acid (18:2 n-6) and α-linolenic acid (18:3 n-3) [2]. From linoleic acid, γ-linolenic and arachidonic acids can be

formed in the body. An intermediate fatty acid in the pathway is eicosatrienoic acid. The pathway is

Linoleic acid (18:2 n-6)
↓
γ-linolenic acid (18:3 n-6)
↓
eicosatrienoic acid (20:3 n-6)
↓
arachidonic acid (20:4 n-6)

The essentiality of linoleic and α-linolenic acids is due to the fact that vertebrates lack enzymes called Δ^{12} and Δ^{15} desaturases, which incorporate double bonds at these positions. These enzymes are found only in plants. Vertebrates are therefore incapable of forming double bonds beyond the Δ^9 carbon in the chain. But given a $\Delta^{9,12}$ fatty acid acquired from the diet, additional double-bond incorporation (desaturation) at Δ^6 can be accomplished. Fatty acid chains can also be elongated by the enzymatic addition of 2 carbon atoms at the carboxylic acid end of the chain. Desaturation and elongation reactions are discussed further in the section on fatty acid synthesis (p. 139), and are illustrated in Figure 6.11.

Most fatty acids have an even number of carbon atoms, the reason for which will be evident from the discussion of fatty acid synthesis. Odd-numbered fatty acids do occur naturally to some extent in some sources. Certain fish, such as medhaden, mullet, and tuna, as well as the bacterium *Euglena gracilis*, contain fairly high concentrations of odd-numbered fatty acids.

Nutritional interest in the n-3 fatty acids has escalated enormously in recent years because of their reported hypolipidemic and antithrombotic effects, the topic of this chapter's "Perspective" section. An n-3 fatty acid of particular interest is eicosapentaenoic acid (20:5 n-3) because it is a precursor of the physiologically important eicosanoids, which are discussed in the following section. Fish oils are particularly rich in these unique fatty acids and are therefore the dietary supplement of choice in research designed to study their effects. Food sources and tissue distribution of a few of the commonly occurring n-3 polyunsaturated fatty acids are shown in Table 6.2.

Eicosanoids: Fatty Acid Derivatives of Physiological Significance

The essentiality of the fatty acids linoleate and α-linolenate is due in part to the fact that some of the longer, more highly unsaturated fatty acids into which they can be converted are necessary (1) for the formation of cell membranes and (2) as precursors of compounds called

TABLE 6.1 Some Naturally Occurring Fatty Acids

Notation	Common Name	Formula	Source
Saturated Fatty Acids			
14:0	Myristic acid	$CH_3-(CH_2)_{12}-COOH$	Coconut and palm nut oils, most animal and plant fats
16:0	Palmitic acid	$CH_3-(CH_2)_{14}-COOH$	Animal and plant fats
18:0	Stearic acid	$CH_3-(CH_2)_{16}-COOH$	Animal fats, some plant fats
20:0	Arachidic acid	$CH_3-(CH_2)_{18}-COOH$	Peanut oil
24:0	Lignoceric acid	$CH_3-(CH_2)_{22}-COOH$	Most natural fats, peanut oil in small amounts
Unsaturated Fatty Acids			
16:1 Δ^9 (n-7)	Palmitoleic acid	$CH_3-(CH_2)_5-CH=CH-(CH_2)_7-COOH$	Marine animal oils, small amount in plant and animal fats
18:1 Δ^9 (n-9)	Oleic acid	$CH_3-(CH_2)_7-CH=CH-(CH_2)_7-COOH$	Plant and animal fats
18:2 $\Delta^{9,12}$ (n-6)	Linoleic acid	$CH_3-(CH_2)_4-CH=CH-CH_2-CH=CH-(CH_2)_7-COOH$	Corn, safflower, soybean, cottonseed, sunflower seed, and peanut oil
18:3 $\Delta^{9,12,15}$ (n-3)	Linolenic acid	$CH_3-(CH_2-CH=CH)_3-(CH_2)_7-COOH$	Linseed, soybean, and other seed oils
20:4 $\Delta^{5,8,11,14}$ (n-6)	Arachidonic acid	$CH_3-(CH_2)_3-(CH_2-CH=CH)_4-(CH_2)_3-COOH$	Small amounts animal fats
20:5 $\Delta^{5,8,11,14,17}$ (n-3)	Eicosapentaenoic acid	$CH_3-(CH_2-CH=CH)_5-(CH_2)_3-COOH$	Marine algae, fish oils
22:6 $\Delta^{4,7,10,13,16,19}$ (n-3)	Docosahexaenoic acid	$CH_3-(CH_2-CH=CH)_6-(CH_2)_2-COOH$	Animal fats as phospholipid component, fish oils

eicosanoids. Eicosanoids are fatty acids comprised of 20 carbon atoms. They include the physiologically potent families of substances called *prostaglandins, thromboxanes,* and *leukotrienes,* all of which are formed from precursor fatty acids by the incorporation of oxygen atoms into the fatty acid chains. Reactions of this sort are often referred to as *oxygenation reactions,* and the enzymes catalyzing the reactions are named *oxygenases.*

The most important fatty acid serving as precursor for eicosanoid synthesis is arachidonate. Its oxygenation follows either of two major pathways: (1) the cyclo-oxygenase pathway, which results in the formation of prostaglandins and thromboxanes; and (2) the lipoxygenase pathway, which produces leukotrienes. The fea-tured enzyme in the cyclo-oxygenase pathway is appropriately called *cyclo-oxygenase.* It receives its name from the fact that, in addition to its catalyzing oxygenation, it causes the cyclization of an internal segment of the arachidonate chain, the hallmark structural feature of the prostaglandins and thromboxanes. Figure 6.1 is an overview of the reactions of the cyclo-oxygenase and lipoxygenase pathways.

Prostaglandins (PG) are 20-carbon fatty acids having a 5-carbon ring in common but displaying modest structural differences among themselves. They are designated PGD, PGE, PGF, PGI, PGG, and PGH. Subscript numbers indicate the number of double bonds, the "2" series being the most important. These compounds,

TABLE 6.2 Dietary Sources and Tissue Distribution of the Major n-3 Polyunsaturated Fatty Acids

Fatty acid series	Major members of series	Tissue distribution in mammals	Dietary sources
n-3	α-linolenic acid 18:3 n-3	Minor component of tissues	Some vegetable oils (soy, canola, linseed, rapeseed) and leafy vegetables
	Eicosapentaenoic acid 20:5 n-3	Minor component of tissues	Fish and shellfish
	Docosahexaenoic acid 22:6 n-3	Major component of membrane phospholipids in retinal photoreceptors, cerebral gray matter, testes, and sperm	Fish and shellfish

along with the thromboxanes, exhibit a wide range of physiologic actions, including the lowering of blood pressure, diuresis, blood platelet aggregation, effects on the immune and nervous systems as well as gastric secretions, and the stimulation of smooth muscle contraction, to name several. They are described as being "hormone-like" in function, but unlike hormones, which originate from a specific gland and whose actions are the same for all their target cells, prostaglandins are widely distributed in animal tissues but affect only the cells in which they are synthesized. They do appear to alter the actions of hormones, often through their modulation of cAMP levels and the intracellular flow of calcium ions.

Certain combinations of prostaglandins and thromboxanes may exhibit antagonistic effects. For example, prostacyclin (PGI_2) is a potent stimulator of adenylate cyclase and thereby acts as a platelet "antiaggregating" factor, since platelet aggregation is inhibited by cAMP. Opposing this action is thromboxane A_2, which inhibits adenylate cyclase and consequently serves as a "proaggregating" force. Another example of opposing actions of the prostaglandins is the vasodilation of blood vessels by PGE_2 and their vasoconstriction by PGF_2.

Certain prostaglandins produce a rise in body temperature (fever), and can cause inflammation and therefore pain. The anti-inflammatory and antipyretic (fever-reducing) activity of aspirin, acetaminophen, and indomethacin is due to their inhibitory effect on cyclo-oxygenase, with the consequent reduction in prostaglandin and thromboxane synthesis.

The 5-lipoxygenase pathway of a leukotriene (LTC_4) formation from arachidonate is shown in Figure 6.1. Although it is not shown in the pathway, LTC_4 is further metabolized to other leukotrienes in the following order:

$$LTC_4 \rightarrow LTD_4 \rightarrow LTE_4 \rightarrow LTF_4$$

The structures of LTA_4 and LTC_4 are shown because these exemplify a leukotriene and a peptidoleukotriene respectively. Notice that LTC_4 is formed from LTA_4 by incorporation of the tripeptide glutathione (γ-glutamyl-cyteinyl-glycine). LTD_4, LTE_4, and LTF_4 are peptidoleukotrienes produced from LTC_4 by peptidase hydrolysis of bonds within the glutathione moiety. Like the prostaglandins, these substances share structural characteristics but are classified within the A, B, C, D, and E series according to their structural differences. The subscript number represents the number of double bonds in the compound.

Leukotrienes have potent biological actions. Briefly, they contract respiratory, vascular, and intestinal smooth muscles. The effects on the respiratory system include constriction of bronchi and increased mucus secretion. These actions, which are known to be expressed through binding to specific receptors, have implicated the leukotrienes as mediators in asthma, immediate hypersensitivities, inflammatory reactions, and myocardial infarction. In fact, one of the major chemical mediators of anaphylactic shock, the so-called slow-reacting substance of anaphylactic shock, or SRS-A, has been found to be a mixture of the peptidoleukotrienes, LTC_4, LTD_4, and LTE_4. Anaphylactic shock is a life-threatening response to chemical substances, primarily histamine, that are released as a result of a severe allergic reaction.

A necessity for eicosanoid formation is an availability of an appropriate amount of free (unesterified) arachidonate. Cellular concentration of the free fatty acid is not adequate, and it must therefore be released from membrane glycerophosphatides by a specific hydrolytic enzyme called *phospholipase A_2*. Structural features of glycerophosphatides are reviewed in the section on phospholipids (p. 120). The most important glycerophosphatides acting as sources of arachidonate in cells are phosphatidylcholine and phosphatidylinositol. When present in these structures, arachidonate normally occupies the *sn*-2 position. Stereospecific numbering (*sn*-) of glycerol-based compounds is discussed in

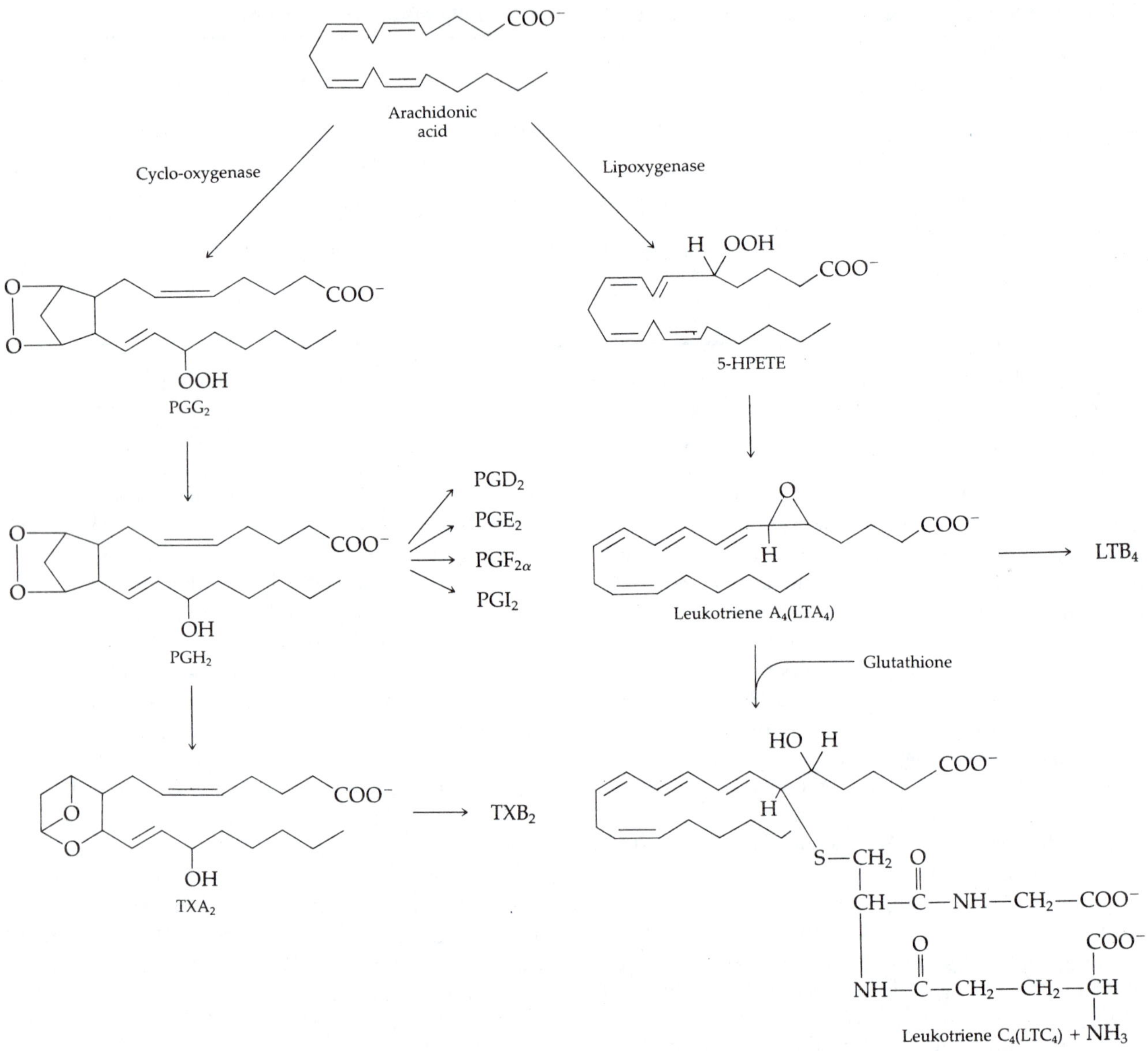

FIGURE 6.1 The formation of prostaglandins, thromboxanes, and leukotrienes from arachidonic acid via cyclo-oxygenase and lipoxygenase pathways. Abbreviations: PG, prostaglandin; TX, thromboxane; 5-HPETE, 5-hydroperoxy-6,8,11,14-eicosatetraenoic acid.

the following section. The release of arachidonate from membrane glycerophosphatides, for eicosanoid synthesis, is influenced by stimuli. These stimuli are of two main types, physiological (specific) and pathological (nonspecific). Physiological stimulation, a natural occurrence, is brought about by stimulatory compounds such as epinephrine, angiotensin II, and antigen–antibody complexes. Pathological stimuli, which result in a more generalized release of all fatty acids from the *sn*-2 position, include mechanical damage, ischemia, and membrane-active venoms.

Table 6.3 lists the precursors, site of synthesis, and physiologic effects of a few of the major eicosanoid groups.

Triacylglycerols (triglycerides)

Most stored body fat is in the form of triacylglycerols, which represent a highly concentrated form of energy. They account for nearly 95% of dietary fat. Structurally they are composed of the trihydroxy alcohol known as *glycerol*, to which are attached three fatty acids by ester

TABLE 6.3 Physiologic Characteristics of Eicosanoids

Eicosanoid Family	Precursor Arachidonate (20:4ω6)	Eicosapentaenoate (20:5ω3)	Site of Synthesis	Mode of Action
Prostacyclins	PGI$_2$	PGI$_3$	Vascular endothelium	Vasodilator Platelet antiaggregator
Thromboxanes	TXA$_2$	TXA$_3$	Platelet	Vasoconstrictor Platelet aggregator
Leukotrienes	LTB$_4$	LTB$_5$	Leukocytes	Chemotaxis

Source: Anderson PA, Sprecher HW. Omega-3 fatty acids in nutrition and health. Dietetic currents. Vol 14, No. 2, 1987. Reprinted with permission of Ross Laboratories, Columbus, OH 43216.

(6B)

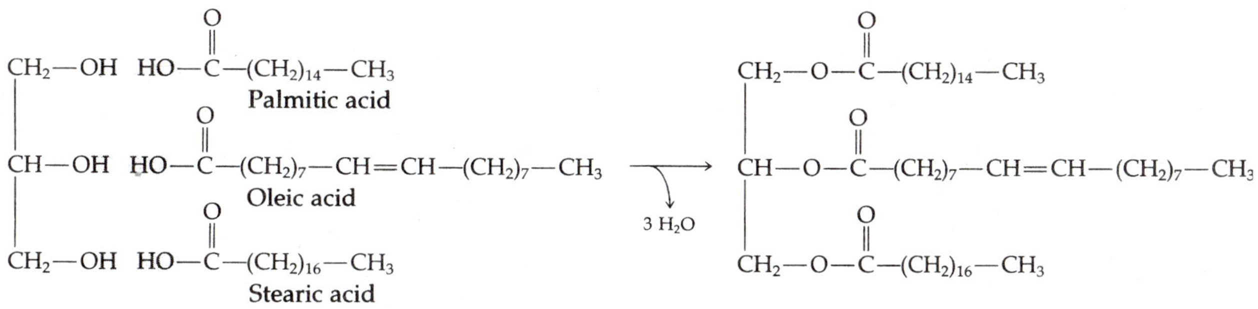

bonds. The fatty acids may all be the same (a simple triacylglycerol) or different (a mixed triacylglycerol). The linking of the fatty acids palmitate, oleate, and stearate to glycerol with the liberation of three water molecules is shown in 6B.

Acylglycerols composed of glycerol esterified to a single fatty acid (a monoacylglycerol) or to two fatty acids (a diacylglycerol) occur in negligible amounts in tissues; however, they are important intermediates in some metabolic reactions and may be components of other lipid classes. They may also occur in processed foods, to which they can be added as emulsifying agents.

The specific glycerol hydroxyl group to which a certain fatty acid is attached is indicated by a numbering system for the three glycerol carbons. This is complicated somewhat by the fact that the central carbon of the glycerol is asymmetric when different fatty acids are esterified at the two end carbon atoms, and may therefore exist in either the D or L form (p. 72). Unfortunately, the same monoacylglycerol may therefore be written in two ways (see 6C). To resolve this ambiguity, a system of nomenclature called *stereospecific numbering (sn)* has been adopted whereby the glycerol is always written as in 6D, with the C-2 hydroxyl group oriented to the left (L) and the carbons, numbered 1 through 3, beginning at the top. Accordingly, 1-monopalmitoyl glycerol (6E) can be drawn in either of the ways shown in 6C. Using this system,

therefore, the naming of the triacylglycerol shown as structure 6B is 1-stearoyl-2-oleoyl-3palmitoyl-L-glycerol.

Triacylglycerols exist as fats or oils at room temperature according to their physical state, which varies according to the structures of the component fatty acids. Those containing a high proportion of relatively short-chain fatty acids or unsaturated fatty acids tend to be liquid (oils) at room temperature. Saturated fatty acids of longer chain length have a higher melting point and exist as solids at ambient temperatures. When used for energy, fatty acids are released in free form (free fatty acids, FFA) from the triacylglycerols in adipose tissue cells by the activity of lipases, and are transported by albumin to various tissues for oxidation.

Sterols and Steroids

This class of lipid is characterized by a four-ring core structure called the *cyclopentanoperhydrophenanthrene*, or *steroid, nucleus*. Sterols are monohydroxy alcohols of steroidal structure, the single commonest being cholesterol. Cholesterol is present only in animal tissues, and it can exist in free form or can be esterified with a fatty acid. Many other sterols are also found in plant tissues. The structure of cholesterol is shown in 6F, along with the numbering system for the carbons in the steroid nucleus.

Meats, egg yolk, and dairy products contain fairly large amounts of cholesterol, and the sterol is an essen-

(6C)

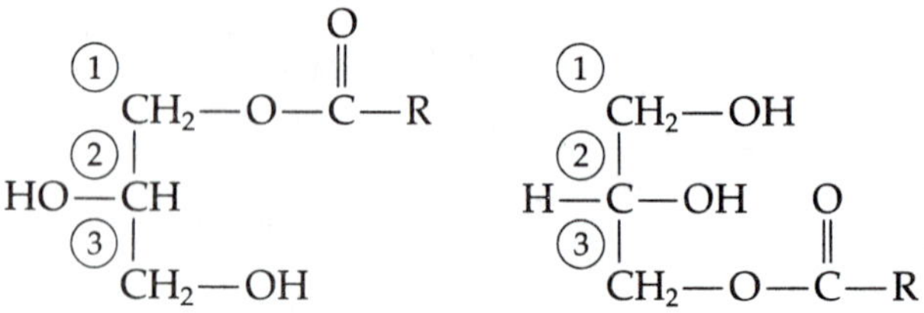

$$CH_2-O-\overset{\overset{\displaystyle O}{\|}}{C}-R$$
$$HO-CH$$
$$CH_2-OH$$

(1) $CH_2-O-\overset{\overset{\displaystyle O}{\|}}{C}-R$
(2) $HO-CH$
(3) CH_2-OH

(1) CH_2-OH
(2) $H-C-OH$
(3) $CH_2-O-\overset{\overset{\displaystyle O}{\|}}{C}-R$

(6D)

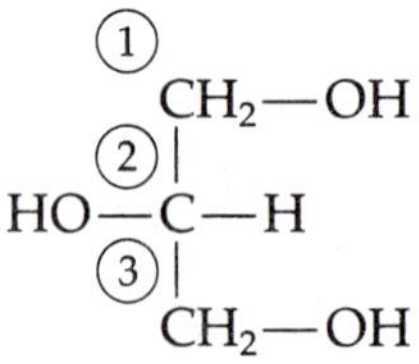

(1) CH_2-OH
(2) $HO-C-H$
(3) CH_2-OH

(6E)

$$CH_2-O-\overset{\overset{\displaystyle O}{\|}}{C}-(CH_2)_{14}-CH_3$$
$$HO-C-H$$
$$CH_2-OH$$

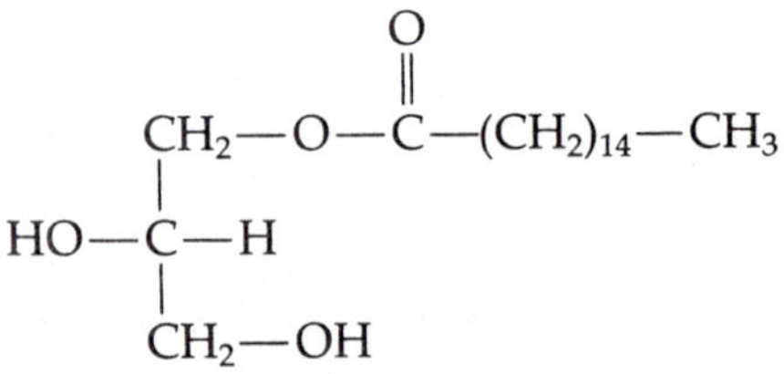

1-monopalmitoyl
glycerol

(6F)

Cholesterol

tial component of cell membranes (p. 6), particularly those comprising nerve tissue. Despite the bad press that cholesterol has garnered over the years because of its alleged implication in cardiovascular disease, it serves as the precursor for many other important steroids in the body. Included among these are the bile acids, steroidal sex hormones such as estrogens, androgens, and progesterone, the adrenocortical hormones, and the vitamin D of animal tissues (cholecalciferol). These steroids differ from one another in the arrangement of double bonds in the ring system, the presence of carbonyl or hydroxyl groups, and the nature of the side chain at C-17. Such structural modifications are all mediated by enzymes that function as dehydrogenases, isomerases, hydroxylases, or desmolases, the latter class removing side chains from the steroid nucleus. The derivation of the various types of steroids from cholesterol is diagrammed in Figure 6.2. Although many physiologically active corticosteroid hormones, sex hormones, and bile acids exist, only representative compounds are shown.

Sterols, together with phospholipids, which will be considered next, comprise only about 5% of dietary lipid.

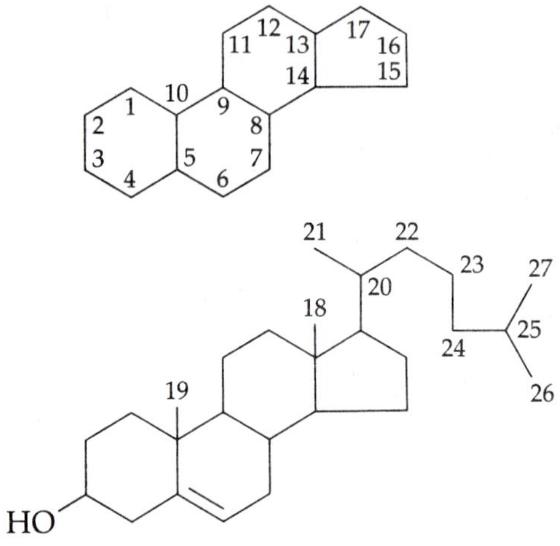

Phospholipids

As the name implies, lipids belonging to this class contain phosphate as a common component. They also possess one or more fatty acid residues. Phospholipids are categorized into one of two groups called *glycerophosphatides* and *sphingophosphatides*, depending on whether their core structure is glycerol or the amino alcohol sphingosine (6I) respectively.

Glycerophosphatides The building block of a glycerophosphatide is *phosphatidic acid*, formed by the esterification of two fatty acids at C-1 and C-2 of glycerol and the esterification of the C-3 hydroxyl with phosphoric acid. The structure in 6G typifies a phosphatidic acid, a term that does not define a specific structure, because different fatty acids may be involved. The convention of the numbering of the glycerol carbon atoms is the same as that for triacylglycerols. The numbering from top to bottom is *sn-1, sn-2, sn-3*, provided the glycerol is written in L-configuration so that the C-2 fatty acid constituent is directed to the left as shown in 6G.

Phosphatidic acids form a number of derivatives with compounds such as choline, ethanolamine, serine, and inositol, each of which possesses an alcohol group through which a second esterification to the phosphate takes place. The compounds are named as the phosphatidyl derivatives of the alcohols, as indicated in 6H. Phosphatidylcholine is probably better known by its common name, *lecithin*.

Glycerophosphatides are very important components of cell membranes. In addition to lending structural support to the membrane, they serve as a source of physiologically active compounds. We have already seen

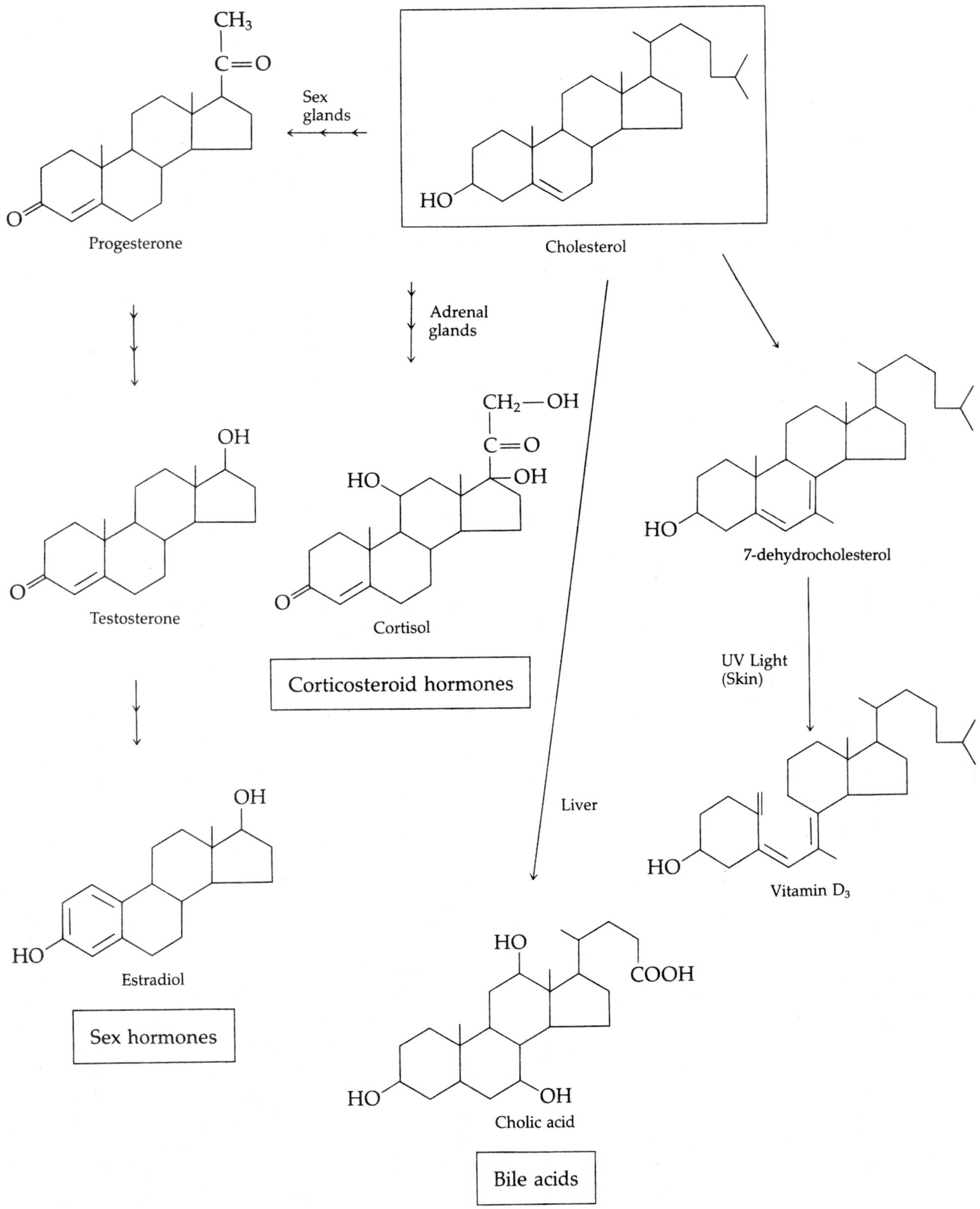

FIGURE 6.2 The formation of physiologically important steroids from cholesterol. Only representative compounds from each category of steroid are shown.

(6G)

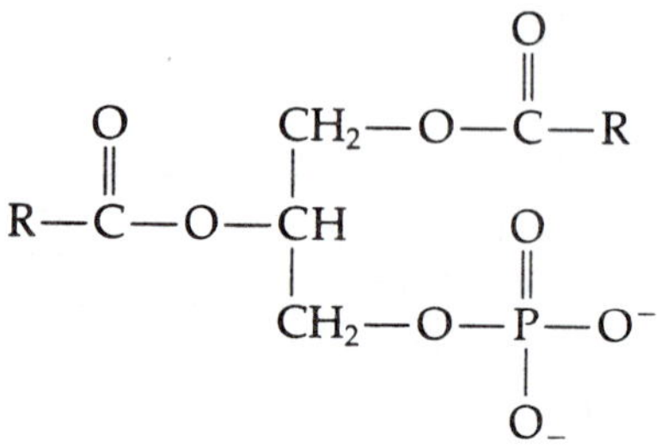

$$
\begin{array}{c}
\qquad\qquad \overset{\displaystyle O}{\overset{\|}{CH_2-O-C-R}} \\[4pt]
\overset{\displaystyle O}{\overset{\|}{R-C-O-CH}} \qquad \overset{\displaystyle O}{\underset{\displaystyle O_-}{\overset{\|}{CH_2-O-P-O^-}}}
\end{array}
$$

(6H)

$$
\begin{array}{c}
\qquad\qquad \overset{\displaystyle O}{\overset{\|}{CH_2-O-C-R}} \\[4pt]
\overset{\displaystyle O}{\overset{\|}{R-C-O-CH}} \qquad \overset{\displaystyle O}{\overset{\|}{CH_2-O-P-O^-}} - - - \\[4pt]
\qquad\qquad\qquad\qquad\quad O_-
\end{array}
$$

$- - - CH_2 - CH_2 - \overset{+}{N}(CH_3)_3$ Phosphatidyl choline

$- - - CH_2 - CH_2 - \overset{+}{N}H_3$ Phosphatidyl ethanolamine

$- - - CH_2 - \underset{\displaystyle COO^-}{CH} - \overset{+}{N}H_3$ Phosphatidyl serine

$- - -$ (inositol ring: HO OH / —OH / HO OH)   Phosphatidyl inositol

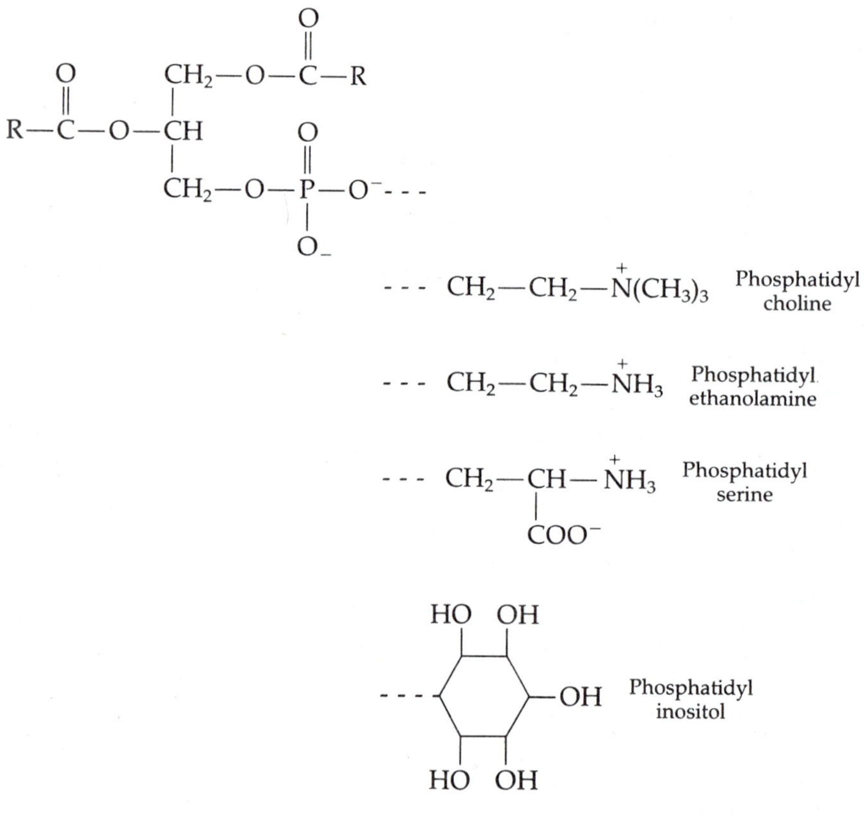

(p. 117) how arachidonate, released on demand from membrane-bound phosphatidylcholine and phosphatidylinositol, is needed for eicosanoid synthesis. Phosphatidylinositol participates in other cell functions as well. For example, it plays a specific role in the anchoring of membrane proteins, when the proteins are covalently attached to lipids. This has been demonstrated by the release of certain membrane proteins when cells are treated with a phosphatidylinositol-specific phospholipase C, which hydrolyzes the ester bond connecting the glycerol to the phosphate. Secondly, certain hydrolytic products of phosphatidylinositol are active in intracellu-

lar signaling and as second messengers in hormone stimulation. A brief discussion of this latter function follows.

Phosphatidylinositol in the plasma membrane can be doubly phosphorylated by ATP, forming phosphatidylinositol-4, 5-bisphosphate. Stimulation of the cell by certain hormones activates a specific phospholipase C, which produces inositol-1,4,5-trisphosphate and diacylglycerol from phosphatidylinositol-4,5-bisphosphate. Both these products function as second messengers in cell signaling [3]. Inositol-1,4,5-trisphosphate causes the release of Ca^{+2} held within membrane-bounded compartments of the cell, triggering the activation of a variety of

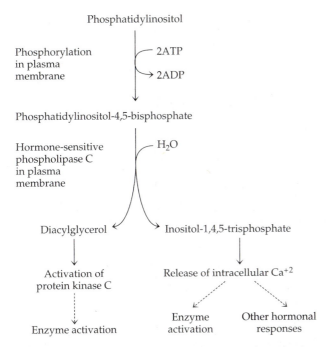

Phosphatidylinositol

Phosphorylation in plasma membrane — 2ATP → 2ADP

Phosphatidylinositol-4,5-bisphosphate

Hormone-sensitive phospholipase C in plasma membrane — H₂O

Diacylglycerol

Inositol-1,4,5-trisphosphate

Activation of protein kinase C

Release of intracellular Ca⁺²

Enzyme activation

Enzyme activation

Other hormonal responses

FIGURE 6.3 Phosphatidylinositol-4,5-bisphosphate, formed in the plasma membrane by phosphorylation of phosphatidylinositol, is hydrolyzed by a specific phospholipase C in response to hormonal signals. Both products of hydrolysis act as intracellular messengers.

Ca^{+2}-dependent enzymes and hormonal responses. Diacylglycerol binds to and activates an enzyme, protein kinase C, which transfers phosphate groups to several cytoplasmic proteins, thereby altering their enzymatic activities. This dual signal hypothesis of phosphatidylinositol hydrolysis is represented in Figure 6.3.

Sphingophosphatides Lipids formed from sphingosine (6I) are categorized into three subclasses: sphingomyelins, cerebrosides, and gangliosides. Of these, only the sphingomyelins are sphingophosphatides, and are described further in this section. The other two subclasses of sphingolipids contain no phosphate, but instead possess a carbohydrate moiety. They are referred to as *glycolipids*, and are discussed in the following section.

Sphingomyelins occur in plasma membranes of animal cells, and are found in particularly large amounts in the myelin sheath of nerve tissues. Their name connotes both their anatomic occurrence and the fact that they are formed from the amino alcohol *sphingosine*, which can be synthesized from palmitic acid and serine (see 6I). The sphingomyelins contain a fatty acid residue attached in amide linkage to the amino group of the sphingosine. The product of this union is called *ceramide*, which in turn is esterified to phosphorylcholine (see 6J).

Phospholipids are more polar than the triacylglycerols and sterols, and therefore tend to attract water molecules, which are also polar. Because of this hydrophilic property, they are commonly expressed on the surface of blood-borne lipid particles, such as chylomicrons (p. 125), thereby stabilizing the particles in the aqueous medium. Furthermore, as a constituent of cell and organelle membranes (p. 4), they serve as a regulator of the passage of water-soluble and fat-soluble materials across the membrane.

Glycolipids

Glycolipids can be subclassified into *cerebrosides* and *gangliosides*. They are so named because they have a carbohydrate component within their structure. Like the phospholipids, their physiologic role is principally structural, contributing little as an energy source. They occur in the medullary sheaths of nerves and in brain tissue, particularly the white matter. As in the case of sphingomyelin, the sphingosine moiety provides the backbone for glycolipid structure. It is attached to a fatty acid by an amide-bond–forming ceramide, as discussed previously. The glycolipids do not contain phosphate.

A cerebroside is characterized by the linking of ceramide to a monosaccharide unit such as glucose or galactose, producing either a glucocerebroside or galactocerebroside.

Gangliosides resemble cerebrosides except that the single monosaccharide unit of the cerebroside is replaced by an oligosaccharide containing various monosaccharide derivatives such as N-acetyl neuraminic acid and N-acetyl galactosamine. Gangliosides are known to be involved in certain recognition events occurring at the cell surface. For example, they provide the carbohydrate determinants of the human blood groups A, B, and O.

DIGESTION

Because fats are insoluble in water, their digestion poses a special problem because the enzymes involved in their digestion require an aqueous environment. However, the surface area of dietary lipid, targeted for digestion, is greatly enhanced by a very efficient emulsification process mediated mainly by the bile salts. Consequently, accessibility of the fat to digestive enzymes is greatly increased by bile salt action.

Triacylglycerols, phospholipids (primarily phosphatidylcholine), and sterols (mainly cholesterol) provide the lipid component of the typical Western diet. Of

(6I)

$$CH_3-(CH_2)_{12}-CH=CH-\overset{\overset{OH}{|}}{CH}-\overset{\overset{}{|}}{\underset{NH_2}{CH}}-CH_2-OH$$

Sphingosine

(6J)

$$CH_3-(CH_2)_{12}-CH=CH-\overset{\overset{OH}{|}}{CH}-\overset{\overset{}{|}}{\underset{\overset{|}{\underset{NH-\overset{\overset{O}{\|}}{C}-R}{}}}{CH}}-CH_2-O-\overset{\overset{O}{\|}}{\underset{\overset{|}{O_-}}{P}}-O-CH_2-CH_2-\overset{+}{N}-(CH_3)_3$$

Sphingomyelin

(R=Fatty acid)

these, triacylglycerols, customarily called *fats*, are by far the major contributor, with a consumption rate of about 150 g daily on the average. Digestive enzymes involved in the breakdown of dietary lipids in the gastrointestinal tract are esterases that cleave the ester bonds within triacylglycerols (lipase), phospholipids (phospholipases), and cholesterol esters (cholesterol esterase).

Most dietary triacylglycerol digestion is completed in the lumen of the small intestine, although the process actually begins in the stomach. Digestive activity at these two sites is attributed to two different forms of lipases: (1) lingual lipase, secreted by serous glands lying beneath the tongue, and (2) pancreatic lipase. Basal secretion of lingual lipase apparently occurs continuously, but can be stimulated by neural (sympathetic agonists), dietary (high fat), and mechanical (sucking and swallowing) factors. Lingual lipase accounts for the limited digestion of fat in the stomach, made possible by the enzyme's particularly high stability at the low pH of the gastric juices. It can readily penetrate milk fat globules without substrate stabilization by bile salts, a feature that makes it particularly important for fat digestion in the suckling infant, whose pancreatic function may not be fully developed. Lingual lipases act preferentially on triacylglycerols containing medium- and short-chain length fatty acids. It preferentially hydrolyzes fatty acids at the *sn*-3 position, releasing fatty acids and 1,2-diacylglycerol as products. This specificity is again advantageous for the suckling infant because in milk triacylglycerols, short- and medium-length fatty acids are usually esterified at the *sn*-3 position.

In order for dietary fat in the stomach to be hydrolyzed by lingual lipase, some degree of emulsification must occur to expose sufficient surface area of the substrate. Muscle contractions of the stomach, and the squirting of the fat through a partially opened pyloric sphincter, produce shear forces sufficient for emulsification. Also, potential emulsifiers in the acid milieu of the stomach include complex polysaccharides, phospholipids, and peptic digests of dietary proteins. However, quantitative hydrolysis and absorption, especially of the long-chain fatty acids, require less acidity, appropriate lipases, more effective emulsifying agents (bile salts), and specialized absorptive cells. These conditions are provided in the lumen of the upper small intestine.

The presence of undigested lipid in the stomach delays the rate of emptying of the stomach contents, presumably by way of the hormone enterogastrone—GIP and secretin (p. 33)—which inhibits gastric motility. Fats therefore have a "high satiety value."

The partially hydrolyzed lipid emulsion leaves the stomach and enters the duodenum as fine lipid droplets. Effective emulsification takes place because as mechanical shearing continues, it is complemented by bile, released from the gallbladder as a result of stimulation by the hormone cholecystokinin (CCK). Bicarbonate is simultaneously released from the pancreas, elevating the pH to a level suitable for pancreatic lipase activity. In combination with triacylglycerol breakdown products, bile salts are excellent emulsifying agents, their effectiveness being due to their *amphipathic* properties, that is, their possessing both hydrophilic and hydrophobic "ends." Such molecules tend to arrange themselves on the surface of small fat particles with their hydrophobic ends turned inward and hydrophilic regions outward toward the water phase. This chemical action, together with the help of peristaltic agitation, converts the fat into small droplets with a greatly increased surface area. These particles can then be readily acted on by pancreatic lipase.

Pancreatic lipase activation is complex, requiring the participation of the protein colipase, calcium ions, and bile salts. Colipase is formed by the hydrolytic activation by trypsin of procolipase, also of pancreatic origin. It contains approximately 100 amino acid residues and possesses distinctly hydrophobic regions that are believed to act as lipid-binding sites [4]. Colipase has been shown to associate strongly with pancreatic lipase and therefore may act as an anchor, or linking point, for attachment of the enzyme to the bile salt-stabilized micelles [5] described later.

The action of pancreatic lipase on ingested triacylglycerols results in a complex mixture of diacylglycerols, monoacylglycerols, and free fatty acids. Its specificity is primarily toward *sn*-1-linked fatty acids and secondarily to *sn*-3 bonds. Therefore, the main path of this digestion progresses from triacylglycerols to 2,3-diacylglycerols to 2-monoacylglycerols. Only a small percentage of the triacylglycerols is hydrolyzed totally to free glycerol. That which does occur probably follows the isomerization of the 2-monoacylglycerol to the 1-monoacylglycerol, which is then hydrolyzed. Esterified cholesterol, meanwhile, undergoes hydrolysis to free cholesterol and a fatty acid, catalyzed by the enzyme cholesterol esterase. The C-2 fatty acid of lecithin is hydrolytically removed by a specific esterase called phospholipase A$_2$, producing lysolecithin and still another free fatty acid.

The products of the partial digestion of lipids, chiefly 2-monoacylglycerols, lysolecithin, cholesterol, and fatty acids, combine with bile salts, forming negatively charged polymolecular aggregates called *micelles*. These have a much smaller diameter (approximately 5 nm) than the unhydrolyzed precursor particles, allowing them access to the intramicrovillus spaces (50 to 100 nm) of the intestinal membrane.

ABSORPTION

Stabilized by the polar bile salts, the micellar particles are sufficiently water soluble to penetrate what is called the *unstirred water layer* bathing the absorptive cells of the small intestine. The absorptive cells are called *intestinal mucosal cells*, or *enterocytes* (p. 30). Micelles interact at the brush border of these cells, whereupon the lipid contents of the micelles diffuse out of the micelles and into the enterocytes, moving down a concentration gradient. Although this process occurs in the distal duo-

denum and the jejunum, the bile salts are not absorbed at this point, but instead are absorbed in the ileal segment of the small intestine. There they are returned to the liver via the portal vein to be resecreted in the bile. This circuit is referred to as the "enterohepatic circulation of the bile salts" (p. 42).

After the absorption of free fatty acids, 2-monoacylglycerols, cholesterol, and lysophosphatidylcholine into the enterocytes, intracellular resynthesis of triacylglycerols, phosphatidylcholine, and cholesterol esters takes place. The process is, however, a function of the chain length of the fatty acids involved. Fatty acids having more than 10 to 12 carbon atoms are first activated by being coupled to coenzyme A by the enzyme acyl CoA synthetase. They are then re-esterified into triacylglycerols, phosphatidylcholine, and cholesterol esters as mentioned earlier. Short-chain fatty acids, those containing fewer than 10 to 12 carbon atoms, in contrast, pass from the cell directly into the portal blood. In the blood, short-chain fatty acids attach to albumin for transport to other tissues for processing. The different fate of the long- and short-chain fatty acids is due to the specificity of the acyl CoA synthetase enzyme for long-chain fatty acids only.

Lipids resynthesized in the enterocytes, together with fat-soluble vitamins, are collected in the cell's endoplasmic reticulum as large fat particles. While still in the endoplasmic reticulum, the particles receive a layer of protein on their surface, which tends to stabilize the particles in the aqueous environment of the circulation, which they eventually enter. The particles are pinched off as lipid vesicles that then fuse with the Golgi apparatus (p. 12). There, carbohydrate is attached to the protein coat, and the completed particles, called *chylomicrons*, are transported to the cell membrane and exocytosed into the lymphatic circulation. Chylomicrons therefore belong to a family of compounds called *lipoproteins*, acquiring their name from the fact that lipid and protein comprise their composition. A review of the lipoproteins is offered in the next section.

The protein portion only, of any lipoprotein, is called the *apolipoprotein*. Apolipoproteins play a very important role in the structural and functional relationship among the lipoproteins, and are discussed in the next section. Key features of intestinal absorption of lipid digestion products are depicted in Figure 6.4.

It should be pointed out that triacylglycerols can also be synthesized from α-glycerophosphate in the enterocytes. This metabolite can be formed either from the phosphorylation of free glycerol or from reduction of dihydroxyacetone phosphate, an intermediate in the pathway of glycolysis (see Figs. 4.7 and 6.12). Tri-

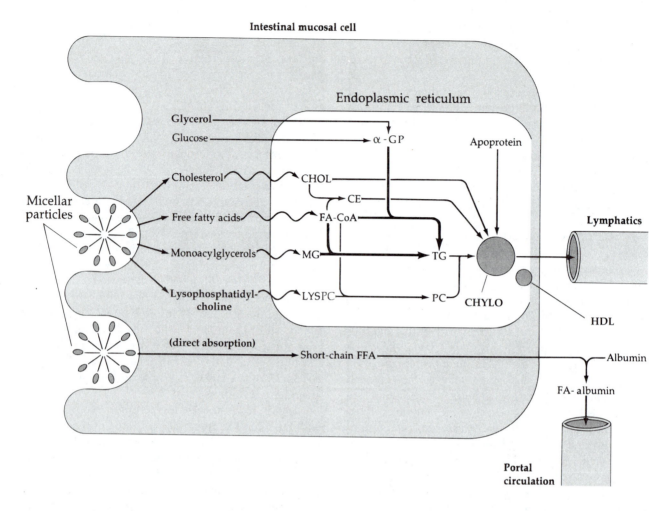

FIGURE 6.4 The uptake of micellar lipid particles by the intestinal mucosal cell, and the reassembly of the lipid components within the endoplasmic reticulum (shown as white area) of the cell. The reassembly of the lipids produces principally chylomicrons, although small amounts of HDL can be formed in this manner. Following their combination with apoproteins, the lipoprotein particles are released into the lymphatic circulation and ultimately the portal blood. Short-chain free fatty acids enter the portal circulation directly, as shown. Abbreviations: CHOL, cholesterol; CE, cholesteryl ester; FA-CoA, CoA activated fatty acids; MG, monoacylglycerol; LYSPC, lysophosphatidyl choline; α-GP, alpha glycerophosphate; CHYLO, chylomicrons; TG, triacylglycerol; PC, phosphatidyl choline.

acylglycerol synthesis by this route is also shown in Figure 6.4.

TRANSPORT

Lipoproteins

Chylomicrons are the primary form of lipoprotein formed from exogenous (dietary) lipids. Lipoproteins other than chylomicrons transport endogenous lipids, which are circulating lipids that do not arise directly from intestinal absorption, but are instead processed through other tissues such as the liver. Several types of

lipoproteins therefore exist, differing in their chemical composition, physical properties, and metabolic function. The role shared by all the lipoproteins, however, is the transport of lipids from tissue to tissue to supply the lipid needs of different cells. The arrangement of the lipid and protein components of a typical lipoprotein particle is represented in Figure 6.5. You can see from the figure that the more hydrophobic lipids are located in the core of the particle, while the relatively more polar proteins and phospholipids are situated on the surface to enhance aqueous stability.

Lipoproteins differ according to the ratio of lipid to protein within the particle as well as having different

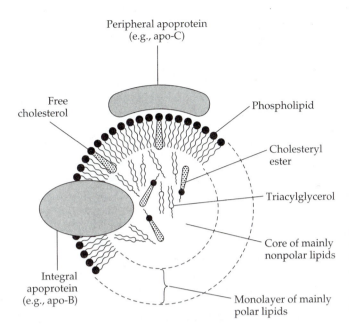

Peripheral apoprotein
(e.g., apo-C)

Free
cholesterol

Phospholipid

Cholesteryl
ester

Triacylglycerol

Core of mainly
nonpolar lipids

Integral
apoprotein
(e.g., apo-B)

Monolayer of mainly
polar lipids

FIGURE 6.5 Generalized structure of a plasma lipoprotein. Note the similarities with the structure of the plasma membrane. A small amount of cholesteryl ester and triacylglycerol are found in the surface layer and a little free cholesterol in the core.

proportions of lipid types: triacylglycerols, cholesterol and cholesterol esters, and phospholipids. Such compositional differences influence the *density* of the particle, and this has become the physical characteristic that is used to differentiate and classify the various lipoproteins. In the order of lowest to highest density, the lipoprotein fractions are chylomicrons, very-low-density lipoproteins (VLDL), low-density lipoproteins (LDL), and high-density lipoproteins (HDL). There is also an intermediate-density particle (IDL), having a density between that of VLDL and LDL. The IDL particles are very short-lived in the bloodstream, however, and have little nutritional or physiological importance. Table 6.4 summarizes several physical and chemical characteristics of the lipoproteins.

Apolipoproteins

In addition to their function of stabilizing the lipoproteins as they circulate in the aqueous environment of the blood, apolipoproteins, the protein components of lipoproteins, have other important functions as well. They confer specificity on the lipoprotein complexes, allowing them to be recognized by specific receptors on cell surfaces. They also stimulate certain enzymatic reactions, which in turn regulate the lipoproteins' metabolic functions.

A series of letters (A to E), with subclasses of each, are now used to identify the various apolipoproteins. For convenience, they are usually abbreviated "apo" followed by the identifying letter; that is, apoA-I, apoB-100, apoC-II, and so on. A partial listing of the

apolipoproteins, together with their molecular weight, the lipoprotein with which they are associated and their postulated physiological function are found in Table 6.5.

Distribution of Lipids

The resynthesized lipid derived from exogenous sources leaves the enterocytes (intestinal mucosal cells) largely in the form of chylomicrons, which then undergo intravascular conversion to chylomicron remnants (structurally similar to VLDL). To some extent, HDL can be synthesized within the enterocytes, and released directly into the mesenteric lymph [6]. The lipoproteins first appear in the lymphatic vessels of the abdominal region and then enter the bloodstream at a slow rate so as to prevent large-scale changes in the lipid content of peripheral blood. Entry of chylomicrons into the blood from the lymph continues for up to 14 hours after consumption of a meal rich in fat. The peak level of lipid in blood plasma usually occurs after one-half to three hours after a meal, and returns to normal within five to six hours.

Chylomicrons and VLDL, which is formed endogenously in the liver, are transported by the blood throughout all tissues in the body while undergoing intravascular hydrolysis at certain tissue sites. This hydrolysis occurs through the action of the enzyme *lipoprotein lipase*, associated with the endothelial cell surface of the small blood vessels and capillaries within adipose and muscle tissue. Its extracellular action on the circulating particles releases free fatty acids and diacylglycerols, which are quickly absorbed by the tissue cells.

TABLE 6.4 Physical and Chemical Properties of Plasma Lipoproteins in Humans

Feature	Chylomicrons	VLDL	IDL	LDL	HDL
Density (g/mL)	< 1.006	< 1.006	1.006–1.019	1.019–1.063	1.063–1.21
Diameter (nm)	80–500	40–80	24.5	20	7.5–12
Lipids (% by weight)	98	92	85	79	50
Cholesterol	9	22	35	47	19
Triglyceride	82	52	20	9	3
Phospholipid	7	18	20	23	28
Apoproteins (% by weight)	2	8	15	21	50
Major	A-I, A-II			A-I A-II	
	B		B	B	B
	C-I, C-II, C-III	C-I, C-II, C-III			
	E	E	E		
Minor		A-I, A-II		C-I, C-II, C-III	C-I, C-II, C-III
					D
					E

Source: Reproduced by permission of Naito, HK. Disorders of lipid metabolism. In Kaplan LA, Pesce AJ. Clinical chemistry. St Louis, 1984, The C.V. Mosby Co.

TABLE 6.5 Apolipoproteins of Human Plasma Lipoproteins

Apolipoprotein	Lipoprotein	Molecular Mass (Da)	Additional Remarks
A-I	HDL, chylomicrons	28,000	Activator of lecithin: cholesterol acyltransferase (LCAT). Ligand for HDL receptor.
A-II	HDL, chylomicrons	17,000	Structure is 2 identical monomers joined by a disulfide bridge. Inhibitor of LCAT?
A-IV	Secreted with chylomicrons but transfers to HDL	46,000	Associated with the formation of triacylglycerol-rich lipoproteins. Function unknown.
B-100	LDL, VLDL, IDL	550,000	Synthesized in liver. Ligand for LDL receptor.
B-48	Chylomicrons, chylomicron remnants	260,000	Synthesized in intestine.
C-I	VLDL, HDL, chylomicrons	7600	Possible activator of LCAT.
C-II	VLDL, HDL, chylomicrons	8916	Activator of extrahepatic lipoprotein lipase.
C-III	VLDL, HDL, chylomicrons	8750	Several polymorphic forms depending on content of sialic acids.
D	Subfraction of HDL	20,000	Function unknown.
E	VLDL, HDL, chylomicrons, chylomicron remnants	34,000	Present in excess in the β-VLDL of patients with type III hyperlipoproteinemia. The sole apoprotein found in HDL$_c$ of diet-induced hypercholesterolemic animals. Ligand for chylomicron remnant receptor in liver and LDL receptor.

Within the muscle cells, the free fatty acids and those derived from the hydrolysis of the absorbed diacylglycerols are primarily oxidized for energy, with only limited use for the resynthesis and storage of triacylglycerols. In adipose tissue, in contrast, the absorbed fatty acids are largely used for the synthesis of triacylglycerols, in keeping with that tissue's storage role. In this manner, chylomicrons and VLDL are cleared rapidly from the plasma in a matter of minutes and a few hours, respectively, from the time they enter the bloodstream. It is the large, triacylglycerol-laden chylomicrons that account for the turbidity of *postprandial* (following a meal) plasma. Because lipoprotein lipase is the enzyme that solubilizes these particles by its lipolytic action, it is sometimes referred to as "clearing factor." That which is left of the chylomicron following this lipolytic action is called a *chylomicron remnant*—a smaller particle relatively less rich in triacylglycerol, but richer in cholesterol. These are removed from the bloodstream by the liver cells by endocytosis following interaction of the remnant particles with specific receptors for apolipoprotein E or B/E on the cells [7]. Nascent VLDL of liver origin also undergoes triacylglycerol stripping by lipoprotein lipase at extracellular sites, resulting in the formation of a transient, intermediate-density lipoprotein (IDL) particle, and finally a cholesterol-rich, low-density lipoprotein (LDL). This is another example of the regulatory function of an apolipoprotein. From Table 6.5 you can see that apoC-

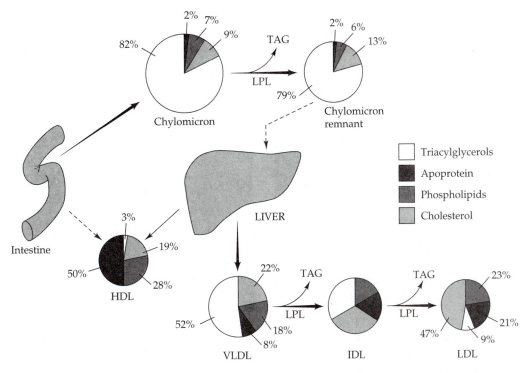

FIGURE 6.6 Conversion pathways of lipoproteins formed from exogenous sources (intestinal absorption) and from endogenous formation (synthesis in liver). Although small amounts of HDL are synthesized within the enterocytes of the small intestine, its major site of synthesis is the liver. Relative particle size of the lipoproteins is shown along with their approximate composition. TAG = triacylglycerols, LPL = lipoprotein lipase.

II, an activator of lipoprotein lipase, is a component of both chylomicrons and VLDL. This accounts for the susceptibility of these particles to lipoprotein lipase action. Figure 6.6 summarizes the formation of, and interconversions among the lipoproteins, along with their lipid–protein composition.

Role of the Liver and Adipose Tissue in Lipid Metabolism

Liver The liver plays a very important role in the body's use of lipids and lipoproteins. Hepatic synthesis of the bile salts, indispensable for digesting and absorbing dietary lipids, is one of its functions. In addition, the liver is the key player in lipid transport, because it is the site of synthesis of lipoproteins formed from endogenous lipids. It is capable of *de novo* synthesis of lipids from nonlipid precursors such as glucose and amino acids. It can also take up and catabolize exogenous lipids delivered to it in the form of chylomicron remnants, repackaging their lipids into HDL and VLDL forms. Nutrient metabolism in the liver is summarized in Figure 6.7. Also shown in Figure 6.7 is a glimpse of the re-

actions by which glucose and amino acids can be converted into lipid. They are included as a reminder to the reader that pathways of lipid, carbohydrate, and protein metabolism are integrated, and cannot stand alone.

In the postprandial state, glucose, amino acids, and short-chain fatty acid concentrations rise in portal blood. In the hepatocyte, glucose is phosphorylated for use, and glycogen is subsequently synthesized until the hepatic stores are repleted. If portal hyperglycemia persists, glucose is converted to fatty acids via acetyl CoA and also to triose phosphates from which the glycerol portion of triglycerides are derived. Amino acids can also serve as precursors for lipid synthesis because they can be metabolically converted to acetyl CoA and pyruvate. The synthesis of fatty acids, triacylglycerols, and glycerophosphatides is described in detail later in this chapter.

In addition to the newly synthesized lipid derived from nonfatty precursors, there is also the exogenous lipid delivered to the liver in the form of chylomicron remnants as well as short-chain fatty acids. The mechanism for the hepatic uptake and hydrolysis of chylomicron remnants is not entirely clear, although these

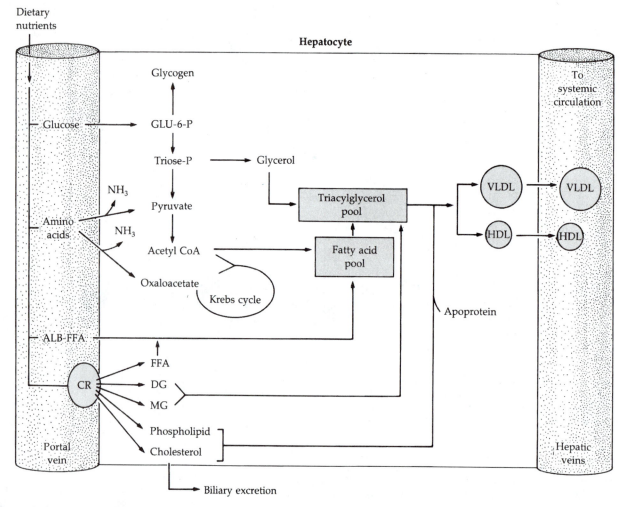

FIGURE 6.7 Fat metabolism in the liver following a meal, showing its relationship to carbohydrate and amino acid metabolism. Abbreviations: ALB-FFA, albumin-bound free fatty acids; CR, chylomicron remnants; DG, diacylglycerols; MG, monoacylglycerols.

particles are believed to first interact, via the apolipoprotein E on their surface, with specific receptors for apoE in the vascular endothelial cells of the organ. The lipid portion of the chylomicron remnant is hydrolyzed in the hepatocyte to free fatty acids, monoacylglycerols and diacylglycerols, glycerol, and cholesterol; but resynthesis of these compounds promptly occurs once again in a manner analogous to the events in the intestinal mucosal cell. Alternatively, the free fatty acids can undergo oxidation for energy (p. 135).

Exogenous free fatty acids of short chain length delivered directly to the hepatic tissue can be used for energy or, following chain elongation, for resynthesis of other lipid fractions. Chylomicron remnant cholesterol and cholesteryl esters may be (1) converted to bile salts and secreted in the bile, (2) secreted into the bile as neu-

tral sterol, or (3) incorporated into VLDL or HDL, and released into the plasma.

Newly synthesized triacylglycerol is combined with phospholipid, cholesterol, and proteins to form VLDL and HDL, which are released into the circulation. The HDL, small and triacylglycerol-poor, relative to the VLDL, possesses phospholipids and cholesterol as its major lipid constituents. Since triacylglycerols can be formed from glucose, hepatic triacylglycerol production is accelerated when the diet is rich in carbohydrate. This results in VLDL overproduction and may account for the occasional transient hypertriacylglycerolemia in normal people when they consume diets rich in simple sugars.

Adipose Tissue Adipose tissue shares with the liver an extremely important role in fat metabolism.

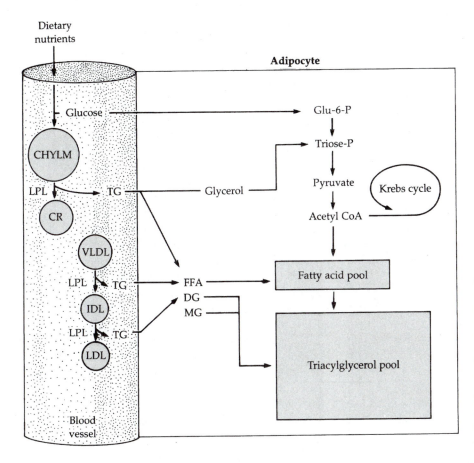

FIGURE 6.8 Fat metabolism in the adipose cell following a meal. The pathways favor the storage of energy as triacylglycerol. Insulin stimulates lipogenesis by promoting the entry of glucose into the cell and by inhibiting the lipase, which hydrolyzes the stored triacylglycerol to free fatty acids and glycerol. Abbreviations: CHYLM, chylomicrons; TG, triacylglycerol; CR, chylomicron remnant; LPL, lipoprotein lipase; FFA, free fatty acids; DG, diacylglycerol; MG, monoacylglycerol.

Unlike the liver, it is not involved in the uptake of chylomicron remnants or the synthesis of endogenous lipoproteins. Adipocytes are instead the major storage site for triacylglycerol, which is in a continuous state of turnover in the cells: lipolysis (hydrolysis), countered by re-esterification. These two processes are not the forward and reverse directions of the same reactions, but are different pathways, involving different enzymes and substrates. Each of the processes are regulated separately by nutritional, metabolic, and hormonal factors, the net effect of which determines the level of circulating fatty acids and the extent of adiposity. Over 85% by volume of the adipose cell consists of a single large globule of fat.

In the fed state, metabolic pathways in adipocytes favor triacylglycerol synthesis. As in the liver, adipocyte triacylglycerol can be synthesized from glucose, a process strongly influenced by *insulin*. The hormone accelerates both the entry of glucose into the adipose cells (the liver does not respond to this action of the hormone) and the availability and uptake of fatty acids through lipoprotein lipase stimulation. Cellular glucose, via its glycolytic breakdown, provides a source of glycerophosphate for re-esterification with the fatty acids to form triacylglycerols. Absorbed monoacylglycerols and diacylglycerols also furnish the glycerol building block for this resynthesis. The lipogenic influence of insulin is further manifested in its inhibitory effect on the intracellular (hormone sensitive) lipase (different from intravascular lipoprotein lipase) that hydrolyzes the stored triacylglycerols. Postprandial fat metabolism is summarized in Figure 6.8. To this point, the discussion has dealt with the role of the liver and adipose tissue in the fed state. In the *fasting* state, shifts in the metabolic scheme occur in these tissues. For example, as blood glucose levels diminish, insulin concentration falls, also causing a shift toward enhanced lipolytic activity in adipose tissue. Free fatty acids derived from adipose tissue circulate in the plasma in association with albumin, and are taken up by the liver and oxidized for energy by way of acetyl CoA formation. In the liver, some of the acetyl CoA is diverted to the production of the ketone bodies (p. 137), which can serve as important energy sources for muscle tissue during fasting. The liver continues the synthesis of VLDL and HDL and releases them into circulation, although these processes are diminished in a fasting situation. Glucose derived from liver glycogen, and free fatty acids transported to the liver from adipose tissue become the major precursors for the synthesis of endogenous VLDL triacylglycerol. As described previously, this lipoprotein then undergoes catabolism to IDL, transiently, and to LDL by lipoprotein lipase activity. Most of the plasma HDL is endogenous and is comprised mostly of phospholipid and cholesterol along with apoproteins, chiefly of the A series.

Metabolism of Lipoproteins

Chylomicrons and chylomicron remnants are normally not present in the blood serum during the fasting state, and the concentration of VLDL is relatively quite low compared to postprandial serum because of VLDL's rapid conversion to IDL and LDL. Therefore, the major lipoproteins in fasting serum are LDL (derived from VLDL), HDL (synthesized mainly in the liver), and a very small amount of VLDL. As discussed earlier, and summarized in Table 6.5, the apolipoproteins may regulate metabolic reactions within the lipoprotein particles, and determine to a great extent how the particles interact with each other and with receptors on specific cells.

The LDL fraction is the major carrier of cholesterol, binding about 60% of the total serum cholesterol. Its function is to transport the sterol to tissues, where it may be used for membrane construction or for conversion into other metabolites such as the steroid hormones. LDL interacts with LDL receptors on cells via its apoB, specifically apoB-100, protein, an event that culminates in the removal of the lipoprotein from the circulation. LDL receptors are located on liver cells as well as on cells of tissues peripheral to the liver, but the liver does not effectively remove the LDL from circulation. The distribution of LDL among tissues may depend on its rate of transcapillary transport as well as on the activity of the LDL receptors on cell surfaces. Once bound to the receptor, the receptor and the LDL particle, complete with its lipid cargo, are internalized together by the cell. In the cell, component parts are then degraded by lysosomal enzymes (see "Perspective" section in this chapter).

The LDL fraction can therefore be thought of as a depositor of cholesterol and other lipids into peripheral cells, including the cells of the vascular endothelium. It follows that a high concentration and activity of LDL have implications in the etiology of cardiovascular disease.

Opposing the LDL's cholesterol-depositing role is the HDL fraction. A significant function of HDL is to remove unesterified cholesterol from cells and other lipoproteins, where it may have accumulated, and return it to the liver for excretion in the bile. Two key properties of HDL are necessary for this process to occur. The first key property is its ability to bind to receptors on both hepatic and extrahepatic cells. Receptors may be specific for HDL, but they also include the LDL receptor to which HDL can bind via its apoE component. In other words, the LDL receptor recognizes both apoE and apoB-100, and is consequently referred to as the *apoB,E receptor*. The implication is that HDL can compete with LDL at its receptor site. The second key property of HDL is mediated through its apo A-1 component, which stimulates the activity of the enzyme lecithin: cholesterol acyltransferase (LCAT). This enzyme forms cholesteryl esters from free cholesterol by catalyzing the transfer of fatty acids from the C-2 position of phosphatidylcholine to free cholesterol. The free cholesterol (recipient) substrate is derived from the plasma membrane of cells, or surfaces of other lipoproteins. Cholesteryl esters resulting from this reaction can then exchange readily among plasma lipoproteins, mediated by a transfer protein called *cholesteryl ester transfer protein*, or CETP. LCAT, therefore, by taking up free cholesterol and producing its ester form, promotes the net transfer of cholesterol out of nonhepatic cells and other lipoproteins. Cholesteryl esters can then be transported directly to the liver in association with HDL or indirectly by LDL, following CETP transfer from HDL to LDL. It will be recalled that either lipoprotein can bind to LDL (apoB,E) receptors. Following their deposition in the liver cells, the esters are hydrolyzed by cholesteryl esterase, and the free cholesterol is excreted in the bile as bile salt (Fig. 6.2). This is the major route of cholesterol excretion from the body.

The net effect of these properties of HDL is the retrieving of cholesterol from peripheral cells and other lipoproteins, and returning it, as its ester, to the liver. The process is referred to as *reverse cholesterol transport*. Its benefit to the cardiovascular system is that by reducing the amount of deposited cholesterol in the vascular endothelium, the risk of fatty plaque formation and atherosclerosis is similarly reduced. This topic is reviewed in the next section.

Lipids, Lipoproteins, and Cardiovascular Disease Risk

Atherosclerosis is a degenerative disease of vascular endothelium. It is marked by an infiltration of the endothelium by lipid material, which then accumulates, eventually occluding the lumen of the blood vessels as the disease progresses. The deposited lipid, known to derive from blood-borne lipids, is called *fatty plaque*. The pathophysiology of atherosclerosis and the role of lipids in its cause have been reviewed [8].

Ever since it was discovered that plaque composition is chiefly lipid, an enormous research effort has been initiated to investigate the possible link between dietary lipid and the development of atherosclerosis. The existence of such a link has come to be called the "lipid hypothesis," which maintains that dietary lipid intake can alter blood lipid levels, which in turn initiate or exacerbate atherogenesis. Following is a brief account of the alleged involvement of certain dietary lipids and fatty acids, and of a genetically acquired apolipoprotein in atherogenesis.

Cholesterol At center stage in the lipid hypothesis controversy is cholesterol, and the effect of manipulations of dietary lipid is generally measured by the extent to which serum cholesterol is raised or lowered. Receiving the greatest attention is not so much the changes in the total cholesterol concentration but how the cholesterol is distributed between its two major transport lipoproteins, LDL and HDL. Since it is commonly and conveniently quantified in clinical laboratories, cholesterol assays can be used to establish LDL–HDL ratios by measuring the amount of cholesterol in each of the two fractions. Since, in the interest of wellness, it is desirable to maintain relatively low serum levels of LDL and relatively high levels of HDL (a low LDL–HDL ratio), the concept of *"good and bad cholesterol"* emerged. The "good" form is that associated with HDL and the "bad" is transported as LDL. It is important to understand, however, that the cholesterol *per se* is not "good" or "bad"; rather, it serves as an indicator of the relative concentrations of LDL and HDL, ratios of which can indeed be good or bad. LDL–HDL ratios are, in fact, determined more reliably by measurements other than cholesterol content. The quantification of apoB (the major LDL apoprotein) and apoA (the primary HDL apoprotein) concentrations by immunological methods, for example, is now widely used.

Among the reasons for cholesterol's "bad press" as it is talked about in connection with cardiovascular disease, is that cholesterol and especially cholesteryl esters are major components of fatty plaque. Contrary to widespread belief, changing the amount of cholesterol in the diet has only a minor influence on blood cholesterol concentration in most people. This is because compensatory mechanisms are engaged, such as HDL activity in scavenging excess cholesterol, and the down-regulation of cholesterol synthesis by dietary cholesterol (discussed in "Synthesis of Cholesterol" section). It is well known, however, that certain individuals respond strongly, and others weakly, to dietary cholesterol (hyper- and hyporesponders). This phenomenon may have a genetic basis, but it is further complicated by the observation that a significant within-person variability exists that is independent of diet. This fact clearly confounds the results of intersubject studies.

Several mechanisms may be considered in trying to account for differences in individual responses to dietary cholesterol: (1) differences in absorption or biosynthesis, (2) differences in the formation of LDL and its receptor-mediated clearance, and (3) differences in its rates of removal and excretion. These considerations have been extensively reviewed [9].

Saturated and Unsaturated Fatty Acids The literature dealing with the effect of dietary fats containing primarily saturated fatty acids (SFA), monounsaturated fatty acids (MUFA), or polyunsaturated fatty acids (PUFA) is as extensive as that related to the feeding of cholesterol itself. Research spanning four decades has generally led to the conclusion that SFAs are hypercholesterolemic and that PUFAs are hypocholesterolemic [10]. Furthermore, it had been assumed that the MUFAs were neutral in this effect, neither increasing nor lowering serum cholesterol. More recent studies have shown, however, that diets rich in MUFA were as effective as PUFA-rich diets in lowering LDL cholesterol and triacylglycerols without significant change in HDL [11,12].

There has also been interest in how carbon-carbon double-bond positions in PUFA are related to their hypocholesterolemic effects. It has been reported that n-3 PUFA were, on an equal-weight basis, more potent than n-6 PUFA in reducing cholesterol [13]. Also, the n-3 PUFA have been found to lower VLDL, and therefore triacylglycerols, more significantly than the n-6 PUFA. In fact, in patients with non–insulin-dependent diabetes mellitus (NIDDM), a disease characterized by high VLDL levels, treatments with dietary supplements of fish oils markedly lowered the VLDL triacylglycerol concentration. Fish oils are particularly rich in n-3 PUFA. Supplementation with n-3 fatty acids can also reduce platelet aggregation, thereby lessening the chance for heart attack and stroke caused by a blocking of blood vessels by coagulation (see "Perspective" section for this chapter).

Saturated fatty acids, which appear to be the major factors causing an increase in serum cholesterol, are lauric (12:0), myristic (14:0), and palmitic (16:0) acids. Stearic acid (18:0), or any fatty acid having fewer than 10 carbon atoms, seemingly has no hypercholesterolemic effect. Chapter 17, Perspective, offers further information on this topic.

Despite years of investigation, the mechanism by which saturated fatty acids elevate serum cholesterol levels has not been conclusively defined. However, they have been alleged to operate in one or more of the following ways: (1) by suppressing the excretion of bile acids, (2) by enhancing the synthesis of cholesterol and LDL, either by reducing the degree of control exerted on the regulatory enzyme HMG-CoA reductase, or by affecting apoB synthesis, or (3) by retarding LCAT activity or receptor-mediated uptake of LDL.

Trans Fatty Acids Double-bonded carbon atoms can exist in either a cis or trans orientation as described on page 114. Most natural fats and oils contain only cis double bonds. The much smaller amount of naturally occurring trans fats are found mostly in the fats of ruminants; for example, in milk fat, which contains 4 to 8% trans fatty acids. Much larger amounts are found in certain margarines and margarine-based products, shortenings, and frying fats as a product of the partial hydrogenation of PUFA. The process of hydrogenation imparts to the product a higher degree of hardness and plasticity, which is more desirable to the consumer and food manufacturer. In the process, however, as hydrogen atoms are catalytically added across double bonds, electronic shifts take place that cause remaining, unhydrogenated cis double bonds to revert to a trans configuration.

The most abundant trans fatty acids in the diet are elaidic acid and its isomers, which are of an 18:1 structure, and it has been reported that diets rich in these fatty acids are as hypercholesterolemic as saturated fatty acids [14]. In fact, serum lipid profiles following feeding of a high trans fatty acid diet may be even more unfavorable than saturated fatty acids because not only are total cholesterol and LDL cholesterol levels elevated, but HDL cholesterol is decreased. The study cited was criticized for using trans elaidic acids obtained by a process not typical of hydrogenation of margarines and shortenings, and also because uncharacteristically large dietary amounts of the trans fatty acids were included in the study diet. However, a more recent study using commonly consumed foods and a large study group, corrob-

orated the former one, suggesting that trans fatty acids can indeed result in the unfavorable serum lipid and lipoprotein profile described [15]. Until the results of additional research are forthcoming, it would seem prudent for those at a high risk of atherosclerosis to avoid a high intake of trans fats.

Lipoprotein a In the 1960s, a genetic variant of LDL was discovered in human serum. The particle differs from normal LDL in that it is attached to a unique marker protein of high molecular weight (513,000 D). The marker protein is currently referred to as *apolipoprotein a, or apo(a)*, and the complete lipoprotein particle is called *lipoprotein a, or Lp(a)*.

At the time of the discovery of Lp(a), it was evident that not all people had the lipoprotein in their serum, and in many of those that did, its concentration was very low compared to other lipoproteins. Consequently, it was dismissed as having little importance. However, interest in Lp(a) was renewed during the following two decades, during which time numerous studies suggested a positive correlation between Lp(a) concentration and atherosclerotic disease.

Structurally, Lp(a) is assembled from LDL and the apo(a) protein. The LDL component of the complex possesses apoB-100 as its only protein component. Linkage of the LDL portion of the particle to apo(a) is through a disulfide bond connecting the two proteins apo(a) and apoB-100. A strong structural homology (similar amino acid sequence) has recently been discovered between apo(a) and plasminogen. Plasminogen is the inactive precursor of the enzyme plasmin, which dissolves blood clots by its hydrolytic action on fibrin. This discovery has stimulated extensive research in the genetics, metabolism, function, and clinical significance of Lp(a).

The physiological function of Lp(a) is not yet defined with certainty, although it is tempting to speculate that its role may be linked to the two functional systems from which the particle was derived, a lipid transport system and the blood-clotting system. It has been proposed that Lp(a) may bind to fibrin clots via its plasminogen-like apo(a), and therefore may deliver cholesterol to regions of recent injury and wound healing.

Numerous epidemiological studies [16] show a positive correlation between Lp(a) concentration and premature myocardial infarction, a blocking of blood vessels in the heart due to clot formation. This has led to the conclusion that Lp(a) may be an independent genetic risk for atherosclerotic disease. One of the many open questions is whether Lp(a) is linked to atherogenesis over an extended period of time because of its

(6K)

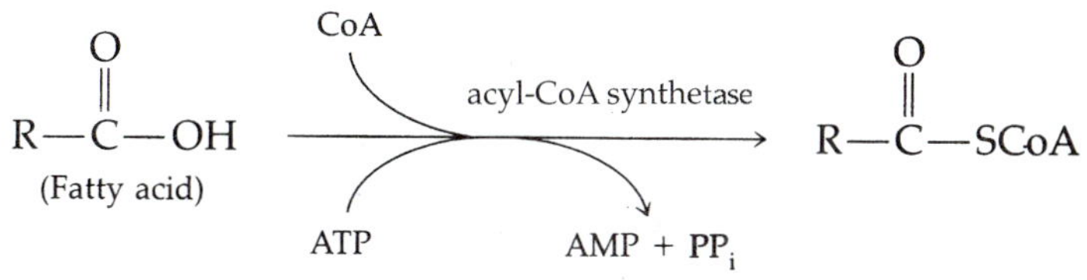

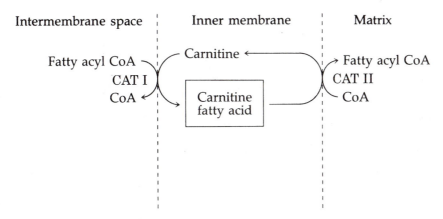

(6L)

lipoprotein properties, or if it plays a role in the sudden development of a clot due to its plasminogen-like apo(a) component binding to fibrin. Perhaps both mechanisms apply.

INTEGRATED METABOLISM IN TISSUES

Catabolism of Triacylglycerols and Fatty Acids

The complete hydrolysis of triacylglycerols yields glycerol and three fatty acids. In the body, this occurs largely through the activity of lipoprotein lipase of vascular endothelium, and through an intracellular lipase that is active in the liver, and particularly active in adipose tissue. The glycerol portion can be used for energy by the liver and by other tissues having activity of the enzyme glycerokinase, through which glycerol is converted to glycerol phosphate. Glycerol phosphate can enter the glycolytic pathway at the level of dihydroxyacetone phosphate, from which point either energy oxidation or gluconeogenesis can occur (Fig. 4.7).

Fatty acids are a very rich source of energy and on an equal-weight basis surpass carbohydrates in this property. This is because fatty acids exist in a more reduced state than that of carbohydrate and therefore undergo a greater extent of oxidation en route to CO_2 and H_2O.

Many tissues are capable of oxidizing fatty acids by way of a mechanism called β-oxidation, which is described next. On entry into the cell of the metabolizing tissue, the fatty acid is first activated by coenzyme A, an energy-requiring reaction catalyzed by cytoplasmic *fatty acyl-CoA synthetase* (see 6K). The reaction actually consumes the equivalent of two ATPs, because the pyrophosphate must also be hydrolyzed to ensure irreversibility of the reaction.

The oxidation of fatty acids is compartmentalized within the mitochondrion. Fatty acids and their CoA derivatives, however, are incapable of crossing the inner mitochondrial membrane, necessitating a membrane transport system. The carrier molecule for this system is *carnitine* (p. 229), which can be synthesized in humans from lysine and methionine, and which is found in high concentration in muscle. The activated fatty acid is joined covalently to carnitine at the cytoplasmic side of the mitochondrial membrane by the transferase enzyme carnitine acyltransferase I (CAT I). A second transferase, acyltransferase II (CAT II), located on the inner face of the inner membrane, releases the fatty acyl CoA and carnitine into the matrix (see 6L).

The oxidation of the activated fatty acid in the mitochondrion occurs via a cyclic degradative pathway, by which two-carbon units in the form of acetyl CoA are cleaved one by one from the carboxyl end. The reactions of β-oxidation are summarized in Figure 6.9.

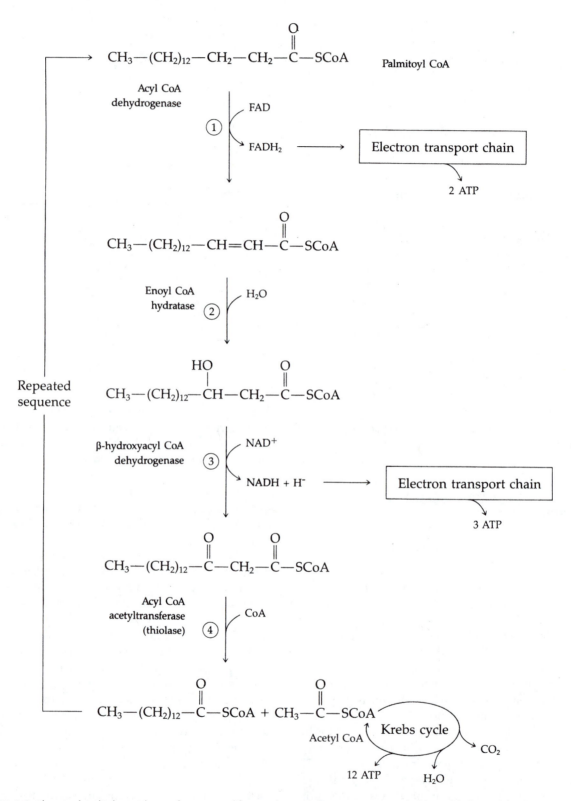

FIGURE 6.9 The mitochondrial β-oxidation of an activated fatty acid using palmitate as an example. The yield of ATPs from the complete oxidation of the fatty acid is indicated. The name of the enzyme catalyzing each reaction is written to the left of each reaction arrow.

The following comments relate to the reactions:

1. The formation of a double bond between the α- and β-carbons, catalyzed by fatty acyl CoA dehydrogenase. There are four such dehydrogenases, each specific for a range of chain lengths. The $FADH_2$ yields its two hydrogens to CoQ and therefore feeds two electrons into the electron transport system (ETS), which, it will be recalled, is also compartmentalized in the mitochondrion. The ETS oxidation of $FADH_2$ yields two ATPs.

2. The unsaturated acyl CoA accepts a molecule of water, a reaction catalyzed by enoyl CoA hydrase, sometimes called *crotonase*.

3. The β-hydroxy group is oxidized to the ketone by the NAD^+-requiring enzyme, β-hydroxyacyl CoA dehydrogenase. The ETS oxidation of the NADH leads to the formation of three ATPs.

4. The β-ketoacyl CoA is cleaved by β-ketothiolase (also called *acyl CoA thiolase*), resulting in the insertion of CoA and cleavage at the β-carbon. The products of this reaction are acetyl CoA and a saturated, CoA-activated fatty acid having two fewer carbons than the original fatty acid. This reaction completes one cycle of the degradative pathway. The entire sequence of reactions is repeated, with two carbons being removed with each cycle.

Energy Considerations in Fatty Acid Oxidation

The activation of a fatty acid actually requires two high-energy bonds per mole of fatty acid oxidized. Each cleavage of a carbon-carbon bond yields 5 ATPs—2 by oxidation of $FADH_2$ and 3 by NADH oxidation via oxidative phosphorylation. The acetyl CoAs produced are oxidized to CO_2 and water in the Krebs cycle, and for each of these oxidized, 12 ATPs (or their equivalent) are produced (p. 92). Using the example of palmitate (16 carbons), the yield of ATP would be summarized as follows:

7 carbon–carbon cleavages	$7 \times 5 =$	35
8 acetyl CoA oxidized	$8 \times 12 =$	96
Total ATPs produced		131
2 ATPs for activation		−2
Net ATPs		129

Nearly one-half of dietary and body fatty acids are unsaturated and therefore must provide a considerable portion of lipid-derived energy. They are catabolized by β-oxidation in the mitochondrion in nearly identical fashion as their saturated counterparts, except for the fact that one fatty acyl CoA dehydrogenase reaction is

not required for each double bond present. This is because the double bond introduced into the saturated fatty acid by the reaction occurs naturally in unsaturated fatty acids. However, the specificity of the enoyl CoA hydrase reaction requires that the double bond be a Δ^2 in order for the hydration to take place, and the "natural" double bond may not occupy this position. For example, after three cycles of β-carbon oxidation, the position of the double bond in what was originally a Δ^9 monounsaturated fatty acid will occupy a Δ^3 position. The presence of a specific enoyl CoA transisomerase then shifts the double bond from Δ^3 to Δ^2, allowing the hydrase and subsequent reactions to proceed. The oxidation of an unsaturated fatty acid results in somewhat less energy production than a saturated fatty acid of the same chain length, since for each double bond present one $FADH_2$-producing fatty acyl CoA dehydrogenase reaction is bypassed, resulting in two less ATPs.

Although most fatty acids metabolized are composed of an even number of carbon atoms, small amounts of fatty acids having an odd number of carbon atoms are also used for energy. β-oxidation occurs as described, with the liberation of acetyl CoA until a residual propionyl CoA remains. The subsequent oxidation of propionyl CoA requires reactions that use the vitamins biotin and B_{12} in a coenzymatic role; see 6M.

Since the succinyl CoA formed in the course of these reactions can be converted into glucose, the odd-numbered fatty acids are therefore uniquely gluconeogenic among all the fatty acids.

Formation of the Ketone Bodies

In addition to its direct oxidation via the Krebs cycle, acetyl CoA may follow a different catabolic route in the liver—a pathway by which the so-called *ketone bodies* (acetoacetate, β-hydroxybutyrate, and acetone) are formed. Acetoacetate and β-hydroxybutyrate are not oxidized further in the liver but instead are transported by the blood to peripheral tissues, where they can be converted back to acetyl CoA, and oxidized via the Krebs cycle. The steps in ketone body formation occur as shown in 6N. Ketone body formation is actually an "overflow" pathway for acetyl CoA use, providing another way for the liver to distribute fuel to peripheral cells. Normally, the concentration of the ketone bodies is very low in the blood, but it may reach very high levels in situations of accelerated fatty acid oxidation combined with low carbohydrate intake or impaired carbohydrate use. Such a situation would occur in diabetes mellitus, starvation, or simply a very low-carbohydrate diet. The inadequate supply of carbohydrate reduces the pool of oxaloacetate, formed mainly from pyruvate, with which the acetyl

(6M)

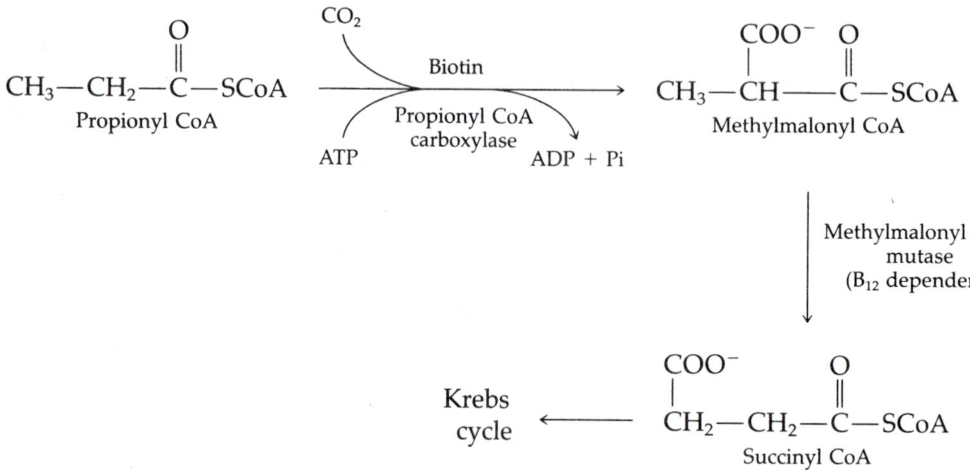

$$CH_3-CH_2-\overset{\overset{\displaystyle O}{\|}}{C}-SCoA$$
Propionyl CoA

$$\xrightarrow[\substack{\text{Propionyl CoA}\\\text{carboxylase}}]{\text{Biotin}}$$

CO$_2$

ATP   ADP + Pi

$$CH_3-\underset{\underset{\displaystyle COO^-}{|}}{CH}-\overset{\overset{\displaystyle O}{\|}}{C}-SCoA$$
Methylmalonyl CoA

Methylmalonyl CoA
mutase
(B$_{12}$ dependent)

Krebs
cycle $\longleftarrow$

$$\underset{\underset{\displaystyle COO^-}{|}}{CH_2}-CH_2-\overset{\overset{\displaystyle O}{\|}}{C}-SCoA$$
Succinyl CoA

(6N)

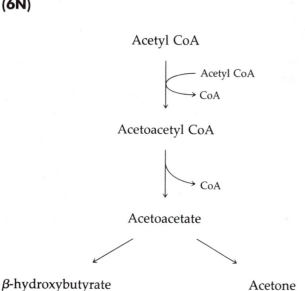

Acetyl CoA

Acetyl CoA
CoA

Acetoacetyl CoA

CoA

Acetoacetate

β-hydroxybutyrate   Acetone

CoA normally combines for Krebs cycle oxidation. As carbohydrate use is diminished, oxidation of fatty acids accelerates in order to provide energy through the production of Krebs cycle substrates (acetyl CoA). This shift to fat catabolism, coupled with reduced oxaloacetate availability, results in an accumulation of acetyl CoA. A sharp increase in ketone body formation follows as would be expected, resulting in the condition known as ketosis.

Ketosis can be dangerous in that it can disturb the body's acid–base balance (two of the ketone bodies are, in fact, organic acids). However, the liver's ability to deliver ketone bodies to peripheral tissues such as the brain is an important mechanism for providing fuel in periods of starvation. It is the lesser of two evils.

Catabolism of Cholesterol

Unlike the triacylglycerols and fatty acids, cholesterol is not an energy-producing nutrient. Its four-ring core structure remains intact in the course of its catabolism and is eliminated as such through the biliary system.

Cholesterol is delivered to the liver chiefly in the form of chylomicron remnants, as well as in the form of LDL and HDL. That which is destined for excretion is hydrolyzed by esterases to the free form, which is secreted into the bile canaliculi directly, or it is first converted into bile acids prior to entering the bile. It is estimated that neutral sterol, most of which is cholesterol, represents about 55%, and bile acids (salts) 45% of total sterol excreted. The key metabolic changes in the cholesterol-to-bile acid transformation are (1) reduction in the length of the hydrocarbon side chain at C-17, (2) addition of a carboxylic acid group on the shortened chain, and (3) addition of hydroxyl groups to the ring system of the molecule. The effect of these reactions is to enhance the water solubility of the sterol, facilitating its excretion in the bile. Cholic acid, the structure of which is shown in Figure 6.2, has hydroxyl groups at C-7 and C-12 in addition to the C-3 hydroxyl of the native cholesterol. The other major bile acids differ from cholic acid only in the number of hydroxyls attached to the ring system. For example, chenodeoxycholic acid has hydroxyls at C-3 and C-7, deoxycholic acid at C-3 and C-12, and lithocholic acid at C-3 only. Other bile acids are formed from the conjugation of these compounds with glycine or taurine, which attach through the carboxyl group of the steroid.

It has already been pointed out that the enterohepatic circulation can return absorbed bile salts to the liver. Bile salts returning to the liver from the intestine

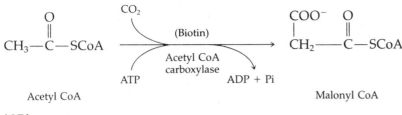

Acetyl CoA   Malonyl CoA

(6P)

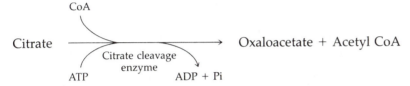

repress the formation of an enzyme catalyzing the rate-limiting step in the conversion of cholesterol into bile acids. If the bile salts are prevented from returning to the liver, the activity of this enzyme increases, thus stimulating the conversion of cholesterol and therefore its excretion. This effect is exploited therapeutically in the treatment of hypercholesterolemia by the use of unabsorbable, cationic resins that bind bile salts in the intestinal lumen and prevent their return to the liver.

Synthesis of Fatty Acids

Aside from linoleic acid and α-linolenic acid, which are essential and must be acquired from the diet, the body is capable of synthesizing fatty acids from simple precursors. An overview of the process is the sequential assembly of a "starter" molecule of acetyl CoA with units of malonyl CoA, the CoA derivative of malonic acid. Ultimately, however, all the carbons of a fatty acid are contributed by acetyl CoA, since malonyl CoA is formed from acetyl CoA and CO_2. This reaction occurs in the cytoplasm. It is catalyzed by acetyl CoA carboxylase, a complex enzyme containing *biotin* as its prosthetic group. The role of biotin in *carboxylation reactions*, such as this one, which involves the incorporation of a carboxyl group into a compound, will be discussed in Chapter 9. ATP furnishes the driving force to attach the new carboxyl group to acetyl CoA (see 6O).

Nearly all the acetyl CoA formed in metabolism occurs in the mitochondria, formed there from pyruvate oxidation (p. 92), from the oxidation of fatty acids (p. 135), and from the degradation of the carbon skeletons of some amino acids (p. 201). The synthesis of fatty acids is localized in the cytoplast, but acetyl CoA as such is not able to pass through the mitochondrial membrane.

The major mechanism for the transfer of acetyl CoA to the cytoplast is by way of its passage across the mitochondrial membrane in the form of citrate. Once in the cytoplast, the *citrate cleavage enzyme* converts the citrate to oxaloacetate and acetyl CoA, a reaction that is essentially the reversal of the citrate synthetase reaction of the Krebs cycle, except that it requires expenditure of ATP (see 6P).

The enzymes involved in fatty acid synthesis are arranged in a complex called the *fatty acid synthase system*. Key components of this complex are the *acyl carrier protein* (*ACP*) (p. 255) and the *condensing enzyme* (*CE*), both of which possess free —SH groups to which the acetyl CoA and malonyl CoA building blocks attach. ACP is structurally similar to CoA (Fig. 9.21) in that they both possess a 4′-phosphopantetheine component that is comprised of *pantothenic acid* coupled to thioethanolamine (which contributes the free —SH group) and phosphate. The free —SH of the condensing enzyme is contributed by the amino acid cysteine.

Before the actual steps in the elongation of the fatty acid chain can begin, the two sulfhydryl groups must be "loaded" correctly with malonyl and acetyl groups. Acetyl CoA is transferred to ACP, with the loss of CoA, to form acetyl ACP. The acetyl group is then transferred again to the —SH of the condensing enzyme, leaving available the ACP—SH, to which malonyl CoA then attaches, again, with the loss of CoA. This loading of the complex can be represented as shown in 6Q.

The extension of the fatty acid chain then proceeds through the following sequential steps, which are also shown schematically in Figure 6.10. The enzymes catalyzing these reactions are also contained in the synthase complex along with ACP and CE. The following are comments on these reactions:

$$
\begin{array}{c}
\text{O} \\
\parallel \\
CH_3-C-SCoA + HS- \boxed{\text{Condensing enzyme}} \\[4pt]
\begin{array}{cc}
COO^- & O \\
| & \parallel \\
CH_2\!\!-\!\!-C-SCoA + HS- \boxed{ACP'}
\end{array}
\end{array}
\longrightarrow
\begin{array}{c}
\text{O} \\
\parallel \\
CH_3-C-S- \boxed{\text{Condensing enzyme}} \\[4pt]
\begin{array}{cc}
COO^- & O \\
| & \parallel \\
CH_2\!\!-\!\!-C-S- \boxed{ACP}
\end{array}
\end{array}
+ 2SCoA
$$

1. The condensation reaction in which the carbonyl carbon of the acetyl group is coupled to C-2 of malonyl ACP with the elimination of the malonyl carboxyl group as CO_2.

2. The β-ketone is reduced, with NADPH serving as hydrogen donor.

3. The alcohol is dehydrated, yielding a double bond.

4. The double bond is reduced to butyryl-ACP, again with NADPH acting as reducing agent.

5. The butyryl group is transferred to the CE, exposing the ACP sulfhydryl site to a second molecule of malonyl CoA.

6. Malonyl ACP forms for a second time.

7. A second condensation reaction takes place, with coupling of the butyryl group on the CE to C-2 of the malonyl ACP. The six-carbon chain is then reduced and transferred to CE in a repetition of steps 2 through 5. A third molecule of malonyl CoA attaches at ACP—SH, and so forth. The completed fatty acid chain is hydrolyzed from the ACP without transfer to the CE.

The normal product of the fatty acid synthase system is palmitate. It can in turn be lengthened by fatty acid *elongation* systems to stearic acid and even longer saturated fatty acids. Elongation occurs by the insertion of 2-carbon units at the carboxylic acid end of the chain. Furthermore, by *desaturation* reactions, palmitate and stearate can be converted to their corresponding Δ^9 monounsaturated fatty acids—palmitoleic and oleic acids, respectively. Fatty acid desaturation reactions are catalyzed by enzymes referred to as *mixed-function oxidases*, so called because two different substrates are oxidized, the fatty acid (by removal of hydrogen atoms to form the new double bond) and NADPH. Oxygen is the terminal hydrogen and electron acceptor.

As pointed out previously, human cells cannot introduce additional double bonds beyond the Δ^9 site because they lack enzymes called Δ^{12} and Δ^{15} desaturases. That is why linoleic acid ($18{:}\Delta^{9,12}$) and α-linolenic acid ($18{:}\Delta^{9,12,15}$) are essential fatty acids. They can be acquired from plant sources because plant cells do have the desaturase enzymes mentioned. Once linoleic acid is acquired, longer, more highly unsaturated fatty acids can be formed from it by the combination of elongation and desaturation reactions. Figure 6.11 illustrates the elongation and desaturation of palmitate and linoleate.

Synthesis of Triacylglycerols (triglycerides)

The biosynthesis of triacylglycerols and glycerophosphatides share common precursors and can be considered together in this section. The precursors are CoA-activated fatty acids and glycerol-3-phosphate, the latter being produced either from the reduction of dihydroxyacetone phosphate or by the phosphorylation of glycerol. These and subsequent reactions of the pathways are shown in Figure 6.12. The *de novo* pathway of lecithin synthesis is the major route; however, the importance of the salvage pathway increases when there is a deficiency of the essential amino acid methionine.

Synthesis of Cholesterol

Nearly all the tissues in the body are capable of synthesizing cholesterol from acetyl CoA, but the two most active synthesizing organs are the liver and the intestinal wall. These two tissues supply over 90% of endogenous plasma cholesterol. The cholesterol production rate, which includes both absorbed cholesterol and endogenously synthesized cholesterol, approximates 1 g/d. The average cholesterol intake is considered to be about 600 mg/d, only about one-half of which is absorbed. Endogenous synthesis therefore accounts for greater than two-thirds of the total cholesterol store.

At least 26 steps are known to be involved in the formation of cholesterol from acetyl CoA. The pathway can be thought of as occurring in three stages: (1) a cytoplasmic sequence by which 3-hydroxy-3 methyl glutaryl CoA (HMG-CoA) is formed from 3 mol of acetyl CoA; (2) the conversion of HMG-CoA to squalene, including the important rate-limiting step of cholesterol synthesis in which HMG-CoA is reduced to mevalonic

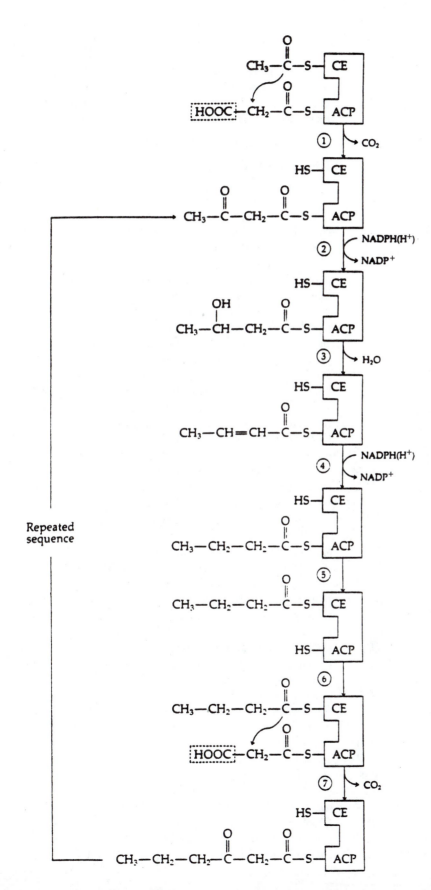

FIGURE 6.10 The steps in the synthesis of fatty acid. CE (condensing enzyme) and ACP (acyl carrier protein) are members of a complex of enzymes referred to as the *fatty acyl synthase system*.

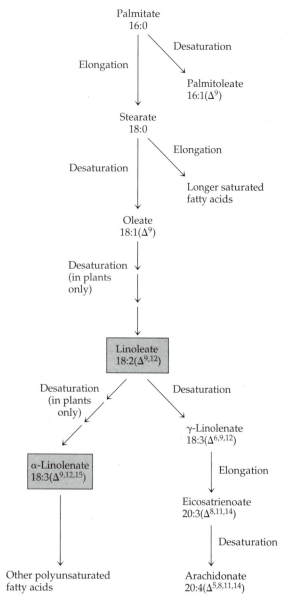

FIGURE 6.11 *Routes of synthesis of other fatty acids from palmitate as precursor. Elongation and desaturation reactions allow palmitate to be converted into longer and more highly unsaturated fatty acids. Mammals cannot convert oleate into linoleate or α-linolenate (shaded in figure). These fatty acids are therefore essential, and must be acquired in the diet.*

acid by HMG-CoA reductase; and (3) the formation of cholesterol from squalene.

As total body cholesterol increases, the rate of synthesis tends to decrease, and this is known to be due to a negative feedback regulation of the HMG-CoA reductase reaction. This suppression of cholesterol synthesis by dietary cholesterol seems to be unique to the liver and is not evident in other tissues to a great extent. The ef-

fect of feedback control of biosynthesis depends to a great extent on the amount of cholesterol absorbed. The suppression is not sufficient to prevent an increase in the total body pool of cholesterol when dietary intake is high. A brief scheme of hepatic cholesterolgenesis and its regulation is shown in Figure 6.13.

REGULATION OF LIPID METABOLISM

The regulation of fatty acid oxidation is closely linked to carbohydrate status. Fatty acids formed in the cytoplast of liver cells can either be converted into triacylglycerols and phospholipids or transported via carnitine into the mitochondrion for oxidation. Carnitine acyl transferase I (see 6L), which catalyzes the transfer of fatty acyl groups to carnitine, is specifically inhibited by malonyl CoA. This, it will be recalled, is the first intermediate in the synthesis of fatty acids, and therefore it is logical that an increase in its concentration would promote fatty acid synthesis while inhibiting fatty acid oxidation. Malonyl CoA increases in concentration whenever the person is well supplied with carbohydrate because excess glucose that cannot be oxidized or stored as glycogen is converted into triacylglycerols for storage, thereby increasing the demands for malonyl CoA. Therefore, glucose-rich cells would not actively oxidize fatty acids for energy. Instead, a switch to fat synthesis (lipogenesis) is stimulated, accomplished in part by inhibition of the entry of fatty acids into the mitochondrion.

Blood glucose levels can affect lipolysis and fatty acid oxidation by other mechanisms as well. Hyperglycemia triggers the release of insulin, which promotes glucose transport into the adipose cell and therefore lipogenesis. The hormone also exerts a pronounced antilipolytic effect. Hypoglycemia results in a reduced intracellular supply of glucose, therefore suppressing lipogenesis. Furthermore, the low level of insulin accompanying the hypoglycemic state would favor lipolysis, with a flow of free fatty acids into the bloodstream. Low glucose levels also stimulate the rate of fatty acid oxidation in the manner described in the section dealing with the ketone bodies. In this case, accelerated oxidation of fatty acids follows the reduction in Krebs cycle activity, which in turn results from inadequate oxaloacetate availability.

The key enzyme for the mobilization of fat is *hormone-sensitive triacylglycerol lipase*, found in adipose tissue cells. Lipolysis is stimulated by such hormones as epinephrine and norepinephrine, adrenocorticotropic hormone (ACTH), thyroid-stimulating hormone (TSH), glucagon,

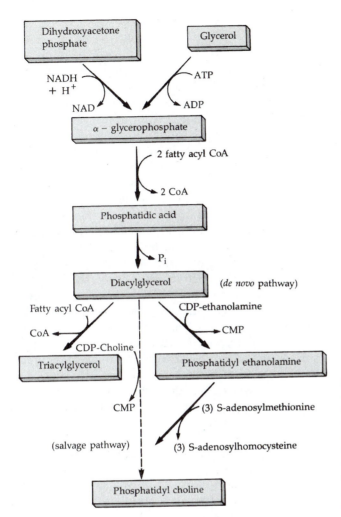

FIGURE 6.12 A schematic summary of the synthesis of triacylglycerols and lecithin showing that precursors are shared. In lecithin formation, three moles of activated methionine (S-adenosylmethionine) introduce three methyl groups in the *de novo* pathway, and choline is introduced as CDP (cytidine diphosphate) choline in the so-called salvage pathway.

growth hormone, and thyroxine. Insulin, as mentioned earlier, antagonizes the effects of these hormones by inhibiting the enzymatic activity.

A very important allosteric enzyme involved in the regulation of fatty acid biosynthesis is acetyl CoA carboxylase, which forms malonyl CoA from acetyl CoA (p. 139). The enzyme, which functions in the cytoplast, is positively stimulated by citrate, and in the absence of this modulator the enzyme is barely active. Citrate is continuously produced in the mitochondrion as a Krebs cycle intermediate, but its concentration in the cytoplast is normally low. However, should mitochondrial citrate concentration increase, the compound can escape to the cytoplast, where it acts as a positive allosteric signal to acetyl CoA carboxylase, thereby increasing the rate of formation of malonyl CoA. Also it may be recalled that citrate is the precursor for cytoplasmic acetyl CoA. Therefore the result of citrate accumulation is that ex-

cess acetyl CoA is diverted to fatty acid synthesis and away from Krebs cycle activity.

Acetyl CoA carboxylase can be modulated *negatively* by palmitoyl CoA, which is the product of fatty acid synthesis. This situation would most likely arise when fatty acid concentrations increase due to insufficient glycerophosphate, with which they must combine to form triacylglycerols. Deficient glycerophosphate levels would likely be due to inadequate carbohydrate availability, and in such a situation, regulation would logically favor fatty acid oxidation rather than synthesis.

A great deal of interest in serum cholesterol levels has been generated because of the alleged correlation of the compound to the predisposition to cardiovascular disease. The regulation of cholesterol homeostasis is associated with its effect on LDL receptor concentration and on the activity of regulatory enzymes such as acyl CoA: cholesterol acyltransferase (ACAT) and hydroxymethyl

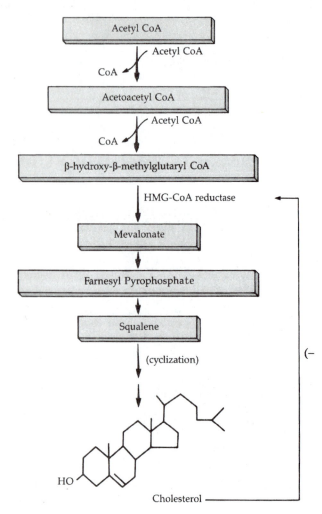

FIGURE 6.13 An overview of the pathway of cholesterol biosynthesis in the hepatocyte indicating the negative regulatory effect of cholesterol on the HMG-CoA reductase reaction.

glutaryl CoA (HMG-CoA) reductase. Cholesterol's feedback suppression of HMG-CoA reductase has already been discussed and is shown in Figure 6.13. The effect of increasing ACAT activity (the conversion of free cholesterol to cholesterol esters) and decreasing the amount of LDL receptors reduces the accumulation of cholesterol in vascular endothelial and smooth muscle cells. Figure 6.14 illustrates these mechanisms of control.

SUMMARY

The hydrophobic character of lipids makes them unique among the major nutrients, requiring special handling in the body's aqueous milieu. Ingested fat must be finely dispersed in the intestinal lumen to present a sufficiently

large surface area for enzymatic digestion to occur. In the bloodstream, reassembled lipid must be associated with proteins to ensure its solubility in that environment while undergoing transport.

The major sites for the formation of lipoproteins are the intestine, which produces them from exogenously derived lipids, and the liver, which forms lipoproteins from endogenous lipid. Central to the processes of fat transport and storage is adipose tissue, which accumulates fat as triacylglycerol when the intake of energy-producing nutrients is greater than the body's caloric requirement. When the energy demand so dictates, fatty acids are released from storage and transported to other tissues for oxidation. The mobilization follows the adipocyte's response to specific hormonal signals that stimulate the activity of the intracellular lipase.

Fatty acids are a rich source of energy. Their mitochondrial oxidation furnishes large amounts of acetyl CoA for Krebs cycle catabolism, and in situations of low carbohydrate intake or use, as in starvation or diabetes, the rate of fatty acid oxidation increases significantly with concomitant acetyl CoA accumulation. This causes a rise in the level of the ketone bodies—organic acids that can be deleterious through their disturbance of acid–base balance but that are also beneficial as sources of fuel to tissues such as muscle and brain in periods of starvation.

Although the lipids are thought of first and foremost as energy sources, some can be identified with intriguing hormone-like functions ranging from blood pressure alteration and platelet aggregation to an enhancement of immunologic surveillance. These potent, bioactive substances are the prostaglandins, thromboxanes, and leukotrienes, all of which are derived from the fatty acids, arachidonate, and certain other long-chain PUFAs.

Dietary lipid has been implicated in atherogenesis, the development of the degenerative cardiovascular disease called *atherosclerosis*. A major consideration in the prevention and control of this disease has been the concentration of cholesterol in the blood serum, and the relative hypocholesterolemic or hypercholesterolemic effect of certain diets. Saturated fatty acids having medium-length chains, and trans unsaturated fatty acids are alleged to be hypercholesterolemic, while mono- and polyunsaturated cis fats tend to lower serum cholesterol.

Fats can be synthesized by cytoplasmic enzyme systems when energy production by carbohydrate is adequate. The synthesis begins with simple precursors such as acetyl CoA and can be triggered by hormonal signals or by elevated levels of citrate, which acts as a regulatory substance. Blood glucose concentration also acts as a

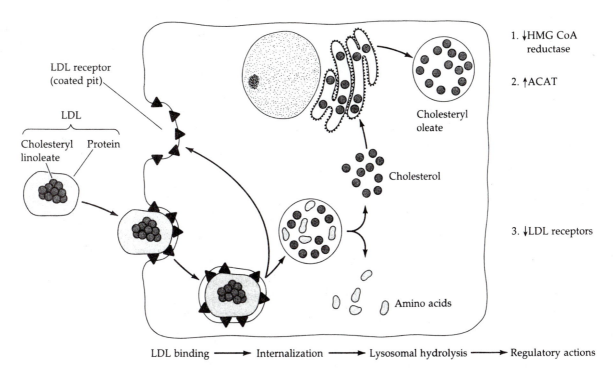

1. ↓HMG CoA
   reductase

2. ↑ACAT

3. ↓LDL receptors

LDL binding ⟶ Internalization ⟶ Lysosomal hydrolysis ⟶ Regulatory actions

FIGURE 6.14 The effect of cholesterol on HMG CoA (hydroxymethyl glutaryl CoA) reductase, ACAT (acyl CoA: cholesterol acyl-transferase and LDL receptor concentration in the regulation of cholesterol homeostasis. (Brown M, Goldstein J. Receptor mediated endocytosis: insights from the lipoprotein receptor system. © The Nobel Foundation 1986.)

sensitive regulator of lipogenesis, which is stimulated when a hyperglycemic state exists.

Protein metabolism will be surveyed in Chapter 7. There, it will be seen that amino acids, like carbohydrates and lipids, can furnish energy through their oxidation, or they can be metabolically converted into other substances of biochemical importance. Once again it should be emphasized that the metabolic pathways of the energy nutrients are linked through common metabolites. Gluconeogenesis, discussed in Chapter 4, illustrates this integration through the formation of carbohydrate from the glycerol moiety of lipids and certain amino acids. Chapter 7 will demonstrate how protein can be converted into fat through common intermediates. "A rose is a rose is a rose" applies quite appropriately to intermediary metabolites. An enzyme acting on acetyl CoA, for example, has no inkling as to whether the substrate was formed through carbohydrate, fat, or protein metabolism—nor does it care!

References

1. Hunter JE, Applewhite TH. Reassessment of trans fatty acid availability in the US diet. Am J Clin Nutr 1991; 54:363–369.

2. Neuringer M, Connor WE. n-3 Fatty acids in the brain and retina: Evidence for their essentiality. Nutr Rev 1986; 44:285–294.

3. Berridge MJ. Inositol triphosphate and diacylglycerol: Two intersecting second messengers. Ann Rev Biochem 1987;56:159–193.

4. Borgstrom B, Erlanson-Albertsson C. Pancreatic colipase. In: Borgstrom B, Brockman HL, eds. Lipases. Amsterdam: Elsevier, 1984;151–183.

5. Verger R. Pancreatic lipase. In: Borgstrom B, Brockman HL, eds. Lipases. Amsterdam: Elsevier, 1984;83–150.

6. Forester GP, Tall AR, Bisgaier CL, Glickman RM. Rat intestine secretes spherical high density lipoproteins. J Biol Chem 1983;258:5938–5943.

7. Borensztajn J, Getz GS, Kotlar TJ. Uptake of chylomicron remnants by the liver: further evidence for the modulating role of phospholipids. J Lipid Res 1988; 29:1087–1096.

8. The Eleventh Annual Arnold O. Beckman Conference in Clinical Chemistry. Atherosclerosis: Metabolism, risk, and control. Clin Chem 1988;34(8B):B1–B135.

9. Beynen AC, Katan MB, and Van Zutphen LFM. Hypo- and hyperresponders: Individual differences in the response of serum cholesterol concentration to changes in diet. Adv in Lipid Res 1987;22:115–171.

10. Jackson RL, Taunton OD, Morrisett JD, Gotto AM Jr. The role of dietary polyunsaturated fat in lowering blood cholesterol in man. Circ Res 1978;42:447–453.

11. Mensink RP, Katan MB. Effect of a diet enriched with monounsaturated or polyunsaturated fatty acids on levels of low-density and high-density lipoprotein cholesterol in healthy women and men. N Engl J Med 1989;321: 436–441.

12. Berry EM, Eisenberg S, Haratz D, et al. Effects of diets rich in monounsaturated fatty acids on plasma lipoproteins—the Jerusalem Nutrition Study: high MU-FAs vs. high PUFAs. Am J Clin Nutr 1991;53:899–907.

13. Connor WE, Lin DS, Harris WB. A comparison of dietary polyunsaturated n-6 fatty acids in humans: Effects upon plasma lipids, lipoproteins, and sterol balance. Arteriosclerosis 1981;1:363a.

14. Mensink RP and Katan MB. Effect of dietary trans fatty acids on high density and low density lipoprotein cholesterol levels in healthy subjects. New Engl J Med 1990; 323:439–445.

15. Troisi R, Willett WC, Weiss ST. trans-Fatty acid intake in relation to serum lipid concentrations in adult men. Am J Clin Nutr 1992;5C:1019–1024.

16. Uterman G. The mysteries of lipoprotein (a). Science 1989;246:904–910.

Suggested Reading

McNamara DJ. Effects of fat-modified diets on cholesterol and lipoprotein metabolism. Ann Rev Nutr 1987; 7:273–290.

This is an interesting summary of the effect of different dietary fats and carbohydrates on cholesterol and lipoprotein metabolism.

Rudney H, Sexton RC. Regulation of cholesterol biosynthesis. Ann Rev Nutr 1986;6:245–272.

This is a review of the regulatory sites of cholesterol biosynthesis and the effect of dietary factors in this regulation.

Budowski P. Omega-3 fatty acids in health and disease. In: Bourne GH, ed. World review of nutrition and dietetics. Basel, Switzerland: Karger, 1988;57:214–274.

The structural aspects, sources, and antithrombotic actions of the omega-3 fatty acids are thoroughly reviewed, along with the eicosanoids and their multiplicity of physiologic functions.

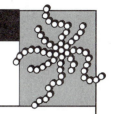

PERSPECTIVE 1

The LDL Receptor

Michael S. Brown, M.D., and Joseph L. Goldstein, M.D., the 1985 Nobel laureates for physiology or medicine, powerfully illuminated for all to see the intimate relationship between the health of the total organism and the functioning of one cellular organelle: the low-density lipoprotein (LDL) receptor.

When these two physicians, one a medical biochemist and the other a medical geneticist, became a team in 1972 at the University of Texas Health Science Center in Dallas, they were seeking the molecular basis for the clinical manifestation of hypercholesterolemia. Beginning with cultured fibroblasts from 77 patients with familial homozygous hypercholesterolemia and then expanding their research through use of various experimental animals, Brown and Goldstein, along with their associates, were able to establish an understanding of normal cholesterol metabolism and the aberrations of this metabolism that result in hypercholesterolemia. The methodic research of Brown and Goldstein revealed the following facts about LDLs and cholesterol metabolism [1].

LDLs bind to normal fibroblasts (and other cells, particularly the hepatocytes and cells of the adrenal gland and ovarian corpus luteum) with high affinity and specificity. In mutant cells, however, the binding is very inefficient. Although deficient binding of LDL is characteristic of all mutant cells, much variation exists in the binding ability among different patients with familial homozygous hypercholesterolemia.

Membrane-bound LDL is internalized by endocytosis made possible by receptors that cluster in coated pits (Fig. 1.16). Figure 1 depicts the fate of the LDL following its binding to the membrane receptor. The receptor, having released its LDL, returns to the surface of the cell, making a round trip into and out of the cell every ten minutes during its twenty-hour life span [2]. The dissociated LDL moves into the lysosome, where its protein and cholesteryl ester components are hydrolyzed by lysosomal enzymes into amino acids and free cholesterol, respectively. The resulting free cholesterol exerts the following regulatory functions. First, by lowering the concentration of receptor mRNA, it suppresses synthesis of LDL receptors so as to prevent further entry of LDL into the cell. Second, it modulates the activity of two microsomal enzymes, 3-hydroxy 3-methylglutaryl CoA reductase (HMG CoA reductase) and acyl CoA: cholesteryl acyl transferase (ACAT). Activity of the HMG CoA reductase, the

rate-limiting enzyme in cholesterol synthesis, is suppressed through decreased transcription of the reductase gene and the concomitant increased degradation of the enzyme. In contrast, ACAT is activated, thereby promoting formation of cholesteryl esters that can be stored as droplets in the cytoplasm of the cell.

Mutant cells unable to bind and/or internalize LDL efficiently and thereby deprived of the cholesterol needed for membrane synthesis must obtain the needed sterol via *de novo* synthesis. In these cells HMG CoA reductase is activated while ACAT is depressed.

LDL receptors interact with apoprotein B-100, the protein carried on the surface of the LDLs. The interaction between the receptors and the apoprotein B-100 is the key to the cell's internalization of the LDL. The number of receptors synthesized by cells varies according to cholesterol requirements.

Purification to homogeneity of the LDL receptor from bovine adrenal cortex and later cloning of the human LDL receptor [3] allowed delineation of the synthesis sequence and the structure of this membrane protein. The LDL receptor has been found to be a transmembrane glycoprotein that, on its way to maturity, undergoes several carbohydrate-processing reactions [4]. As the molecular weight of the receptor increases through the addition of carbohydrate moieties to its precursor, the mobility of the receptor decreases. The decreased mobility of the receptor is due more to a change in the conformation of the protein than to its increase in weight [2].

Five domains of the LDL receptor have been identified and are depicted in Figure 2. Domain 1, which is furthest from the membrane and contains the NH_2 terminal of the receptor protein, is rich in cysteine residues. These residues allow the formation of many disulfide bonds that give stability to the molecule. Many of the other amino acid residues in this cysteine-rich domain have negatively charged side chains. This first domain, then, could be the binding site for apoprotein B-100, with its positively charged lysine and arginine residues. These positively charged residues of this apoprotein are known to be crucial for receptor binding.

The second domain, made up of 350 amino acids, is the possible location for the N-linked glycosylation that occurs during the maturation process of the receptor protein. Domain 3 is located immediately outside the plasma membrane and is the site of the O-linked

PERSPECTIVE 1 (continued)

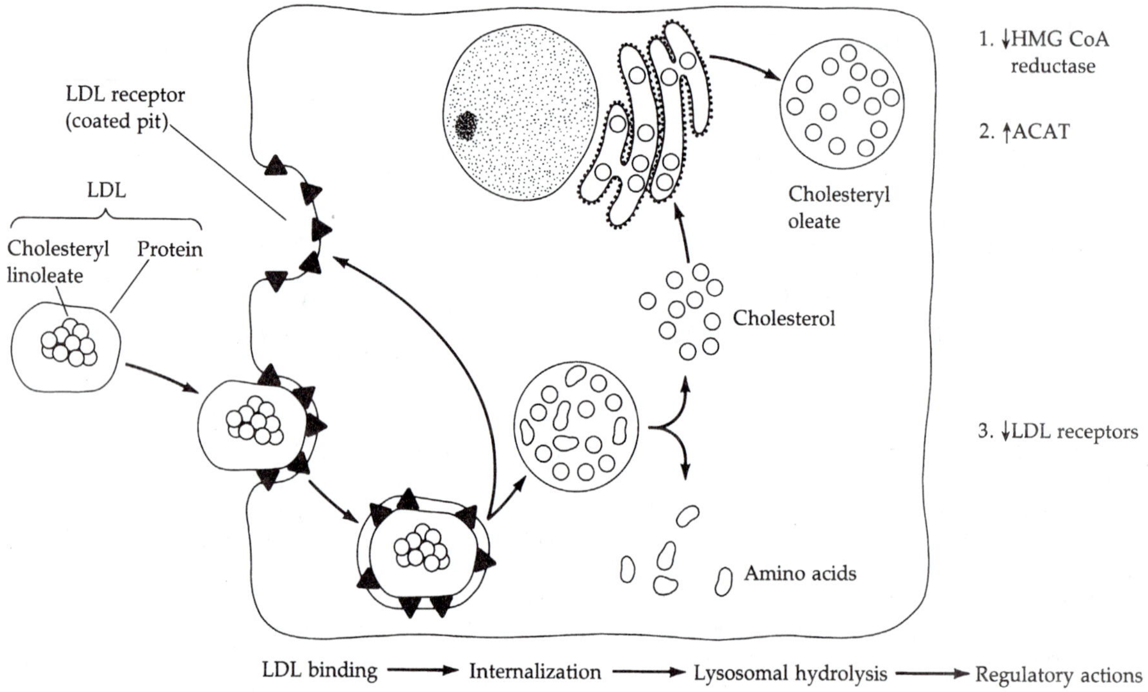

FIGURE 1 Sequential steps in the LDL receptor pathway. Abbreviations: LDL, low-density lipoprotein; HMG CoA reductase, 3-hydroxy-3-methylglutaryl CoA reductase; and ACAT, acyl CoA: cholesterol acyltransferase. (Brown M, Goldstein J. Receptor mediated endocytosis: Insights from the lipoprotein receptor system. Proceedings of Nation Academy of Sciences USA 1979;76:3330. Reprinted with permission.)

glycosylation. This glycosylation, too, occurs during the maturation process of the receptor. The fourth domain is made up of 22 hydrophobic amino acids that, because of their affinity for lipids, are able to span the plasma membrane. The final domain is the COOH terminal end of the protein and projects into the cytoplast. This tail enables the receptors to move laterally, thereby mediating the clustering of the receptors in the coated pits.

Along with the delineation of the structure of the normal LDL receptor, knowledge of the structural defects existing in mutants has developed. Although a gene on chromosome 19 encodes the protein of the LDL receptor, the mutations of the gene are not always the same [2,5,6]. How the normal functioning of the receptor is affected depends on what particular domain(s) of the receptor has undergone mutation. Of the 110 familial hypercholesterolemia homozygotes studied, 10 different abnormal forms of the LDL receptors have been identified [2]. These identified mutations can be divided into four classes:

Class 1, in which no receptors are synthesized

Class 2, in which precursors of the receptors are synthesized but then are not processed properly and fail to move into the Golgi apparatus

Class 3, in which the precursors for the LDL receptors are synthesized and processed but the processing is faulty, thereby preventing the receptors from binding LDL normally

Class 4, mutations that allow production of receptors that reach the surface of the cell and bind LDL but are unable to cluster in the coated pits.

Maturation of the LDL receptor precursor proteins, like other proteins synthesized on the endoplasmic reticulum of the cell, occurs in the cell's Golgi apparatus. Here in the Golgi apparatus the LDL receptors are targeted for their final destination (p. 12). Incomplete or improper processing can prevent the receptor from reaching its proper destination on the plasma membrane.

Relatively few people (1 in 1 million) are homozygous for familial hypercholesterolemia, but many people carry one mutant gene for the disease (1 in 500).

PERSPECTIVE 1 (continued)

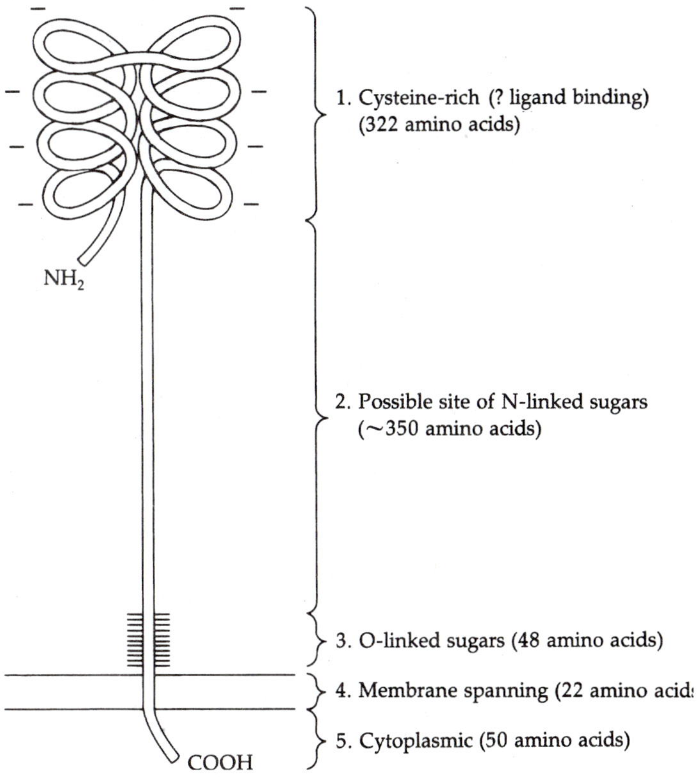

1. Cysteine-rich (? ligand binding)
   (322 amino acids)

2. Possible site of N-linked sugars
   (~350 amino acids)

3. O-linked sugars (48 amino acids)

4. Membrane spanning (22 amino acids)

5. Cytoplasmic (50 amino acids)

FIGURE 2 An illustration of the five domains in the structure of the human LDL receptor. (Yamamoto T et al. The human LDL receptor: A cysteine-rich protein with multiple alu sequences in its mRNA. Cell 1984;39:27–36, copyright © Cell Press. Reprinted with permission.)

Knowledge of the mechanisms of the disease can be of tremendous benefit in treatment of the latter individuals [2]. Although it is still unclear just how hypercholesterolemia leads to development of atherosclerosis [7], there is little doubt about a causal relationship.

Reducing serum cholesterol through drug therapy can cause an increased transcription for LDL receptors by the one normal gene in the heterozygotes, and serum cholesterol can be normalized. Drug therapy includes both bile acid-binding resins, which increase fecal removal of cholesterol, and HMG-CoA reductase inhibitors, which reduce cholesterol synthesis in the liver.

Many people who exhibit no clear-cut genetic defect also are found to possess an inadequate number of LDL receptors. In this population group, nutrition could be the environmental factor, leading to decreased production of LDL receptors. A diet high in saturated fats and cholesterol appears to be one of the culprits.

References

1. Goldstein JL, Brown MS. Familial hypercholesterolemia. In: Stanbury J, Wyngaarden J, Fredreickson D, Goldstein J, Brown M, eds. The metabolic basis of inherited diseases, 5th ed. New York: McGraw-Hill, 1983;672–712.

2. Brown MS, Goldstein JL. A receptor-mediated pathway for cholesterol homeostasis. Science 1986;232:34–47.

3. Yamamoto T, Davis CG, Brown MS, et al. The human LDL receptor: a cysteine-rich protein with multiple Alu sequences in its mRNA. Cell 1984;39:27–38.

4. Cummings RD, Kornfeld S, Schneider W, et al. Biosynthesis of N- and O-linked oligosaccharides of the low density lipoprotein receptor. J Biol Chem 1983;258:15261–15273.

5. Francke U, Brown MS, Goldstein JL. Assignment of the human gene for the low density lipoprotein receptor to chromosome 19: synteny of a receptor, a ligand, and a genetic disease. Proc Natl Acad Sci USA 1984;81:2826–2830.

6. Tolleshaug H, Hobgood KK, Brown MS, Goldstein L. The LDL receptor locus in familial hypercholesterolemia: Multiple mutations disrupt transport and processing of a membrane receptor. Cell 1983;32:941–951.

7. Ross R. The pathogenesis of atherosclerosis—an update. N Engl J Med 1986;314:488–500.

PERSPECTIVE 1 (continued)

Suggested Reading

Brown MS, Goldstein JL. A receptor-mediated pathway
for cholesterol homeostasis. Science 1986; 232:34–47.

This is a superb step-by-step review of the research resulting in the delineation of the LDL receptor, its mechanisms of cholesterol homeostasis, and the therapeutic
implications of these mechanisms.

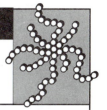

PERSPECTIVE 2

The Possible Role of Omega-3 (n-3) Polyunsaturated Fatty Acids in the Prevention of Heart Disease

Heart disease, cancer, and strokes are, in that order, the first, second, and third leading causes of morbidity and mortality in the United States. Most cases of heart disease and stroke are brought on by arterial thrombosis, which occludes the flow of blood through the vessel and deprives the tissue of needed oxygen. Although the precise etiology of thrombosis is still unclear, the aggregation of platelets, a normal hemostatic (clotting) mechanism, is implicated in the process. The term *atherosclerosis* is commonly used to describe the excessive adhesion of aggregating platelets along an arterial wall accompanied by the deposition of fat. The term *fatty plaque* is used to describe this concurrent accumulation of cells and fat, which is responsible for the narrowing of the arterial lumen.

The factors that initiate the events that lead to plaque formation are not fully understood but may be related to any inflammatory process or injury to the arterial endothelial cells and/or underlying smooth-muscle cells. This can lead to the normal platelet response to aggregate at the site of injury in an effort to plug the damaged area. The adhering platelets secrete a growth factor that stimulates the outgrowth of underlying myoepithelial cells, which then begin to protrude into the lumen. Through receptors for apolipoprotein B, these cells ingest lipoprotein particles and accumulate cholesterol and triacylglycerols, transforming themselves into fat-engorged foam cells. Finally, connective tissue intersperses the plaque, which in advanced situations can become calcified and consequently adds rigidity to the occlusion. Plaque formation and thrombosis can therefore be thought of as an overly aggressive hemostatic process that in turn may be caused by an imbalance among platelet aggregatory and antiaggregatory chemical mediators.

Important in platelet aggregation and function are the eicosanoids (20 carbon compounds), which are metabolically derived from arachidonic acid (20:4 n-6), eicosatrienoic acid (20:3 n-6), and eicosapentaenoic acid (20:5 n-3) by the cyclo-oxygenase pathway. These compounds include the prostaglandin and thromboxane series—potent, bioactive agents that modulate numerous biological functions. Their precursor, arachidonate, is released from specific membrane phospholipid pools, primarily phosphatidyl choline and phosphatidyl isositol, in response to certain stimuli. The specific biological function of each eicosanoid depends on the type of cell being stimu-

lated. Central to the biochemical control of the platelet proaggregatory and antiaggregatory balance is the rate of synthesis of prostaglandin I_2 (PGI_2, or prostacyclin) and PGI_3, relative to that of thromboxane A_2 (TXA_2). Prostacyclin is formed primarily in endothelial tissue such as that of arterial wall structure. It has platelet antiaggregatory activity. This effect is countered by the potent proaggregatory function of TXA_2 produced within the platelets themselves. The synthetic pathways of these antagonistic eicosanoids are shown in Figure 1.

Although it was recognized as early as the 1950s that a negative correlation existed between the ingestion of fish or fish oils and the incidence of heart attacks, it was the later observations of Dyerberg [1] that sparked considerable interest in the relationship [2]. The epidemiologic data on Greenland Eskimos, reported in those studies, clearly showed fewer per capita deaths from heart disease and a 10-fold lower incidence of infarction and stroke. Systematic analyses revealed much lower serum cholesterol, TG, VLDL, and LDL, and higher HDL among those in this population compared to Danish Eskimos, who consume typical Western-type diets. The Danish subjects showed a more "normal" serum lipid profile and were more subject to symptoms of ischemic heart disease. The Greenland Eskimos consume considerably more seafood than their Danish counterparts, averaging 500 g/d, which provide 30 to 40 g of oil. The ratio of n-3 polyunsaturated fatty acids (PUFAs) to n-6 PUFAs in fish oils is very high (4:1) compared to vegetable oils and other animal fats, a fact that leads to the consideration that n-3 fatty acids may be a factor in reducing plaque development. Subsequently it became clear that the n-3 PUFAs were substituting for arachidonic acid in platelet phospholipid pools. This was reflected in a bleeding tendency of the Greenland Eskimos, indicating reduced platelet aggregation and suggesting that less TXA_2 and more PGI_2 may be involved. The following data show relative percentages of PUFA concentrations in platelet lipids as well as the bleeding times of Eskimo and Danish subjects [3].

	Eskimo	Dane
Arachidonic acid (20:4 n-6; AA)	8.5	22.1
Eicosapentaenoic acid (20:5 n-3; EPA)	8.0	0.5
Docosahexaenoic acid (22:6 n-3; DHA)	5.8	1.5
Bleeding time (min)	8.1	4.7

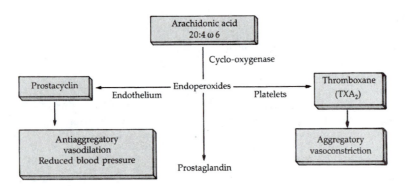

FIGURE 1 Formation of antagonistic eicosanoids from arachidonate.

The antiatherogenic properties of the n-3 fatty acids therefore are due in part to their interference with platelet aggregation. But other investigators have found that fish oil consumption can also dramatically reduce serum lipids. The following data illustrate a comparison of the effects of fish oil and vegetable oil consumption (30 ml/d) on serum lipids (mg/dL) of hyperlipidemic subjects [4]. The same study showed a marked decline in apoB levels relative to that of apoA-1 among subjects on a fish oil diet.

	Control	Fish Oil	Vegetable Oil
Cholesterol (total)	285	199	235
Triacylglycerol (total)	374	137	258
Cholesterol (VLDL)	80	18	46
Triacylglycerol (VLDL)	304	69	177

Among the mechanisms proposed for the lipid-lowering properties of the n-3 PUFA are suppressed fatty acid and triacylglycerol synthesis, inhibition of apolipoprotein synthesis and assembly, and the enhancement of lipoprotein receptor activity. These are only speculative explanations, and a clearer understanding awaits further research.

Perhaps the most plausible explanation for the correlation between high n-3 fatty acid diets and re-

duced incidence of atherogenesis and thrombosis relates to a decrease in TXA_2 production, together with only minimally suppressed concentrations of PGI_2. Further support for the concept that a favorable shift in the balance of these aggregatory–antiaggregatory factors is involved is found in the activity of their analogs, TXA_3 and PGI_3. Both of these substances can be produced directly from the n-3 fatty acid EPA (eicosapentanoic acid). However, while TXA_3 is only a weak agonist of TXA_2, with minimal aggregatory properties, the prostacyclin PGI_3 is significantly bioactive as a platelet antiaggregatory factor.

In summary, the n-3 PUFA found in high concentration in fish oils can displace arachidonic acid from platelet phospholipid stores, thereby reducing available substrate for TXA_2 synthesis.

The n-3s do not appear to significantly reduce endothelial PGI_2, which is antiaggregatory, and in fact they promote the production of its potent agonist, PGI_3, further improving the prostacyclin–thromboxane balance. Included also in the antithrombotic mode of action of the n-3s is their capacity to reduce markedly serum lipid levels in hyperlipemic subjects. The review by Herold and Kinsella [5] summarizes the knowledge dealing with the physiologic effects of the n-3 PUFAs and how they relate to human health and nutrition.

PERSPECTIVE 2 (continued)

References

1. Dyerberg J. Platelet-vessel wall interaction: Influence of diet. Philos Trans Soc Lond 1981;94:373–387.
2. Bang HO, Dyerberg J. Personal reflections on the incidence of ischaemic heart disease in Oslo during the Second World War. Acta Med Scand 1981; 210:245–248.
3. Dyerberg J. Linolenate-derived polyunsaturated fatty acids and prevention of atherosclerosis. Nutr Rev 1986;44:125–134.
4. Phillipson BE, Rothrock DW, Connor WE, Harris WS, Illingworth DR. Reduction of plasma lipids, lipoproteins, and apoproteins by dietary fish oils in patients with hypertriglyceridemia. N Engl J Med 1985;312:1210–1216.
5. Herold PM, Kinsella JE. Fish oil consumption and decreased risk of cardiovascular disease: A comparison of findings from animal and human feeding trials. Am J Clin Nutr 1986;43:566–598.

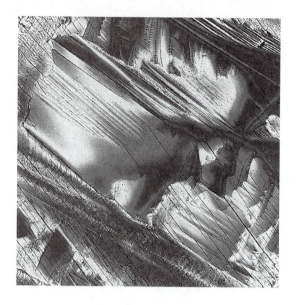

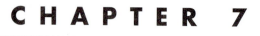

PROTEIN

Photo: Photomicrograph of crystallized glutamine

The importance of protein in nutrition and health cannot be overemphasized. It is quite appropriate that the Greek word chosen as a name for this nutrient is *proteos*, meaning "primary," or "taking first place." Proteins are essential nutritionally because of their constituent amino acids, which the body must have in order to synthesize its own variety of proteins and nitrogen containing molecules that make life possible. Each body protein is unique in the characteristics and pattern of sequencing of the amino acids that comprise its structure.

In a review of protein and amino acid metabolism, an appropriate focus is the functional characteristics of various body proteins and their constituent amino acids, which allows conceptualization of amino acid metabolism in the body as a whole. Also needed is an examination of amino acid metabolism in specific organs and tissues because the enzymes and receptors necessary for certain metabolic pathways are not present in all cells of the body.

The molecular architecture and activity of living cells are largely dependent on proteins, which make up over half of the solid content of cells and which show great variability in size, shape, and physical properties. Their physiologic roles also are quite variable, and because of this variability, a categorization of proteins according to their functions can be helpful in the study of human metabolism. This type of categorization demonstrates the body's dependence on properly functioning proteins and provides a basis for understanding the significance of protein structure.

FUNCTIONAL CATEGORIES

Enzymes

Enzymes exist in vast numbers and are necessary for sustaining life. These protein molecules are constructed so that they combine selectively with other molecules in the cell, thereby catalyzing chemical reactions. Most human physiologic processes require enzymes for promotion of chemical changes that could not otherwise occur. Some examples of physiologic processes dependent on enzyme function include digestion, tissue energy production, blood coagulation, and excitability and contractibility of neuromuscular tissue.

Peptide Hormones

Peptide hormones control many body functions, often by regulating the synthesis or activity of enzymes. Numerous peptide hormones exist, but some that have particular significance for nutrition and human metabolism include insulin, glucagon, parathyroid hormone (PTH), thyroid hormones, adrenocorticotropic hormone (ACTH), somatotropin (growth hormone), and vasopressin (also known as antidiuretic hormone, ADH).

Structural Proteins

Proteins with structural roles include both the contractile proteins of the muscles and the fibrous proteins found in connective tissue and in skin, hair, and nails. Contractile proteins of primary importance are actin and myosin, while the main fibrous protein is collagen. Other fibrous proteins of importance are elastin and keratin.

Transport Proteins

Transport proteins are a diverse group of proteins that combine with other substances in the blood to provide a mode of transport for the substances. Of particular importance among these transport proteins are albumin, transthyretin (formerly called *prealbumin*), hemoglobin, ceruloplasmin, transferrin, and retinol-binding protein. Some of these proteins are discussed further in this chapter under the heading "Plasma Proteins and Nitrogen-Containing Compounds," page 164.

Immunoproteins

Immunoproteins may also be referred to as *immunoglobulins* (Ig) or *antibodies* (Ab). Immunoglobulins are produced by plasma cells derived from B-lymphocytes, a type of white blood cell. Immunoglobulins function by binding to antigens and inactivating them. Antigens typically consist of foreign substances such as bacteria or viruses that have entered the body. By complexing with antigens, immunoglobulin–antigen complexes can be recognized and destroyed through reactions with either complement proteins produced primarily by the liver, or cytokines, produced by white blood cells such as T-

helper cells and macrophages. In addition, the process of phagocytosis by white blood cells such as macrophages and neutrophils also destroys foreign antigens.

BASIC STRUCTURE AND ORGANIZATION

The functional role of protein is determined by its basic structure and organization. The primary, secondary, and tertiary structures of proteins illustrate their three key levels of organization. Some proteins have an additional fourth level of organization, the quaternary structure.

Primary Structure

The primary structure of a protein is the sequencing and strong covalent bonding of amino acids occurring as the polypeptide chain is synthesized on the ribosomes. The primary structure of a protein is shown in Figure 7.1. The various amino acids making up the polypeptide are labeled in sequence and represent the primary structure. The side chain of one amino acid differs from that of another amino acid, thus making each amino acid different. Polypeptide backbones do not differ between polypeptide chains. The side chains of the amino acids of the polypeptide chain or chains making up the total protein molecule account for the differences among proteins. Moreover, the side chains affect the coiling and folding of a protein on itself to (in effect) help determine the final form of the protein molecule.

Secondary Structure

The secondary structure of the protein is achieved through weaker bonding, such as hydrogen bonding, than that which characterizes the primary structure. Weak repeating linkages between nearby amino acids account for this second level of protein organization.

One type of secondary structure of proteins is the α-helix, which is formed by a coiling of the polypeptide chain on itself with interactions occurring at every fourth peptide linkage (Fig. 7.2a). Varying degrees of the alpha helix appear in widely divergent proteins, depending on their function. In those regions where it occurs, the α-helix provides some rigidity to that portion of the molecule.

Another type of secondary protein structure is the β-conformation, or pleated sheet. In this structure, the polypeptide chain is fully stretched out with the side chains positioned either up or down. The stretched polypeptide can fold back on itself with its segments packed together, as shown in Figure 7.2b. Both this

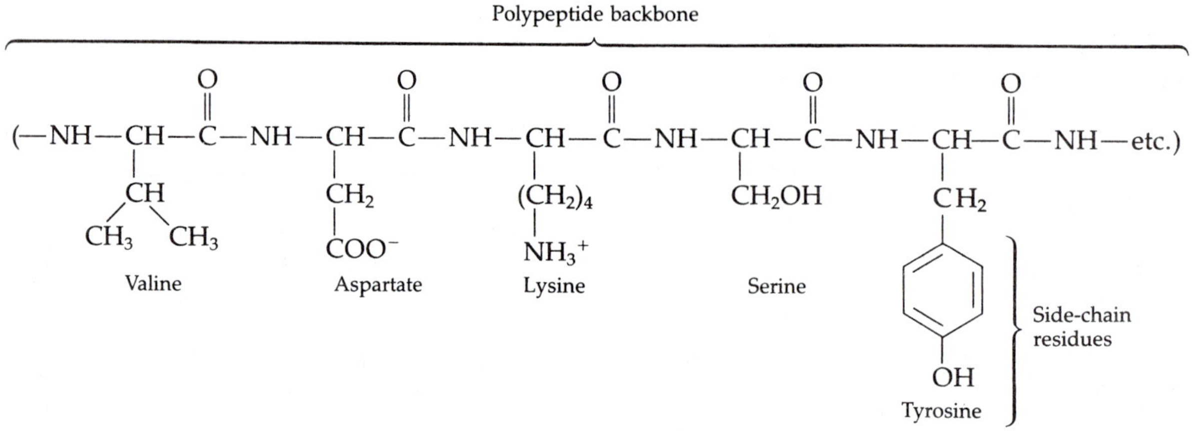

Polypeptide backbone

FIGURE 7.1 The primary structure of proteins.

structure and the α-helix are quite stable and provide strength and rigidity to proteins. These two secondary structures are particularly abundant in proteins with structural roles such as collagen, elastin, and keratin.

The random coil is the third type of secondary structure (Fig. 7.2c). No real stability exists in this structure due to the presence of certain amino acids whose side chains interfere with one another. The interference can be due to the large size of the side chains or the fact that the side chains are carrying similar charges. Proline is an example of an amino acid that, regardless of its location in the peptide chain, cannot participate with other amino acids in forming an α-helix. Whenever proline occurs in the chain, a twist or loop will occur, thereby interrupting the helical form. Table 7.1 shows the structure of proline as well as the other amino acids.

Tertiary Structure

The third level of organization in proteins is the tertiary structure. This structure results from interactions occurring among amino acid residues that are located at considerable linear distances from each other along the peptide chain. These interactions produce the binding and looping of the protein molecule, the result of which can be seen in Figure 7.3. Interactions producing this third level of organization include the (1) clustering together of hydrophobic amino acids toward the center of the protein molecule, (2) electrostatic attraction of oppositely charged amino acid residues, and (3) strong covalent bonding between cysteine residues where the SH groups are oxidized to form disulfide bridges ($-S-S-$). Other weaker attractions among

amino acid residues may also occur along the chain. Taken together, these interactions among the amino acid residues determine the protein's overall shape and, therefore, the particular function of the protein in the cell.

Quaternary Structure

The final level of protein organization, quaternary structure, involves anywhere from two to several polypeptide chains. Proteins with a quaternary structure most commonly are composed of either two or four polypeptide chains, and the aggregate formed is called an *oligomer*. The polypeptides making up the oligomer are commonly termed *subunits* and are held together by hydrogen bonds and electrostatic salt bridges. Oligomeric proteins are particularly important in intracellular regulation because the subunits can assume different spatial orientations relative to each other and in so doing change the properties of the oligomer. Hemoglobin (Fig. 7.4), an oligomer with four subunits, illustrates this point. Each subunit of hemoglobin can bind 1 mol of oxygen. Rather than acting independently, however, the subunits cooperate by conformational changes so as to enhance the affinity of hemoglobin for oxygen in the lungs and to increase its ability to unload oxygen in the peripheral tissues. Other very important oligomers, such as regulatory enzymes, similarly undergo conformational changes on interaction with substrate molecules. In so doing, they enhance the formation of enzyme–substrate complexes whenever the concentration of substrate presented to the cell begins to increase or inhibit the formation of complexes when the substrate concentration falls to a low level.

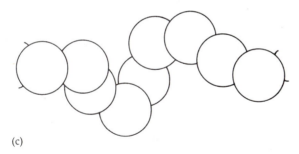

(a)

(b)

(c)

FIGURE 7.2 The secondary structure of proteins: (a) the α helix, (b) the β-pleated sheet, and (c) the random coil.

AMINO ACID CLASSIFICATION

The distinctive characteristics of the side chains of the amino acids making up a polypeptide bestow on a protein its structure, and consequently its functional role in the body. These same distinctive characteristics determine whether certain amino acids can be synthesized in the body or must be ingested. Furthermore, these characteristics program the various amino acids for their specific metabolic pathways in the body. The differences among the side chains of the amino acids that are commonly found in body proteins are shown in Table 7.1.

Over 30 years ago Rose [1] identified the amino acids found in proteins as nutritionally essential (indispensable) or nutritionally nonessential (dispensable). At that time only eight amino acids were found to be essential for adult humans: leucine, isoleucine, valine, lysine, tryptophan, threonine, methionine, and phenylalanine. Histidine was later added to the list of essential amino acids for both children and adults [2]. Arginine may also be essential. Identifying amino acids strictly as dispensable or indispensable, however, is an inflexible classification that allows no gradations, even with decidedly different and/or changing physiologic circumstances. Jackson [3] followed by Laidlaw and Kopple [4] suggested that amino acids be classified according to their functional role (Table 7.2). Table 7.2 illustrates that amino acids that are normally nonessential may become essential under certain physiologic conditions.

DIGESTION AND ABSORPTION

Digestion

Ingested proteins serve as sources of the essential amino acids and are the primary source of the additional nitrogen needed for the synthesis of the nonessential amino acids and nitrogen-containing compounds. Dietary sources of protein include animal products such as meat, poultry, fish, and dairy products, with the exception of butter, sour cream, and cream cheese. Plant products such as grains, grain products, legumes, and vegetables also provide protein. A discussion of protein quality is found at the end of this chapter, page 188. Endogenous proteins presented to the digestive tract represent another source of amino acids and nitrogen to the body. Endogenous proteins include desquamated mucosal cells, which generate about 50 g protein per day, and digestive enzymes and glycoproteins, which generate about 17 g protein per day and are derived from digestive secretions of the salivary glands, stomach, intestine, biliary tract, and pancreas. Some of these endogenous proteins, which may total 60 to 70 g per day, may be digested and provide amino acids available for absorption [5–7]. Digestion of protein and absorption of amino acids are crucial for protein nutriture and metabolism.

Although macronutrient digestion is covered in Chapter 2, this chapter outlines digestion solely with respect to protein. The digestion of exogenous protein begins in the stomach, with the action of hydrochloric acid in gastric juice. Hydrochloric acid release is stimulated by a variety of compounds including the hormone gastrin, the neuropeptide gastrin-releasing peptide (GRP),

TABLE 7.1 Structural Classification of α-amino Acids Present in Proteins

Amino Acids

1. *With aliphatic side chains*

Glycine (Gly)

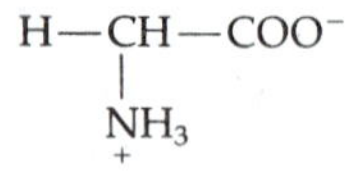

$$H-\underset{\underset{+}{NH_3}}{CH}-COO^-$$

Alanine (Ala)

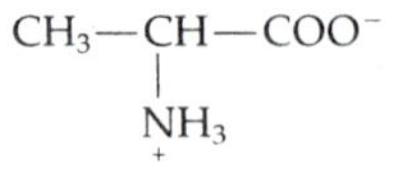

$$CH_3-\underset{\underset{+}{NH_3}}{CH}-COO^-$$

Valine (Va)

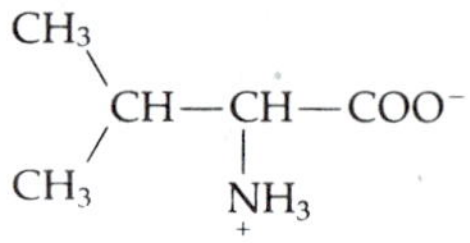

$$\underset{CH_3}{\overset{CH_3}{\diagdown}}CH-\underset{\underset{+}{NH_3}}{CH}-COO^-$$

Leucine (Leu)

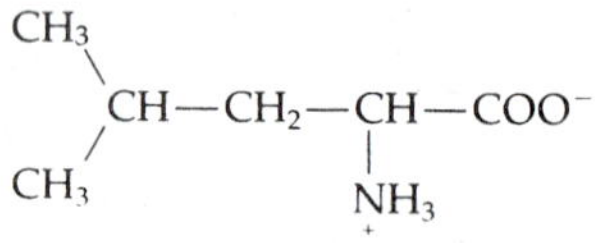

$$\underset{CH_3}{\overset{CH_3}{\diagdown}}CH-CH_2-\underset{\underset{+}{NH_3}}{CH}-COO^-$$

Isoleucine (Ile)

$$\overset{CH_3}{\underset{\underset{CH_3}{|}}{\overset{|}{CH_2}}}CH-\underset{\underset{+}{NH_3}}{CH}-COO^-$$

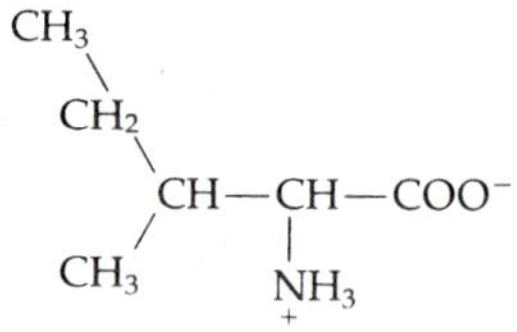

2. *With side chains containing hydroxylic (OH) groups[a]*

Serine (Ser)

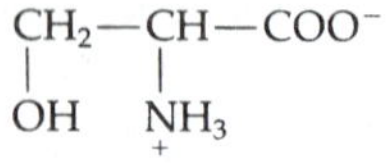

$$\underset{OH}{CH_2}-\underset{\underset{+}{NH_3}}{CH}-COO^-$$

Threonine (Thr)

$$CH_3-\underset{OH}{CH}-\underset{\underset{+}{NH_3}}{CH}-COO^-$$

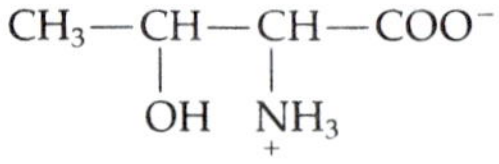

3. *With side chains containing sulfur atoms*

Cysteine (Cys)

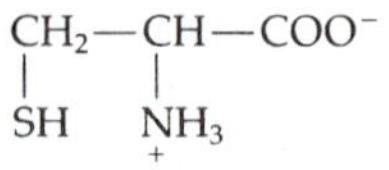

$$\underset{SH}{CH_2}-\underset{\underset{+}{NH_3}}{CH}-COO^-$$

Methionine (Met)

$$\underset{S-CH_3}{CH_2}-CH_2-\underset{\underset{+}{NH_3}}{CH}-COO^-$$

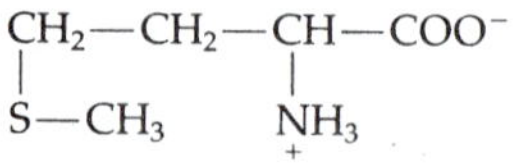

4. *With side chains containing acidic groups or their amides*

Aspartic acid (Asp)

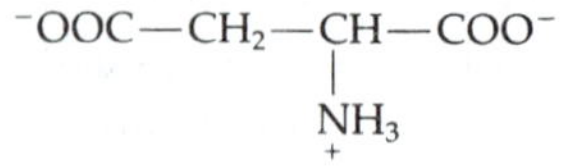

$$^-OOC-CH_2-\underset{\underset{+}{NH_3}}{CH}-COO^-$$

Glutamic acid (Glu)

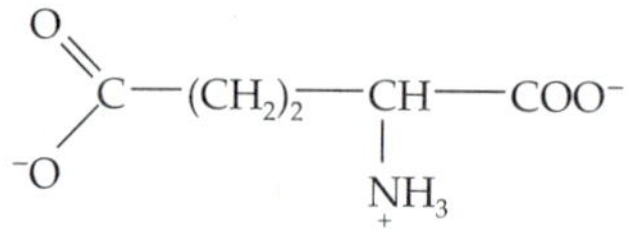

$$\underset{^-O}{\overset{O}{\diagdown}}C-(CH_2)_2-\underset{\underset{+}{NH_3}}{CH}-COO^-$$

Asparagine (Asn)

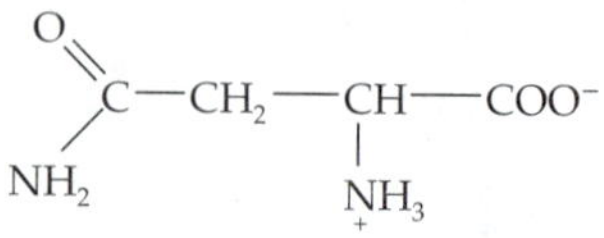

$$\underset{NH_2}{\overset{O}{\diagdown}}C-CH_2-\underset{\underset{+}{NH_3}}{CH}-COO^-$$

Glutamine (Gln)

$$\underset{NH_2}{\overset{O}{\diagdown}}C-(CH_2)_2-\underset{\underset{+}{NH_3}}{CH}-COO^-$$

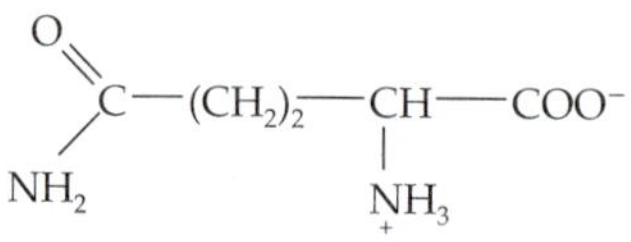

5. *With side chains containing basic groups*

Arginine (Arg)

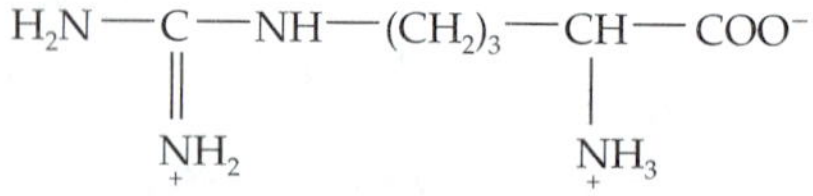

$$H_2N-\underset{\underset{+}{NH_2}}{\overset{\|}{C}}-NH-(CH_2)_3-\underset{\underset{+}{NH_3}}{CH}-COO^-$$

Lysine (Lys)

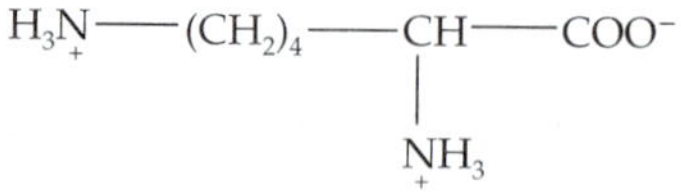

$$\underset{+}{H_3N}-(CH_2)_4-\underset{\underset{+}{NH_3}}{CH}-COO^-$$

Histidine (His)

$$\underset{\underset{H}{N=C-NH}}{HC=C}-CH_2-\underset{\underset{+}{NH_3}}{CH}-COO^-$$

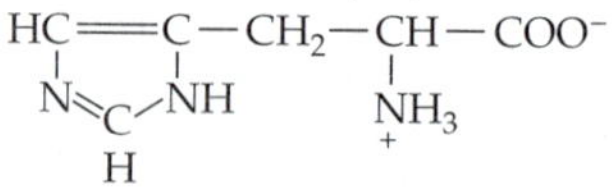

6. *With side chains containing aromatic ring*

Phenylalanine (Phe)

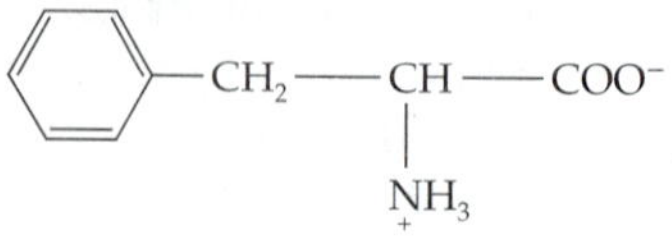

$$-CH_2-\underset{\underset{+}{NH_3}}{CH}-COO^-$$

Tyrosine (Tyr)

$$HO-\bigcirc-CH_2-\underset{\underset{+}{NH_3}}{CH}-COO^-$$

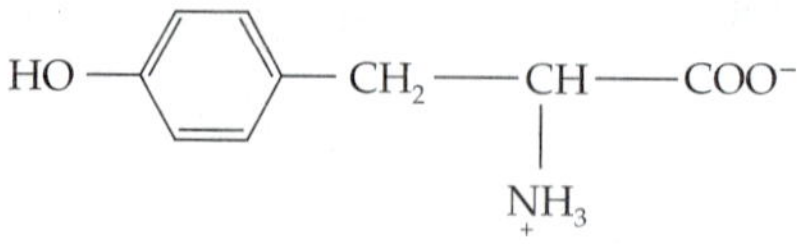

Tryptophan (Trp)

$$-CH_2-\underset{\underset{+}{NH_3}}{CH}-COO^-$$

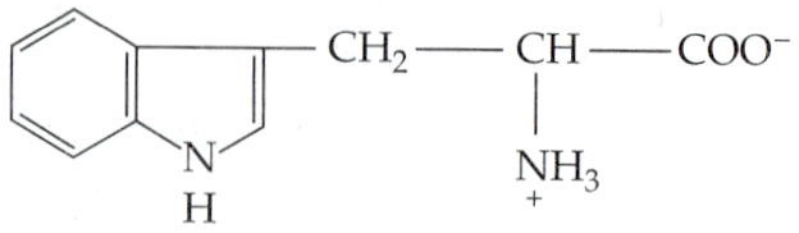

TABLE 7.1 Structural Classification of α-amino Acids Present in Proteins (*continued*)

Amino Acids

7. *Imino acid*
   Proline (Pro)

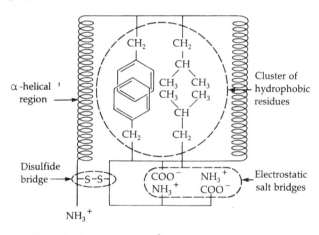

8. *Amino acids formed posttranslationally*
   Cystine (Cys-S-S-Cys)

$^-OOC-CH-CH_2-S-S-CH_2-CH-COO^-$

with NH_3^+ groups

Hydroxylysine (Hyl)

$CH_2-CH-CH_2-CH_2-CH-COO^-$

Hydroxyproline (Hyp)

3-methylhistidine (3-meHis)

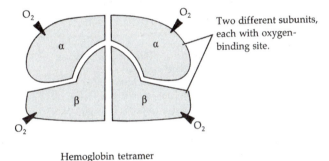

ᵃAlthough tyrosine contains a hydroxylic group, it is classified as an amino acid containing aromatic rings (see Group 6). Also the hydroxylic group on threonine is phenolic in character.

FIGURE 7.3 Tertiary structure of proteins.

FIGURE 7.4 Quaternary structure of proteins.

by acetylcholine, and by histamine. Hydrochloric acid denatures the quaternary, tertiary, and secondary structures of protein and begins the activation of pepsinogen to pepsin. Pepsin, once formed, is catalytic against pepsinogen as well as other proteins. Pepsin functions as an endopeptidase at a pH < 3.5 to hydrolyze peptide bonds in proteins or polypeptides. Pepsin attacks peptide bonds adjacent to the carboxyl end of a relatively wide variety (that is, pepsin has low specificity) of amino acids including leucine, methionine, aromatic amino acids consisting of phenylalanine, tyrosine, and tryptophan, and the dicarboxylic amino acids glutamate and aspartate. The end products of gastric protein digestion with pepsin include primarily large polypeptides along with some oligopeptides and free amino acids. These end products in an acid chyme are emptied through the pyloric sphincter into the duodenum for further digestion and serve to stimulate the release of regulatory peptides such as secretin and cholecystokinin (CCK) from the mucosal endocrine cells. Secretin and CCK are carried by the blood to the pancreas where the acinar cells are stimulated to secrete alkaline pancreatic juice along with digestive proenzymes.

Digestive proenzymes or zymogens secreted by the pancreas, and responsible on activation for protein and polypeptide digestion, include trypsinogen, chymotrypsinogen, procarboxypeptidases A and B, proelastase, and collagenase. Pancreatic zymogen secretion is stimulated by hormones such as cholecystokinin and also appears to be regulated by luminal dietary protein [5]. Within the small intestine, trypsinogen is converted to trypsin by enteropeptidase (an endopeptidase for-

TABLE 7.2 Functional Classification of Amino Acids

I. Indispensable amino acids (negative nitrogen balance results whenever there is a deficiency)
  A. *Totally indispensable:* lysine and threonine. No metabolic precursor can substitute for these amino acids; omission from diet can lead to serious nutritional and metabolic effects.
  B. *Carbon skeleton indispensable amino acids:* histidine, isoleucine, leucine, methionine, phenylalanine, tryptophan, and valine. The keto or hydroxy acid of each amino acid can be converted into its respective amino acid through transamination.
II. Conditionally indispensable amino acids: cysteine, tyrosine. Cysteine and tyrosine can reduce the requirements for the indispensable amino acids methionine and phenylalanine, respectively. Furthermore, under certain conditions cysteine and tyrosine may become indispensable themselves.
III. Acquired indispensable amino acids (may become indispensable in immaturity, in states of metabolic disorder, and/or during severe stress):
  A. *Possibly indispensable during immaturity:* cysteine and tyrosine. These two amino acids may become indispensable in the neonate.
  B. *Possibly indispensable due to genetic disorders or acquired disease states:* cysteine, tyrosine, arginine, and citrulline[a]
  C. *Possibly indispensable due to extended periods of large intakes of amino acids* (e.g., TPN): cysteine, tyrosine, arginine; possibly citrulline[a] and taurine[b]
IV. Completely dispensable amino acids (extensively synthesized in the body and not essential components of the diet): alanine, glutamic acid, aspartic acid, glycine, serine, proline, glutamine, asparagine

[a]Citrulline is not used in protein synthesis, but along with arginine, it plays a critical role in the urea cycle. Both citrulline and arginine may become essential in disease states where hyperammonemia occurs (urea cycle disorders).
[b]Taurine, like citrulline, is not used in protein synthesis but normally occurs in high concentrations in the body. A deficiency of taurine has been indicated in abnormal retinal functioning, particularly among young children who have been maintained for long periods on total parenteral nutrition (TPN).
Source: Adapted from Laidlaw SA. Indispensable amino acids. Nutrition & the M.D. 1986;12:3.

merly known as *enterokinase*), which is secreted from the intestinal brush border in response to CCK and secretin. Once trypsin is formed, it can act on more trypsinogen as well as on chymotrypsinogen to yield active proteolytic enzymes. Trypsin and chymotrypsin are both endopeptidases. Trypsin is specific for peptide bonds adjacent to dibasic amino acids (lysine and arginine). Excess free trypsin generated from trypsinogen also acts by negative feedback to inhibit pancreatic cell trypsinogen synthesis, thereby regulating pancreatic zymogen secre-

tion [5]. Chymotrypsin is specific for peptide bonds adjacent to aromatic amino acids (phenylalanine, tyrosine, and tryptophan), as well as for methionine, asparagine, and histidine. Both elastase, an endopeptidase derived from proelastase, and collagenase hydrolyze polypeptides into smaller fragments such as oligopeptides and tripeptides. Procarboxypeptidases are converted to carboxypeptidases by trypsin and serve as exopeptidases. These exopeptidases attack peptide bonds at the C-terminal end of polypeptides to release free amino acids. Carboxypeptidases are zinc-dependent enzymes, specifically requiring zinc at its active site. Carboxypeptidase A hydrolyses peptides with C-terminal aromatic neutral or aliphatic neutral amino acids. Carboxypeptidase B cleaves dibasic amino acids from the C-terminal, generating free dibasic amino acids as end products.

Several peptidases are produced by the brush border of the small intestine, including the ileum, enabling peptide digestion and amino acid absorption to occur in the distal small intestine. Aminopeptidases varying in specificity cleave amino acids from the N-terminal end of oligopeptides. Dipeptidlyaminopeptidases, some of which are magnesium dependent, hydrolyze N-terminal amino acids from dipeptides. Tripeptidases specific for selected amino acids are also found on the intestinal brush border and hydrolyze tripeptides to yield a dipeptide and a free amino acid. Some tripeptides, such as trileucine, undergo brush border hydrolysis, while other tripeptides such as triglycine or proline-containing peptides are absorbed intact and are hydrolyzed within the intestinal cell [6–11]. Amino acids (an end product of protein digestion) have also been shown to inhibit the activity of brush border peptidases (end product inhibition) [7]. Table 7.3 outlines the process of protein digestion.

In addition to being found on the brush border, peptidases are also found within the cytoplasm of intestinal mucosal cells. These peptidases function intracellularly to hydrolyze peptides that have been absorbed intact into the intestinal cell. Thus, the end products of protein digestion within the gastrointestinal tract are peptides, principally dipeptides and tripeptides, and free amino acids. Yet once within the enterocyte, amino acids represent the end product of protein digestion.

Brush Border Absorption

Amino acid absorption occurs along the entire small intestine, but sites of maximal absorption of peptides and their component amino acids differ. In general, most amino acids are absorbed in the proximal small intestine. Less than 5% of ingested nitrogen or up to about 10 g protein is excreted daily in the feces [5]; under normal cir-

TABLE 7.3 Some Enzymes Responsible for Digestion of Protein

Zymogen	⟶	Enzyme	Site of Activity	Substrate (Peptide Bonds Adjacent to)
Pepsinogen	HCl or ⟶ Pepsin	Pepsin	Stomach	Most amino acids, including aromatic, dicarboxylic, leu, met
Trypsinogen	Enteropeptidase ⟶ or Trypsin	Trypsin	Intestine	Dibasic amino acids
Chymotrypsinogen	Trypsin ⟶	Chymotrypsin	Intestine	Aromatic amino acids, met, asn, his
Procarboxypeptidases	Trypsin ⟶	Procarboxypeptidase A B	Intestine	C-terminal neutral amino acids C-terminal dibasic amino acids
—		Aminopeptidases	Intestine	N-terminal amino acids

cumstances colonic bacterial proteases have little effect on protein digestion and amino acid absorption [7].

Multiple energy-dependent transport systems with overlapping specificity for amino acids have been demonstrated in the intestinal brush border. Both sodium-dependent and sodium-independent transport systems exist. Figure 7.5 represents a schematic of sodium-dependent amino acid transport [12]. As shown in Figure 7.5, sodium binds to the carrier first and appears to increase the affinity of the carrier for the amino acid. Next, a sodium–amino acid–cotransporter complex forms. This step is followed by a conformational change in the complex that results in the delivery of the sodium and amino acid into the cytoplasm of the enterocyte. Sodium is pumped out of the cell by Na^+/K^+- ATPase.

Transport systems for amino acids are designated using a lettering system with a further distinction that uppercase letters be used for sodium dependence and lowercase letters be used for sodium independence [8,13]; however, not all systems follow this rule. Carrier systems (Table 7.4) are thought to be present in enterocytes for (1) the dibasic amino acids lysine and arginine plus cystine and ornithine, (2) the dicarboxylic amino acids aspartate and glutamate, as well as (3) the neutral amino acids. In fact, several neutral transport systems are thought to exist in the brush border of the intestine. Some of the different brush border amino acid transport systems include the L, NBB or B, IMINO, y+, and PHE systems [8]. Not all systems, however, have been identified in humans. The L system—an exception to the letter ruling—is sodium independent, and its preferred substrates are leucine and other neutral amino acids. The B system, formerly called the NBB system, transports neutral amino acids such as threonine and alanine.

The IMINO system transports proline across the brush border. Both the B and IMINO systems are sodium dependent. The y+ system is sodium independent and transports dibasic amino acids. In the presence of sodium, however, neutral amino acids can competitively inhibit the y+ system and participate in exchange reactions with the dibasic substrates [14]. The PHE system transports phenylalanine and methionine and is sodium dependent.

Competition between amino acids for transport by a common carrier has been documented. In addition, regulation (both induced *de novo* synthesis of specific amino acid carriers and decreased carrier synthesis) of transport carriers has been shown, and helps to ensure adequate absorptive capacity [14].

The affinity (K_m) of a carrier for an amino acid is influenced by both the hydrocarbon mass of the amino acid's side chain and by the net electrical charge of the amino acid. As the hydrocarbon mass of the side chain increases, affinity increases [7,15]. Thus, the branched-chain amino acids typically are absorbed faster than smaller amino acids. Neutral amino acids also tend to be absorbed at higher rates than dibasic or dicarboxylic amino acids. Essential amino acids are absorbed faster than nonessential amino acids, with methionine, leucine, isoleucine, and valine being the most rapidly absorbed [15]. The most slowly absorbed amino acids are the two dicarboxylic amino acids, glutamate and aspartate, both of which are nonessential [15].

Ingesting free, crystalline L-amino acids is thought by many athletes to be superior to ingesting natural foods containing protein for muscle protein synthesis. However, amino acids using the same carrier system compete with each other for absorption. Thus, ingesting one or a particular group of amino acids that use the same carrier

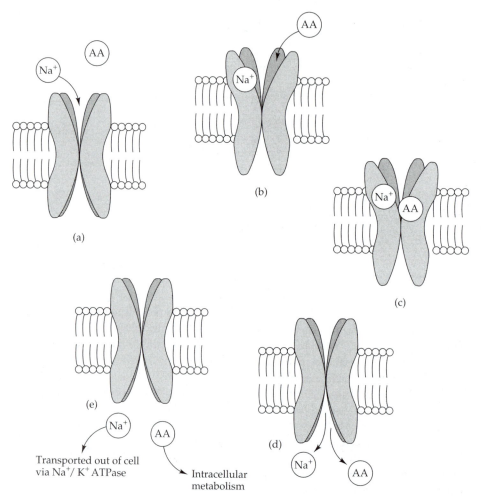

FIGURE 7.5 Conceptual schematic of a membrane-bound sodium-dependent amino acid carrier. a. In the "preferred random" binding model, amino acid AA transport is favored when the activator sodium ion (Na+) binds preferentially to the transporter. b. Initial binding of the sodium ion increases the affinity of the extracellularly oriented cotransporter binding site for subsequent amino acid attachment. c. A sodium/amino acid/cotransporter complex is formed. d. A conformational change of the complex results in delivery of the sodium ion and the amino acid into the cytoplasm of the cell. e. The translocated sodium ion is transported out of the cell by the sodium/potassium adenosine triphosphatase (Na+/K+ ATPase) transporter to maintain the electrochemical gradient, whereas the amino acid is metabolized within the cell. *(Souba WW, Pacitti AJ. How amino acids get into cells: mechanisms, models, menus, and mediators. J Parent and Enter Nutr. 1992;16:569–578. © by The American Society of Parenteral and Enteral Nutrition.)*

system may create, depending on the amount ingested, a competition between the amino acids for absorption. The result may be such that the amino acid present in highest concentration is absorbed, but also may impair the absorption of the other less concentrated amino acids carried by that same system. Thus, amino acid supplements may result in impaired or imbalanced amino acid absorption. Furthermore, absorption of peptides (which are obtained from digestion of natural protein-containing foods) is more rapid than absorption of an equivalent mixture of free amino acids. And nitrogen assimilation following ingestion of protein-containing foods is supe-

rior to that following ingestion of free amino acids. In other words, free amino acids have no absorptive advantage. Moreover, the supplements are typically expensive, taste terrible, and may cause gastrointestinal distress.

Peptide transport into the enterocyte occurs by transport systems different from those which transport amino acids. The number of transport systems for peptides has not been determined. Sodium has been shown to be required for one of the carrier systems that transports both dipeptides and tripeptides [8]. Affinity of the carrier for the peptide appears to be influenced by stereoisomerism, length of side chain of the N-terminal amino acid, substi-

TABLE 7.4 Systems Transporting Amino Acids Across the Intestinal Cell

Intestinal Amino Acid Transport Systems	Sodium Required	Examples of Substrates Carried
L	No	Leucine, other neutral amino acids
B	Yes	Threonine, alanine, other neutral amino acids
IMINO	Yes	Proline
y+	No	Dibasic amino acids
PHE	Yes	Phenylalanine, methionine
A	Yes	Alanine, other short-chain, polar amino acids
ASC	Yes	Alanine, cysteine, serine, other 3- and 4-carbon amino acids
asc	No	Same substrates as ASC

tutions on the N- and C-terminals, as well as by the number of amino acid residues in the peptide [6–8,16–19].

Peptide transport is thought to represent the primary system for amino acid absorption. Sixty-seven percent of amino acids are absorbed in the form of small peptides, with the remaining 33% absorbed as free amino acids [20].

Basolateral Absorption

The transport of the amino acids through the basolateral membrane of the enterocyte into the interstitial fluid appears to be the same as the transport of amino acids across the membrane of nonepithelial cells [8,21]. Some of the basolateral transport systems include (1) the L system, which is sodium independent and broadly selective for leucine and other neutral amino acids; (2) the y+ system, also sodium independent, specific for dibasic amino acids; (3) the A system, which is sodium dependent and specific for short-chain, polar, neutral amino acids such as alanine; and (4) the ASC (sodium-dependent) and asc (sodium-independent) systems, which both transport three- and four-carbon neutral amino acids including alanine, serine, and cysteine. Diffusion and sodium-independent transport are thought to be the primary modes of basolateral membrane transport in the enterocyte. Sodium-dependent pathways are quantitatively important when the amino acid concentrations are low in the gut lumen. Active transport into the enterocytes is necessary to provide the enterocyte with amino acids for its own maintenance [21].

Intestinal Amino Acid Use and Absorption into Extraintestinal Tissues

Once transported across the basolateral membrane of the enterocyte into interstitial fluid, amino acids enter the capillaries of the villi and eventually the portal vein for transport to the liver. Most peptides that have been absorbed intact into the intestinal cell undergo hydrolysis by proteases present within the cytoplasm of the enterocyte. Thus, primarily free amino acids are found in portal circulation. Occasionally, however, small oligopeptides can be found in splanchnic circulation and are thought to have entered circulation by paracellular or intercellular routes, that is, passing through tight junctions of mucosal cells or by transcellular endocytosis [22]. Hydrolysis of these peptides may occur by peptidases or proteases in the plasma, at the cell membrane especially the liver, kidney, and muscle, or intracellularly in the cytosol and in various organelles [19,22].

Not all amino acids, however, are transported out of the intestinal cell and into circulation. Many of the amino acids absorbed following protein ingestion are used along the villus for protein synthesis. Within the intestinal cell, amino acids may be used to synthesize (1) new proteins such as apoproteins necessary for lipoprotein formation, new digestive enzymes, and hormones; or (2) nitrogen-containing compounds such as glutathione, which functions along with the selenium-dependent enzyme glutathione peroxidase to destroy hydrogen peroxides (H_2O_2) and other toxic compounds. Amino acid metabolism within the enterocytes includes synthesis of nonessential amino acids such as (1) proline (synthesized from glutamate), and (2) alanine (synthesized through transamination with glutamate, although alanine transamination with aspartate also occurs within the intestinal cell). In addition, four other nitrogen-containing compounds are synthesized within the enterocyte: (1) citrulline is synthesized within the intestinal cell from ornithine and carbamoyl phosphate; (2) ornithine along with (3) urea is synthesized from arginine metabolism in intestinal cells; and lastly, (4) carbamoyl phosphate is synthesized from ammonia and CO_2 in mucosal epithelial cells. Citrulline, once made, is released into blood and then typically taken up by the kidney, which has a high capacity for arginine synthesis.

Glutamine is thought to have trophic effects on the gastrointestinal mucosa cells and is used by intestinal cells as a primary source of energy. This role of glutamine in the gastrointestinal tract has prompted several companies to add or enrich enteral nutrition products with glutamine. Glutamine is being added also to parenteral (intravenous) nutritional mixtures and used for hospitalized patients. Glutamine catabolism generates both ammonia, which enters portal blood, and glutamate, which can undergo subsequent transamination to generate α-ketoglutarate, an intermediate in the Krebs

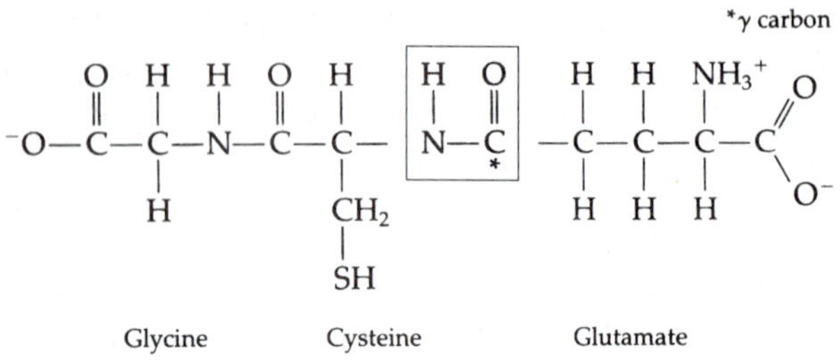

FIGURE 7.6 The structure of glutathione (GSH).

cycle. The amino nitrogen, from glutamine metabolism as well as from aspartate and glutamate metabolism, is primarily used to generate alanine. Alanine then leaves the intestinal cell and enters portal blood. These reactions are shown later in this chapter in Figures 7.15 and 7.16.

Although some amino acids are used by the enterocytes, most amino acids are transported from the intestinal cell by the portal vein to the liver. Amino acid transport into liver cells (hepatocytes) occurs by some carrier systems similar to those within the intestinal basolateral membrane. Additional systems also transport amino acids into the liver. The sodium-dependent N system transports glutamine and histidine into hepatocytes [14,23]. Hormones, cytokines such as interleukin-1, and tumor necrosis factor alpha have been shown to influence amino acid transport. System A in hepatocytes, for example, is induced by glucagon [14], and provides amino acid substrates for gluconeogenesis. Extrahepatic tissues such as the kidneys are also thought to transport amino acids by systems similar to those described for the intestinal basolateral membrane. However, an additional system, the γ-glutamyl cycle proposed by Meister [24,25], is thought to be important in transporting amino acids through membranes of renal tubular cells, erythrocytes, and perhaps neurons.

In the γ-glutamyl cycle, glutathione acts as a carrier of selected neutral amino acids into cells. Glutathione, found in most cells of the body, is a tripeptide consisting of glycine, cysteine, and glutamate. As shown in Figure 7.6, an unusual peptide linkage occurs in glutathione between the γ-carboxyl group of glutamate and the α-amino group of cysteine. In the γ-glutamyl cycle (Fig. 7.7), glutathione reacts with γ-glutamyl transpeptidase located in cell membranes to form a γ-glutamyl enzyme complex. The glutamate part of the glutathione molecule remains with the enzyme complex; cysteinylglycine is released into the cell cytoplasm and is eventually cleaved into its constituent amino acids by a cytosolic peptidase. The γ-glutamyl enzyme complex functions

by binding to a neutral amino acid at the cell surface and carries it via a γ-carboxyl peptide linkage into the cell. Within the cell, γ-glutamyl cyclotransferase can cleave the peptide bond between the neutral amino acid and the γ-carbon of glutamate. Glutathione is resynthesized within the cell from cysteine, glutamate, and glycine in a series of energy-dependent reactions; the neutral amino acid that has just been released within the cell may function in the synthesis of new proteins or nitrogen-containing molecules or may be catabolized. An overview of amino acid metabolism is shown in Figure 7.8 and will be referred to throughout the chapter.

AMINO ACID METABOLISM

The liver is the primary site for the uptake of most of the amino acids following ingestion of a meal. The liver is thought to monitor the absorbed amino acids and to adjust the rate of their metabolism according to the needs of the body [5]. For example, essential amino acid intakes in excess of needs or requirements result in increased hepatic degradative enzyme activity against the amino acid present in excess. Moreover, increased synthesis of the degradative enzymes and reduced enzyme catabolism occurs following ingestion of protein-containing meals [5].

Of the amino acids entering the liver, 57% are typically catabolized. About 20% of the amino acids entering the liver are used in the synthesis of both proteins, such as enzymes that will remain in the liver (14%) and proteins that will be released into the plasma (6%) [5]. Amino acids released into systemic circulation represent approximately 23% of the total and consist of primarily the branched-chain amino acids (BCAAs): isoleucine, leucine, and valine [5].

Hepatic Amino Acids

20% protein synthesis $\begin{cases} 14\% \text{ remains in liver} \\ 6\% \text{ released into blood} \end{cases}$

57% catabolized

23% released as free amino acids into blood

Plasma Proteins and Nitrogen-Containing Compounds

The liver cells, like other body cells, synthesize and retain many of the proteins it makes especially enzymes; other proteins, however, are released into the plasma. The concentration of total protein in human plasma typically ranges up to 7.5 g/dL. The proteins found in

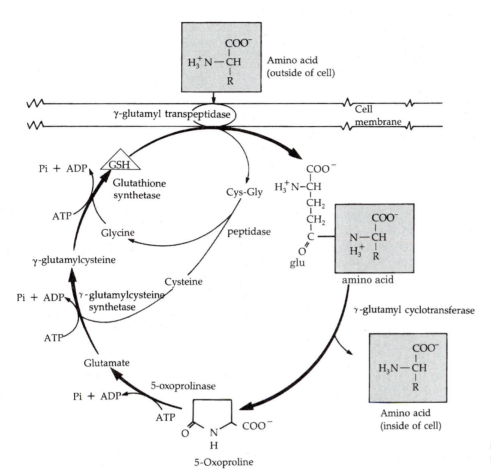

FIGURE 7.7 The γ-glutamyl cycle for transport of amino acids.

plasma consist of primarily glycoproteins, but also include simple proteins and lipoproteins.

Indicators of Visceral Protein Status Several of the proteins in the plasma are used to assess an individual's protein status, specifically visceral (internal organ) protein status. Albumin, the most abundant of the plasma proteins, is synthesized by the liver and is used quite extensively as an indicator of visceral protein status. Albumin functions in the plasma to maintain oncotic pressure as well as to transport nutrients such as vitamin B_6; minerals including zinc, calcium, and small amounts of copper; nutrients such as fatty acids; and the amino acid tryptophan. Some drugs and hormones such as the thyroid hormones are also transported by albumin. Because of albumin's relatively long half-life (about 14 to 18 days), it is not as good or as sensitive an indicator of visceral protein status as some of the other plasma proteins.

Other proteins synthesized by the liver and released into plasma include transthyretin (formerly called *prealbumin*) and retinol-binding protein (complexed together and involved with retinol and thyroid hormone transport), blood-clotting proteins, and globulins. There are several classes of globulins. α_1-globulins include various glycoproteins and high-density lipoproteins (HDL). α_2-globulins include various glycoproteins, haptoglobin for free hemoglobin transport, ceruloplasmin for copper transport and oxidase activity, prothrombin for blood coagulation, and very low density lipoproteins (VLDL). β-globulins include transferrin for iron and other mineral transport and low-density lipoprotein (LDL). γ-globulins include immunoglobulins or antibodies. Transthyretin and retinol-binding protein have relatively short half-lives (about two days and 12 hours respectively) and thus are more sensitive indicators of changes in visceral protein status than albumin.

Nitrogen-containing compounds or molecules (Fig. 7.8 and Table 7.5) can also be synthesized from amino acids. For example, *glutathione* is found in most cells of

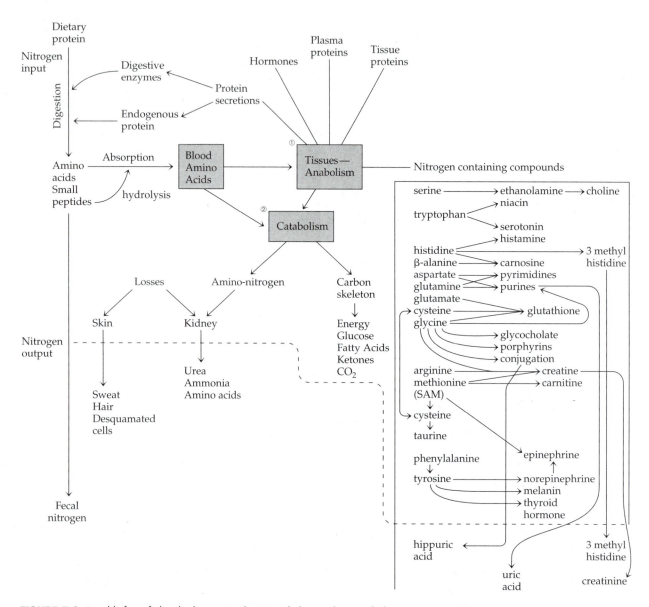

FIGURE 7.8 Possible fate of absorbed amino acids: (1) anabolism and (2) catabolism.

the body. It is synthesized from glycine, cysteine, and glutamate, and functions both in the γ-glutamyl cycle and with glutathione peroxidase (p. 383) to protect cells from, for example, hydrogen peroxides (H_2O_2) and lipid hydroperoxides (LOOHs). Glutathione is also used to synthesize leukotriene (LT) LTC_4. *Carnitine*, another nitrogen-containing compound, is needed for the transport of long-chain fatty acids into the mitochondria for oxidation. Carnitine may also be involved in branched-chain amino acid metabolism as well as immune function [26]. Carnitine is found preformed in foods such as beef and pork. Carnitine is absorbed in

the proximal small intestine by sodium-dependent active transport. Approximately 54 to 87% of carnitine intake is absorbed. Carnitine may also be synthesized in the body from lysine, which has been methylated using methyl groups derived from methionine. Iron and vitamins B_6, C, and niacin participate in the synthesis of carnitine (shown on p. 230) [26]. Synthesis of carnitine occurs in several tissues, including the liver and kidney, but not muscle. Muscle, however, represents the primary carnitine pool. Carnitine homeostasis is maintained principally by the kidney, with greater than 84% of filtered carnitine being reabsorbed. Carnitine defi-

TABLE 7.5 Sources of Nitrogen for the Nitrogen-Containing Compounds

Nitrogen-Containing Compound	Constituent Amino Acids
Glutathione	Cys, gly, glu
Carnitine	Lys, met
Creatine	Arg, gly, met
Carnosine	His, β-ala

ciency results in impaired energy metabolism [26]; however, carnitine deficiency is quite rare. Advertisements marketing carnitine supplements to help one burn fat or give one energy are making false claims. *Creatine*, a key component of the energy compound creatine phosphate, is synthesized initially in the kidney where arginine and glycine react to form guanidinoacetic acid. This compound is then methylated in the liver, using methionine (as SAM, S-adenosyl methionine) as a methyl donor. Creatine is phosphorylated in muscle by ATP to form creatine phosphate. *Carnosine*, derived from histidine and beta alanine, functions in nerve transmission and possibly as a neurotransmitter and activator of myosin ATPase.

Another group of nitrogen-containing compounds derived in part from amino acids are *purine and pyrimidine bases* (Fig. 7.8). A brief review of purine and pyrimidine synthesis and degradation follows.

The synthesis of the nitrogen-containing bases of nucleotides occurs for the most part *de novo* in the liver. Synthesis of the pyrimidines uracil, cytosine, and thymine, is initiated by the formation of carbamoyl phosphate from glutamine, CO_2, and ATP. The enzyme carbamoyl phosphate synthetase II catalyzes this reaction in the cytoplasm and is distinct from carbamoyl phosphate synthetase I, which is needed in the initial step of urea synthesis and is found in the mitochondria. Carbamoyl phosphate reacts with the amino acid aspartate to form N-carbamoylaspartate. Aspartate transcarbamoylase catalyzes the reaction, which is the committed step in pyrimidine biosynthesis. Synthesis of the pyrimidine bases is illustrated in Figure 7.9. Once uridine monophosphate (UMP) is formed, UMP may react with other nucleoside di- and triphosphates. The formation of d-thymidine monophosphate (dTMP) from deoxyuridine monophosphate (dUMP) should be noted particularly. ATP can phosphorylate dTMP to form dTTP. In the synthesis of DNA, dTTP (deoxythymidine triphosphate) replaces UTP, uridine triphosphate.

Purines, adenine and guanine, are synthesized *de novo* as nucleoside monophosphates by sequential addition of carbons and nitrogens to ribose-P that has orig-

inated from the hexose monophosphate shunt. As shown in Figure 7.10a, ribose 5-P reacts with ATP to form phosphoribosyl pyrophosphate (PRPP). Glutamine donates a nitrogen to form 5-phosphoribosylamine. This step represents the committed step in purine nucleotide synthesis. Next in a series of reactions nitrogen and carbon atoms from glycine are added, formylation occurs by methenyl tetrahydrofolate (THF, a form of the B vitamin folate), another nitrogen atom is donated by the amide group of glutamine, and ring closure occurs. Another set of reactions occurs and involves the addition of carbons from CO_2 and from N^{10} formyl THF (from folate), and a nitrogen from aspartate. Thus, the purine ring as shown in Figure 7.10b is derived from amino acids, including glutamine, glycine, and aspartate, as well as from folate and CO_2.

The formation of individual purine bases and nucleotides is shown in Figure 7.10c. Inosine monophosphate (IMP) is used to synthesize adenosine monophosphate (AMP) and guanosine monophosphate (GMP). AMP and GMP are phosphorylated to ADP and GDP respectively by ATP. The deoxyribotides are formed at the diphosphate level by converting ribose to deoxyribose, thereby producing dADP and dGDP. ADP can be phosphorylated to ATP via oxidative phosphorylation; the remaining nucleotides are phosphorylated to their triphosphate form by ATP. Purine nucleotides can also be synthesized by the salvage pathways, whereby purine bases react with PRPP to form the mononucleotides.

Degradation of pyrimidines involves the sequential hydrolysis of the nucleoside triphosphates to mononucleotides, nucleosides, and finally to free bases. This process can be accomplished in most cells by lysosomal enzymes. During catabolism of pyrimidines, the ring is opened with the production of CO_2 and ammonia from the carbamoyl portion of the molecule. The ammonia can be converted to urea and excreted. Malonyl CoA and methylmalonyl CoA, produced from the remainder of the ring, follow their normal metabolic pathways, therefore requiring no special excretion route.

Purines are progressively oxidized primarily in the liver, yielding hypoxanthine, xanthine, and uric acid. Xanthine dehydrogenase or oxidase, molybdenum- and iron-dependent enzymes, catalyze these two reactions shown in Figure 7.11. Uric acid normally is excreted in the urine; however, about 200 mg uric acid is excreted daily into the digestive tract [27]. Under pathologic conditions such as gout or with renal failure, the uric acid may accumulate in the blood and deposit in and around joints. Furthermore, under conditions of oxygen deprivation, as with a myocardial infarction or intestinal ischemia, xanthine dehydrogenase may be converted to

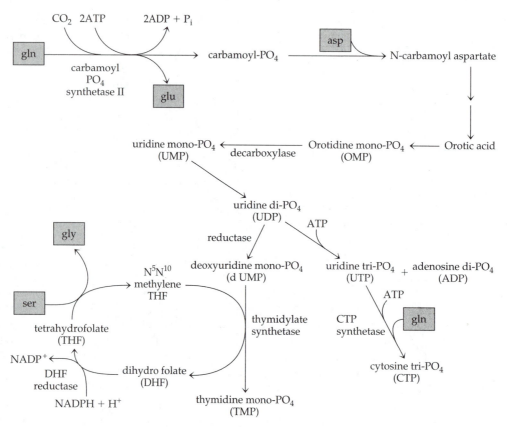

FIGURE 7.9 Pyrimidine synthesis.

xanthine oxidase. Reperfusion of the tissue with oxygen can result in increased hydrogen peroxide and free radical concentrations. Hydrogen peroxide and free radicals may further damage the injured tissues. Research involving introduction of enzymes and antioxidant nutrients to help minimize tissue damage with reoxygenation is ongoing.

**Sources of Amino Acids for Metabolism:
Plasma Amino Acids and Amino Acid Pool(s)**

The liver releases 23% of ingested amino acids without metabolism and of this amount 70% of the free amino acids leaving the liver via the plasma are the branched-chain amino acids (BCAAs) [5]. The BCAAs are primarily taken up and transaminated by the skeletal muscles and, to a lesser extent, by tissues such as the heart, brain, and kidneys. Transferases needed in the first step of BCAA catabolism are limited in the liver. Hepatic transferases increase in response to glucocorticoid (cortisol) release, which occurs in situations such as stress, trauma, burns, and sepsis. Insulin release, triggered primarily by a rise in blood glucose concentration that occurs following meals, may dramatically decrease plasma BCAA concentrations by promoting tissue, especially muscle, BCAA uptake.

Following protein-containing meals, plasma amino acid concentrations rise steadily for several hours, then return to basal concentrations. In basal situations or between meals, plasma amino acid concentrations are relatively stable and are species specific; however, there is variability (large coefficients of variation) among people with respect to absolute concentrations of specific amino acids in the plasma [28].

Amino acids circulating in the plasma and found within cells arise from digestion and absorption of dietary protein as well as from the breakdown of existing body tissues. These amino acids of endogenous source intermingle with exogenous amino acids to form a "pool" in the plasma along with some smaller pools in various tissues of the body. The total pool is estimated at 100 g [5]. Munro and Crim [5] suggest that adults synthesize 250 to 300 g of protein daily. Reuse of endogenous amino acids is thought to represent the primary source of amino acids needed for protein synthesis.

Despite differences in protein intake and rate of degradation of tissue protein, the pattern of the amino

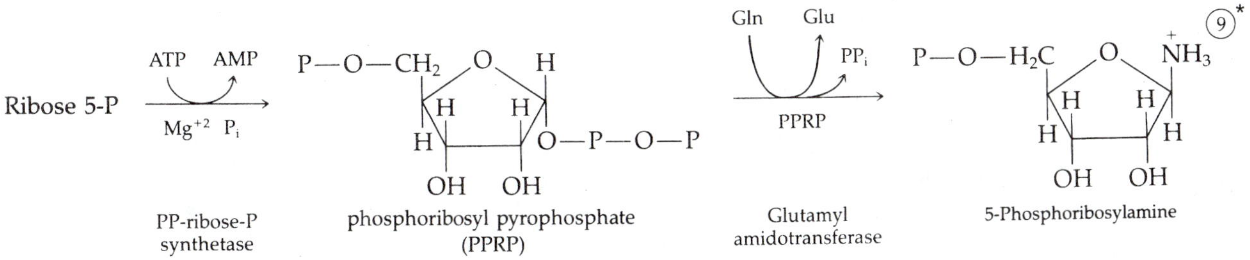

a. Biosynthesis is initiated by reaction between PPRP and glutamine (Gln) as shown above.

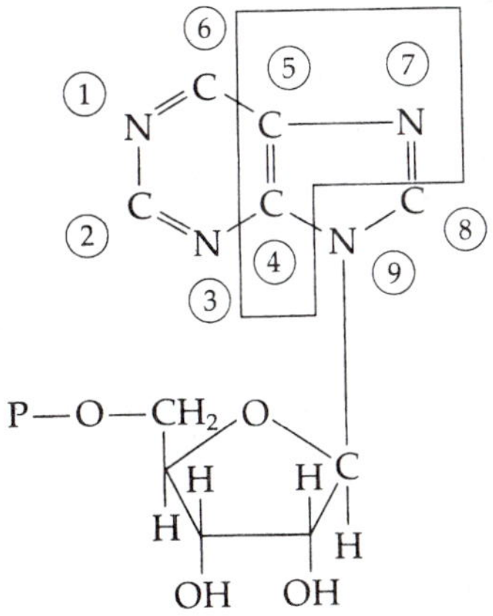

*Nitrogen ⑨ is donated by amide group from *glutamine*. Donors of other atoms in order of introduction:

a. *Glycine*: N ⑦ and C ④ and ⑤ introduced as single unit.

b. *Formate*: C ⑧ donated via N^{10} formyl THF (tetrahydrofolic acid)

c. *Glutamine* amide group: N ③

d. *Respiratory CO_2 as "active CO_2"*: C ⑥

e. *Aspartic acid*: N ①

f. *Formate*: C ② via N^{10} formyl THF

b. Sources of carbon and nitrogen atoms in purine ring.

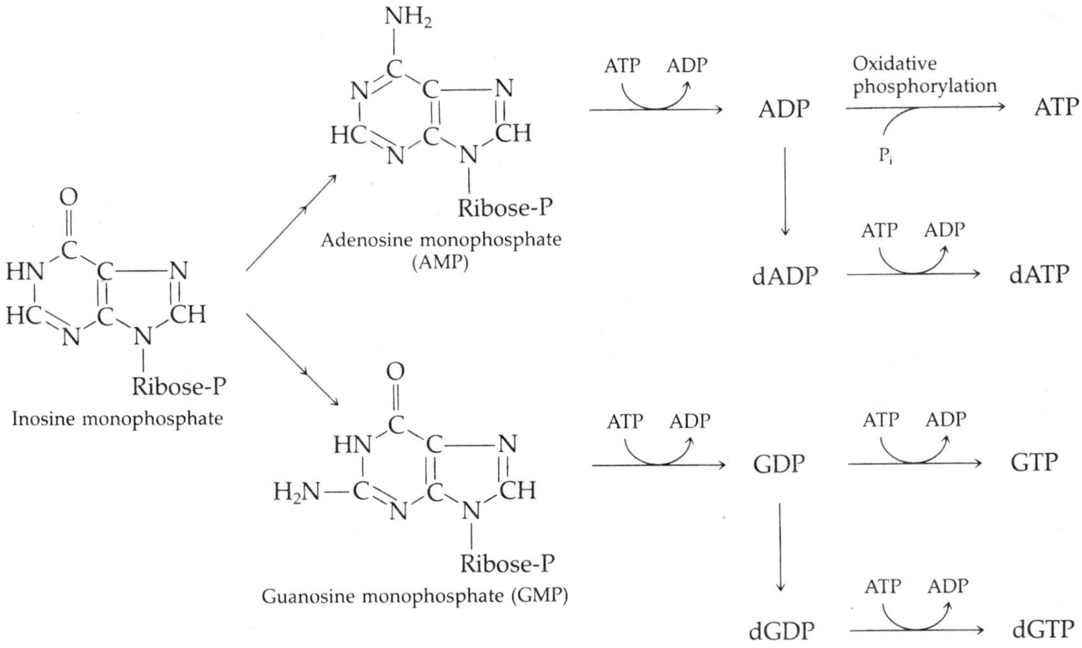

c. Formation of individual purine bases and nucleotides.

FIGURE 7.10 Synthesis of purines and sources of carbon and nitrogen atoms.

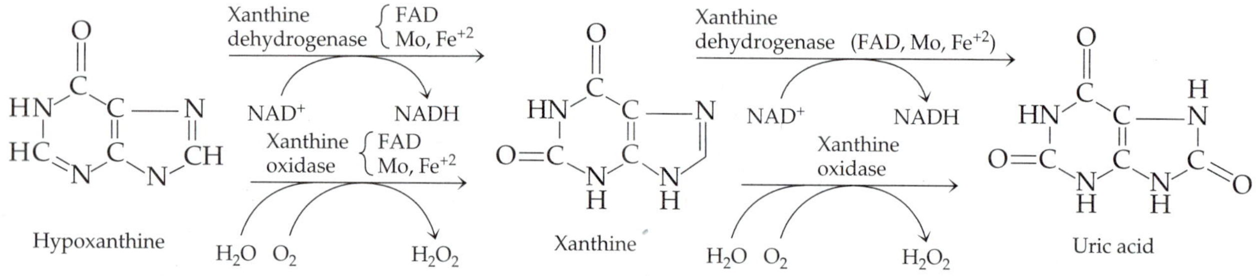

FIGURE 7.11 Purine catabolism yields uric acid.

acids in the free amino acid pool appears to remain relatively constant, although the pattern is quite different from that found in body proteins. The total amount of the essential amino acids found in the pool is less than that of the nonessential amino acids. The essential amino acids found in greatest concentration are lysine and threonine, both of which are totally indispensable (Table 7.2). Of the nonessential amino acids, those found in greatest concentration are alanine, glutamate, aspartate, and glutamine. Harper [2] believes that the nonessential amino acids may function to conserve the essential amino acids, with the exception of lysine and threonine, through the reamination of α-keto acids of the essential amino acid. An α-keto acid is simply an amino acid

$$(^-OOC-CH-(CH_2)_2-COO^-)$$
$$\underset{NH_3^+}{|}$$

with its amino group, NH_3, replaced by a keto group,

$$\underset{\|}{\overset{O}{-C-}}, (^-OOC-\underset{\|}{\overset{O}{C}}-(CH_2)_2-COO^-)$$

The amino acids within the pool, regardless of source, are metabolized in response to various stimuli [29]. Amino acids in excess of need for synthesis of protein and/or nitrogen-containing compounds, are likely to be oxidized by way of their conversion into potential energy sources (glucose, fatty acids, ketones). In addition, some amino acids appear to affect cholesterol synthesis and/or blood cholesterol concentrations [30].

Amino Acid Catabolism

Transamination and Deamination Usually, the first step in the metabolism of amino acids is the removal of the amino group from the amino acid. Amino acids can undergo either transamination or deamination to remove amino groups. In the transamination reaction shown in Figure 7.12, the amino group from the amino acid leucine is being transferred to α-ketoglutarate, an α-keto acid. Transamination reactions typically require vitamin B_6 in its coenzyme form, pyridoxal phosphate (PLP). Figure 7.12 also shows the deamination of the amino acid threonine by threonine dehydratase to form α-ketobutyrate (another α-keto acid) and ammonium. When essential amino acids are transaminated or deaminated, the removed amino group (or ammonia) can be used for the synthesis of dispensable amino acids or can be used to synthesize urea, which is then excreted from the body.

The most active aminotransferases in cells are alanine aminotransferase (ALT) (formerly called *glutamate pyruvate transaminase* and abbreviated GPT) and aspartate aminotransferase (AST) (formerly called *glutamate oxaloacetate transaminase* and abbreviated GOT). These aminotransferases involve three key amino acids, alanine, glutamate, and aspartate; require PLP for activity; and are found in varying concentrations in different tissues. For example, AST is found in higher concentrations in the heart than the liver, muscle, and other tissues. In contrast, ALT is found in higher concentrations in the liver than the heart, but is also found in moderate amounts in the kidney and small amounts in other tissues. Normal serum concentrations of these enzymes are low; however, with trauma or disease to an organ, serum enzyme concentrations rise and serve as an indicator of which organ has been damaged and the severity of the organ damage. Reactions catalyzed by ALT and AST are shown in Figure 7.13. ALT transfers amino groups from alanine to an α-keto acid (such as α-ketoglutarate) forming pyruvate and another amino acid (such as glutamate), respectively. AST transfers amino groups from aspartate also to an α-keto acid (such as α-ketoglutarate), yielding oxaloacetate and another amino

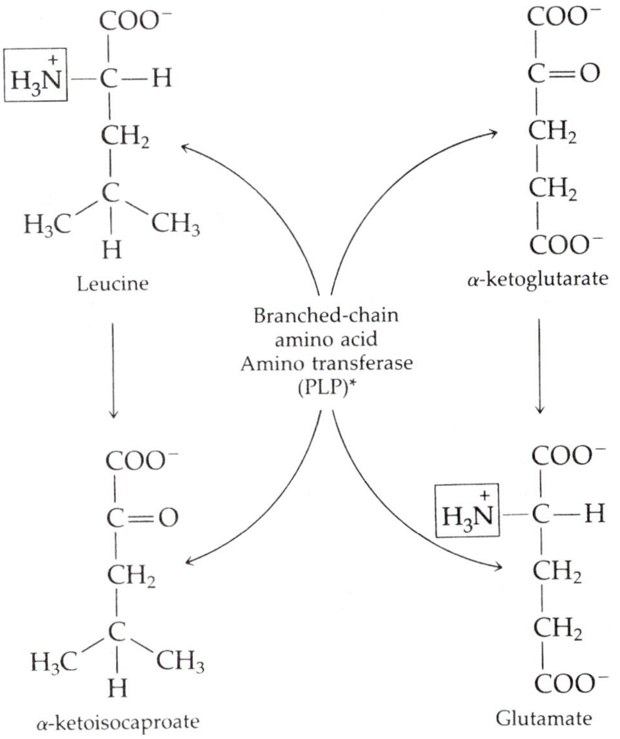

(a) Transamination reaction

(Chemical structures: Leucine + α-ketoglutarate → α-ketoisocaproate + Glutamate, via Branched-chain amino acid Amino transferase (PLP)*)

(a) *Transamination reaction*: Amino transferases transfer an amino group from an amino acid to an α-keto acid. *PLP, pyridoxal phosphate.

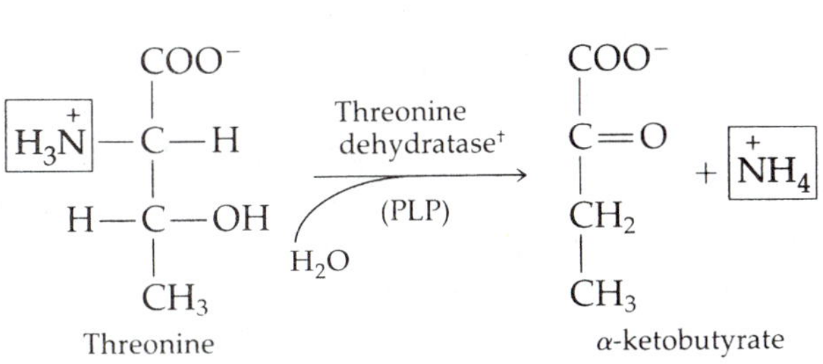

(b) Deamination reaction

(Chemical structures: Threonine → α-ketobutyrate + NH_4^+, via Threonine dehydratase† (PLP), H_2O)

(b) *Deamination reaction*. †The enzyme is called *dehydratase* rather than *deaminase* because the reaction proceeds by loss of elements of water.

FIGURE 7.12 The transamination and deamination of selected amino acids.

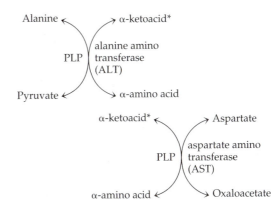

*Typically α-ketoglutarate to generate glutamate on transamination with alanine or aspartate.

FIGURE 7.13 Transfer of an amino group from alanine (top) and aspartate (bottom) to form other amino acids from their respective alpha keto acids.

---

acid (glutamate) respectively. These reactions are reversible. Because glutamate and α-ketoglutarate readily transfer and/or accept amino groups, these compounds play central roles in amino acid metabolism and in the excretion of ammonia and α-amino nitrogen.

The Roles of Glutamate, Glutamine, Alanine, and Aspartate *Glutamate* is the major amino acid in-

volved in the transfer of α-amino nitrogen from the amino group of amino acids into urea. Ammonia or ammonium ions (NH_4^+) from amino acid transamination or deamination can combine with glutamate to form the amide *glutamine* (Fig. 7.14). This reaction is catalyzed by glutamine synthetase and requires ATP and magnesium (Mg^{+2}) or manganese (Mn^{+2}). Glutamine synthesis occurs within all tissues, especially the muscle and lungs, and carries out of the cell the generated ammonia [31].

Glutamine freely leaves tissues, and travels principally to the liver, kidney, or intestine, but also to organs such as the pancreas [31]. Glutamine is used as an energy source by the enterocyte; in fact, the gastrointestinal tract is thought to be the principal organ of glutamine utilization [31]. Glutamine is also thought to have trophic effects on the mucosal cells. In the liver, glutamine is an important donor of nitrogen for the synthesis of purine nucleotide bases. In the liver and kidney, glutamine can be catabolized by *glutaminase*, which removes the amide nitrogen to yield glutamate and ammonia (Fig. 7.15). Free ammonia, generated by bacterial cleavage of urea or from bacterial degradation of amino acids in the digestive tract and subsequently absorbed, can also be extracted by the liver from portal blood. In the absorptive state or during periods of alkalosis, liver glutaminase activity increases, yielding ammonia for the urea cycle. Within the mitochondria of liver cells in the first step of the urea cycle, ammonia typically reacts with CO_2, 2 mol of ATP, and Mg^{+2}, and with the enzyme carbamoyl phosphate synthetase I generates carbamoyl phosphate. In an acidotic state, the use of glutamine for the urea cycle diminishes and the liver releases glutamine for transport to and uptake by the kidney [32].

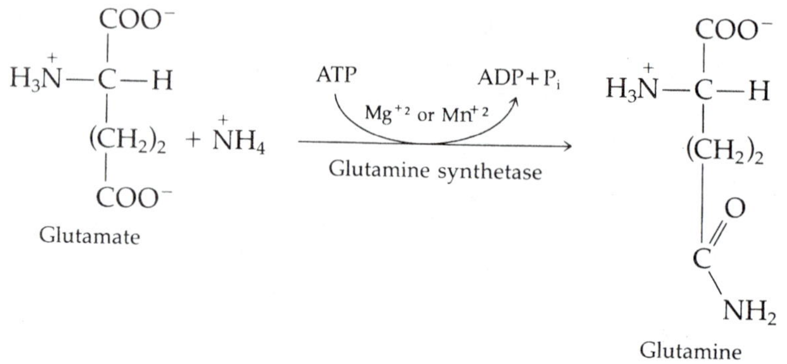

FIGURE 7.14 The synthesis of glutamine from glutamate and ammonium ion.

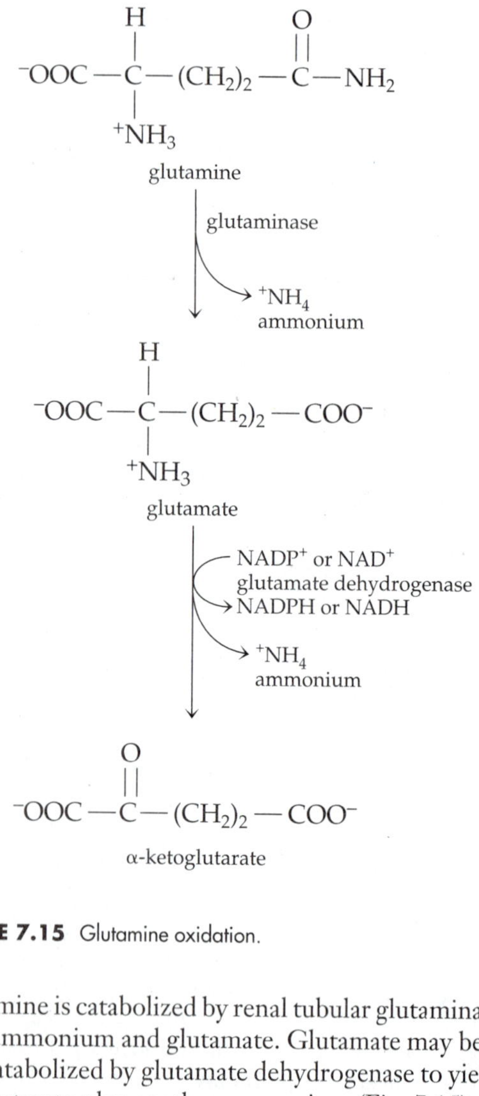

FIGURE 7.15 Glutamine oxidation.

Glutamine is catabolized by renal tubular glutaminase to yield ammonium and glutamate. Glutamate may be further catabolized by glutamate dehydrogenase to yield α-ketoglutarate plus another ammonium (Fig. 7.15). Ammonium is in equilibrium with cell ammonia and H$^+$.

Ammonia, which is lipid soluble, may diffuse into the urine and react with H$^+$ to form ammonium for excretion. Renal glutaminase activity and ammonium excretion increase with acidosis and decrease with alkalosis [32].

Alanine is also important in the transfer of amino groups generated from the catabolism of amino acids in tissues such as the skeletal muscle. For example, amino groups generated from BCAA transamination can combine with α-ketoglutarate to form glutamate or can combine with glutamate to form glutamine. Glutamate may also transfer its amino group to pyruvate, generated from glucose metabolism, to form alanine (Fig. 7.16) [33]. Both glutamine and alanine are released in relatively large proportions from skeletal muscle. Alanine may travel to the liver, where it may undergo transamination to generate glutamate and pyruvate (used for glucose synthesis) (the cycle is referred to as the *alanine* or *glucose alanine cycle*, see Fig. 7.16 and see Fig. 8.9). Glutamate may be degraded subsequently to yield ammonia for the urea cycle. Transamination of alanine produces glutamate from α-ketoglutarate. In a reaction catalyzed by AST, the glutamate can be transaminated with oxaloacetate, which becomes *aspartate* (Fig. 7.13). Aspartate is used in the synthesis of pyrimidines and purines (Fig. 7.8), and is one of the amino acids directly involved in urea generation by the urea cycle.

The Urea Cycle Figure 7.17 reviews key compounds of the urea cycle and shows its relationship with amino acids and the Krebs cycle. The regulation of the urea cycle was recently reviewed by Morris [34]. High concentrations of arginine increase the synthesis of N-acetylglutamate (NAG), which is needed for the synthesis of carbamoyl phosphate in the mitochondria. NAG is required as an allosteric activator to allow ATP binding. As indicated in the previous section, carbamoyl phosphate is formed from ammonia and CO$_2$

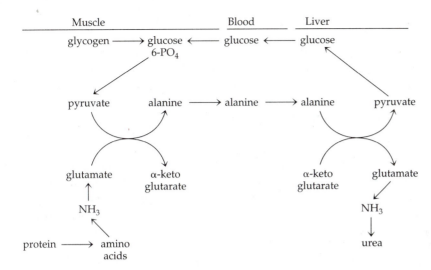

FIGURE 7.16 The alanine–glucose cycle: alanine generation in muscle, glucose generation in liver.

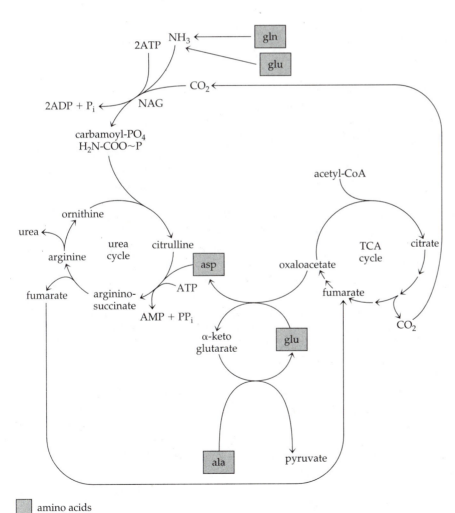

☐ amino acids

FIGURE 7.17 Interrelationships of amino acids and the urea and TCA cycles in the liver.

in a reaction catalyzed by mitochondrial carbamoyl phosphate synthetase I (CPS-I) and using 2 mol ATP and Mg^{+2}. Carbamoyl phosphate reacts with ornithine in the mitochondria, using the enzyme ornithine transcarbamoylase (OTC) to form citrulline. Citrulline in turn inhibits OTC activity. Aspartate reacts with citrulline once it has been transported into the cytosol. This step, catalyzed by argininosuccinate synthetase, is the rate-limiting step of the cycle. ATP (two high-energy bonds) and Mg^{+2} are required for the reaction, and argininosuccinate is formed. Argininosuccinate, arginine, and $AMP + PP_i$ inhibit the enzyme. Argininosuccinase in the cytosol cleaves argininosuccinate to form fumarate and arginine. Both fumarate and arginine can inhibit argininosuccinase activity. Argininosuccinase is found in a variety of tissues throughout the body, especially the liver and kidney. Urea is formed and ornithine is reformed from the cleavage of arginine by arginase, a manganese-requiring enzyme. Arginase activity is inhibited by both ornithine and lysine and may become rate limiting under conditions that limit manganese availability or that alter its affinity for manganese [34].

Overall, the urea cycle uses four high-energy bonds. Oxidations in the Krebs cycle coupled with phosphorylation through the electron transport chain can provide the ATP required for urea synthesis. The urea molecule derives one nitrogen from ammonia, a second nitrogen from aspartate, and its carbon from CO_2. Once formed, urea typically travels via the blood to the kidneys for excretion in the urine; however, up to about 25% of urea may be secreted from the blood into the intestinal lumen, where it may be degraded by bacteria to yield ammonia [35].

Activities of urea cycle enzymes fluctuate with diet and hormone concentrations. For example, with low-protein diets or with acidosis, urea synthesis (the amount of mRNA for each of the enzymes) diminishes and urinary urea nitrogen excretion decreases significantly. In the healthy individual with a normal protein intake, blood urea nitrogen (BUN) concentrations range from 8 to 20 mg/dL, and urinary urea nitrogen represents about 80% of total urinary nitrogen. Glucocorticoids and glucagon typically increase mRNA for the urea cycle enzymes [34].

Several urea cycle enzyme-deficient disorders have been characterized. Defects in any one of the enzymes of the urea cycle are possible. Urea cycle enzyme defects typically result in high levels of blood ammonia (hyperammonemia), and necessitate a nitrogen-restricted diet, which may be coupled with supplements of carnitine or single amino acids, among other compounds.

The Carbon Skeleton Once an amino group has been removed from an amino acid, the remaining molecule is referred to as a *carbon skeleton* or *α-keto acid*. This carbon skeleton (Fig. 7.8) can either be used for energy after further degradation to a Krebs cycle intermediate or the carbon skeleton, depending on the original amino acid from which it was derived, can be used for synthesis of glucose, fatty acids, or ketones. Such different fates of amino acids typically occur when people are not receiving sufficient energy or carbohydrate in the diet. Moreover, these reactions are accelerated by high glucagon-to-insulin ratios and by glucocorticoids such as cortisol. Oxaloacetate from aspartate and asparagine, and pyruvate from alanine, glycine, serine, cysteine, and tryptophan contribute to glucose production in the liver, although gluconeogenesis may also occur in the kidney. In times of excess energy and protein intakes coupled with adequate carbohydrate intake, the carbon skeleton of amino acids may be used to synthesize fatty acids. Figure 7.18 shows the general fates of amino acid carbon skeletons with respect to key intermediates of metabolism.

Hepatic Metabolism of Aromatic and S-Containing Amino Acids Aromatic and sulfur (S)-containing amino acid catabolism typically occurs in the liver. In end-stage liver disease, the inability of the liver to take up and catabolize these amino acids is evidenced by the increased plasma concentrations of both the aromatic and the S-containing amino acids. The metabolism of phenylalanine, tyrosine, and tryptophan, as well as methionine will be reviewed briefly and is outlined in Figures 7.8 and 7.19.

The first step in the degradation of phenylalanine is specific to the liver and to a smaller extent, the kidney. Phenylalanine is converted to tyrosine by the hepatic enzyme *phenylalanine hydroxylase* or monooxygenase. This enzyme is iron dependent, and vitamin C and tetrahydrobiopterin are required for the reaction. A genetic absence or deficient activity of phenylalanine hydroxylase results in the genetic disorder *phenylketonuria* (PKU) and necessitates a phenylalanine restricted diet. Further catabolism of tyrosine is not specific to the liver; however, the reactions occur primarily in the liver and yield many compounds significant to metabolism. Tyrosine hydroxylase, a copper dependent enzyme, catalyzes the first step in tyrosine metabolism to generate 3,4 hydroxyphenylalanine (L-dopa). Subsequent reactions yield the catecholamines (dopamine, norepinephrine, and epinephrine, see Fig. 7.25), as well as melanin, a pigment in the skin. In the thyroid gland, tyrosine is taken up and used with iodine

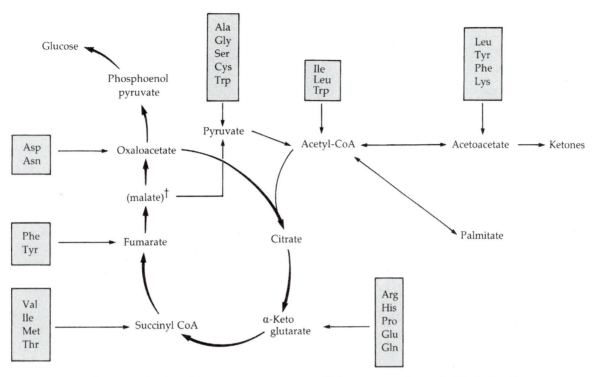

FIGURE 7.18 The fate of amino acid carbon skeletons. Ketogenic: Leu; Partially ketogenic and glucogenic: Phe, Ile, Trp, Tyr, Lys; Glucogenic: Ala, Gly, Cys, Ser, Thr, Asp, Asn, Glu, Gln, Arg, Met, Val, His, Pro.

to synthesize thyroid hormones. Degradation of phenylalanine and tyrosine yield fumarate and acetoacetate (Fig. 7.18).

Another aromatic amino acid principally metabolized by the liver is tryptophan. The first step in tryptophan metabolism yields N-formylkynurenine. The enzyme tryptophan oxygenase is iron dependent. Further metabolism of N-formylkynurenine yields many compounds, including picolinic acid (a possible binding ligand for minerals), niacin as nicotinamide adenine dinucleotide (NAD$^+$), and the nonessential amino acid alanine. Alanine formed from tryptophan can be transaminated to pyruvate. Degradation of tryptophan also yields acetyl CoA (Fig. 7.18).

The metabolism of methionine, a S-containing essential amino acid, also occurs to a large extent in the liver. A major role of methionine in the body, other than for protein synthesis, is as a donor of methyl groups. The enzyme required for this methyl donor role, methionine adenosyl transferase, is present in abundance in the liver. Methionine adenosyl transferase catalyzes the conversion of methionine to S-adenosyl methionine (SAM) in an ATP-requiring reaction. SAM is the principal methyl donor in the body and is required for the synthesis of carnitine, creatine, epinephrine, purines,

and nicotinamide. The removal of or donation of the methyl group from SAM yields the compound S-adenosyl homocysteine (SAH). SAH can then be converted to homocysteine. Homocysteine can either be converted back to methionine in a vitamin B$_{12}$ (as methylcobalamin), folate (as 5-methyl THF), and betaine-dependent reaction, or homocysteine can react with serine, and in a series of vitamin B$_6$–PLP-dependent reactions, can be converted into the nonessential amino acid cysteine. Cysteine is required for the synthesis of both protein and glutathione. Cysteine may be further metabolized to form cystine and another amino acid, taurine. Taurine is not involved in protein synthesis, but is important in vision (retina), in membrane stability, as a bile salt taurocholate, and may function as an inhibitory neurotransmitter [4,36]. Genetic defects in methionine metabolism have been documented and include homocystinuria, due to defects in cystathionine synthase activity, and cystathioninuria due to cystathionase inactivity. Both defects necessitate a methionine-restricted diet. Methionine degradation typically yields succinyl CoA (Fig. 7.18).

Several other reactions of amino acid metabolism are common to tissues throughout the body. Some of these reactions are presented in Figure 7.8. For example,

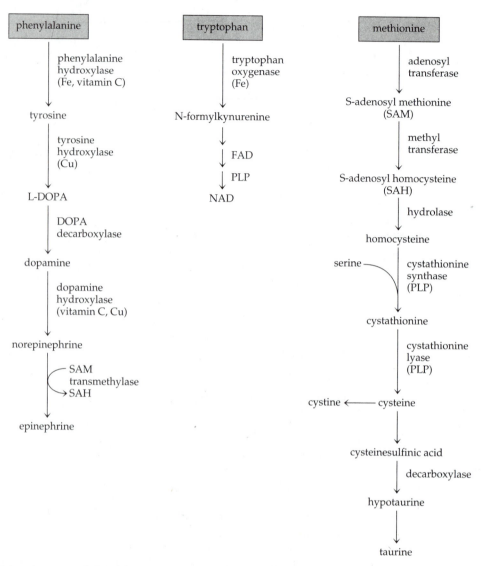

FIGURE 7.19 Selected reactions of phenylalanine, tyrosine, tryptophan, and methionine metabolism.

serine may be converted to glycine in a folate- and vitamin B₆-requiring reaction; glycine is principally converted to serine in the kidney. Glycine is needed for the synthesis of creatine, porphyrin, and the bile salt glycocholate. Serine is used for the synthesis of ethanolamine. Arginine and glutamate may be metabolized to form proline, arginine is also used for creatine synthesis. Histidine may be catabolized to form glutamate, or may combine with β-alanine to generate carnosine (a nitrogen-containing compound). Through a vitamin B₆-dependent decarboxylation reaction, histamine can also be formed from histidine.

INTERORGAN "FLOW" OF AMINO ACIDS AND ORGAN-SPECIFIC METABOLISM

From the plasma, tissues extract amino acids for synthesis of nonessential amino acids, protein, nitrogen-containing compounds, glucose, fatty acids, ketones, or for energy production, depending on the person's nutritional status. A brief review of the flow of amino acids between selected organs and organ-specific amino acid metabolism follows. Amino acid metabolism in selected organs is shown pictorially in

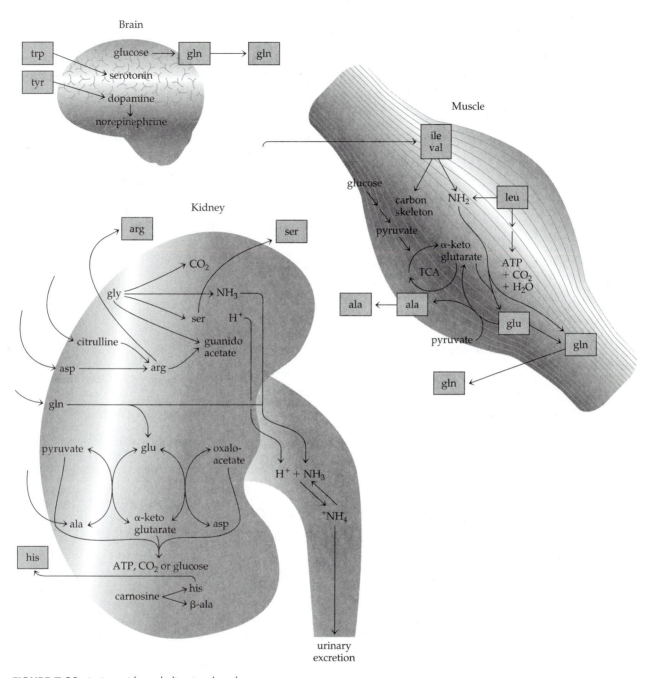

FIGURE 7.20 Amino acid metabolism in selected organs.

Figure 7.20 and is reviewed and shown in detail by Jungas et al. [37].

Skeletal Muscle

Uptake of amino acids by the skeletal muscles readily occurs following ingestion of a protein-containing meal.

After meals, skeletal muscles typically experience a net protein synthesis. The BCAAs, or possibly just leucine, are thought to induce protein synthesis within the skeletal muscle [33,38]. The mechanism by which leucine directly influences protein synthesis has not been elucidated. Leucine's ability to stimulate insulin secretion, a promoter of protein synthesis along with growth hor-

TABLE 7.6 Amino Acids Classified According to Pattern of Metabolism in Skeletal Muscle

Amino Acids	Pattern of Metabolism
1. Alanine Glutamine	Synthesized *de novo* and released
2. Arginine Cysteine Glycine Histidine Lysine Methionine Phenylalanine Proline Serine Threonine Tryptophan Tyrosine	Not oxidized, released as intact amino acids or their keto analogs on proteolysis
3. Leucine	Used as energy source
4. Aspartic acid Asparagine Glutamic acid Isoleucine Valine	Mainly converted to glutamine. Some oxidized for energy, some converted to lactate, and remainder released as intact amino acids or keto analogs on proteolysis

Source: Adapted from Goldberg A, Chang TW. Regulation and significance of amino acid metabolism in skeletal muscle. Fed Proc 1978;37:2301.

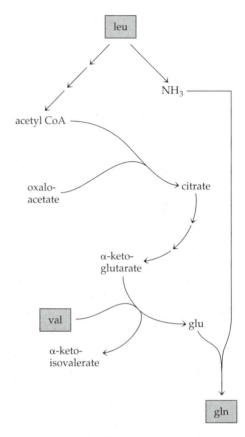

FIGURE 7.21 Proposed pathway for synthesis of glutamine from leucine and valine in the muscle.

mone, may play a role [39]. Leucine or its metabolites may also impede proteolysis, but data are conflicting [33,39].

Muscle, as well as the heart, kidney, diaphragm, and other organs possess BCAA transferases, located in both the cytosol and mitochondria. The transferases transaminate the three BCAAs. Degradation of the BCAAs does not proceed unless the α-keto acids formed are decarboxylated (irreversible reaction) by the branched-chain α-keto acid dehydrogenase complex. This enzyme complex is found in the mitochondria of many tissues, including liver, muscle, heart, kidney, intestine, and the brain. The enzyme complex is highly regulated and is similar to pyruvate dehydrogenase in that it requires thiamin in its coenzyme form TDP/TPP, niacin as NADH, Mg^{+2} and CoA from pantothenic acid. A genetic defect diminishing branched-chain α-keto acid dehydrogenase complex activity results in maple syrup urine disease (MSUD). MSUD necessitates a diet restricted in leucine, isoleucine, and valine intakes.

A great deal of interest in protein metabolism within the skeletal muscle was generated through the discovery that during starvation the amounts of the various amino acids released from the muscle could not reflect proteolysis alone. In particular, much more alanine and glutamine were appearing in the blood than could be at-

tributed to muscle protein content. Transamination of the BCAAs occurs primarily with α-ketoglutarate to form glutamate, which may either donate its amino group to pyruvate to form alanine or may incorporate free ammonia to form glutamine [33]. The relative amounts of glutamine and alanine produced depend largely on the concentration of ammonia within the tissue; high ammonia concentrations promote glutamine synthesis and decrease alanine production [33].

Table 7.6 classifies the amino acids according to their pattern of metabolism in the muscle. Six amino acids (leucine, aspartate, asparagine, glutamate, valine, and isoleucine) are catabolized in the skeletal muscle. Five of the six amino acids, all but leucine, are mainly converted to glutamine. Glutamine can be produced from any two amino acids that are capable of being oxidized in the muscle. Figure 7.21 depicts the synthesis of glutamine from the oxidation of valine and leucine.

Thus, following transamination, the branched-chain α-keto acids may remain within muscle for further oxidation or may be transported bound to albumin in the blood to other tissues for reamination or for further catabolism [39]. Complete oxidation of valine yields succinyl CoA while the end products of isoleucine catabolism are succinyl CoA and acetyl CoA (Fig. 7.18). Complete oxidation of leucine results in acetyl CoA and acetoacetate formation (Fig. 7.18).

Leucine is the only amino acid that is completely oxidized in the muscle for energy. Leucine, a totally ketogenic amino acid, is oxidized in a manner similar to fatty acids, and its oxidation results in the production of 1 mol of acetyl CoA and 1 mol of acetoacetate. During fasting, leucine rises to high levels in the blood and muscle, while the capacity of the muscle to degrade leucine increases concurrently. By supplying the muscle with the equivalent of 3 mol of acetyl CoA per molecule of leucine oxidized, the latter produces energy for the muscle while simultaneously inhibiting pyruvate oxidation and therefore stimulating lactate release from the muscles [38]. Thus, the oxidation of leucine spares essential gluconeogenic precursors. Pyruvate, along with lactate, can be returned to the liver, the former either being transported as pyruvate per se or (more likely) being converted to alanine for transport.

Alanine, the other amino acid that is synthesized in the muscle, is released in relatively large quantities from muscle in the basal state as well as with starvation [33]. Alanine is believed to arise by amination of pyruvate (derived from glucose catabolism). The amino group source may be from an amino group released from BCAA transamination, or from the transamination of pyruvate by glutamate (Fig. 7.16) [33,39]. The amino acids being oxidized in the muscle transfer their amino groups to α-ketoglutarate to form glutamate, which in turn transfers its amino group to pyruvate to form alanine [33,39]. The increase in transamination of α-ketoglutarate is believed to be the stimulus for the synthesis of both alanine and glutamine [33], the production of which provides a means for ridding the muscle of toxic ammonia.

Both alanine and glutamine can be carried from the muscle by the blood to one or more organs of the body (liver, kidney, intestine), where the amino or amide groups respectively can be removed, converted to excretory products, and excreted. Alanine taken up by the liver can be converted to glucose, which can then be released into the blood, and subsequently taken up again and used by muscle (alanine, glucose alanine, or alanine glucose cycle). This cycle (Fig. 7.16) serves to transport nitrogen to the liver for conversion to urea. Other amino acids released in lesser quantities from muscle (forearm and/or leg) in a postabsorptive state include phenylalanine, methionine, lysine, arginine, histidine, tyrosine, proline, tryptophan, threonine, and glycine [40,41].

Further studies investigating the effects of meals containing all three energy nutrients on amino acid uptake and output by muscle are needed.

Indicators of Muscle Mass and Muscle Catabolism
Urinary excretion of creatinine and 3-methylhistidine are used as indicators of the amount of existing muscle mass and the rate of muscle degradation, respectively. Creatinine is a reflection of muscle mass because it is the degradation product of creatine, which makes up approximately 0.3 to 0.5% of muscle mass by weight [5]. Although a muscle component, creatine is a nitrogen-containing compound synthesized by the kidney and liver. Once synthesized, creatine is transported to the muscle where it is phosphorylated by ATP. The product of this phosphorylation, creatine phosphate or phosphocreatine, acts as a storehouse for high-energy phosphate. Creatine and creatine phosphate slowly but spontaneously cyclize due to nonreversible, nonenzymatic dehydration, thereby forming creatinine. Once formed, creatinine leaves the muscle, passes across the glomerulus of the kidney, and is excreted in the urine. Small amounts of creatinine may be excreted into the gut, and like urea, metabolized by bacterial flora [42]. Creatinine clearance is frequently used as a means of estimating kidney function.

Figure 7.22a depicts the phosphorylation of creatine and the spontaneous cyclization of phosphocreatine into creatinine. Figure 7.22b shows how phosphocreatine replenishes ATP in a muscle that is rapidly contracting. The creatinine excreted in the urine reflects about 1.7% of the total creatine pool per day, but because of the variation in muscle content of creatine (0.3 to 0.5%), creatinine cannot be used to make an accurate determination of muscle mass [5].

On proteolysis, 3-methylhistidine (shown in Table 7.1) is released and is a nonreusable amino acid because the methylation of histidine occurs post-translationally. Because 3-methylhistidine is found primarily in actin, this compound has been used to estimate muscle protein degradation. Excretion of the compound is used as an index of muscle degradation. However, actin is widely distributed in the body, including tissues such as the intestine and platelets, which have high turnover rates. Therefore, the urinary excretion of 3-methylhistidine provides an index of protein breakdown in many tissues in the body [5,43].

Kidneys

Studies in humans as well as animals suggest that the kidneys preferentially take up a number of amino acids including, for example, glycine, alanine, glutamine, glu-

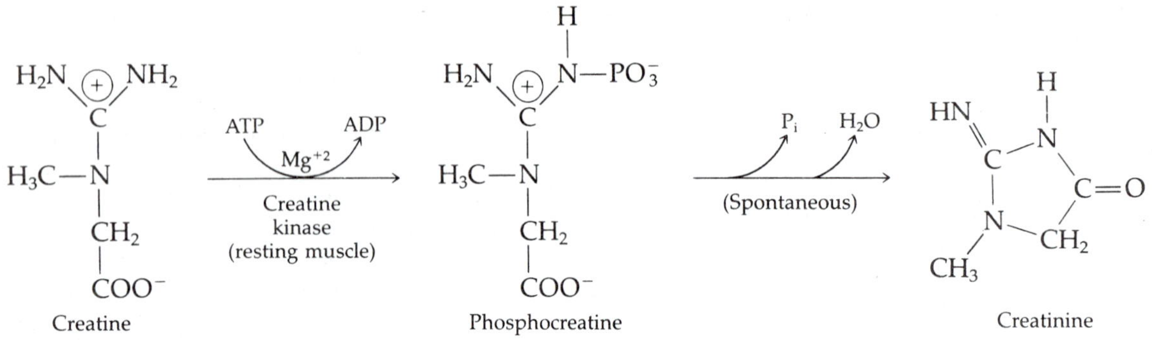

(a) Conversion of creatine to phosphocreatine in the muscle and its spontaneous cyclization to creatinine.

$$\text{Phosphocreatine} + \text{ADP} \xrightarrow[\substack{\text{Creatine} \\ \text{kinase} \\ \text{(active muscle)}}]{\text{Mg}^{+2}} \text{Creatine} + \text{ATP}$$

(b) Synthesis of ATP from ADP and phosphocreatine during contractile activity.* Creatine kinase catalyzes the reaction in both directions (a and b).

*ATP in muscle can suffice for only a fraction of a second, but phosphocreatine stored in the muscle and possessing a higher phosphate group transfer potential than ATP, transfers a phosphoryl group to ADP, thereby forming ATP and providing energy for muscular activity.

FIGURE 7.22 Creatinine metabolism.

tamate, and aspartate. Metabolism of amino acids within the kidney (Fig. 7.20) includes (1) the synthesis of serine from glycine, (2) glycine catabolism, (3) histidine synthesis from carnosine degradation, (4) arginine synthesis from aspartate and citrulline that was released from the intestinal cells, and (5) guanidoacetate formation from arginine and glycine for creatine synthesis. The kidney is considered to be the major site for arginine, histidine, and serine production.

In addition, the kidney is the only organ besides the liver that has the enzymes necessary for gluconeogenesis. α-Ketoacids formed from the transamination or deamination of amino acids brought to the kidney can be used for glucose production or can be used for energy. Renal metabolism of amino acids becomes particularly significant during fasting. Gluconeogenesis can raise the amount of glucose available to the body for energy, while the ammonia (formed from deamination of amino acids, especially glutamine) can help normalize the pH of the blood, which typically decreases with fasting. Acidosis occurs with fasting because of the resulting rise in ketone concentration in the blood. There is also a loss of sodium and potassium as these minerals are excreted in the urine along with the ketones. Renal glutamine uptake for ammonia production during periods of acidosis

(or low bicarbonate concentrations) is increased, while uptake by the intestine, liver, and other organs is diminished [32]. Ammonia generated from amino acids, especially glutamine deamination, enters the filtrate and combines with H^+ ions to form ammonium ions which cannot be reabsorbed, and thus are excreted in the urine. The loss of the H^+ from the body serves to increase pH from an acidotic state toward a normal value of about 7.35–7.45.

The role of the kidney in nitrogen metabolism cannot be overemphasized because of the organ's responsibility in ridding the body of nitrogenous wastes that have accumulated in the plasma. Moreover, enzymes particularly active in the kidney and involved in removal of nitrogenous compounds from the body include the amino transferases, glutamate dehydrogenase, and glutaminase, all of which catalyze the removal of ammonia from glutamate and glutamine. Kidney glomeruli act as filters of blood plasma, and all constituents in plasma move into the filtrate with the exception of plasma protein. (Some albumin normally moves into the filtrate but is reabsorbed by the proximal tubular cells.) Essential nutrients such as sodium (Na^+), amino acids, and glucose are actively reabsorbed, as the filtrate moves through the tubules. Many other substances are not actively reab-

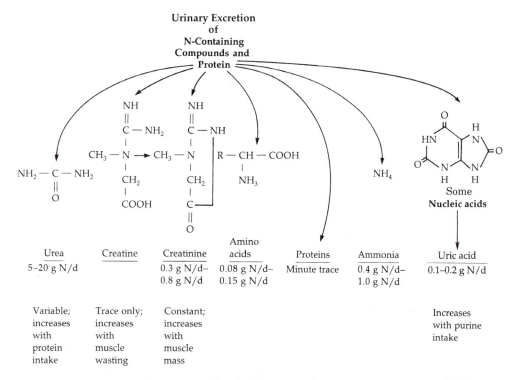

FIGURE 7.23 Nitrogenous wastes in normal urine. *(Reproduced with permission from W.C. McMurray, Essentials of Human Metabolism, 2/e, 1983, Harper & Row, p. 261.)*

sorbed, and if they move into the tubular cells they must either move along an electrical gradient or move osmotically with water. The amount of these substances that enters the tubular cells, then, depends on how much water moves into the cells and how permeable the cells are to the specific substances. The cell membranes are relatively impermeable to urea and uric acid, while membranes are particularly impermeable to creatinine, none of which is reabsorbed.

Figure 7.23 shows the normal range of nitrogenous wastes found in the urine. About 80% of nitrogen is lost in the urine as urea under normal conditions. Additional nitrogen may be lost through the skin as urea, and the loss of hair and skin cells also results in insensible nitrogen losses. In acidotic conditions, as occur with fasting, urinary urea nitrogen losses decrease and the percentage of nitrogen lost as urea also decreases. Urinary ammonia excretion rises in absolute terms as well as in percentage terms.

Brain and Accessory Tissues

Because the brain has the capacity for active transport of the indispensable amino acids, neurons have access to a higher concentration of these amino acids than is found in the plasma. The brain has transport systems for neutral, dibasic, and dicarboxylic amino acids, and as in other cells, competition occurs between amino acids for uptake by a common carrier system.

Amino Acids Used in Neurotransmitter Synthesis
The uptake of two aromatic amino acids, tryptophan and tyrosine, by the brain is particularly important because these amino acids act as precursors for a variety of neurotransmitters or modulators of nerve function. Tryptophan is used to synthesize serotonin (5-OH tryptamine), an excitatory neurotransmitter (Fig. 7.24). Tyrosine is used to synthesize dopamine, norepinephrine, and epinephrine, referred to as *catecholamines*, because they are derivatives of catechol (Fig. 7.25).

Other amino acids also function as neurotransmitters in the brain. Glycine and taurine are thought to function as inhibitory neurotransmitters. Aspartate is thought to act as an excitatory neurotransmitter in the central nervous system (CNS); aspartate is derived chiefly from glutamate through AST activity common in neural tissue.

Neurotransmitters are stored in the nerve axon terminal as vesicles or granules until stimuli arrive to cause their release. After their action on the cell membranes, the neurotransmitters are inactivated. The fastest mechanism for inactivation is uptake of the neurotransmitter by adjacent cells, where mitochondrial monoamine oxidase (MAO) remove the amine group. Each of the cate-

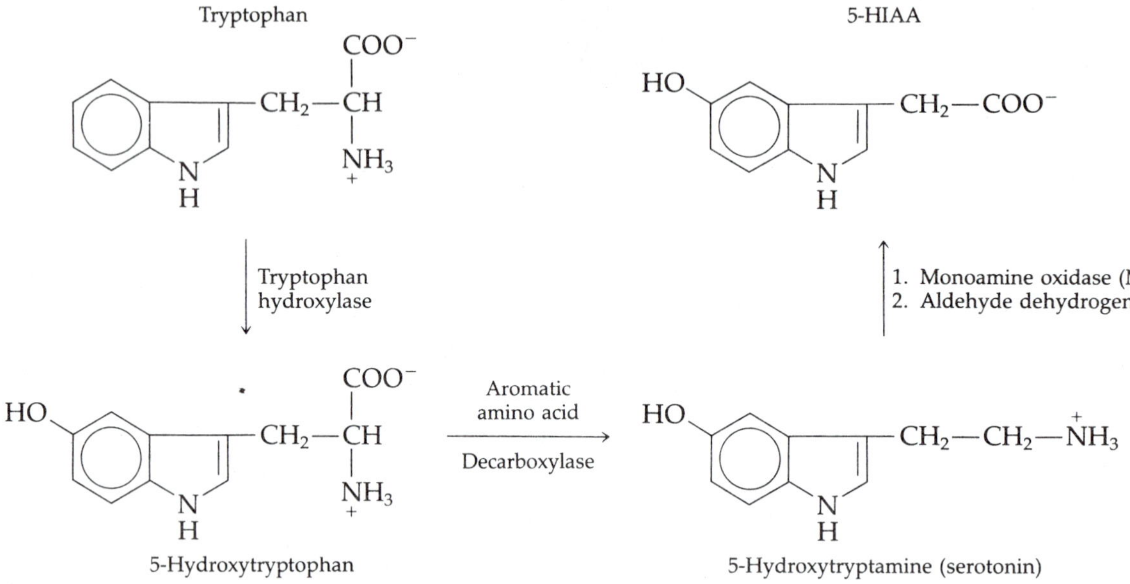

FIGURE 7.24 Serotonin synthesis from tryptophan.

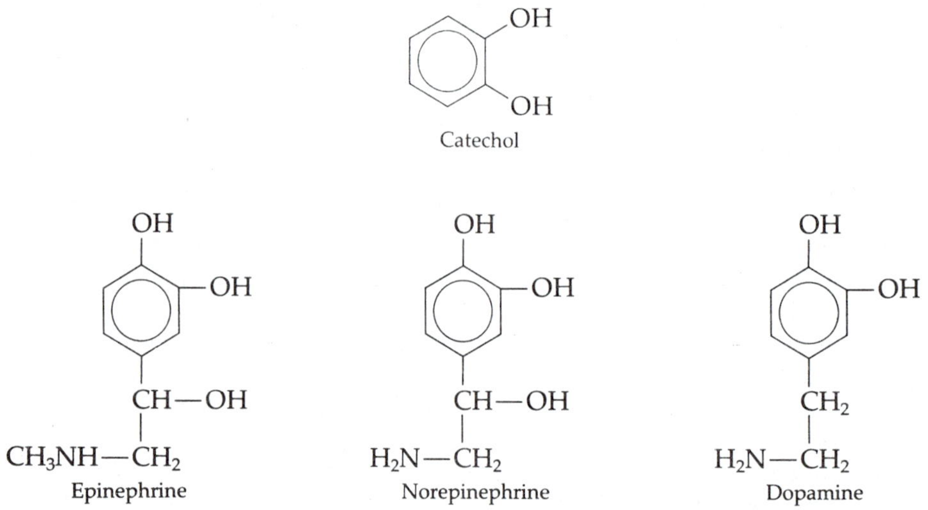

FIGURE 7.25 The catecholamines.

cholamines (dopamine, norepinephrine, epinephrine) as well as serotonin can be inactivated by MAO. A slower mechanism of inactivation requires that the catecholamines be carried by the blood to the liver where they are methylated by catechol-O-methyltransferase (COMT).

Foods also contain amines, especially tyramine [44]. Tyramine is formed from tyrosine that has been decarboxylated. Another food amine is dopamine. Both dopamine and tyramine are inactivated in the body by MAO. Generally aged cheeses (cheddar, camembert,

stilton, boursalt), yeast extracts, and Brewer's yeast are very high in tyramine. Smoked, salted, or pickled fish such as herring or cod, as well as dry sausage, including salami, pepperoni, corned beef, and bologna, are high in tyramine. Foods moderately high to high in tyramine include meat extracts; tenderizers; red wines, including chianti, vermouth, sherry and burgundy; and cheeses such as blue, natural brick, brie, gruyere, mozzarella, parmesan, romano, and roquefort. Broad beans (fava, Chinese pea pods), chocolate, large amounts of caffeine, liver (chicken or beef), and selected fruits may also con-

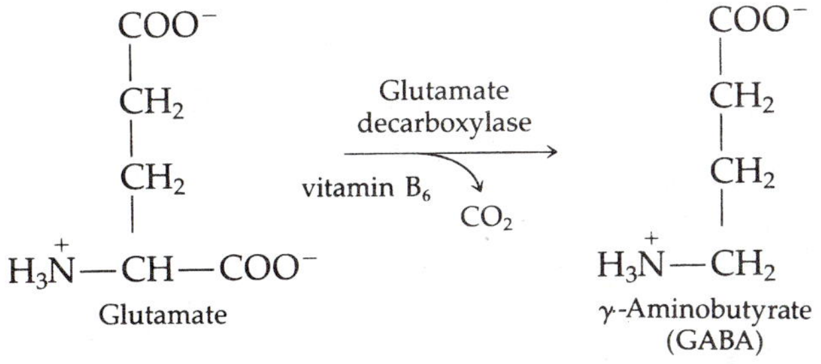

FIGURE 7.26 GABA synthesis.

tain high amounts of tyramine [44]. Consumption of these foods ordinarily presents no problem to individuals because the tyramine or dopamine may be quickly inactivated by MAO. However, there are a group of drugs known as MAO inhibitors. These drugs are used in the treatment of depression, hypertension (high blood pressure), or certain cancers. MAO inhibitors prevent MAO from catabolizing both amines in diet and catecholamines made endogenously. The problem arises when people on MAO inhibitors eat foods high in tyramine. High dietary tyramine coupled with endogenous norepinephrine may result in excessive vasoconstriction, manifested as acute hypertension or a hypertensive crisis. Individuals on MAO-inhibitor drugs are counselled against ingesting foods high in tyramine.

Glutamate has several functions in the brain. With respect to neurotransmitters, glutamate may act as an excitatory neurotransmitter in the brain. Secondly, glutamate is needed in the brain for the synthesis of γ-amino butyric acid (GABA), which functions as an inhibitory neurotransmitter. GABA is believed to be the neurotransmitter for cells that exert inhibitory effects on other cells in the central nervous system (CNS). The conversion of glutamate to GABA involves the removal of the α-carboxyl group of glutamate by the enzyme glutamate decarboxylase in a vitamin B_6–(PLP)-dependent reaction (Fig. 7.26). Glutamate uptake by the brain is typically low; thus, synthesis of glutamate from glucose represents the primary source of brain glutamate.

Glutamate is of significance to the brain not just as a neuromodulator or for the synthesis of GABA, but also as a means of ridding the brain of ammonia. The starting point for glutamate metabolism is the synthesis in neurons of α-ketoglutarate from glucose that has been transported from the blood across the blood–brain barrier. α-ketoglutarate can be converted to glutamate via reductive amination. Whenever excessive ammonia is present in the brain, glutamine is formed through the action of glutamine synthetase, which is highly active in neural tissues (Fig. 7.14). Glutamine is freely diffusible and can move easily into the blood or cerebrospinal fluid, thereby allowing the removal of 2 mol of toxic ammonia from the brain. Any condition that causes an unusual elevation of blood ammonia can interfere with the normal handling of amino acids by the brain. Treatment of hepatic encephalopathy (dysfunction of the brain, due to liver disease, that characteristically results in elevated blood ammonia concentrations) is aimed at normalizing the effects of altered amino acid metabolism on the CNS.

Neuropeptides The CNS abounds in peptides, termed *neuropeptides*. Many of the same peptides that were mentioned in Chapter 2 with respect to digestion and that were found associated with the intestinal tract are also found associated with the CNS. These neuropeptides are of varying lengths and possess a variety of functions. Some peptides act as hormone-releasing factors, such as ACTH involved with cortisol release; some have endocrine effects, such as somatotropin or growth hormone; some have modulatory actions on transmitter functions, mood, or behavior, such as the enkephalins. The enkephalins and endorphins, although similar to natural opiates, possess a wide range of functions including affecting pain sensation, blood pressure and body temperature regulation, governance of body movement, secretion of hormones, control of feeding, and modulation of learning ability [45].

The neurosecretory cells of the hypothalamus are foremost in the secretion of the neuropeptides. Those that have hormone action move out of the axons of the nerve cells into the pituitary from which they are secreted. This linkage between the nervous system and pituitary is of great significance in the overall control of metabolism due to the fact that the pituitary gland is primary in coordinating the various endocrine glands scattered throughout the body.

The neuropeptides are believed to be synthesized from their constituent amino acids via the DNA-coding, messenger RNA (mRNA), ribosomes, and transfer RNA (tRNA) system. Because the nucleus and ribosomes are found in the cell body and dendrites, the peptides must travel to the end of the axon to be stored in vesicles for future release. The neuropeptides are stored as inactive precursor polypeptides. The release of the active peptide, therefore, involves not only exocytosis of the neurotransmitter but also cleavage of its precursor. Because the precursor is not resynthesized from the active peptide, the neuropeptide, after performing its function at the membrane, is hydrolyzed to its constituent amino acids. The overall process can be outlined as follows:

$$\text{Precursor peptide} \xrightarrow[\text{(cleavage)}]{\text{amino acids}} \text{active peptide} \longrightarrow$$

$$\text{exocytosis of neuropeptide} \xrightarrow[\text{(hydrolysis)}]{} \text{amino acids}$$

SYNTHESIS AND CATABOLISM OF TISSUE PROTEINS

The constancy of the amino acid pool(s), both in size and pattern, under a variety of conditions suggests that the concentration of each amino acid is regulated [46]. The pool(s) serves as the connecting link between two cycles of nitrogen metabolism: balance (intake versus output of nitrogen) and turnover (protein synthesis versus degradation). These two cycles operate somewhat independently, but if either cycle gets out of balance the other is affected to some degree. For example, during growth, protein synthesis exceeds degradation. At the same time, nitrogen intake exceeds excretion, resulting in a positive nitrogen balance. The increase in protein turnover, however, is much greater than is reflected by the change in nitrogen balance. The amino acid pool(s), regulated in some manner, is acting as ballast between protein turnover and nitrogen balance. The most important component regulating the pool(s) is the rate of amino acid oxidation, which is sensitive to a surplus or deficit of specific amino acids [46]. In fact, the initial response to inadequate intakes of amino acids or nitrogen is a decreased rate of amino acid oxidation [47,48]. Subsequently, synthesis of specific proteins diminish within selected tissues or organs, such as liver transport proteins or muscle proteins [47].

When the body is considered as a whole, it is estimated that synthesis and degradation (turnover) account for 15 to 20% of resting energy expenditure [46]. For each cellular protein, there is a specific and characteristic rate of synthesis [43]. The degradative regulation of specific proteins has not been elucidated. Rates of protein turnover vary among tissues, as is evidenced in the more rapid turnover of visceral protein as compared with skeletal muscle. Turnover of protein is under independent control, and the rates of synthesis and degradation can be quite high under certain circumstances. Growth and febrile conditions are examples of such circumstances; it is the small difference between the rates of synthesis and degradation that permits protein accre-

tion during growth but results in protein loss during fevers [46].

Some of the control sites for protein synthesis include the nucleus, cytoplasm, and membrane. The cellular protein to be synthesized is determined by specific mRNA produced in the nucleus under hormonal (steroid or peptide) influence. The rate at which the protein is synthesized is affected by (1) the amount of mRNA, (2) the ribosome number (amount of ribosomal RNA, rRNA), and (3) the activity of the ribosomes (rapidity of translation, or peptide formation) [46]. Obviously, the amino acids must be all present and in the appropriate concentrations to charge the tRNA. Degradation of proteins, either made intracellularly or brought into the cell by endocytosis, may be cytoplasmic or lysosomal. Amino acids generated from protein degradation may be reused to synthesize new proteins, degraded for energy, or used to synthesize glucose, ketones, or fatty acids depending on the person's nutritional status.

Although food intake and the nutritional status of the organism affect the rate of protein turnover, their effect is believed to be indirect. Food, or its lack, exerts an influence on protein synthesis and degradation through changes in hormone balance [43,46]. Hormone balance is particularly sensitive to changes in plasma amino acid concentrations. The secretion of insulin, glucagon, growth hormone, and glucocorticoids increases in response to elevated concentrations of selected amino acids. Therefore, the protein component of food intake, up to a certain threshold level, appears to be of particular importance. When this threshold level of protein (or plasma amino acids) has been reached, however, any further increase in intake has little or no effect on the rate of protein synthesis, probably because of the counterregulatory effects of the various hormones being secreted. It is believed that this threshold level for protein intake corresponds roughly to dietary protein requirements [46].

In general, protein synthesis and positive nitrogen balance are promoted by insulin, while the counterregulatory hormones, glucagon, catecholamines, and glucocorticoids have an opposite effect, promoting protein degradation and a negative nitrogen balance. Growth hormone, although counterregulatory, is an anabolic agent, like insulin. Prostaglandins and thyroid hormones also are affected by dietary nutrient intakes, and can promote changes in protein turnover. The effects of a hormone on protein turnover, however, may differ depending on the tissue.

The constant degradation of intracellular proteins is of prime importance to the life of the cells because it ensures a flux of proteins (amino acids) through the cytosol that can be used for cellular growth and/or maintenance [49]. The proteases responsible for protein degradation in the cell include lysosomal proteases and cytosolic proteases. Lysosomes, with their digestive enzymes, represent the primary means of protein digestion. Lysosomes are found in all mammalian cell types with the exception of the erythrocyte. The lysosomal proteases include endopeptidases and exopeptidases known as *cathepsins*. Numerous cathepsins have been isolated; some examples include cathepsins B, H, L, and D, each with varying specificities [50,51]. The lysosome is responsible for degradation of extracellular proteins brought into the cell by endocytosis, and for intracellular protein degradation under conditions of nutrient deprivation [50,52]. In nutritionally (amino acid) deprived cells, autophagic vacuoles containing the intracellular protein form and fuse with lysosomes. The protein in turn is completely digested by the lysosomal proteases; the process is often referred to as *macroautophagy* and is enhanced by glucagon and suppressed by insulin [51,53].

Although autophagy (self-consumption of a cell or the internalization and digestion of cytosol, endoplasmic reticulum and whole organelles into vacuoles or autophagosomes) [50] is not observed in the well-nourished cell, some degradation of intracellular proteins by the lysosomal autophagic enzyme system typically occurs. This slow, continuous degradation of intracellular proteins by lysosomes is referred to as *basal* autophagy or *microautophagy* [49,50,53]. Microautophagy needs some mechanism by which selected intracellular proteins could enter the lysosomes more rapidly than other proteins. The conformation of intracellular proteins as a determinant of intracellular degradation rates has been proposed [50,51]. For example, compact proteins with hydrophobic groups on the interior would not be as susceptible to degradation as larger, more hydrophobic proteins [51]. In the liver, microautophagy may function in the degradation of proteins with long half-lives and that are not good substrates for other proteolytic pathways [52]. A merger of the lysosomal and cytosolic ubiquitin systems has also been postulated. While several mechanisms have been theorized, one of the ubiquitin enzymes, E_1, is thought to be required for accelerated degradation of cellular proteins in lysosomes. For example, cellular proteins preferentially targeted for lysosomal degradation may first need to be conjugated to ubiquitin [54]. The contributions of lysosomal and cytosolic pathways in proteolysis varies depending on the cell type and the physiological status [52].

The role of cytosolic proteases including the ubiquitin system in protein degradation has been only recently recognized. Most proteins with short half-lives are degraded by cytosolic ATP-dependent pathways that may or may not require ubiquitin conjugation [52]. How specific proteins are selected by the proteolytic system is not fully understood, but the major component of selectivity appears to reside within the structural properties of the protein [50]. The structure can either increase or decrease the vulnerability of the protein to the degradative system. Newly synthesized proteins that have not yet been integrated into their appropriate cell location are particularly vulnerable to degradation. Whether or not these proteins can escape degradation seems to depend largely on their primary structure and consequently on their final conformation and function. Abnormal or aberrant proteins appear to be recognized and degraded rapidly, but certain normal proteins also undergo rapid degradation. Some normal proteins with extremely short half-lives are the regulatory enzymes, which need to be adjusted quickly in response to appropriate stimuli such as excess substrate.

Characteristics of short-lived proteins include large size, acidic pH values, hydrophobicity, and rapid inactivation by a low pH or high temperature [50]. Rapidly degraded proteins may also possess a common amino acid sequence. Rogers et al. [55] have developed the PEST hypothesis, based on the observation that proteins with particularly short half-lives contain regions rich in proline (P), glutamic acid (E), serine (S), and threonine (T) and surrounded by regions of positively charged amino acids [54,55]. However, neither the mechanism by which the PEST signal targets proteins for degradation, nor the system that recognizes the signal, have been identified [54]. In the ubiquitin system, proteins that are to be degraded are ligated to the polypeptide ubiquitin in an ATP-requiring reaction [50]. Ubiquitin protein conjugases have been identified in both the cytosol and the nucleus [54]. Once ligated, a multienzyme complex degrades the ubiquitinated proteins in a series of reactions; following proteolysis, ubiquitin is released for reuse [54].

Signals in proteins for ubiquitin-mediated degradation include N-terminal recognition. Specificity of binding by E_3alpha, an ubiquitin protein ligase of the ubiquitin protein degradation system, to selected N-terminal amino acid residues has been demonstrated [54]. E_3 has two distinct sites that interact with specific N-terminal residues. Proteins with valine, methionine, glycine, alanine, serine, threonine, and cysteine residues at their N-terminal position are relatively stable [56]. In contrast, proteins with N-terminal leucine, glutamate, histidine, tyrosine, glutamine, aspartate, asparagine, phenylalanine, leucine, tryptophan, lysine, and arginine are typically unstable, with short half-lives [54,56]. Proteins with acetylated N-termini are not degraded by the ubiquitin system [54].

The requirement for energy for protein catabolism is a paradox that has been recognized for over thirty years [51]. ATP-dependent proteases have been demonstrated in the cytosolic degradation system. Waxman and Goldberg [57] based on their work with an ATP-dependent protease found in *Escherichia coli*, have shown that this enzyme is activated by both ATP and by substrate proteins, and that the two have an additive effect. When the protein is activated by ATP, it will degrade various small hydrophobic peptides that are bound to its active site, but concomitant hydrolysis of the ATP molecule does not occur. When substrate protein activates the protease, it evidently does so by binding to two sites on the enzyme: the active site, which has a preference for specific amino acid sequences and a regulatory site, which somehow recognizes that the protein is unfolded and vulnerable. When activated by both ATP and a substrate protein, the enzyme is believed to undergo a distinct structural change that enhances its capacity for peptide cleavage and also causes hydrolysis of ATP. A protein that binds itself to both sites of the enzyme can induce its own destruction, but other proteins that are unable to bind the enzyme at both sites will remain unaffected. Furthermore, the adenosine diphosphate (ADP) produced as a result of the proteolysis acts as an inhibitor of continued hydrolysis, thereby helping to prevent excessive proteolysis once the enzyme has been activated. Should an analogous mechanism exist in mammalian cells, this scheme could go far in explaining not only the observed heterogeneous selectivity of protein catabolism but also the function of ATP in this catabolic process [58].

PROTEIN INTAKE AND PROTEIN QUALITY

Dietary protein is required by humans because it contributes to the body's supply of indispensable amino acids and to its supply of nitrogen for the synthesis of the dispensable amino acids. The quality of a protein depends to some extent on its digestibility, but primarily on its indispensable amino acid composition. Both the specific amounts and proportions of these amino acids are important to the quality of a protein.

Recommended Protein Intake

Although many factors influence the protein requirements of humans, the quality of the protein(s) consumed is paramount. Factors impinging on protein requirements other than the quality of the protein include growth and body size, physiologic state, and level of energy intake. The influence of energy intake on protein requirement is particularly significant. Excess energy intake fosters nitrogen retention, whereas insufficient calories from carbohydrate and/or fat mandate the oxidation of some protein to supply energy needs. The promotion of nitrogen retention by a high caloric intake appears to have been a factor in estimating human requirements for the indispensable amino acids [59–61]. The high caloric intake, causing weight gain of experimental subjects, may have permitted nitrogen equilibrium at an amino acid intake lower than the actual requirement [60]. Most of the information about requirements of indispensable amino acids and the relationship between these amino acids and protein need has been provided through nitrogen balance studies in adults and children, and growth studies in infants. Nitrogen balance studies involve the measurement and summation of nitrogen losses from the body when (1) nitrogen intake is at or near a predicted adequate amount, and (2) nitrogen intake is less than (including protein-free nitrogen) and greater than a predicted adequate amount. Nitrogen losses are measured in the urine (U), feces (F), and skin (S). Nitrogen losses are subtracted from nitrogen intake (I_n):

$$\text{Nitrogen balance} = I_n - [(U - U_e) + (F - F_e) + S]$$

The subscript e (as U_e and F_e) shown in the equation stands for *endogenous* (also called *obligatory*) and refers to losses of nitrogen that occur when the subject is on a nitrogen free diet.

The factorial method has also been used to determine protein needs. As with nitrogen balance studies, the factorial method involves the measurement and summation of all losses of nitrogen from the body when the diet is devoid of protein. These losses represent endogenous (obligatory) nitrogen losses. Obligatory nitrogen losses from adults typically range from 41 to 59 mg nitrogen per kg body weight, with an average of about 55 mg nitrogen per kg body weight. Obligatory protein losses range from 0.26 to 0.43 g protein per kg body weight, with an average of about 0.34 g protein per kg body weight.

Recommendations for protein intakes include a coefficient of variation and may also include estimates of efficiency of utilization. A summary of the current estimates of indispensable amino acid requirements at different ages is given in Table 7.7, while Figure 7.27 illustrates the relationship between these amino acid re-

TABLE 7.7 A Summary of the Estimates of Amino Acid Requirements at Different Ages, as Proposed in 1985 by Food and Agriculture Organization, World Health Organization, United Nations [61]

Amino Acid	Infants (3 to 4 months)	Children (2 years)	School boys (10 to 12 years)	Adults
Histidine	28[a]			(8–12)
Isoleucine	70	31	28	10
Leucine	161	73	44	14
Lysine	103	64	44	12
Methionine and cystine	58	27	22	13
Phenylalanine and tyrosine	125	69	22	14
Threonine	87	37	28	7
Tryptophan	17	12.5	3.3	3.5
Valine	93	38	25	10
Total	714	352	216	84

[a]Values are mg/kg/day.

Reprinted with permission from Recommended Dietary Allowances: 10th Edition. Copyright 1989 by the National Academy of Sciences. Courtesy of the National Academy Press, Washington, D.C.

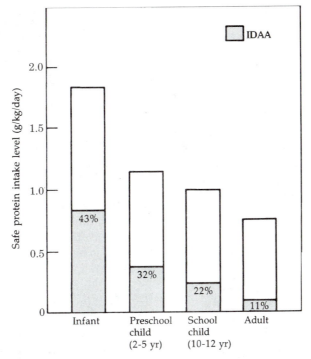

FIGURE 7.27 The relationship between protein and indispensable amino acid needs. The currently accepted percentage of protein requirements that should be provided by indispensable amino acids (IDAA) ranges from 43% in infants to 11% in adults.

quirements and total protein need. Figure 7.27 makes clear the currently accepted concept that maintenance of existing body tissue is much less dependent on protein quality than is growth. There is an inconsistency, however. Although the growth component in the older school-aged child appears to be only a small consideration in total protein need, protein quality still assumes much more importance in this group than in the adult [61,62].

The many difficulties associated with the nitrogen balance method, both in logistics and interpretation, have led Young et al. [60, 61] and numerous other researchers [63–66] to use a continuous, stable isotope infusion technique for estimating amino acid requirements in human adults. Their results from studies of adult requirements for leucine, valine, lysine, and threonine suggest that adult needs for indispensable amino acids are two to three times greater than the currently accepted levels and even higher than the levels presently postulated for children 10 to 12 years of age. Should further research prove this supposition to be fact, an adult's need for the indispensable amino acids in relation to total protein may nearly approximate that of the preschool child. The indispensable amino acids would need to provide 33% (rather than the present 11 to 19%) of the adult protein requirement. Calculations of human protein requirements are described in references 62 and 66.

Evaluation of Protein Quality

Although the potential quality of a protein resides in its content of indispensable amino acids, its true quality depends on the availability of these amino acids to the human body. Nevertheless, the most commonly used method for estimating protein quality is the chemical score, which considers only potential quality.

Chemical Score Chemical score (or amino acid score) involves a comparison of the test protein with whole egg protein (considered to have a score of 100) or with an ideal reference pattern of amino acids. In the 1989 RDA [67], amino acid requirement patterns have been calculated for various population groups; that is, requirements of individual indispensable amino acids (in mg) for each population group have been divided by the corresponding recommended intake of protein (in grams). The chemical score of a food protein, as the name implies, is a chemical evaluation of its quality and can be calculated as follows:

$$\text{Score of test protein} = \frac{\begin{array}{c}\text{content of each indispensable amino acid}\\\text{in food protein (mg/g protein)}\end{array}}{\begin{array}{c}\text{content of same amino acid in reference}\\\text{protein or reference pattern (mg/g protein)}\end{array}}$$

The amino acid with the lowest score in relation to the reference pattern becomes the first limiting amino acid; the one with the next lowest score is the second limiting amino acid; and so on. Table 7.8 gives the amino acid pattern in whole egg, and the amino acid requirement reference pattern for adults. Comparison of the quality of different food proteins against the standard of whole-egg protein can be valuable but probably is not nearly so important to adequate protein nutriture as their comparison with reference patterns for the various population groups. The indispensable amino acids that appear to be relatively more difficult to obtain in the mixed American diet are lysine, the sulfur-containing

TABLE 7.8 Amino Acid Reference Patterns [67]

Indispensable Amino Acids	Whole-Egg Pattern	Requirement Pattern for Adults
	mg amino acid/g protein	
Histidine	22	(11)+
Isoleucine	54	13
Leucine	86	19
Total sulfur amino acids (met and cys[a])	57	17
Total aromatic amino acids (phe and tyr[a])	93	19
Lysine	70	16
Threonine	47	9
Tryptophan	17	5
Valine	66	13
Total indispensable amino acids[b] (without histidine)	490	111

[a]Cysteine and tyrosine are considered "conditionally indispensable" because they spare methionine and phenylalanine.
[b]Value is imputed. Requirement for histidine has not been quantified beyond infancy but probable requirement is estimated to be between 8–12 mg/kg body wt/d for adults. Reprinted with permission from Recommended Dietary Allowances: 10th Edition. Copyright 1989 by the National Academy of Science. Courtesy of the National Academy Press, Washington, D.C.

amino acids (methionine and cysteine), threonine, and tryptophan [67].

Biological Value Biological evaluation of protein use is tedious and time consuming, and requires a living organism. Biological value (BV) of proteins most often is determined in experimental animals, but it can be determined in humans as well through use of the following equation:

$$\text{BV of test protein} = \frac{I - (F - F_0) - (U - U_0)}{I - (F - F_0)} \times 100$$

where I is intake of nitrogen; F is fecal nitrogen; F_0 is endogenous fecal nitrogen when subjects are maintained on a nitrogen free diet; U is urinary nitrogen; and U_0 is endogenous urinary nitrogen when subjects are maintained on a nitrogen-free diet.

BV is a measure of nitrogen retained for growth and/or maintenance and is expressed as a percentage of nitrogen absorbed:

$$\text{BV} = (\text{nitrogen retained/nitrogen absorbed}) \times 100$$

Proteins exhibit a higher BV when fed at levels below the amount necessary for nitrogen equilibrium. As intake of protein approaches or exceeds adequacy, retention decreases.

Protein Efficiency Ratio Protein efficiency ratio (PER) represents the gain in body weight on a test protein divided by the grams of protein consumed.

$$PER = \frac{\text{gain in body weight (in grams)}}{\text{grams of protein consumed}}$$

Young growing animals are typically placed on a standard diet with about 10% (by weight) of the diet as test protein. Weight gain is measured for a specific time period and compared to the amount of the protein consumed.

The PER for casein is 2.5, thus rats gain 2.5 g of weight for every 1 g of casein consumed. PER is used in nutrition labeling such that if the PER is ≥ 2.5, then 45 g protein is considered as meeting 100% US RDA. If the PER is < 2.5, then 65 g protein is needed to meet 100% US RDA.

Net Protein Utilization Another biological measure of protein quality that includes an evaluation of protein digestibility as well as of content of indispensable amino acids is net protein utilization or use (NPU). NPU measures retention of food nitrogen rather than retention of absorbed nitrogen and is calculated from the following equation:

$$NPU = I - (F - F_0) - (U - U_0)/I$$

Although NPU can be measured in humans through nitrogen balance studies in which two groups of well-matched experimental subjects are used, a more nearly accurate measurement is made on experimental animals through direct analysis of the animal carcasses. In either case, one experimental group is fed the test protein, while the other group receives an isocaloric, protein-free diet. When experimental animals are used as subjects, carcasses can be analyzed for nitrogen directly (total carcass nitrogen, or TCN) or indirectly at the end of the feeding period. The indirect measurement of nitrogen is made by water analysis. Given the amount of water removed from the carcasses, an approximate nitrogen content of lean body mass can be calculated:

$$NPU = \frac{\text{TCN on test protein} - \text{TCN on protein-free diet}}{\text{g nitrogen consumed}}$$

Net Dietary Protein Calories The net dietary protein calories percentage (NDpCal%) is particularly helpful in evaluation of human diets in which the protein-to-calorie ratio may vary greatly:

$$NDpCal\% = \text{protein kcal}/$$
$$\text{total kcal intake} \times 100 \times NPUop$$

(NPUop is NPU when protein is fed above the minimum requirement for nitrogen equilibrium.)

Munro et al. [68] introduced a simple method by which the adequacy of a food protein can be roughly estimated. By calculating the percentage of calories provided by the recommended protein intake when adequate energy is supplied, one can estimate the percentage of protein calories that should be found in a food used as a primary protein source. For instance, the protein and energy RDA [67] for a 25-year old, 79 kg male are 63 g protein (79 kg × 0.8 g/kg body weight [67]) and 2900 kcal. To calculate kcal from protein, 63 g protein × 4 kcal/g = 252 kcal from protein. Then to determine percentage total kcal from protein, 252 kcal from protein/ 2900 total kcal recommended × 100 = 8.7% kcal provided by dietary protein. Any food, therefore, used as a primary source of protein and energy, but providing less than 8.7% of its calories as protein is probably unable to meet maintenance needs for indispensable amino acids. Foods particularly suspect are cassava flour (1.8 kcal from protein/100 kcal flour) and plantain (3.1 kcal from protein/100 kcal plantain). Both these foods are known to be staples in some of the developing countries.

Knowledge of the chemical scores of a variety of proteins permits certain proteins to be combined so that their amino acid patterns become complementary. For the vegan, this knowledge is particularly valuable. Legumes, with their high content of lysine but low content of sulfur-containing amino acids, complement the grains, which are more than adequate in methionine and cysteine but which are limited in lysine.

The lacto-ovo vegetarian should have no problems with protein adequacy because when milk and eggs are combined, even in small amounts, with plant foods, the indispensable amino acids are supplied in adequate amounts. One exception is the combination of milk with legumes. Although milk contains more methionine and cysteine per gram of protein than do the legumes, it still fails to meet the standard of the ideal pattern for the sulfur-containing amino acids.

The formula for vegan protein balance is as follows: 60% of protein from grains, 35% from legumes, 5% from leafy greens [69]. The 70 kg adult man whose RDA for protein is 56 g could obtain his needed indispensable amino acids by consuming

- 4 servings (4 slices) whole-grain bread
- 5 servings (2 1/2 cups) grain from oatmeal, brown rice, cracked wheat
- 1 serving (1/4 cup) nuts or seeds
- 2 1/2 servings (1 1/4 cups) beans or (2 cups soy milk and 1/3 cup navy beans)
- 4 servings (2 cups) vegetables, two of which are leafy greens

Plant protein foods contribute about 65% of the per capita supply of protein world-wide, and about 32% in North America [70].

SUMMARY

Proteins in foods become available for use by the body after they have been broken down into their component amino acids. Nine of these amino acids are considered essential; therefore, the quality of dietary proteins correlates with its content of these indispensable amino acids.

An important concept in protein metabolism is the amino acid pool(s), which contains amino acids of dietary origin plus those contributed by the breakdown of body tissue. The amino acids comprising the pool(s) are used in a variety of ways: (1) for synthesis of new proteins for growth and/or replacement of existing body proteins, (2) for production of important nonprotein nitrogen-containing molecules, and (3) for oxidation as a source of energy.

The liver is the primary site of amino acid metabolism but no clear picture of the body's overall handling of nitrogen can emerge without consideration of amino acid metabolism in a variety of tissues and organs. Of particular significance is the metabolism of the branched-chain amino acids in the skeletal muscle and the production of the ammonium ion in the kidney. In addition, current research on neuropeptides spotlights the importance of amino acid metabolism in neural tissue.

Of the nonessential amino acids, glutamate assumes particular importance because of its versatility in overall metabolism of the amino acids. Glutamate and its α-keto acid make possible many crucial reactions in various metabolic pathways for amino acids. An appreciation for the functions performed by glutamate makes one realize that the connotation of "dispensable" as applied to this amino acid may be misleading.

Protein metabolism is particularly responsive to hormonal action, and this action can vary according to the tissue effect. Protein metabolism as regulated by

hormonal action is particularly significant during periods of stress (see "Perspective" section).

Protein plays many roles in the body: it provides structure, it can be used as a source of energy, and many protein molecules, such as enzymes and neuropeptides, serve in a regulatory capacity. Because of its contribution to both energy production and synthesis of regulatory molecules, protein provides an excellent transition from the energy-producing nutrients to those with regulatory functions.

References Cited

1. Rose WC. The amino acid requirements of adult man. Nutr Abstr Rev 1957;27:631–643.
2. Harper AE. Dispensable and indispensable amino acid relationships. In: Blackburn GL, Grant JP, Young VR, eds. Amino acids. Boston: Wright, PSG, 1983:105–121.
3. Jackson AA. Amino acids: Essential and non-essential. Lancet 1983;1:1034–1037.
4. Laidlaw SA, Kopple JD. Newer concepts of the indispensable amino acids. Am J Clin Nutr 1987;46:593–605.
5. Munro HN, Crim MC. The proteins and amino acids. In: Shils ME, Olson JA, Shike M, eds. Modern nutrition in health and disease, 8th ed. Philadelphia: Lea and Febiger, 1994:1–35.
6. Silk DBA, Grimble GK, Rees RG. Protein digestion and amino acid and peptide absorption. Proc Nutr Soc 1985;44:63–72.
7. Alpers DH. Digestion and absorption of carbohydrates and proteins. In: Johnson LR. Physiology of the gastrointestinal tract. New York: Raven Press, 1987: 1469–1487.
8. Hopfer U. Membrane transport mechanisms for hexoses and amino acids in the small intestine. In: Johnson LR. Physiology of the gastrointestinal tract. New York: Raven Press, 1987:1499–1526.
9. Adibi SA, Morse EL. The number of glycine residues which limits intact absorption of glycine oligopeptides in human jejunum. J Clin Invest 1977;60:1008–1016.
10. Adibi SA, Morse EL, Masilamani SS, Amin PM. Evidence for two different modes of tripeptide disappearance in human intestine. J Clin Invest 1975;56:1355–1363.
11. Craft IL, Geddes D, Hyde CW, Wise IJ, Matthews DM. Absorption and malabsorption of glycine and glycine peptides in man. Gut 1968;9:425–437.
12. Souba WW, Pacitti AJ. How amino acids get into cells: Mechanisms, models, menus, and mediators. JPEN 1992;16:569–578.
13. Christensen HN. Naming plan for membrane transport systems for amino acids. Neurochemical Res 1984; 9:1757–1758.
14. Kilberg MS, Stevens, BR, Novak DA. Recent advances in mammalian amino acid transport. Ann Rev Nutr 1993; 13:137–165.

15. Adibi SA, Gray S, Menden E. The kinetics of amino acid absorption and alteration of plasma composition of free amino acids after intestinal perfusion of amino acid mixtures. Am J Clin Nutr 1967;20:24–33.

16. Steinhardt HJ, Adibi SA. Kinetics and characteristics of absorption from an equimolar mixture of 12 glycyl-dipeptides in human jejunum. Gastroenterology 1986; 90:577–582.

17. Grimble GK, Rees RG, Keohane PP, Cartwright T, Desreumaux M, Silk DBA. Effect of peptide chain length on absorption of egg protein hydrolysates in the normal human jejunum. Gastroenterology 1987;92:136–142.

18. Grimble GK, Keohane PP, Higgins BE, Kaminski MV, Silk DBA. Effect of peptide chain length on amino acid and nitrogen absorption from two lactalbumin hydrolysates in the normal human jejunum. Clin Sci 1986;71:65–69.

19. Vazquez JA, Daniel H, Adibi SA. Dipeptides in parenteral nutrition: From basic science to clinical applications. Nutr Clin Prac 1993;8:95–105.

20. Zaloga GP. Physiologic effects of peptide-based enteral formulas. Nutr Clin Prac 1990;5:231–237.

21. Stevens BR, Kaunitz JD, Wright EM. Intestinal transport of amino acids and sugars: Advances using membrane vesicles. Ann Rev Physiol 1984;46:417–433.

22. Gardner MLG. Gastrointestinal absorption of intact proteins. Ann Rev Nutr 1988;8:329–350.

23. Kilberg MS, Handlogten ME, Christensen HN. Characteristics of an amino acid transport system in rat liver for glutamine, asparagine, histidine and closely related analogs. J Biol Chem 1980;255:4011–4019.

24. Meister A. Amino acids and glutathione. Proc Biochem Symp 1982:5–27.

25. Meister A, Anderson ME. Glutathione. Ann Rev Biochem 1983;52:711–760.

26. Tanphaichitr V, Leelahagul P. Carnitine metabolism and carnitine deficiency. Nutr 1993;9:246–254.

27. Sorensen LB. Degradation of uric acid in man. Metabolism 1959;8:687–703.

28. Scriver CR, Gregory DM, Sovettes D, Tissenbaum G. Normal plasma free amino acid values in adults: The influence of some common physiological variables. Metabolism 1985;34:868–873.

29. Young VR, Bier DM. A kinetic approach to determination of human amino acid requirements. Nutr Rev 1987;45:289–298.

30. Kurowska EM, Carroll KK. Hypercholesterolemic responses in rabbits to selected groups of dietary essential amino acids. J Nutr 1994;124:364–370.

31. Souba WW. Glutamine: A key substrate for the splanchnic bed. Ann Rev Nutr 1991;11:285–308.

32. Krebs HA, Baverel G, Lund P. Effect of bicarbonate on glutamine metabolism. Internl J Biochem 1980;12:69–73.

33. Goldberg AL, Chang TW. Regulation and significance of amino acid metabolism in skeletal muscle. Fed Proc 1978;37:2301–2307.

34. Morris SM. Regulation of enzymes of urea and arginine synthesis. Ann Rev Nutr 1992;12:81–101.

35. Walser M, Bodenlos LJ. Urea metabolism in man. J Clin Invest 1959;38:1617–1626.

36. Gaull GE, Pasantes-Morales H, Wright CE. Taurine in human nutrition: Overview. In: Taurine: Biological actions and clinical perspectives. New York: Liss, 1985:3–21.

37. Jungas RL, Halperin ML, Brosnan JT. Quantitative analysis of amino acid oxidation and related gluconeogenesis in humans. Physiol Rev 1992;72:419–448.

38. Goldberg AL. Factors affecting protein balance in skeletal muscle in normal and pathological states. In: Blackburn GL, Grant JP, Young VR, eds. Amino acids. Boston: Wright, PSG, 1983:201–211.

39. Harper AE, Miller RH, Block KP. Branched chain amino acid metabolism. Ann Rev Nutr 1984;4:409–454.

40. Abumrad NN, Rabin D, Wise KL, Lacy WW. The disposal of an intravenously administered amino acid load across the human forearm. Metabolism 1982; 31:463–470.

41. Wahren J, Felig P, Hagenfeldt L. Effect of protein ingestion on splanchnic and leg metabolism in normal man and in patients with diabetes mellitus. J Clin Invest 1976;57:987–999.

42. Jones JD, Burnett PC. Creatinine metabolism in humans with decreased renal function: Creatinine deficit. Clin Chem 1974;20:1204–1212.

43. Reeds PJ, James WPT. Protein turnover. Lancet 1983;1:571–574.

44. McCabe BJ. Dietary tyramine and other pressor amines in MAOI regimens: A review. J Am Diet Assoc 1986; 86:1059–1064.

45. Bloom FE. Neuropeptides. Sci Am 1981;245:148–168.

46. Waterlow JC. Protein turnover with special reference to man. Q J Exp Physiol 1984;69:409–438.

47. Young VR, Marchini JS, Cortiella J. Assessment of protein nutritional status. J Nutr 1990;120:1496–1502.

48. Benevenga NJ, Gahl MJ, Blemings KP. Role of protein synthesis in amino acid catabolism. J Nutr 1993; 123:332–336.

49. Wheatley DN. Intracellular protein degradation: Basis of a self-regulating mechanism for the proteolysis of endogenous proteins. J Theor Biol 1984;107:127–149.

50. Beynon RJ, Bond JS. Catabolism of intracellular protein: Molecular aspects. Am J Physiol 1986;251:C141–152.

51. Ballard FJ, Gunn JM. Nutritional and hormonal effects on intracellular protein catabolism. Nutr Rev 1982: 40:33–42.

52. Dice JF. Peptide sequences that target cytosolic proteins for lysosomal proteolysis. Trends Biol Sci 1990; 15:305–309.

53. Mortimore GE, Poso AR. Intracellular protein catabolism and its control during nutrient deprivation and supply. Ann Rev Nutr 1987;7:539–564.

54. Hershko A, Ciechanover A. The ubiquitin system for protein degradation. Ann Rev Biochem 1992;61:761–807.

55. Rogers S, Wells R, Rechsteiner M. Amino acid sequences common to rapidly degraded proteins: The PEST hypothesis. Science 1986;234:364–368.

56. Bachmair A, Finley D, Varshavsky A. In vivo half-life of a protein is a function of its amino-terminal residue. Science 1986;234:179–186.

57. Waxman L, Goldberg AL. Selectivity of proteolysis: Protein substrates activate the ATP-dependent protease (La). Science 1986;232:500–503.

58. Goldberg AL. The mechanism and functions of ATP-dependent proteases in bacterial and animal cells. Eur J Biochem 1992;203:9–23.

59. Rose WC. The amino acid requirements of adult man. Nutr Abstr Rev 1957;27:631–643.

60. Young VR, Bier DM. A kinetic approach to determination of human amino acid requirements. Nutr Rev 1987;45:289–298.

61. Young VR. 1987 McCollum award lecture: Kinetics of human amino acid metabolism: Nutritional implications and some lessons. Am J Clin Nutr 1987;46:709–725.

62. Energy and protein requirements. Report of a joint FAO/WHO/UN expert consultation. WHO technical report series 724. Geneva: World Health Organization, 1985.

63. Mequid MM, Matthews DE, Bier DM, Meredith CN, Soeldner JS, Young VR. Leucine kinetics at graded leucine intakes in young men. Am J Clin Nutr 1986;43:770–780.

64. Mequid MM, Matthews DE, Bier DM, Meredith CN, Young VR. Valine kinetics at graded valine intakes in young men. Am J Clin Nutr 1986;43:781–786.

65. Ahao K, Wen A, Meredith CN, Matthews DE, Bier DM, Young VR. Threonine kinetics at graded threonine intakes in young men. Am J Clin Nutr 1986;43:795–802.

66. Meredith CN, Wen A, Bier DM, Matthews DE, Young VR. Lysine kinetics at graded lysine intakes in young men. Am J Clin Nutr 1986;43:787–794.

67. Food and Nutrition Board, National Research Council: Recommended dietary allowances, 10th ed. Washington, DC: National Academy Press, 1989.

68. Munro HN, Crim MC. The proteins and amino acids. In: Shils ME, Young VR, eds. Modern nutrition in health and disease. 7th ed. Philadelphia: Lea and Febiger, 1988;1–37.

69. Robertson L, Flinder C, Godfrey B. Laurel's Kitchen—A handbook for vegetarian cookery and nutrition. Petaluma, CA: Nilgiri Press, 1984.

70. Young VR, Pellett PL. Plant proteins in relation to human protein and amino acid nutrition. Am J Clin Nutr 1994;59(suppl):1203S–1212S.

Additional References

A. E. Harper Symposium on Emerging Aspects of Amino Acid Metabolism. J Nutr 1994;124:1491S–1532S.

Murray RK, Granner DK, Mayes PA, Rodwell VW. Harper's biochemistry, 23rd ed. Norwalk CT: Appleton and Lange, 1993.

McGilvery RW. Biochemistry, a functional approach, 3rd ed. Philadelphia: Saunders, 1983.

McMurray WC. Essentials of human metabolism, 2nd ed. Philadelphia: Harper & Row, 1983.

Montgomery R, Dryer RL, Conway TW, Spector AA. Biochemistry, a case-oriented approach, 4th ed. St. Louis: Mosby, 1983.

Newsholme EA, Leech AR. Biochemistry for the medical sciences. New York: Wiley, 1984.

Pike RL, Brown ML. Nutrition: an integrated approach, 3rd ed. New York: Wiley, 1984.

Stryer L. Biochemistry, 3rd ed. San Francisco: Freeman, 1988.

Suggested Readings

Beynon RJ, Bond JS. Catabolism of protein: Molecular aspects. Am J Physiol 1986;251:C141–152.
This is an excellent review on the different mechanisms by which protein may be catabolized in the cell.

Visek WJ. Arginine and disease states. J Nutr 1985;115:532–541.

Visek WJ. Arginine needs, physiological state and usual diets. A reevaluation. J Nutr 1986;116:36–46.
These articles address the role of arginine and address the question of the essentiality or lack of essentiality of arginine for adults.

Blackburn GL, Grant JP, Young VR, eds. Amino acids: Metabolism and medical applications. Boston: Wright, PSG, 1983.
This is a compilation of papers presented at an international symposium on amino acid metabolism. Results of research on numerous aspects of amino acid metabolism are included.

Bloom FE. Neuropeptides. Sci Am 1981; 245:148–168.
This is a lucid introduction to the very complicated subject of neuropeptides. The illustrations are excellent and easy to follow despite the complexity of the subject.

Goldberg AL, Chang Tse Wen. Regulation and significance of amino acid metabolism in skeletal muscle. Fed Proc 1978;39:2301–2307.
This article offers a concise but in-depth explanation of amino acid metabolism in the skeletal muscle.

Waterlow JC. Protein turnover with special reference to man. Q J Exp Physiol 1984; 69:409–438.
This is an inclusive review of current knowledge regarding protein turnover in various tissues of the body as well as in the body as a whole.

Young VR. 1987 McCollum award lecture: Kinetics of human amino acid metabolism: Nutritional implications and some lessons. Am J Clin Nutr 1987; 46:709–725.
This article offers an excellent discussion of data generated from nitrogen-balance studies and a comparison of estimated amino acid requirements for adults as determined by N-balance studies and by continuous isotope diffusion.

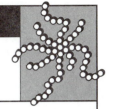

PERSPECTIVE

Protein Turnover: Starvation Versus Stress

Protein turnover is continuous, and the two processes comprising turnover, synthesis and degradation, approximately balance one another in the healthy adult. Whole-body turnover in humans is correlated to one's metabolic mass ($W^{0.75}$); daily turnover of protein is calculated to be approximately 4.6 g/kg body weight. For the average 70-kg male, turnover of whole-body protein would approximate 320 g daily [1].

Individual body proteins, however, vary in their turnover rate; the half-life of a protein can range from only a few minutes to several months [2]. Furthermore, neither the turnover rate of an individual protein nor that of total body protein remains constant. The rate of synthesis and degradation can be influenced by a variety of factors related to nutrition, including immediate food intake, previous diet, and overall nutrition status [1]. Another factor unrelated to nutrition but exerting the greatest influence on protein turnover is stress, whether it be injury (including surgery, trauma, burns) or infection or sepsis (the presence of pathogenic micro-organisms or their toxins in the blood and/or body tissues).

Study of the effect of overall nutrition on protein turnover has revealed that malnutrition decreases general protein synthesis in two ways: (1) mRNA is reduced and (2) the rate of peptide bond synthesis (or RNA "activity") is decreased. It is suggested that the amount of mRNA may vary with the level of immediate food intake, whereas a change in peptide synthesis could be due to the influence of previous food intake.

Malnutrition to the point of starvation is characterized by a definite decrease in protein synthesis. Even those proteins with very rapid turnover, such as plasma proteins, are synthesized at a rate 30 to 40% below normal. In muscle, protein synthesis rates drop even lower. However, protein degradation rates decrease concurrently so that in chronic starvation daily losses of nitrogen become quite small. For example, a person fully adapted to starvation can survive at a cost of 3 to 4 g of his or her body protein per day [3].

The principal mechanism of adjustment to starvation is a change in hormone balance. In particular, there is a sharp decrease in insulin production. In addition, the muscle and adipocytes become somewhat resistant to the action of insulin so that whatever insulin is circulating is ineffective in promoting of cellular nutrient uptake for protein synthesis and lipogenesis. Decreased insulin activity, coupled with increased synthesis of counterregulatory hormones such as glucagon, promotes fatty acid mobilization from adipose tissue, production of ketones, and the availability of amino acids for gluconeogenesis. The glucocorticoids are important in gluconeogenesis because they promote catabolism of muscle protein to provide substrates for gluconeogenesis. However, an increased adjustment to starvation is characterized by a decrease in the secretion of glucocorticoids. An additional hormonal change facilitating adjustment to starvation includes decreased synthesis of tri-iodothyronine (T_3, a thyroid hormone), which thus results in a lowered metabolic rate.

In the initial stages or first few days of fasting or starvation, glycogen in the liver is depleted. Muscles undergo proteolysis. Urinary 3-methylhistidine excretion increases to reflect myofibrillar protein catabolism. Muscles undergoing proteolysis also release a mixture of amino acids containing relatively high alanine and glutamine concentrations. Alanine is a preferred substrate for gluconeogenesis, and serves to stimulate the secretion of the gluconeogenic hormone glucagon. Alanine released from muscle is taken up by the liver, where the nitrogen is removed and converted to urea for excretion by the kidney, and the pyruvate formed can enter the gluconeogenic pathway. Glucose formed in the liver may be released into the blood for cellular uptake and metabolism. Glutamine released from muscles circulates in the blood for uptake and metabolism primarily by the gastrointestinal (GI) tract and kidney. Glutamine uptake by the liver diminishes and coupled with adaptive changes, hepatic glutamine synthesis is increased and urea synthesis diminishes. These hepatic changes help to direct glutamine to the kidneys for maintenance of acid–base balance.

As fasting or starvation continues, tissues continue to use fatty acids and glucose for energy, but also begin to use ketones formed in the liver from fatty acid oxidation. A decrease in protein catabolism and gluconeogenesis occurs concurrently with the brain's and other tissues' adaptation to ketones as a source of energy. Glutamine metabolism in the kidney increases as starvation continues and acidosis occurs. Within the kidney, glutamine catabolism generates ammonia, which serves to help correct the acidosis.

Figure 1 illustrates how adaptation to starvation allows the conservation of body protein. Because less carbohydrate is required by the body, less protein must

PERSPECTIVE (continued)

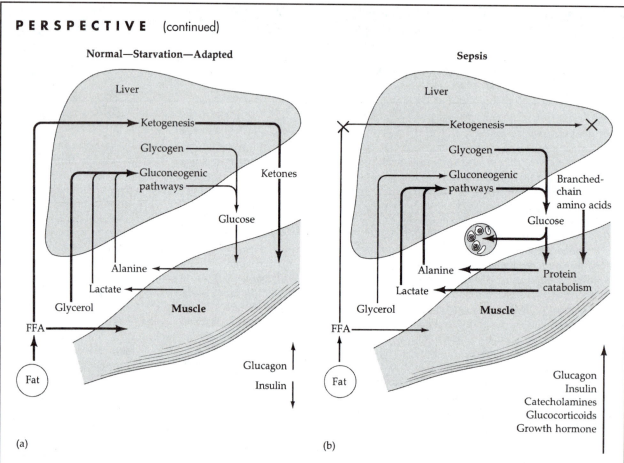

FIGURE 1 Gluconeogenesis during starvation and sepsis. During starvation (a), fat mobilization and ketogenesis provide energy, thereby sparing body protein and decreasing gluconeogenesis. In contrast, sepsis (b) causes stimulation of gluconeogenesis and inhibition of ketogenesis. Body protein is catabolized with no sparing effects from ketones. Fat mobilization occurs but to a lesser extent than with starvation. Increased responses during starvation and sepsis are shown by the heavy arrows. *(Beisel WR, Wannemacher RW. Gluconeogenesis, ureagenesis and ketogenesis during sepsis. J Parent Enter Nutr 1980;4:278. © by The American Society of Parental and Enteral Nutrition.)*

be broken down for gluconeogenesis. Amino acids resulting from proteolysis of muscle tissue can be used for the synthesis of crucial visceral proteins such as plasma proteins, which have more rapid turnover rates than muscle. It is estimated that under normal conditions visceral protein has a turnover rate three times greater than that of muscle protein [4].

Figure 1 demonstrates the change in hormone balance and the shift in fuel sources that occur in severe stress such as with trauma, surgery, burns, or sepsis. With sepsis as well as with trauma, surgery, and burns, glucocorticoids (primarily cortisol), catecholamines (such as epinephrine), and glucagon release increase (Fig. 1). The synthesis and release of cytokines also increase. Cytokines are low-molecular-weight peptides that evoke a number of varied reactions in the body and are used by primarily immune cells to communi-

cate with each other. Cytokines such as interleukin-1 (IL-1) and tumor necrosis factor (TNF) produced from macrophages in part mediate proteolysis and the hormonal response [5]. Inflammation, in contrast, involves cytokines such as IL-1, interleukin-6 (IL-6), TNF-alpha, interleukin-8 (IL-8), and interferon gamma (IFN-gamma).

An increase in protein turnover accompanies surgery, sepsis, burns, and trauma situations. Glucocorticoids, in part, are thought to stimulate hepatic protein synthesis. Proteins that are synthesized in the liver during these stress situations include primarily a group of proteins referred to as *acute phase reactants* (APR) or *acute phase response proteins* (APRP). Examples of APRP are (1) haptoglobin, which binds free hemoglobin (hemoglobin not in the red blood cell and released by hemolysis of the red blood cell); (2) cerulo-

P E R S P E C T I V E   (continued)

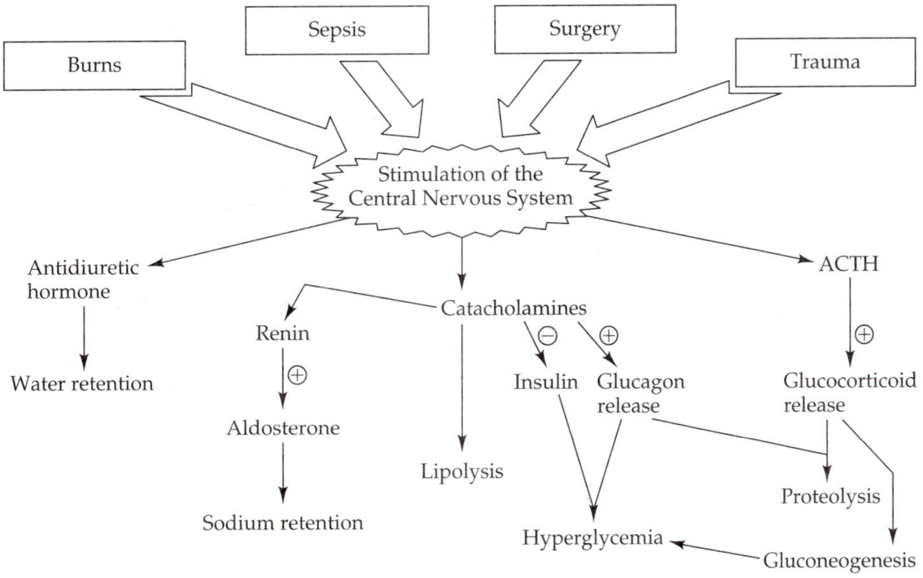

FIGURE 2 Metabolic stress response.

plasmin, a copper containing protein with oxidase activity; (3) alpha 2 macroglobulin, which activates macrophages among other white blood cells; (4) alpha 1 antitrypsin, which minimizes further tissue damage associated with phagocytosis of micro-organisms; (5) fibrinogen, which is required for blood coagulation; (6) C-reactive protein, which stimulates phagocytosis by white blood cells and activates complement proteins, which are needed for antibody-induced destruction of micro-organisms; and (7) alpha 1 acid glycoprotein, necessary for wound healing.

The increased rate of synthesis of protein with sepsis and other stress situations, however, is insignificant when compared with the rate of degradation. Protein catabolism predominates and provides amino acid substrates for glucose production via gluconeogenesis. Moreover, a delay in or the lack of enteral (meaning by way of or into the gastrointestinal tract) nutrition, which may accompany severe stress situations, may also result in the atrophy of intestinal mucosa and contribute to the risk of sepsis through possible translocation of bacteria or toxins [6]. The rate of glutamine production and release from muscle is not thought to meet the intestinal cells' need for glutamine during catabolic states [6–8].

With stress events, as with starvation, adipose tissue undergoes lipolysis. Although the body can partially defend itself against starvation through conservation of energy and adaptation to ketosis, it has no such de-

fense against injury, trauma, surgery, and/or infection. Unlike during starvation, ketogenesis is inhibited by insulin during sepsis, burns, injury or trauma, and surgery. Thus proteolysis continues with degradation exceeding synthesis. Each gram of nitrogen lost can be translated into the breakdown of approximately 30 g hydrated lean tissue [2].

Although insulin secretion increases with stress, the glucagon-to-insulin ratio favors glucagon, tissues become resistant to insulin action, and hyperglycemia (high blood glucose concentrations) persists. In addition, cortisol concentrations may remain elevated in the blood for prolonged periods following severe trauma or stress events and contribute to proteolysis and hyperglycemia. Interleukin-1 has also been shown to induce proteolysis with sepsis, although the mechanism of action is unknown [6].

Additional hormonal changes, illustrated in Figure 2, include the release of aldosterone, which promotes renal sodium and fluid reabsorption, thus increasing blood volume. Antidiuretic hormone (ADH) inhibits diuresis (urination) to also effect an increase in blood volume. Both aldosterone and ADH help restore circulation if it has been depressed by shock or loss of blood fluids by hemorrhage. The hormones thus help diminish total fluid losses, which may be high with skin loss from burns or with increased dermal losses from fever.

It has been suggested [2] that the body places a high priority on wound repair and host defense, gam-

PERSPECTIVE (continued)

bling that convalescence will occur before depletion of tissues becomes a threat to survival. Adaptation to stress is crucial and is characterized by changes such as the normalization of glucocorticoids and other hormones, diminished catabolism of mucle protein, and normalization of blood glucose.

References Cited

1. Waterlow JC. Protein turnover with special reference to man. Q J Exp Physiol 1984;69:409–438.
2. Kinney JM, Elwyn DH. Protein metabolism and injury. Ann Rev Nutr 1983;3:433–466.
3. Tepperman J, Tepperman HM. Metabolic and endocrine physiology, 5th ed. Chicago: Year Book Medical, 1987.
4. Anon. Measuring human muscle protein synthesis. Nutr Rev 1989; 47:77–79.
5. Hasselgren P, Fischer JE. Cytokines and protein metabolism. In: Gussler JD, ed. Cytokines in critical illness. Columbus, OH: Ross Laboratories, 1992:39–46.
6. Souba WW. Glutamine: A key substrate for the splanchnic bed. Ann Rev Nutr 1991;11:285–308.
7. Askanazi J, Carpentier YA, Michelsen CB, et al. Muscle and plasma amino acids following injury. Ann Surg 1980;192:78–85.
8. Lacey JM, Wilmore DW. Is glutamine a conditionally essential amino acid? Nutr Rev 1990;48:297–309.

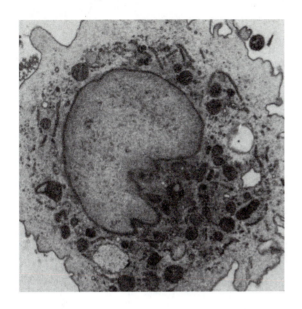

INTEGRATION AND REGULATION OF METABOLISM

Photo: A phagocytic cell (macrophage)

Chapters 4, 6, and 7 featured carbohydrate, lipid, and protein metabolism at the level of the individual cell, with emphasis on metabolic pathways common to nearly all eukaryotic cells. We also discussed in those chapters how the pathways are regulated at the level of certain regulatory enzymes by substrate availability, allosteric mechanisms, and covalent modification such as phosphorylation.

For their significance to be fully appreciated, metabolic pathways, and the specific metabolic roles of different organs and tissues, must be viewed in the context of the whole organism. Therefore this chapter will examine (1) how the major organs and tissues interact through integration of their metabolic pathways, and (2) hormonal regulation of these metabolic processes in maintaining homeostasis. The pathways themselves are not reproduced again in this chapter, but when appropriate, the reader will be referred to pertinent sections in previous chapters where the pathways are described.

INTERRELATIONSHIP OF CARBOHYDRATE, LIPID, AND PROTEIN METABOLISM

If ingested in sufficient amounts, any of the three energy-producing nutrients—carbohydrate, fat, and protein (amino acids)—can provide the body with its needed energy on a short-term basis. Within certain limitations, anabolic interconversion among the nutrients also occurs. For example, certain amino acids can be synthesized in the body from carbohydrate or fat, and conversely, most amino acids can serve as precursors for carbohydrate or fat synthesis. The considerable metabolic interconversion among the nutrients is illustrated as an overview in Figure 8.1. Not evident from Figure 8.1, but very important to recall, is that the Krebs cycle is an *amphibolic pathway*, mean-

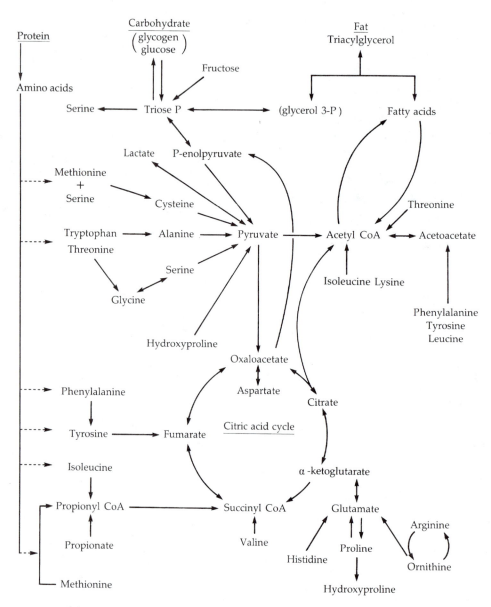

FIGURE 8.1 Interconversion of the macronutrients.

ing that it functions not only in the oxidative catabolism of carbohydrates, fatty acids, and amino acids, but also provides precursors for many biosynthetic pathways, particularly gluconeogenesis (p. 93). Along with pyruvate, several Krebs cycle intermediates, including α-ketoglutarate, succinate, fumarate, and oxaloacetate can be formed from the carbon skeletons of certain amino acids, and can function as gluconeogenic precursors.

The fact that animals can be fattened on a predominantly carbohydrate diet is evidence of the apparent ease by which carbohydrate can be converted into fat. However, it is believed that in the human, lipogenesis

from glucose may be much less efficient than previously proposed [1]. Glucose is the precursor for both the glycerol and the fatty acid components of triacylglycerols. The glycerol portion can be formed from dihydroxyacetone phosphate (DHAP), a 3-carbon intermediate in glycolysis (see Fig. 4.7). Reduction of DHAP by glycerol 3-phosphate dehydrogenase and NADH produces glycerol 3-phosphate, to which CoA-activated fatty acids attach in the course of triacylglycerol synthesis (see Fig. 6.12). A most significant reaction linking glucose metabolism to fatty acid synthesis is the reaction of the pyruvate dehydrogenase complex, which converts pyru-

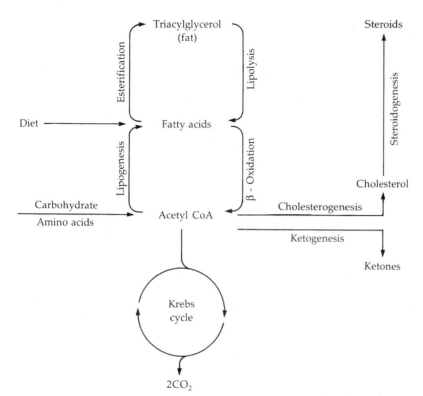

FIGURE 8.2 Overview of lipid metabolism, emphasizing the central role of acetyl CoA.

vate to acetyl CoA by dehydrogenation and decarboxylation. Acetyl CoA is the starting material for the synthesis of long-chain fatty acids as well as a variety of other lipids (Fig. 8.2) (see also "Synthesis of Fatty Acids," p. 139).

Although carbohydrate can be converted into both the glycerol and fatty acid components of fat, only the glycerol portion of fat can be converted to carbohydrate. The conversion of fatty acids into carbohydrate is not possible because *the pyruvate dehydrogenase reaction is not reversible.* This prevents the direct conversion of acetyl CoA, the sole catabolic product of even-numbered carbon fatty acids, into pyruvate for gluconeogenesis. In addition, gluconeogenesis from acetyl CoA as a Krebs cycle intermediate also cannot occur. This is because for every two carbons in the form of acetyl CoA entering the cycle, two carbons are lost by decarboxylation in early reactions of the pathway (see Fig. 4.10). Therefore, there can be no net conversion of acetyl CoA to pyruvate or to the gluconeogenic intermediates of the cycle. Consequently, acetyl CoA produced from whatever source must be used for energy, lipogenesis, cholesterogenesis, or ketogenesis.

Although fatty acids having an even number of carbons are degraded exclusively to acetyl CoA, and therefore are not glucogenic (gluconeogenic) for the reasons mentioned, fatty acids possessing an odd number of

carbon atoms are partially glucogenic. This is because propionyl CoA ($CH_3-CH_2-COSCoA$), ultimately formed by β-oxidation, is carboxylated and rearranged to succinyl CoA, a glucogenic Krebs cycle intermediate (see 6M, p. 138).

The glycerol portion of all triacylglycerols is glucogenic, entering the glycolytic pathway at the level of DHAP (see Figure 4.7). Following its release from triacylglycerol by lipase hydrolysis, glycerol can be phosphorylated to glycerol 3-phosphate by glycerokinase, then oxidized to DHAP by glycerol 3-phosphate dehydrogenase (8A).

(8A)

$$CH_2-OH \xrightarrow[\text{ATP ADP}]{} CH_2-OH \xrightarrow[\text{NAD}^+ \text{NADH}]{} CH_2-OH$$
$$CH-OH \qquad\qquad CH-OH \qquad\qquad C=O$$
$$CH_2-OH \qquad\qquad CH_2-O-P \qquad\qquad CH_2-O-P$$
Glycerol   Glycerol 3-P   DHAP

During the fasting state, when fat catabolism is accelerated, this conversion assumes greater importance in maintaining a normal level of blood glucose.

Metabolism of the amino acids gives rise to a variety of amphibolic intermediates, some of which produce glucose while others produce the ketone bodies via their conversion to acetyl CoA or acetoacetyl CoA (see 6N,

p. 138). Those amino acids that can be used for production of glucose are termed *glucogenic*, and those producing ketones are called *ketogenic*. Because they can be catabolized to acetyl CoA or acetoacetyl CoA, ketogenic amino acids are therefore potentially lipogenic. Several amino acids are both glucogenic and ketogenic, meaning that their carbon skeletons can give rise to both glucose and fats. Only the amino acids leucine and lysine are purely ketogenic. These amino acids cannot be gluconeogenic precursors. The dispensable glucogenic amino acids are usually interconverted with carbohydrate, but like the ketogenic amino acids, they also can be converted (however, indirectly) into fatty acids via acetyl CoA. The fatty acids, however, cannot be converted into the glucogenic amino acids for the same reason that fatty acids cannot form glucose, namely the irreversibility of the pyruvate dehydrogenase reaction. Although entirely possible, the conversion of the glucogenic amino acids into fat is rather uncommon. Only when protein is supplying a high percentage of the calories would one expect glucogenic amino acids to be used in fat synthesis. Leucine and lysine, along with those amino acids that are partially ketogenic, will give rise directly to acetyl CoA, but the reversal of the process—that is, the synthesis of these amino acids from acetyl CoA—is impossible. All the amino acids producing acetyl CoA directly (isoleucine, threonine, phenylalanine, tyrosine*, lysine, and leucine) are indispensable.

The interconversion of the energy-producing nutrients appears to be skewed toward providing the organism with an energy source that can be easily stored (fat), thereby providing for times when food is not readily available.

Energy released by the catabolic processes of the major nutrients must be shared by the energy-requiring synthetic pathways discussed earlier. On reaching the cells, the energy-producing nutrients can be catabolized to produce phosphorylative energy (ATP) and/or reductive energy (NADH, NADPH, $FADH_2$). Alternatively, they may be synthesized into more complex organic compounds and/or macromolecules that become cellular components. For synthesis of a cellular component to occur, however, chemical energy must be provided. Therefore when the cell places priority on the synthesis of a particular component, this synthesis is accomplished at the expense of another substance being catabolized. The common energy pool within a cell is finite, and all anabolic and endergonic processes must compete for this energy. For example, when the liver needs to pro-

duce more glucose by reversing glycolysis (that is, gluconeogenesis), it cannot simultaneously synthesize lipids and proteins. Instead, some of the existing cellular proteins or lipids are hydrolyzed, and the resulting amino acids or fatty acids are oxidized to generate the NADH and ATP needed for gluconeogenesis. Likewise, when hepatic lipogenesis occurs, glucose must be used so as to produce the NADPH and ATP necessary for the conversion of acetyl CoA to fatty acids.

The final common catabolic pathway for carbohydrate, fat, and protein is the Krebs cycle and oxidative phosphorylation via the electron transport chain (Figs. 4.10 and 3.14). In addition to releasing energy, these mitochondrial processes are crucial for many other metabolic sequences:

• CO_2 produced by oxidation of acetyl CoA is a source of cellular carbon dioxide for carboxylation reactions that initiate fatty acid synthesis and gluconeogenesis (pp. 93, 139). This CO_2 also supplies the carbon of urea and certain portions of the purine and pyrimidine rings (Figs. 7.9, 7.10, 7.17).

• Intermediates in the cycle allow cross-linkages between lipids, carbohydrate, and protein metabolism, as illustrated in Figure 8.1. Particularly notable intermediates are α-ketoglutarate and oxaloacetate. Another interrelationship not shown in Figure 8.1 is that between heme and an intermediate of the Krebs cycle, succinyl CoA. The initial step in heme biosynthesis is the formation of δ-aminolevulinic acid from "active" succinate and glycine.

• Cycle intermediates—citrate, isocitrate, and malate—intermesh with lipogenesis. Citrate can move from the mitochondria into the cytoplast where citrate cleavage enzyme cleaves it into oxaloacetate and acetyl CoA, the initiator of fatty acid synthesis. Isocitrate and malate, in the presence of $NADP^+$-linked decarboxylating enzymes, may provide a portion of the NADPH† required for reductive stages of fatty acid synthesis.

Acetyl CoA resulting from catabolism of carbohydrate and fat enters the Krebs cycle in combination with oxaloacetate. Some of the protein breakdown products also enter the cycle as acetyl CoA, but many enter as α-ketoacids. In any event, the oxidative degradation of the product(s) transfers hydrogen from the product(s) to flavin adenine dinucleotide (FAD) fixed in the membranes of the mitochondria or to the mobile NAD^+

*Tyrosine is formed by hydroxylation of phenylalanine; therefore, its carbon skeleton cannot be synthesized in the body but must be obtained from food.

†A large portion of the NADPH is formed in the hexose–monophosphate shunt, an alternate pathway in the anaerobic oxidation of glucose.

molecules. Any FADH$_2$ produced is reoxidized by the coenzyme Q of the electron transport chain. The NADH formed, however, may transfer its hydrogen to the electron transport chain, or its reducing equivalents can be shuttled out of the mitochondria, to be used in reductive syntheses (for example, in gluconeogenesis). A key factor in determining the direction taken by NADH will be the ADP/ATP ratio. High ADP levels, which signify low energy reserves, will stimulate oxidative phosphorylation, thereby causing NADH to be drawn into the electron transport chain [2]. High ATP levels will inhibit oxidative phosphorylation, and cause NADH to be used for reductive syntheses.

THE CENTRAL ROLE OF THE LIVER IN METABOLISM

Each tissue and organ of the human body has a specific function that is reflected in its anatomy and its metabolic activity. For example, skeletal muscle uses metabolic energy to perform mechanical activity, the brain uses energy to pump ions against concentration gradients in the transfer of electrical impulses, and adipose tissue serves as a depot for stored fat, which on release provides fuel for the rest of the body. Central to these processes is the liver. It plays the key role of processor and distributor in metabolism, furnishing by way of the bloodstream a proper combination of nutrients to all the other organs and tissues. It warrants special attention in a discussion of tissue-specific metabolism.

Figures 8.3, 8.4, and 8.5 illustrate the fate of glucose 6-phosphate, amino acids, and fatty acids, respectively, that enter the liver from the bloodstream. In these figures, anabolic pathways are shown pointing upward, catabolic pathways, down, and distribution to other tissues horizontally. The pathways indicated are described in detail in Chapters 4, 6, and 7, which deal with carbohydrate, lipid, and protein metabolism respectively.

Glucose entering the hepatocytes is phosphorylated by glucokinase to glucose 6-phosphate. Other dietary monosaccharides (fructose, galactose, and mannose) are also phosphorylated and rearranged to glucose 6-phosphate. Figure 8.3 shows the possible metabolic routes available to glucose 6-phosphate.

It is likely that liver glycogenesis occurs primarily from gluconeogenic precursors delivered to the hepatocytes from peripheral tissues rather than through glucose directly [3] (see also Fig. 4.4). This finding is referred to again in the following section.

Figure 8.4 reviews the particularly active role of the liver in amino acid metabolism. The liver is the site of

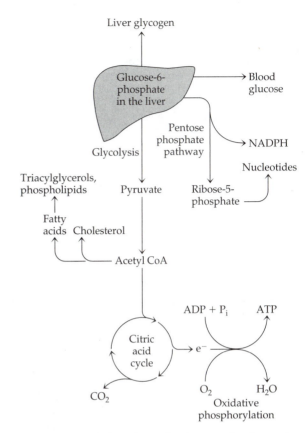

FIGURE 8.3 Metabolic pathways for glucose 6-phosphate in the liver. Here and in Figures 8.4 and 8.5, which follow, anabolic pathways are shown pointing upward, catabolic pathways downward, and distribution to other tissues horizontally.

synthesis of many different proteins, both structural and plasma-borne, from amino acids. Amino acids can also be converted into nonprotein products such as nucleotides, hormones, and porphyrins. Amino acids can be transaminated and degraded to acetyl CoA and other Krebs cycle intermediates, and these can in turn be oxidized for energy or converted to glucose or fat. Glucose formed from gluconeogenesis can be transported to muscle for use by that tissue, and synthesized fatty acids can be mobilized to adipose tissue for storage or used as fuel by muscle. Hepatocytes are the exclusive site for the formation of urea, the major excretory form of amino acid nitrogen.

The fate of fatty acids entering the liver is represented in Figure 8.5. Fatty acids can be assembled into liver lipids or released into the circulation as plasma lipoproteins. In humans, most fatty acid synthesis takes place in the liver rather than in adipocytes. Adipocytes store triacylglycerols arriving from the liver primarily in the form of plasma VLDLs, and from the lipoprotein li-

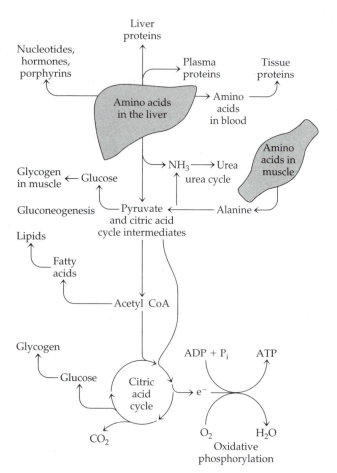

FIGURE 8.4 Pathways of amino acid metabolism in the liver.

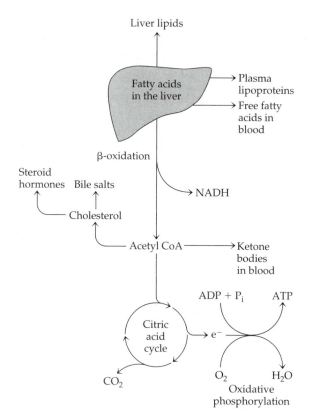

FIGURE 8.5 Pathways of fatty acid metabolism in the liver.

pase action on chylomicrons (p. 127). Under most circumstances, fatty acids are the major oxidative fuel in the liver. Acetyl CoA not used for energy can be used for the formation of the ketone bodies, which are very important fuels for certain peripheral tissues such as the brain and heart muscle, particularly during prolonged fasting.

TISSUE-SPECIFIC METABOLISM DURING THE FEED–FAST CYCLE

Carbohydrate and Fat Metabolism

The extent to which different organs are involved in carbohydrate and fat metabolism varies within the feed–fast cycles that underlie the eating habits of the human being. Food consumption often occurs at a level 100 times greater than the basal caloric requirement, allowing us to survive from meal to meal without nibbling continuously. Excess calories are stored as glycogen and fat, and these can be used as needed.

A feed–fast cycle can be divided into states, or phases: (1) the fed state, lasting about 3 hours after the ingestion of a meal; (2) the postabsorptive or early fasting state, occurring during a time span of from 3 to about 12 to 16 hours following the meal; (3) the fasting state, lasting up to two days without additional intake of food; and (4) the starvation state, marked by prolonged food deprivation of several weeks' duration. Clearly, in a normal eating routine only the fed and early fasting states apply. Time frames of the phases cited are only approximate, and are strongly influenced by factors such as activity level, the caloric value and nutrient composition of the meal, and the subject's metabolic rate.

The Fed State Figure 8.6 depicts the fed state and the disposition of ingested glucose by the various tissues. The red blood cells (RBCs) and the central nervous system (CNS) have no metabolic mechanisms by which glucose can be converted into energy stores; glucose available to these tissues is oxidized immediately to produce energy. In the liver, in contrast, some of the glucose can be converted directly to glycogen. Contrary to the conventional view of liver glycogenesis, however, research indicates that most of the liver glycogen is

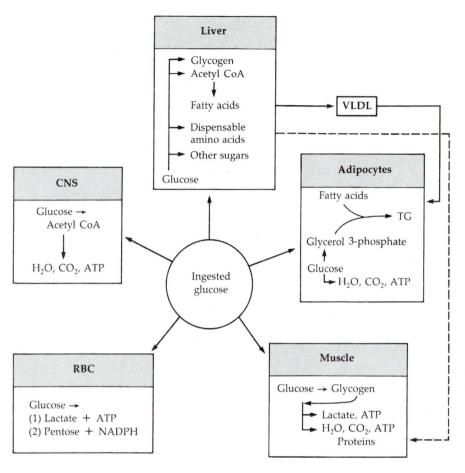

FIGURE 8.6 Flow of substrates in the fed state between liver, CNS, adipose tissue, muscle, and erythrocytes. *(Zakim D, Boyer T. Integration of energy metabolism by the liver. In: Hepatology: A textbook of liver disease, edited by M. Greene. Philadelphia: WB Saunders, 1982:77. Reprinted with permission.)*

synthesized indirectly from gluconeogenic precursors (pyruvate and lactate) returning to the liver from the periphery rather than directly from glucose entering the liver via the portal vein [3]. The reason why glucose is not used well as a direct precursor of glycogen has been attributed to the low phosphorylating activity of the liver at physiological concentrations of glucose [4].

The liver is the first tissue to have the opportunity to use dietary glucose. In the liver, glucose can be converted indirectly into glycogen, and when available glucose or its gluconeogenic precursors exceed the glycogen storage capacity of the liver, excess glucose can be metabolized in a variety of ways. This is shown in Figure 8.3 and in somewhat more detail in Figure 8.6. The conversion of glucose to fatty acids and dispensable amino acids is important because both represent the storage of glucose carbon. The potential conversion of excess glucose to fatty acids is particularly crucial because these fatty acids, along with those removed from the chylomicrons and VLDL by lipoprotein lipase, can be stored in the adipose tissue, thereby providing a ready

source of fuel for most body tissues during the postabsorptive and fasting states.

Some exogenous glucose—that is, that coming from the intestine—escapes the liver, and circulates to other tissues. The brain and other tissues of the central nervous system are almost solely dependent on glucose as an energy source. Other major users of glucose include (1) the RBCs, which, lacking mitochondria, convert it glycolytically to lactate for the small amount of energy the cell requires, and also use it as a source of NADPH via the hexosemonophosphate shunt; (2) adipose tissue, which can use it to some extent as a precursor for both the glycerol and fatty acid components of triacylglycerols, although, in the human, most triacylglycerol is synthesized by the liver, and transported to the adipose tissue; and (3) muscle, which uses glucose for the synthesis of glycogen. With the exception of the RBCs, all the tissues included in Figure 8.6 actively catabolize glucose for energy via the Krebs cycle.

In considering fat delivery to the tissues, it is necessary to differentiate between exogenous and endogenous

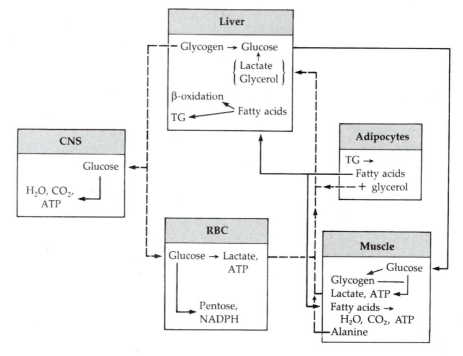

FIGURE 8.7 The primary postabsorptive flow of substrates between the liver, CNS, adipose tissue, muscle, and erythrocytes. (Modified from Zakim D, Boyer T. Integration of energy metabolism by the liver. In: Hepatology: A textbook of liver disease, edited by M. Greene. Philadelphia: WB Saunders, 1982:78. With permission.)

fat. Dietary fat, except for short-chain fatty acids, enters the bloodstream as chylomicrons, which are promptly acted on by lipoprotein lipase from the vascular endothelium, releasing free fatty acids and glycerol. Chylomicron remnants remaining from this hydrolysis are taken up by the liver, and their lipid contents transferred to the very low density lipoprotein fraction. The fatty acids are taken up by the adipocytes, re-esterified with glycerol to form triacylglycerols, and stored as such as large fat droplets within the cells.

Postabsorptive or Early Fasting State With the onset of the postabsorptive state, tissues can no longer derive their energy directly from ingested glucose and other nutrients but must begin to depend on other sources of fuel. During the short period of time marking this phase (a few hours after eating), hepatic glycogenolysis is the major provider of glucose as fuel to other tissues. The synthesis of glycogen and triacylglycerols is diminished, and the *de novo* synthesis of glucose (gluconeogenesis) begins to help maintain blood glucose levels. Lactate, formed in and released by RBCs and muscle tissue, becomes an important carbon source for hepatic gluconeogenesis. The alanine–glucose cycle, in which carbon in the form of alanine returns to the liver from muscle cells, also becomes important. Conversion of alanine to pyruvate by transamination is the first step in the gluconeogenic conversion of alanine.

Glucose provided to the muscle by the liver comes primarily from the recycling of lactate and alanine, and to a lesser extent, from hepatic glycogenolysis. Muscle glycogenolysis provides glucose as fuel only for those muscle cells in which the glycogen is stored, because muscle lacks the enzyme glucose 6-phosphatase. Glucose, once phosphorylated in the muscle, is trapped there.

The brain and other tissues of the CNS are extravagant consumers of glucose, oxidizing it for energy and releasing no gluconeogenic precursors in return. Therefore, the rate of glucose use is greater than that of gluconeogenesis, and the stores of liver glycogen begin to diminish rapidly. In the course of an overnight fast, nearly all reserves of liver glycogen and most of the muscle glycogen have been depleted. Figure 8.7 shows the shifts of metabolic pathways occurring in the tissues during the postabsorptive state.

The Fasting State The postabsorptive state evolves into the fasting state after 48 hours of no food intake. Particularly notable in the liver is the *de novo* glucose synthesis (gluconeogenesis) occurring in the wake of glycogen depletion. Amino acids from muscle protein breakdown provide the chief substrate for gluconeogenesis, although the glycerol from lipolysis and the lactate from anaerobic metabolism of glucose also are used to some extent.

The shift to gluconeogenesis during prolonged fasting is signaled by the secretion of the hormone glucagon and the glucocorticosteroid hormones in response to low levels of blood glucose. Proteins are hydrolyzed in muscle cells at an accelerated rate to provide the glucogenic amino acids. Of all the amino acids, only leucine and lysine cannot contribute at all to gluconeogenesis because, as noted previously, these amino acids are totally ketogenic in nature. However, ketogenic amino acids released by muscle protein hydrolysis serve a purpose as well. Since they are converted into ketones—that is, acetyl CoA, acetoacetyl CoA, or acetoacetate—they allow the brain, heart, and skeletal muscle to adapt to the use of these substrates should the nutritive state continue to deteriorate into a state of frank starvation.

The fasting state is accompanied by large daily losses of urinary nitrogen, in keeping with the high rate of gluconeogenic conversion of muscle protein to provide substrates for hepatic gluconeogenesis.

The Starvation State If the fasting state persists, and progresses into a starvation state, a metabolic fuel shift occurs again in an effort to spare body protein. This new priority is justified by the vital physiological importance of body proteins. Proteins that must obviously be conserved for life to continue include antibodies, needed to fight infection, enzymes, which catalyze life-sustaining reactions, and hemoglobin, for the transport of oxygen to tissues. The protein-sparing shift at this point is from gluconeogenesis to lipolysis, as the fat stores become the major supplier of energy. The blood level of fatty acids increases sharply, and these replace glucose as the preferred fuel of heart, liver, and skeletal muscle tissue that oxidize them for energy. The brain cannot use fatty acids for energy because fatty acids cannot cross the blood–brain barrier. However, the shift to fat breakdown also releases a large amount of glycerol, which becomes the major gluconeogenic precursor, rather than amino acids. This assures a continued supply of glucose as fuel for the brain.

Eventually, the use of Krebs cycle intermediates for gluconeogenesis depletes the supply of oxaloacetate. Low levels of oxaloacetate, coupled with the rapid production of acetyl CoA from fatty acid catabolism, causes acetyl CoA to accumulate, favoring the formation of acetoacetyl CoA and the ketone bodies. Ketone body concentration in the blood then rises (ketosis) as these fuels are exported from the liver, which cannot use them, to skeletal muscle, heart, and brain, which oxidize them instead of glucose. As long as ketone bodies are maintained at a high level by hepatic fatty acid oxidation, the need for glucose and gluconeogenesis is reduced, thereby sparing valuable protein. Figure 8.8 illustrates the changes in energy metabolism that occur in various tissues during fasting and starvation states.

Survival time in starvation, therefore, depends on the quantity of fat stored before starvation. Stored triacylglycerols in the adipose tissue of an individual of normal weight and adiposity can provide enough fuel to sustain basal metabolism for about three months. A very obese adult could probably endure a fast of more than a year, but physiological damage and even death could result from the accompanying extreme ketosis. When fat reserves are gone, the degradation of essential protein begins, leading to loss of liver and muscle function, and ultimately, to death [5].

Amino Acid Metabolism

Organ interactions in amino acid metabolism, illustrated in Figure 8.9, are largely coordinated by the liver [6]. The pathways shown undergo regulatory adjustments after consumption of a meal containing protein.

In the fed state, absorbed amino acids pass into the liver, where the fate of most of them is determined in relation to needs of the body; amounts in excess of need are degraded. Only the branched-chain amino acids (BCAAs) are not regulated by the liver according to the body's need. Instead, the BCAAs pass to the periphery, going primarily to the muscles and adipose tissue, where they may be metabolized. Of particular interest is the fate of the BCAAs reaching the muscle. These amino acids are usually much in excess of need for muscle protein synthesis. It is believed that the excess is used for synthesizing the dispensable amino acids that are needed for the protein synthesis spurt that occurs after a protein meal.

The liver is the site of urea synthesis, the primary mechanism for disposing of the excess nitrogen derived from amino acids used for energy or gluconeogenesis. The liver is the primary site for gluconeogenesis, where α-ketoacids (amino acids from which the amine group has been removed) serve as the chief substrate. During fasting, gluconeogenesis becomes a very important metabolic pathway in the regulation of plasma glucose levels. Liver gluconeogenesis is supplemented by that occurring in the kidney during prolonged fasts. Kidney gluconeogenesis is accompanied by the formation and excretion of ammonia.

The importance of the liver to the functioning of the muscle during the fasting state or very vigorous exercise is exemplified in the alanine–glucose cycle (Fig. 7.16). Alanine, formed in the muscle, results primarily from pyruvate that is transaminated with glutamate. The pyruvate is formed mainly from muscle glycogenolysis

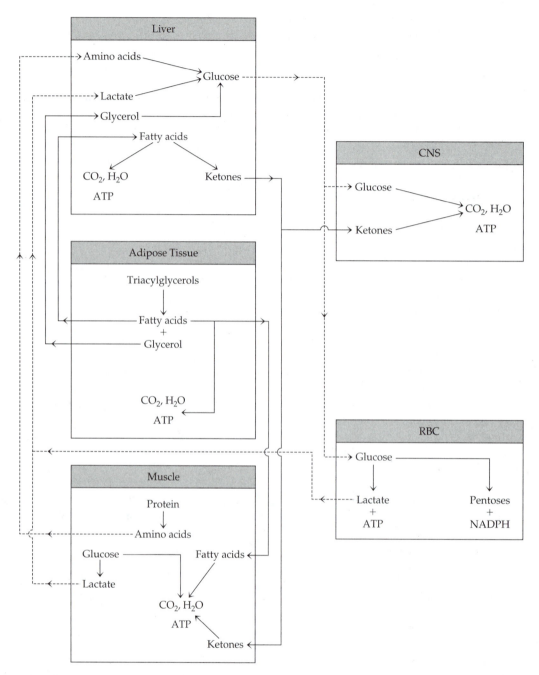

FIGURE 8.8 Flow of substrates among the liver, brain and CNS, adipose tissue, muscle, and red blood cells during fasting and starvation states. Broken lines indicate major substrate flow during fasting of about two days' duration. Solid lines reflect predominant substrate flow during the starvation state. Notice the shift to fatty acid and glycerol export from adipose tissue, and the increased use of fatty acids and ketones as fuel, during starvation, by brain and muscle.

but may also have been recycled from the liver. The alanine thus formed provides a disposal route for the nitrogen produced from catabolism of muscle amino acids. Alanine returning to the liver is transaminated with α-ketoglutarate, re-forming pyruvate. The transaminated nitrogen enters the urea cycle while the pyruvate is converted once again to glucose through the gluconeogenic pathway. The glucose can then be returned to muscle for energy, thereby completing the cycle. Alanine can also be formed in intestinal mucosal cells by transamination

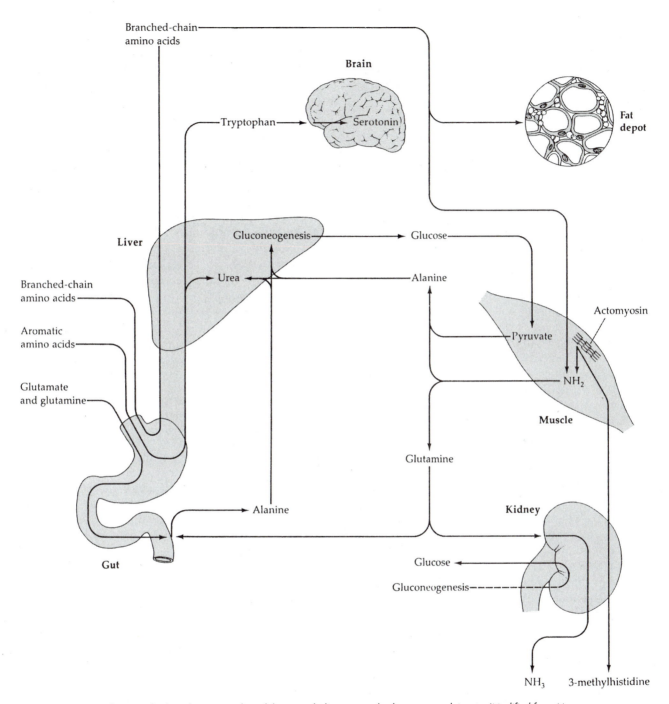

FIGURE 8.9 Interchanges of selected amino acids and their metabolites among body organs and tissues. *(Modified from Munro HN. Metabolic integration of organs in health and diseases. J. Parenteral and Enteral Nutr 1982;6:271–279, © Am Soc of Parenteral and Enteral Nutrition. With permission.)*

involving pyruvate, thereby serving as a carrier of amino acid nitrogen from that site to the liver.

Glutamine also plays a central role in the transport and excretion of amino acid nitrogen (p. 171). Many tissues, including the brain, combine ammonia, released primarily by the glutamate dehydrogenase reaction, with glutamate to form glutamine. The reaction is catalyzed by glutamine synthetase. In the form of glutamine, ammonia can then be carried to the liver or kidneys for excretion as urea or ammonium ion, respectively. In those tissues, glutamine is acted on by the enzyme glutaminase, releasing the ammonia for excretion, and re-forming glutamate. An overview of organ cooperativity in these and other aspects of amino acid metabolism is illustrated in Figure 8.9. See Chapter 7 for a more detailed discussion of amino acid metabolism in general.

SYSTEM INTEGRATION AND HOMEOSTASIS

Integration of the metabolic processes, as outlined in the preceding sections, allows the "constancy of the internal milieu" of humans and other multicellular organisms that was described by the French physiologist Claude Bernard about a century ago. This integration of metabolism at the cellular and the organ and tissue levels, which is essential for the survival of the entire organism, receives its direction via body systems. Through the integration of body systems, communication is made possible among all parts of the body.

The three major systems that direct activities of the cells, tissues, and organs to ensure their harmony with the whole organism are the nervous, endocrine, and vascular systems [2]. The *nervous system* is considered the primary communication system because it not only has receiving mechanisms to assess the body's status in relation to its environment but also has transmitting processes to relay appropriate commands to various tissues and organs. The nervous system can inform the body of such conditions as hunger, thirst, pain, and lack of oxygen. This allows organs to adjust to external changes, and appropriate behavior by the whole organism may be initiated. Tepperman and Tepperman [7] compare the nervous system to an elaborate system of telegraphy that has a "wire" connection from the source of message initiation to the place where message reception has its needed effect.

The *endocrine system* [7] is compared to a wireless system that transmits messages via highly specialized substances called *hormones*. The endocrine system depends on the vascular system to carry messages to target tissues. The *vascular system* is the primary transport mechanism for the body, not only delivering specialized chemical substances but also carrying oxygen, organic nutrients, and minerals from the external environment to the cells throughout the body [2]. It also transports the waste products of metabolism from the cells, carrying them to the lungs and/or kidneys for elimination.

The concentration of solutes in the blood must be regulated within a narrow range. Among the most prominent sentinel cells that monitor and regulate solute concentration are those that synthesize and secrete hormones. Although hormone synthesis and secretion occur primarily in the endocrine system, considerable overlap exists between the endocrine system and CNS. With the recent discovery of a variety of neuropeptides and recognition of the hormonal action of many of these peptides, it has become apparent that the CNS and endocrine system are functionally interdependent [7,8].

Tissues and cells that respond to hormones are called the "target" tissues and cells of the hormones. These hormone-responsive cells have been preprogramed by the process of differentiation to respond to the presence of hormones by acting in a predictable way. Not only do hormone-responsive cells respond to hormones via specific receptors, but their metabolic pathways also can be affected by the concentration of circulating substrates [7]. Hormone-responsive cells live in a complex and continually changing environment of fuels and ions. Their ultimate response to these changes is the net result of both hormonal and non-hormonal information brought to them by the extracellular fluids in which they are bathed [7].

Endocrine Function in Fed State

Endocrine organs are distributed throughout the body, and most of these organs are involved primarily with nutrient ingestion, that is, the gastrointestinal (GI) tract. Interspersed among the absorptive and exocrine secretory cells of the upper GI tract are the highly specialized endocrine cells. These cells present a sensor face to the lumen, and secrete granule-stored hormones into the bloodstream [7]. Each of these cells is stimulated to secrete by a different combination of chemical messages. Chemical messages include, for example, glucose, amino acids, fatty acids, and alkaline or acid pH. Hormones secreted by these stimulated GI cells (GIP, CCK, gastrin, secretin) (Table 2.1, p. 33) then enter the bloodstream, and sensitize appropriate cells of the endocrine pancreas for response to the approaching nutrients. The primary action of the GI hormones, secreted in response to a mixed diet, is to amplify the response of the pancreatic islet β-cells to glucose [7].

Insulin, secreted by the β-cells, is the hormone primarily responsible for the direction of energy metabolism during the fed state (Fig. 8.6). Its effects can be categorized as (1) very fast, occurring in a matter of seconds; (2) fast, occurring in minutes; (3) slower, occurring in minutes to several hours; (4) slowest, only occurring after several hours or even days. An example of a *very fast action* of insulin is membrane changes stimulated by the hormone. These changes occur in specific cells where glucose entry depends on membrane transport (see "Perspective," Chapter 1). The *fast action* of insulin involves the activation or inhibition of many enzymes, with anabolic actions being accentuated. For example, glycogenesis, lipogenesis, and protein synthesis become paramount (Fig. 8.6), while a coordinated inhibition of opposing catabolic actions occurs. Several metabolic effects of insulin and the corresponding target enzymes involved are listed in Table 8.1. Insulin favors glycogenesis through the activation of a phosphatase that dephosphorylates phosphorylase and glycogen synthetase. This dephosphorylation activates glycogen synthetase while inhibiting the phosphorylase that initiates glycogenolysis (p. 96). The fast effect of insulin on protein synthesis is not as clear-cut as its influence on lipogenesis and glycogenesis. Nevertheless, protein synthesis is promoted and appears related to stimulation of the translation process [7].

One *slower action* of insulin involves a further regulation of enzyme activity. This regulation is accomplished through the selective induction or repression of enzyme synthesis. The induced enzymes are the key rate-limiting enzymes for anabolic reaction sequences, while the repressed enzymes are those crucial to control of opposing catabolic reactions. An example of selective induction is the effect of insulin on glucokinase activity. Insulin increases the synthesis of glucokinase by promoting transcription of the glucokinase gene. Another slower action of insulin is its stimulation of cellular amino acid influx. The *slowest effect* of insulin is its promotion of growth through mitogenesis and cell replication [7]. The passage of a cell through its various phases before it can replicate is a relatively slow process that requires 18–24 hours for completion. Its complexity precludes a significant rate increase in the overall process.

Endocrine Function in Postabsorptive or Fasting State

Metabolic adjustments that occur in response to food deprivation operate on two time scales: *acutely*, measured in minutes (such adjustments can be seen in a postabsorptive state), and *chronically*, measured in hours and days (adjustments occurring during fasting or starvation). In contrast to the fed state, in which insulin is the hormone primarily responsible for the direction of energy metabolism, the body deprived of food requires a variety of hormones to regulate its fuel supply.

Figure 8.7 depicts the postabsorptive state wherein hepatic glycogenolysis is providing some glucose to the body, while increased use of fatty acids for energy is de-

TABLE 8.1 Metabolic Effects of Insulin and Its Action on Specific Enzymes

Metabolic Effect	Target Enzyme
↑Glucose uptake (muscle)	↑Glucose transporter
↑Glucose uptake (liver)	↑Glucokinase
↑Glycogen synthesis (liver, muscle)	↑Glycogen synthase
↓Glycogen breakdown (liver, muscle)	↓Glycogen phosphorylase
↑Glycolysis, acetyl CoA production (liver, muscle)	↑Phosphofructokinase-1 ↑Pyruvate dehydrogenase complex
↑Fatty acid synthesis (liver)	↑Acetyl CoA carboxylase
↑Triacylglycerol synthesis (adipose tissue)	↑Lipoprotein lipase

creasing the glucose requirement of cells. Also, gluconeogenesis is being initiated, with lactate and glycerol serving as substrates.

Hepatic glycogenolysis is initiated through the action of glucagon, secreted by the α-cells of the endocrine pancreas, and of epinephrine (adrenaline) and norepinephrine, synthesized primarily in the adrenal medulla and sympathetic nerve endings, respectively. Epinephrine is considerably more potent in this metabolic action than norepinephrine, which mainly functions as a neurotransmitter. Epinephrine and norepinephrine are called the *catecholamine hormones* because they are derivatives of the aromatic alcohol catechol. Although influencing hepatic glycogenolysis somewhat, the catecholamines exert their effect primarily on the muscles [9]. The action of glucagon and the catecholamines is mediated through cAMP and protein kinase phosphorylation. (This mechanism is described in the section on glycogenolysis in Chapter 4; see also Figure 4.6.) Through the action of glucagon on the liver, phosphorylase and glycogen synthetase are phosphorylated, in direct opposition to the action of insulin; consequently phosphorylase is activated and glycogen synthetase is inhibited. As a result, glycogen is broken down, giving rise to glucose 6-phosphate, which then can be hydrolyzed by the specific liver phosphatase (glucose 6-phosphatase) to produce free glucose.

In contrast, muscle glycogenolysis, stimulated by the catecholamines, provides glucose only for the muscles in which the glycogen has been stored. This is because muscle tissue lacks glucose 6-phosphatase and cannot release free glucose into the circulation. The catecholamines, however, do raise the blood glucose indirectly because they stimulate the secretion of glucagon and also inhibit the uptake of blood glucose by the muscles [9].

Glycogenolysis can occur within minutes, and meets an acute need for raising the blood glucose level.

However, because so little glycogen is stored in the liver (approximately 60 to 65 g), blood glucose cannot be maintained over a prolonged period. In prolonged glucose deprivation such as occurs during fasting, the liver employs another mechanism for supplying the body with glucose, namely gluconeogenesis. Although lactate and glycerol serve as substrates for gluconeogenesis, the primary substrates are the amino acids derived from protein tissues, principally from muscle mass. Gluconeogenesis is fostered by the same hormones that initiate glycogenolysis (glucagon and epinephrine), but the amino acids needed as substrate are made available through the action of the glucocorticoids secreted by the adrenal cortex. Glucocorticoid hormones stimulate gluconeogenesis. Alanine, generated in the muscle from other amino acids and from pyruvate by transamination, and serving as the principal gluconeogenic substrate, also acts as a stimulant of gluconeogenesis via its effect on the secretion of glucagon. In fact, alanine is the prime stimulator of glucagon secretion by α-cells that have been sensitized to the action of alanine by the glucocorticoids [2].

Low levels of circulating insulin not only decrease the use of glucose but also promote lipolysis and a rise in free fatty acids. Contributing to this effect is the increase in glucagon during the fasting period. Glucagon raises the level of cyclic AMP in adipose cells, and the cyclic AMP then activates a lipase that hydrolyzes stored triacylglycerols [9]. The muscles, inhibited by the catecholamines from taking up glucose, now begin to use fatty acids as the primary source of energy. This increased use of fatty acids by the muscles represents an important adaptation to fasting. Growth hormone and the glucocorticoids foster this adaptation because they, like the catecholamines, inhibit in some manner the use of glucose by the muscles [7,9].

As starvation is prolonged, less and less glucose is used, thereby reducing the amount of protein that must be catabolized to provide substrate for gluconeogenesis. As glucose use decreases, hepatic ketogenesis increases and the brain adapts to the use of ketones (primarily β-hydroxybutyrate) as a partial source of energy. After three days of starvation, about one-third of the energy needs of the brain are met by ketones, and with prolonged starvation, ketones become the major fuel source for the brain [9]. Under conditions of continued carbohydrate shortage, ketones are oxidized by the muscles in preference not only to glucose but also to fatty acids. During starvation, the use of ketones by the muscles as the preferred source of energy spares protein, thereby prolonging life. Although Figure 8.8 depicts fuel metabolism during starvation, it does not show some of the

TABLE 8.2 Fuel Metabolism in Starvation

Fuel Exchanges and Consumption	Amount Formed or Consumed in 24 Hours (grams)	
	Day 3	Day 40
Fuel use by the brain		
Glucose	100	40
Ketones	50	100
Fuel mobilization		
Adipose tissue lipolysis	180	180
Muscle protein degradation	75	20
Fuel output of the liver		
Glucose	150	80
Ketones	150	150

Source: Adapted from Stryer L. Biochemistry. 3rd ed. New York: Freeman 1988:640.

adjustments in energy substrates that occur when starvation is prolonged. These adjustments are shown in Table 8.2. As mentioned previously, the duration of starvation compatible with life depends to large degree on depot fat status.

SUMMARY

Animal survival depends on a constant internal environment maintained through specific control mechanisms. Controls, operative at all levels (cellular, organ, and system), integrate energy metabolism and permit the adaptation of the body to a wide variety of environmental conditions. Primary in the promotion of cooperation among the tissues and organs that allows adaptation to varying conditions are the nervous, endocrine, and vascular systems. In normal operation of these systems, metabolic pathways may be stimulated, maintained, or inhibited, depending on the conditions imposed on the body. Recognizing the metabolic pathways unique to the liver, and the hormones secreted solely by the endocrine pancreas, shows why these two organs are crucial to homeostasis and therefore to life.

References Cited

1. Role of fat and fatty acids in modulation of energy exchange. Nutr Rev 1988;46:382–384.
2. McMurray WC. Essentials of human metabolism, 2nd ed. Philadelphia: Harper & Row, 1983.
3. McGarry JD, Kuwajima M, Newgard CB, et al. From dietary glucose to liver glycogen: The full circle round. Ann Rev Nutr 1987;7:51–73.

4. Foster DW. From glycogen to ketones and back. Banting Lecture 1984. Diabetes 1984;33:1188–1199.

5. Lehninger AL, Nelson DL, Cox MM. Principles of biochemistry, 2d ed. New York: Worth, 1993:757–758.

6. Monroe HN. Metabolic integration of organs in health and diseases. J Parenteral and Enteral Nutr 1982; 6:271–279.

7. Tepperman J, Tepperman HM. Metabolic and endocrine physiology. 5th ed. Chicago: Year Book, 1987.

8. AJ Turner, ed. Neuropeptides and their peptidases. New York: VCH, 1987.

9. Stryer L. Biochemistry, 3rd ed. New York: Freeman, 1988:627–646.

Suggested Reading

Tepperman J, Tepperman HM. Metabolic and endocrine physiology, 5th ed. Chicago: Year Book, 1987.

This is a well-illustrated, easy-to-read explanation of the regulatory role of the endocrine system in human metabolism.

Harris RA, Crabb DW. Metabolic interrelationships. In: Textbook of biochemistry with clinical correlations, 3rd ed. (Devlin TM, ed.). New York: Wiley, 1992:576–606.

This integration of human metabolic pathways is written primarily for the medical student. Information is presented so as to be relevant for the health practitioner.

Additional Reference

The following reference was used for background information.

Zakim D. Integration of energy metabolism by the liver. In: Green M, Greene H, eds. The role of the gastrointestinal tract in nutrient delivery. New York: Academic Press, 1984;3:157–181.

This publication is a compilation of papers presented at the Bristol Myers Symposia, December 1 and 2, 1983, Washington, DC.

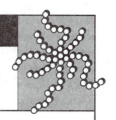

PERSPECTIVE 1

Diabetes: Metabolism Out of Control

Diabetes is no longer considered to be one disease but is believed to be a group of diseases differing in etiology, biochemical features, and natural history. Diabetes mellitus is currently classified as insulin-dependent diabetes mellitus, ketosis prone (IDDM), and as non-insulindependent diabetes mellitus (NIDDM). The current theories on the etiology and characteristics of these two classifications of diabetes are given in Figure 1.

Diabetes is generally characterized by a relative lack of insulin, but the acute insulin deprivation often occurring in the ketosis-prone type of diabetes (Figure 1) emphasizes the crucial role of insulin in the regulation of metabolism. An absence of insulin not only inhibits the use of glucose by muscles and adipose tissue but also sets into motion a sequence of events that, without effective intervention, will result in coma and death of the affected animal or human.

Insulin has a variety of actions on metabolism, most of which have the effect of lowering blood glucose. Such actions include decreasing hepatic glucose output, while increasing glucose oxidation, glycogen deposition, lipogenesis, protein synthesis, and cell replication. In the absence of insulin, all the hormones favoring catabolism and the raising of blood glucose operate without opposition. The direction of metabolism in response to these catabolic hormones is that seen in Figure 8.8, which depicts the body's adaptation to fasting. In diabetes, however, the responses are much more violent than those occurring in the body's adaptation to fasting or starvation, during which the purpose is maintenance of a blood glucose level sufficient to meet the crucial demands of the CNS and RBCs. The unrestrained action of the catabolic hormones in the absence of insulin, along with the dramatically decreased use of glucose caused by an insulin lack, results in aberrations in metabolism. Not only is carbohydrate, fat, and protein metabolism affected, but water and electrolyte imbalance occurs also. A summary of the metabolic events set into motion by an absence of insulin is given in Figure 2.

Hyperglycemia, the hallmark of diabetes, which is due to decreased glucose use and increased hepatic glucose output, results in an osmotic diuresis that proves fatal if uninterrupted (Fig. 2). The water and electrolytes lost through this diuresis leads to a dehydration compounded by increased insensible water loss due to the hyperpnea of metabolic acidosis. Metabolic acidosis results from the excessive ketogenesis occurring in the liver.

Peripheral circulatory failure, a consequence of severe hemoconcentration, leads to tissue hypoxia with a consequent shift of the tissues to anaerobic metabolism. Anaerobic metabolism raises the concentration of lactic acid in the blood, thereby worsening the metabolic acidosis.

The ketonuria along with glucosuria associated with acidosis causes an excessive loss of sodium (Na^+) from the body; loss of this extracellular cation further compromises body water balance. A net loss of potassium (K^+), the chief intracellular cation, accompanies increased protein catabolism and cellular dehydration, both of which characterize uncontrolled diabetes.

Figure 8.6, showing the normal flow of substrates following food intake and secretion of insulin, emphasizes the positive effect of insulin on anabolism and its inhibition of catabolic pathways. Figure 2, in contrast, shows metabolism out of control when the inhibiting effect of insulin is lacking and conservation of energy is impossible. Diabetes is a vivid negative example that emphasizes the integration of metabolism and the importance of metabolic regulation (homeostasis) to continuance of life.

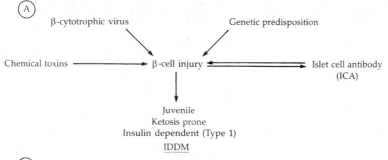

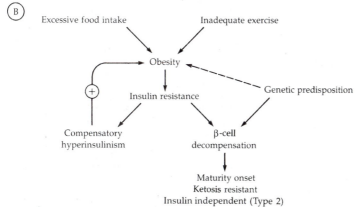

FIGURE 1 Overview of present theories of diabetes mellitus etiology. Ⓐ depicts the factors impinging on the development of diabetes mellitus that requires exogenous insulin. This type of diabetes presently is most commonly designated as insulin dependent diabetes mellitus (IDDM). Ⓑ illustrates the interaction of factors that may result in non–insulin-dependent diabetes mellitus (NIDDM).

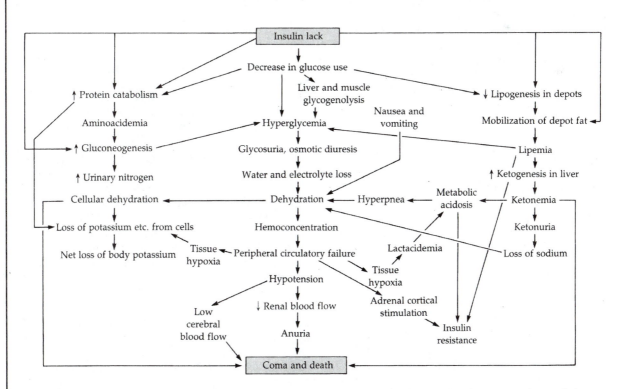

FIGURE 2 Composite summary of pathophysiology of diabetic acidosis. Particularly striking are the aberrations in the metabolism of carbohydrates, lipids, and protein caused by an insulin lack and the interconnections among these altered metabolic pathways. (Tepperman D, Tepperman H. Metabolic and endocrine physiology. 5th ed. Chicago: Year Book, 1987:284.)

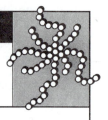

of Ethanol, and Associated Metabolic Alterations

Ethanol (ethyl alcohol) is a purely exogenous compound in humans, consumed in the form of alcoholic beverages such as beer, wines, and distilled liquors. Excessive consumption of ethanol can lead to the condition of alcoholism, defined by the National Council on Alcoholism as that which is capable of producing pathological changes. Alcoholism is a serious socioeconomic and health problem, exemplified by the fact that in the United States, alcohol-related liver disease is the sixth leading cause of death [1].

Ethanol is readily absorbed throughout the entire gastrointestinal tract. It is transported unaltered in the bloodstream and then oxidatively degraded in tissues, primarily the liver, first to acetaldehyde, and then to acetate. In tissues peripheral to the liver, as well as in the liver itself, the acetate is subsequently converted to acetyl CoA and oxidized via the Krebs cycle. At least three enzyme systems are capable of ethanol oxidation: (1) alcohol dehydrogenase (ADH), (2) the microsomal ethanol-oxidizing system (MEOS; or the cytochrome P-450 system), and (3) catalase, in the presence of hydrogen peroxide. Of these, the catalase–H_2O_2 system is the least active of the three, probably accounting for less than 2% of *in vivo* ethanol oxidation. Therefore, it will not be discussed further. Nearly all ingested ethanol is oxidized by hepatic alcohol dehydrogenase and hepatic microsomal cytochrome P-450 systems.

The Alcohol Dehydrogenase (ADH) Pathway

ADH is a soluble enzyme functioning in the cytoplasm of liver cells. It is an ordinary NAD^+-requiring dehydrogenase, and it is known to be able to oxidize ethanol to acetaldehyde.

$$CH_3-CH_2-OH + NAD^+ \overset{ADH}{\longleftrightarrow} CH_3-CHO + NADH + H^+$$
$$\text{ethanol} \qquad\qquad \text{acetaldehyde}$$

The NADH formed by the reaction can be oxidized by mitochondrial electron transport, by way of the NADH shuttle systems (p. 88), thereby giving rise to ATP formation by oxidative phosphorylation. The K_m of alcohol dehydrogenase for ethanol is approximately 1 mM, or about 5 mg/dL. This means that at that cellular concentration of ethanol, ADH is functioning at one-half of its maximum velocity. At concentrations three or four times the K_m, the enzyme is saturated

with the ethanol substrate and is catalyzing at its maximum rate. It follows that any ethanol present in the cell in excess of the $4 \times K_m$ level cannot be oxidized by ADH. (K_m is reviewed in Chapter 1, in the section dealing with enzymes.) There is, of course, no "normal" concentration of ethanol in the cells or bloodstream. The so-called toxic level of blood ethanol, however, is considered to be in the range of 50–100 mg/dL. The high lipid solubility of ethanol allows it to enter cells passively with ease, and if its cellular concentration reaches a level even a third or a fourth of that in blood, ADH would be saturated by the substrate and would be functioning at its maximum velocity. The excess, or "spillover," ethanol must then be metabolized by alternate systems, the most important of which is the microsomal ethanol oxidizing system, described next. Another factor forcing a shift to the microsomal metabolizing system is a depletion of NAD^+, brought about by the high level of activity of ADH. The microsomal system does not require NAD^+ for its oxidative reactions.

The Microsomal Ethanol Oxidizing System (MEOS)

Despite its name, the microsomal ethanol oxidizing system (MEOS) is able to oxidize a wide variety of compounds in addition to ethanol. These include fatty acids, aromatic hydrocarbons, steroids, and barbiturate drugs. The oxidation occurs through a system of electron transport, similar to the mitochondrial electron transport system described in detail in Chapter 3. Since MEOS is microsomal, and is associated with the smooth endoplasmic reticulum, it is sometimes referred to as the "microsomal electron transport system." Another distinction of the system is its requirement for a special cytochrome called *cytochrome P-450*, which acts as an intermediate electron carrier. Cytochrome P-450 is not a singular compound but exists as a family of structurally related cytochromes, the members of which share the property of absorbing light having a wavelength of 450 nanometers.

Ethanol oxidation by MEOS is linked to the simultaneous oxidation of NADPH by molecular oxygen. Since two substrates are therefore oxidized concurrently, the enzymes that are involved in the oxidations are commonly called mixed-function oxidases. One oxygen atom of the oxygen molecule is used to oxidize

PERSPECTIVE 2 (continued)

NADPH to NADP+, and the second oxidizes the ethanol substrate to acetaldehyde. Both oxygen atoms are reduced to H_2O, and therefore two H_2O molecules are formed in the reactions. Microsomal electron transport of the MEOS is shown as the reaction scheme that follows. Acting as carriers of electrons from NADPH to oxygen are FAD, FMN, and a cytochrome P-450 system.

An important feature of the MEOS is that certain of its enzymes, including the cytochrome P-450 units, are *inducible* by ethanol. This means that ethanol, particularly at higher concentrations, can stimulate (induce) the synthesis of these substances. The result is that the hepatocytes can metabolize the ethanol much more effectively, thereby establishing a state of metabolic *tolerance*. Compared to a normal (nondrinking or light-drinking) subject, an individual in a state of metabolic tolerance to ethanol can ingest larger quantities of the substance before showing the effects of intoxication. In effect, he or she is "tolerant" to it. When enzyme induction occurs, however, it can also accelerate the metabolism of other substances metabolized by the microsomal system. In other words, tolerance to ethanol induced by heavy drinking can also render a person tolerant to other substances as well as ethanol.

Biochemical and Metabolic Alterations

The well-known consequences of alcoholism—fatty liver, hepatic disease (cirrhosis), lactic acidosis, and metabolic tolerance—can be explained by the manner in which ethanol is metabolized. Basically, the consequences of excessive alcohol intake are explainable by metabolic effects of (1) acetaldehyde toxicity, (2) elevated NADH/NAD+ ratio, (3) metabolic competition, and (4) induced metabolic tolerance.

Acetaldehyde Toxicity Both the ADH and the MEOS routes of ethanol oxidation produce acetaldehyde, which is believed to exert direct adverse effects on metabolic systems. For example, acetaldehyde is able to attach covalently to proteins forming protein adducts. Should the adduct involve an enzyme, the activity of that enzyme could be impaired.

Acetaldehyde has also been shown to impede the formation of microtubules in liver cells and to cause the development of perivenular fibrosis, either of which is believed to initiate the events leading to cirrhosis. These and other possible adverse effects of acetaldehyde are reviewed by Lieber [2].

It was once thought that alcoholic cirrhosis was caused by malnutrition, as the drinker satisfied his or her caloric needs with the "empty" calories of alcohol at the expense of those of a nutritionally balanced diet. In view of the effect of high levels of acetaldehyde on hepatocyte structure and function, however, it is now known that chronic overindulgence can cause cirrhosis in the absence of nutritional deficiency, and even if the alcohol is coingested with an enriched diet [3].

High NADH/NAD+ Ratio The oxidation of ethanol increases the concentration of NADH at the expense of NAD+, therefore elevating the NADH/NAD+ ratio. This is because both ADH and acetaldehyde dehydrogenase use NAD+ as cosubstrate. NADH is an important regulator of certain dehydrogenase reactions. Its rise in concentration represents an overproduction of reducing equivalents, which in turn acts as a signal for a metabolic shift toward reduction, namely hydrogenation. Such a shift can account for fatty liver and lactic acidemia, which often accompany alcoholism. For example, lactic acidemia can be attributed in part to the direct effect of NADH in shifting the lactate dehydrogenase (LDH) reaction toward the formation of lactate. The reaction, shown as follows, is driven to the right by the high concentration of NADH:

$$\text{Pyruvate} + \text{NADH} \underset{\text{LDH}}{\rightleftharpoons} \text{lactate} + \text{NAD}^+$$

Lipids accumulate in most tissues in which ethanol is metabolized, resulting in fatty liver, fatty myocardium, fatty renal tubules, and so on. The mechanism appears to involve both increased lipid synthesis and decreased lipid removal, and is explained in part by the increased NADH/NAD+ ratio. As NADH accumulates,

PERSPECTIVE 2 (continued)

it slows dehydrogenase reactions of the Krebs cycle, such as the iso-citrate dehydrogenase and αketoglutarate dehydrogenase reactions, thereby slowing the overall activity of the cycle. This results in an accumulation of citrate, which positively regulates acetyl CoA carboxylase. Acetyl CoA carboxylase converts acetyl CoA into malonyl CoA by the attachment of a carboxyl group. It is the key regulatory enzyme for the synthesis of fatty acids from acetyl CoA (p. 139). The high ratio of $NADH/NAD^+$ therefore directs metabolism away from Krebs cycle oxidation and toward fatty acid synthesis.

Also contributing to the lipogenic effect of alcoholism is the NADH effect on the glycerophosphate dehydrogenase (GPDH) reaction. The reaction, shown as follows, favors the reduction of dihydroxyacetone phosphate (DHAP) to glycerol 3-phosphate if NADH concentration is high.

$$
\begin{array}{ccc}
CH_2-OH & & CH_2-OH \\
| & & | \\
C=O \ +NADH \ \rightleftharpoons_{GPDH} & CH_2-OH \ +NAD^+ \\
| & & | \\
CH_2-O-P & & CH_2-O-P \\
DHAP & & \text{Glycerol 3-P}
\end{array}
$$

Glycerol 3-phosphate provides the glycerol component in the synthesis of triacylglycerols. Therefore, a high $NADH/NAD^+$ ratio stimulates the synthesis of both the fatty acids and glycerol components of triacylglycerols, contributing to the cellular fat accumulation that develops in alcoholism.

The glutamate dehydrogenase (GluDH) reaction also is affected by a rise in NADH concentration, resulting in impaired gluconeogenesis. The GluDH reaction is extremely important in gluconeogenesis because of the role it plays in the conversion of amino acids into their carbon skeletons by transamination, and the release of their amino groups as NH_3. A shift in the reaction toward glutamate by NADH, shown as follows, depletes the availability of α-ketoglutarate, which is the major acceptor of amino groups in the transamination of amino acids.

$$
\begin{array}{cc}
\textit{Glutamate} & \textit{α-ketoglutarate} \\
COO^- & COO^- \\
| & | \\
CH-NH_3^+ + NAD^+ \rightleftharpoons_{GluDH} & C=O + NADH \\
| & | \quad +NH_3 \\
CH_2 & CH_2 \\
| & | \\
CH_2-COO^- & CH_2-COO^-
\end{array}
$$

Substrate Competition A well-established nutritional problem associated with excessive alcohol metabolism is a deficiency of vitamin A. There are probably two aspects of ethanol interference on normal metabolism that can account for this problem. One of these is the effect of ethanol on retinol dehydrogenase, the cytoplasmic enzyme that converts retinol to retinal. Retinol dehydrogenase is thought to be identical to ADH, and therefore ethanol competitively inhibits the hepatic conversion of retinol to retinal [4]. Retinal is required for the synthesis of photopigments used in vision.

Induced Metabolic Tolerance As explained earlier, ethanol can induce enzymes of the MEOS, causing an increased rate of metabolism of substrates oxidized by this system. Retinol, like ethanol, spills over into the MEOS when ADH is saturated and NAD^+ stores are low due to heavy ingestion of ethanol. Ethanol induction of retinol-metabolizing enzymes then can occur. The specific component of the MEOS that is known to be induced by a heavy consumption of ethanol has been designated cytochrome P-450IIE1[2]. Although induction accelerates the hepatic oxidation of retinol, the oxidation product is not retinal but other polar, inert products of oxidation. The hepatic depletion of retinol can therefore be attributed to its accelerated metabolism, secondary to ethanol induction of a metabolizing enzyme. In effect, the alcoholic subject becomes tolerant to vitamin A, necessitating a higher dietary intake of the vitamin in order to maintain normal hepatocyte concentrations.

In summary, ethyl alcohol might be thought of as a "Jekyll and Hyde" among our commonly ingested substances. This Perspective, with its focus on the effects of alcohol at high intake levels, has clearly emphasized the negative. But it is only fair to remind the reader that a low to moderate intake of alcohol has been reported to have beneficial effects, particularly in its ability to improve plasma lipid profiles, and reduce cardiovascular disease risk. The adage that moderation is the key to a healthy lifestyle certainly applies in this case.

P E R S P E C T I V E   (continued)

References Cited

1. US Bureau of the Census: Statistical abstract of the United States, 1975. Washington, DC: US Government Printing Office, 1975.
2. Lieber CS. Biochemical and molecular basis of alcohol-induced injury to liver and other tissues. N Engl J Med 1988;319:1639–1650.
3. Lieber CS. Pathogenesis and early diagnosis of alcoholic liver injury. N Engl J Med 1978;298:888–893.
4. Thomson AD, Majumdor SK. The influence of ethanol on intestinal absorption and utilization of nutrients. Clin Gastroenterol 1981;10:263–293.

THE REGULATORY NUTRIENTS

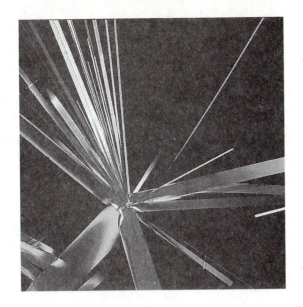

CHAPTER 9

THE WATER-SOLUBLE VITAMINS

Vitamin C (ascorbic acid)

Thiamin

Riboflavin

Niacin

Pantothenic Acid

Biotin

Folic Acid

Vitamin B₁₂

Vitamin B₆

For each vitamin, the following subtopics are discussed:
Sources
Digestion (when applicable)
Absorption and Transport
Functions and Mechanisms of Action
Interactions with Other Nutrients
   (when applicable)
Metabolism and Excretion
Recommended Dietary Allowance
Deficiency
Toxicity
Assessment of Nutriture

Photo: Photomicrograph of crystallized thiamin

The early part of the twentieth century marks the most exciting era in the history of nutrition science. It was during this time that the discovery of vitamins, or "accessory growth factors," began. Researchers found that for life and growth, animals required something more than a chemically defined diet consisting of purified carbohydrate, protein, fat, minerals, and water. The first of these dietary essentials discovered was an antiberiberi substance isolated from rice polishings by Funk, a Polish biochemist. Funk gave it the name *vitamine* because the substance was an amine and necessary for life. Very shortly thereafter McCollum and Davis extracted a factor from butter fat that they called *fat-soluble A* to distinguish it from the water-soluble antiberiberi substance. These two essential factors became known as *vitamine A* and *vitamine B*. As each additional vitamin was discovered, it was assigned a letter; the *e* on *vitamine* was dropped to give the general name *vitamin* because only a few of the essential substances were found to be amines.

As the chemical structure of a vitamin became known through its isolation and synthesis, it was given a chemical name. When the chemical name was assigned, it was assumed that the name applied to one substance with one specific activity. Now it is evident that a vitamin may have a variety of functions and that vitamin activity may be found in several closely related compounds known as *vitamers*. An excellent example of this is vitamin A, which has several seemingly unrelated functions and encompasses not only retinol but also retinal and retinoic acid.

Vitamins can be defined as essential organic compounds required in very small amounts (micronutrients) that are involved in fundamental functions of the body, such as growth, maintenance of health, and metabolism. Because these substances must be supplied wholly or partially by the diet, their discovery came about because of their *absence* in the diet. Although in the case of a deficiency the clinician should be able to recognize the syn-

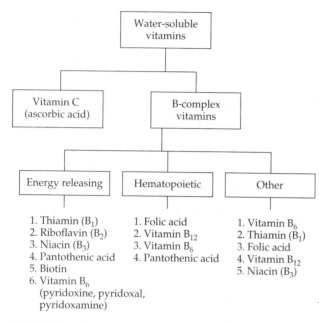

FIGURE 9.1 The water-soluble vitamins.

given, when precise information is available, to structure, sources, absorption (also digestion, where applicable), transport, functions and mechanisms of action, metabolism and excretion, recommended dietary allowance, deficiency, toxicity, and assessment of nutriture. Specific interrelationships with other nutrients are also noted for selected vitamins. Table 9.1 contains a summary of the discovery, functions, deficiency syndrome, sources, and the recommended dietary allowance or estimated safe and adequate daily dietary intake of each of the water-soluble vitamins. Appendix A provides the 1989 RDA for all nutrients and for all age groups.

Suggested Reading

McCollum EV. A history of nutrition. Boston: Houghton Mifflin, 1957.

drome caused by a lack of the vitamin, it is more relevant in this country of abundant and varied food supply for the nutrition professional to think in terms of what a specific vitamin does rather than what disease it prevents. Unfortunately, it is often impossible to directly relate the function of the vitamin to its deficiency syndrome.

Vitamins, for the most part, are not related chemically, and differ in their physiologic roles. The broad classifications of water-soluble vitamins and fat-soluble vitamins are made because of certain properties common to each group. The fat-soluble vitamins are discussed in Chapter 10. The body handles the water-soluble vitamins differently from the way it handles the fat-soluble vitamins. They are absorbed into portal blood, in contrast to fat-soluble vitamins and, with the exception of cyanocobalamin (vitamin B_{12}), they cannot be retained for long periods by the body. Any storage occurring results from their binding to enzymes and transport proteins. Water-soluble vitamins are excreted in the urine whenever plasma levels exceed renal thresholds.

Water-soluble vitamins, with the exception of vitamin C (ascorbic acid), are members of the B complex. Most of the B-complex group can be further divided according to general function: energy releasing or hematopoietic. Other vitamins cannot be classified this narrowly because of their wide range of functions. Figure 9.1 shows the classification of vitamins.

In this chapter, discussions of the vitamins are grouped similarly. For each vitamin, consideration is

VITAMIN C (ASCORBIC ACID)

The human being is one of the few mammals unable to synthesize ascorbic acid or vitamin C. Other animals that require vitamin C include primates, flying mammals (such as bats), guinea pigs, and birds belonging to the order passeriformes [1]. Animals that require an exogenous source of ascorbic acid lack gulonolactone oxidase, the last enzyme needed for ascorbic acid synthesis. The pathway and structure of the vitamin are shown in Figure 9.2.

Sources

The best food sources of vitamin C include papaya, oranges, orange juice, cantaloupe, cauliflower, broccoli, brussels sprouts, green peppers, grapefruit, grapefruit juice, kale, lemons, and strawberries.

Absorption and Transport

Absorption of ascorbate occurs primarily by active transport. Transport systems for ascorbate are saturable and dose dependent [2–5]. Simple diffusion or carrier-mediated transport may also contribute to a small extent to uptake of the vitamin from the mouth and stomach [2,3,5]. Prior to absorption, ascorbate may be oxidized (two electrons and two protons are removed) to form dehydroascorbate (Figs. 9.3 and 9.4) which may be absorbed by passive diffusion [1]. Absorption of dehydroascorbate is thought to be better than absorption of ascorbate [4,5]. Within the intestinal cells (but also other cells), dehydroascorbic acid is generally rapidly reduced

Table 9.1 The Vitamins: Discovery, Functions, Human Deficiency Syndromes, Food Sources, and Recommended Intake

Water-Soluble Vitamins

Vitamin	Discovery	Coenzymes	Biochemical or Physiologic Function	Deficiency Syndrome or Symptoms	Good Food Sources in Rank Order	1989 RDA[a]
Thiamin (vitamin B$_1$)	Casimir Funk (1912)	Thiamin diphosphate (TDP) or thiamin pyrophosphate (TPP)	Oxidative decarboxylation of α-keto acids and 2-keto sugars	*Beriberi*, muscle weakness, anorexia, tachycardia, enlarged heart, edema	Yeast, pork, sunflower seeds, legumes	1.1 mg 1.5 mg
Riboflavin (vitamin B$_2$)	Kuhn, Szent-György, and Wagner-Jaunergy (1933)	Flavin adenine dinucleotide (FAD); flavin mononucleotide (FMN)	Electron (hydrogen) transfer reactions	*Cheilosis*, glossitis, hyperemia and edema of pharyngeal and oral mucous membranes, angular stomatitis, photophobia	Beef liver, braunschweiger sausage, lean sirloin steak, mushrooms, ricotta cheese, nonfat milk, oysters	1.3 mg 1.7 mg
Niacin (vitamin B$_3$) (nicotinic acid, nicotinamide)	Elvehjem et al. (1937)	Nicotinamide adenine dinucleotide (NAD); nicotinamide adenine dinucleotide phosphate (NADP)	Electron (hydrogen) transfer reactions	*Pellagra*, diarrhea, dermatitis, mental confusion, or dementia	Tuna, beef liver, chicken breast, beef, halibut, mushrooms	15 mg 19 mg
Pantothenic acid	R. J. Williams (1933)	Coenzyme A	Acyl transfer reactions	Deficiency very rare: numbness and tingling of hands and feet, vomiting, fatigue	Widespread in foods; exceptionally high amounts in egg yolk, liver, kidney, yeast	4–7 mg[b]
Biotin	Szent-György (1940)	N-carboxybiotinyl lysine	CO_2 transfer reactions; carboxylation reactions	Deficiency very rare, usually induced by ingestion of large	Synthesized by microflora of digestive tract;	30–100 μg[b]

Table 9.1 *(continued)*

Water-Soluble Vitamins

Vitamin	Discovery	Coenzymes	Biochemical or Physiologic Function	Deficiency Syndrome or Symptoms	Good Food Sources in Rank Order	1989 RDA[a]
				amounts of raw egg whites containing avidin; anorexia, nausea, glossitis, depression, dry, scaly dermatitis	yeast, liver, kidney	
Vitamin B_6 (pyridoxine, pyridoxal, pyridoxamine)	Szent-György, Kuhn (1938)	Pyridoxal phosphate (PLP)	Transamination and decarboxylation reactions	Dermatitis, glossitis, convulsions	Sirloin steak, navy beans, potato, salmon, banana	1.6 mg 2.0 mg
Folic acid (folacin)	Mitchell et al. (1941)	Derivatives of tetrahydrofolic acid $N^{5,10}$ methylidyne THFA N^{10} formyl THFA N^5 formimino THFA $N^{5,10}$ methylene THFA N^5 methyl THFA	One-carbon transfer reactions	Megaloblastic anemia, diarrhea, fatigue, depression, confusion	Brewer's yeast, spinach, asparagus, turnip greens, lima beans, beef liver	180 μg 200 μg
Vitamin B_{12} (cobalamin)	Riches, Folkers, et al. (1948)	Methylcobalamin, adenosyl cobalamin (cobalamides)	Methylation of homocysteine to methionine; conversion of methylmalonyl CoA to succinyl CoA	Megaloblastic anemia, degeneration of peripheral nerves, skin hypersensitivity, glossitis	Meat, fish, shellfish, poultry, milk	2.0 μg
Ascorbic acid (vitamin C)	Szent-György[c] (1928) King[c] (1932)	None	Antioxidant, cofactor of hydroxylating enzymes involved in synthesis of collagen, carnitine, norepinephrine	Scurvy, loss of appetite, fatigue, retarded wound healing, bleeding gums, spontaneous rupture of capillaries	Papaya, orange juice, cantaloupe, broccoli, brussels sprouts, green peppers, grapefruit juice, strawberries	60 mg

[a]Adults aged 19–50 years, females and males respectively.
[b]Estimated Safe and Adequate Daily Dietary Intake.
[c]Szent-György and King are considered to be codiscoverers of vitamin C.

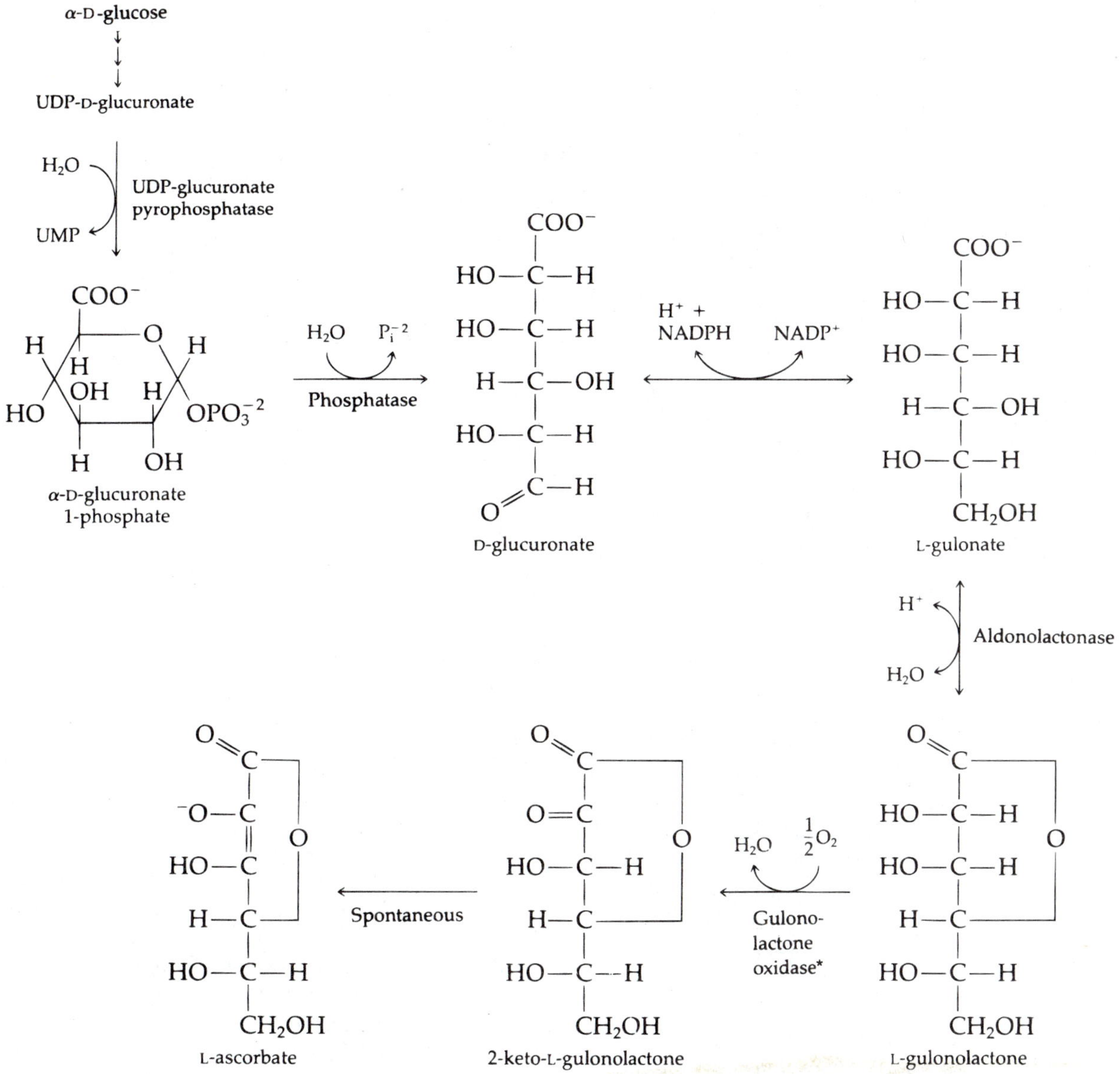

FIGURE 9.2 Synthesis of ascorbic acid. Primates lack the gulonolactone oxidase* that catalyzes the final enzymatic reaction.

back to ascorbic acid (Fig. 9.3) by the enzyme dehydro-ascorbate reductase, which requires reduced glutathione (GSH). During the reduction of dehydroascorbate, glutathione is oxidized (GSSG).

Most absorption of vitamin C occurs in the distal portion of the small intestine, with the degree of absorption decreasing with increased vitamin intake. Absorption can vary from 16% at high intakes (approximately 12g) to 98% at low intakes (<20 mg) [4]. Over a range of usual intakes from food (20 to 120 mg/day), the average, overall absorption is around 80 to 95%

[2,6,7]. Unabsorbed vitamin C may be metabolized by intestinal flora.

Factors that may impair the absorption of vitamin C include pectin (14.2 g/day) and zinc (9.3 mg/day) [2,7]. The degree of absorption as suggested by the urinary excretion of vitamin C appears to be adversely affected by both pectin and zinc; however, the mechanism of action has not been elucidated and the use of urinary vitamin C excretion as a measure of absorption is not standard [2,7]. In the gastrointestinal tract, a high iron concentration present with vitamin C may result in the

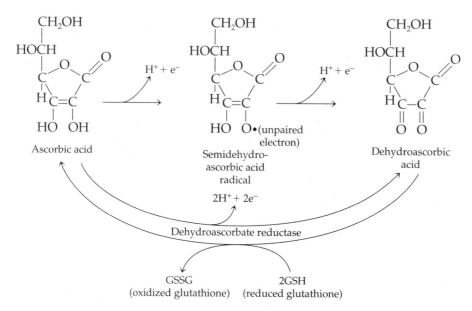

FIGURE 9.3 The interconversion of ascorbate and dehydroascorbate.

oxidative destruction of the vitamin yielding diketogulonic acid (Fig. 9.4) and other products without vitamin C activity [2].

Transport of vitamin C across the basolateral membrane of the intestinal cell occurs by sodium-independent carrier-mediated transport systems. Absorbed ascorbic acid is transported in the plasma in free form. Ascorbate readily equilibrates with the body pool of the vitamin [6,7]. The size of the pool varies with intake. Albumin may also transport some ascorbate and dehydroascorbate in the plasma. About 5% of plasma vitamin C is in the form of dehydroascorbate [8].

Ascorbate moves freely into body cells, but the concentration is much greater in some tissues than in others. The highest concentration of vitamin C is found in the adrenal gland (30 to 40 mg/100 g wet tissue), with the cortex having a higher concentration than the medulla. Other tissues with particularly high concentrations are the pituitary gland and the eye [6,7]. Ascorbate is thought to be actively transported into the adrenal and pituitary glands [7]. Intermediate levels of vitamin C are found in the liver, lungs, pancreas, and leukocytes or white blood cells, while smaller amounts occur in the kidneys, muscles, and red blood cells [6]. Dehydroascorbate formed from oxidation of ascorbate is also taken up by red blood cells, lymphocytes, and neutrophils [7]. Dehydroascorbic acid may be reduced back to ascorbic acid within the cells (Fig. 9.3).

Tissue concentrations of vitamin C usually exceed the plasma level by three to ten times, the degree of concentration depending on the specific tissue. Tissue concentration and plasma level are related to each other, and both are related to intake until intake exceeds about 90 mg/day [6].

Functions and Mechanisms of Action

Despite its uncomplicated structure, vitamin C has a very complex functional role in the body. The response of susceptible organisms to a deficiency and replenishment of vitamin C has been carefully observed, and the biochemical reactions in which vitamin C may participate have been identified. However, no unequivocal mechanisms of action have been established. The only functional role of the vitamin to be categorically established is its ability to prevent and/or cure scurvy [5]. In this role, however, it affects to some extent every body function [9]. For example, normal development of cartilage, bone, and dentine depends on an adequate supply of vitamin C. In addition, the basement membrane lining the capillaries, the "intracellular cement" holding together the endothelial cells, and the scar tissue responsible for wound healing all require the presence of vitamin C for their formation and maintenance.

Antioxidant and Pro-oxidant Activity Ascorbic acid acts as a reducing agent (or stated differently, it is an antioxidant in that it reverses oxidation). During oxidation, electrons are freed and taken up by an acceptor molecule [9]. Reducing agents or antioxidants may reverse oxidation by donating electrons and hydrogen

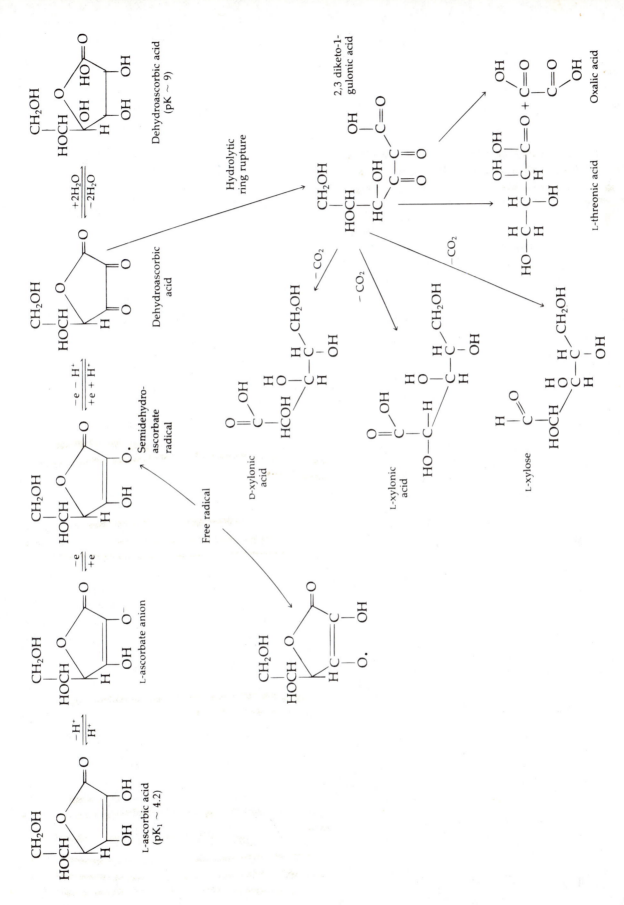

FIGURE 9.4 Postulated biochemical steps in metabolism of ascorbic acid. (Mark Levine, "New Concepts in the Biology and Bio-chemistry of Ascorbic Acid." Reprinted, by permission of the New England Journal of Medicine 314:892–902, 1986.)

228

ions. As an antioxidant, ascorbate (AH⁻) may react with a variety of free radicals and reactive oxygen species. Examples of free-radical and reactive oxygen species include OH (hydroxy radical), O_2^- (superoxide radical), H_2O_2 (hydrogen peroxide), and HO_2 (hydroperoxyl radical). Free radicals are generated by reactive oxygen species and are formed during normal cellular metabolism. Once formed, free radicals attack phospholipids and protein embedded in membranes. For example, aqueous peroxyl radicals induce oxidation of low-density lipoproteins (with implications for increased risk of cardiovascular disease) and oxidation and hemolysis of red blood cell membranes, among others [10,11].

Some examples of reactions involving ascorbate as an antioxidant include [12]:

$$\text{Ascorbate (AH}^-) + \text{OH} \longrightarrow$$
$$\text{semidehydroascorbate radical (A}^-) + H_2O$$

$$\text{Ascorbate (AH}^-) + O_2^- + H^+ \longrightarrow$$
$$\text{semidehydroascorbate radical (A}^-) + H_2O_2$$

$$\text{Ascorbate (AH}^-) + H_2O_2 \longrightarrow$$
$$\text{semidehydroascorbate radical (A}^-) + H_2O$$

Semidehydroascorbate radical (Figs. 9.3 and 9.4) may also be referred to as *ascorbyl* or *monodehydroascorbate radical*. Two semidehydroascorbate radicals typically react to form ascorbate and dehydroascorbate.

$$2 \text{ semidehydroascorbate radicals} \longrightarrow$$
$$\text{ascorbate + dehydroascorbate}$$

Frei [11] reported that ascorbate can effectively react, in aqueous solutions such as blood, with oxidants before their initiation of oxidative damage to lipids. The role of vitamin C and other antioxidants as a defense against oxidative damage to the cell is discussed in the "Perspective" section at the end of Chapter 10.

Although ascorbate is a powerful reducing agent and may be the preferred reductant in certain oxidation–reduction reactions, its action may be nonspecific. Passmore [9] suggested that the function of ascorbate in the cells may be to balance or to set the redox potential (that is, relative states of oxidation or reduction) of other cellular water-soluble substances.

Regeneration of ascorbic acid from semidehydroascorbate radical and from dehydroascorbate is crucial. Reductases are found in most tissues to reduce the semidehydroascorbate radical to ascorbate [8]. Glutathione in its reduced state (GSH) and niacin as NADH or NADPH function in this capacity [5,12]. Examples of some reactions that regenerate ascorbate include [12]:

$$2 \text{ semidehydroascorbate radical (A}^-) + 2GSH \longrightarrow$$
$$2 \text{ ascorbate (AH}^-) + GSSG$$

$$\text{Dehydroascorbate (A)} + 2GSH \longrightarrow$$
$$\text{ascorbate (AH}^-) + GSSG$$

$$2 \text{ semidehydroascorbate radical (A}^-) + NADH + H^+$$
$$\longrightarrow 2 \text{ ascorbate (AH}^-) + NAD^+$$

$$2 \text{ semidehydroascorbate radicals} \longrightarrow$$
$$\text{ascorbate + dehydroascorbate}$$

As a pro-oxidant, vitamin C can reduce transition metals, cupric ions (Cu^{+2}) to cuprous (Cu^{+1}), and ferric ions (Fe^{+3}) to ferrous (Fe^{+2}).

$$\text{Ascorbate (AH}^-) + Fe^{+3} \text{ or } Cu^{+2} \longrightarrow$$
$$\text{semidehydroascorbate radical (A}^-) + Fe^{+2} \text{ or } Cu^{+1}$$

The products—Fe^{+2} and Cu^{+1}—generated from these reactions can proceed to cause cell damage through the generation of reactive oxygen species and free radicals. Examples of some of these reactions include

$$Fe^{+2} \text{ or } Cu^{+1} + H_2O_2 \longrightarrow Fe^{+3} \text{ or }$$
$$Cu^{+2} + OH^- + OH$$

$$Fe^{+2} \text{ or } Cu^{+1} + O_2 \longrightarrow Fe^{+3} \text{ or } Cu^{+2} + O_2^-$$

Collagen Synthesis Ascorbate functions in a number of hydroxylation reactions. Two hydroxylation reactions requiring vitamin C are necessary for collagen formation. For the collagen molecule to aggregate into its triple-helix configuration, selected proline residues on newly synthesized collagen alpha chains must be hydroxylated. Formation of the triple helix is very important because it is in this configuration that the procollagen is secreted from the fibroblast and osteoblast [1,13]. The importance of the lysine hydroxylation is not as clear, but hydroxylysyl residues permit cross-linking of collagen and other posttranslational modifications, such as glycosylation and phosphorylation [1]. Some investigators have also reported that, aside from the hydroxylation reactions, vitamin C influences messenger RNA (mRNA) levels needed for collagen synthesis [1].

Hydroxylations of proline and lysine are both catalyzed by dioxygenases. Dioxygenase enzymes catalyze reactions in which both atoms of O_2 become incorporated into the product(s). The reactions (Fig. 9.5) involve alpha-ketoglutarate, such that one oxygen atom is incorporated into the new carboxyl group of succinate and the other is found in the other substrate. Prolyl hydroxylase and lysyl hydroxylase both require iron bound as a cofactor. Silicon may be needed for maximal prolyl hydroxylase activity. During the hydroxylation reactions, the iron is oxidized; it is converted from a ferrous (+2) state to a ferric (+3) state. Ascorbate functions as the reductant, thereby reducing iron back to its ferrous state (+2).

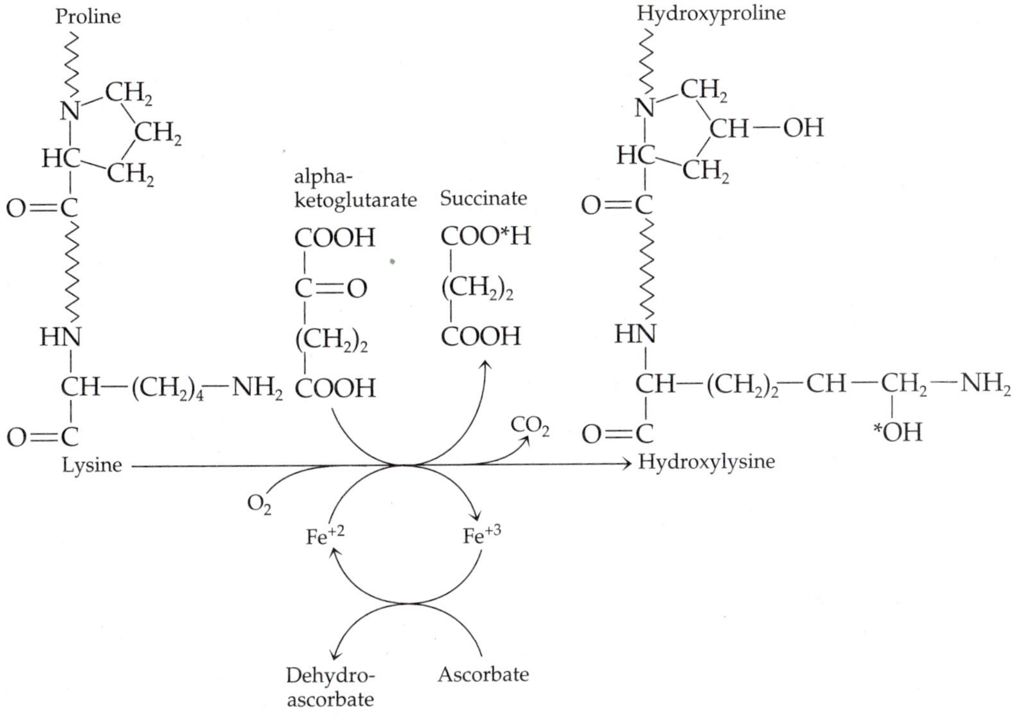

FIGURE 9.5 Ascorbate functions in the hydroxylation of peptide-bound proline and lysine in procollagen. The reaction is driven by alpha-ketoglutarate decarboxylation. One atom of oxygen* appears in the hydroxyl group of the product and the other in succinate.

Carnitine Synthesis Ascorbate is implicated in two reactions required for the synthesis of carnitine from trimethyllysine [14], as shown in Figure 9.6. The iron-containing enzyme trimethyllysine dioxygenase (or hydroxylase) catalyzes the conversion of trimethyllysine to 3-hydroxy trimethyllysine. The iron-containing enzyme 4-butyrobetaine dioxygenase (or hydroxylase) catalyzes the conversion of 4-butyrobetaine to carnitine. These reactions involving ascorbate are hydroxylations that require alpha-ketoglutarate and are almost identical to those for proline and lysine hydroxylation depicted in Figure 9.5. Vitamin C is the preferred reducing agent in carnitine synthesis; however, other substances may be able to replace the ascorbate [5,14]. Sufficient production of carnitine is of significance in fat metabolism because carnitine is essential for the transport of long-chain fatty acids from the cell cytoplasm into the mitochondrial matrix, where β-oxidation occurs. Additional information regarding carnitine can be found on p. 166.

Tyrosine Synthesis and Catabolism Tyrosine is generated from phenylalanine hydroxylation via phenylalanine mono-oxygenase (or hydroxylase), an iron-dependent enzyme. The reaction (Fig. 9.7) occurs in the liver and kidney and requires O_2 and tetrahydro-

biopterin, which is converted to dihydrobiopterin. Vitamin C is thought to function in the regeneration of tetrahydrobiopterin from dihydrobiopterin [15].

Another hydroxylation in which ascorbate participates occurs in the metabolism of tyrosine (Fig. 9.7). Ascorbate is a preferred reductant for the copper-dependent p-hydroxyphenylpyruvate hydroxylase or dioxygenase, the enzyme necessary for the conversion of p-hydroxyphenylpyruvate to homogentisate [1]. Vitamin C is thought to protect the enzyme from inhibition by its substrate [5]. The conversion of homogentisate to 4-maleylacetoacetate is catalyzed by the iron-dependent homogentisate dioxygenase and also requires vitamin C (Fig. 9.7).

Neurotransmitter Synthesis A more direct involvement of ascorbate in enzyme activity is thought to occur with two Cu^{+1}-dependent mono-oxygenases, dopamine mono-oxygenase and peptidylglycine alpha-amidating mono-oxygenase. Mono-oxygenases catalyze reactions in which only one atom of O_2 becomes incorporated into the product(s). Neither of these enzymes is alpha-ketoglutarate dependent. In the case of dopamine mono-oxygenase, which converts dopamine to norepinephrine (Figs. 9.7 and 9.8), it is believed that ascorbate

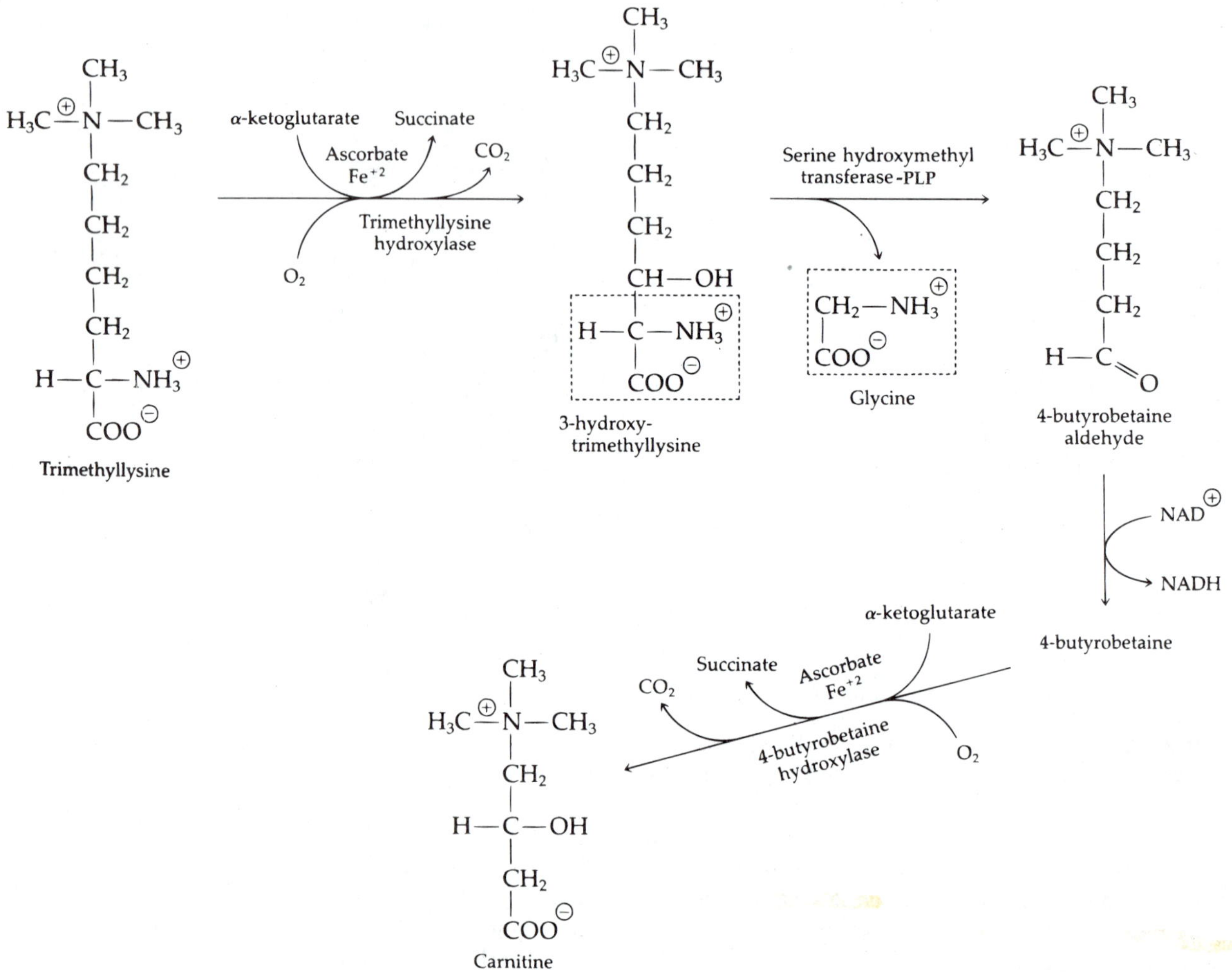

FIGURE 9.6 Role of ascorbate in the synthesis of carnitine.
(McGilvery RW. Biochemistry: A functional approach. 3rd ed. Philadelphia: Saunders, 1983. Reprinted with permission.)

may donate a hydrogen (be oxidized) to semidehydroascorbate radical with subsequent reduction to dehydroascorbate [1,5,16]. The hydrogen donated from ascorbate is thought to be used to reduce the atom of oxygen, not incorporated into the dopamine, to water. The copper atom in the enzyme is thought to act as an intermediate, accepting electrons from ascorbate as it is reduced to the cuprous ion and subsequently transferring these electrons to oxygen as it is reoxidized back to the cupric ion [5].

Ascorbate is thought to keep the copper in peptidylglycine alpha-amidating mono-oxygenase in its reduced state (Fig. 9.9). In the reaction catalyzed by peptidylglycine alpha-amidating mono-oxygenase, the carboxyl-terminal residue is oxidatively cleaved through use of molecular oxygen. The cleavage is not a simple hydrolytic cleavage of a peptide bond because the

amino group is retained as a terminal amide while the rest of the oxidized residue is released as glyoxylate (Fig. 9.9). Although most of the substrate peptides for this enzyme have a terminal glycine residue, the enzyme is also active with peptides terminating in other amino acids. Many of the amidated peptides resulting from this reaction, which has been shown to occur in, for example, the pituitary and adrenal glands, are active as hormones, hormone-releasing factors, or neurotransmitters. Examples include bombesin or gastrin-releasing peptide (GRP), calcitonin, cholecystokinin (CCK), corticotropin-releasing factor, gastrin, growth hormone-releasing factor, oxytocin, and vasopressin [1,15]. If ascorbate is the favored reductant for the required amidating enzyme, then the vitamin assumes an important, although indirect, role in many regulatory processes.

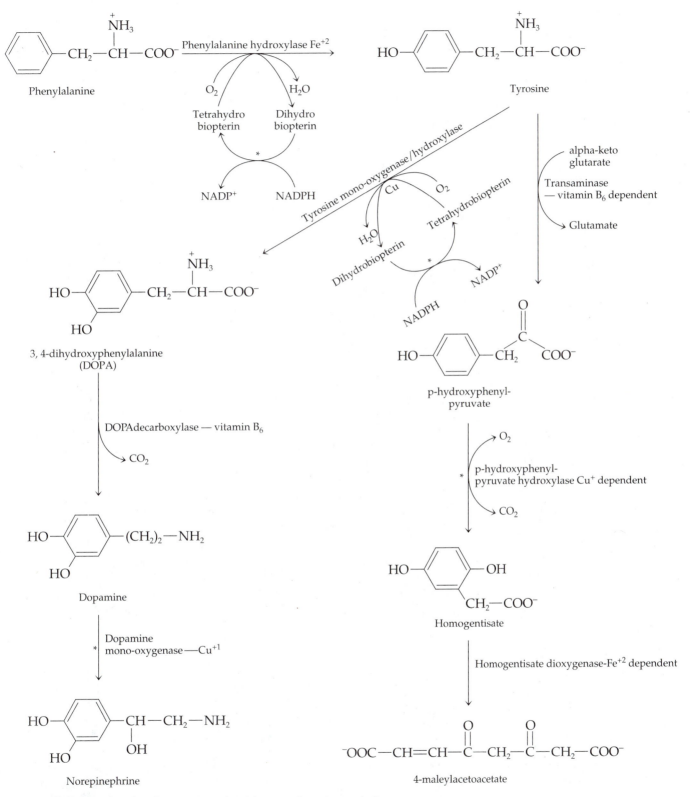

FIGURE 9.7 The roles of vitamin C* in phenylalanine and tyrosine metabolism.

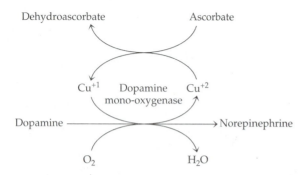

FIGURE 9.8 The role of vitamin C in the dopamine mono-oxygenase catalyzed reaction.

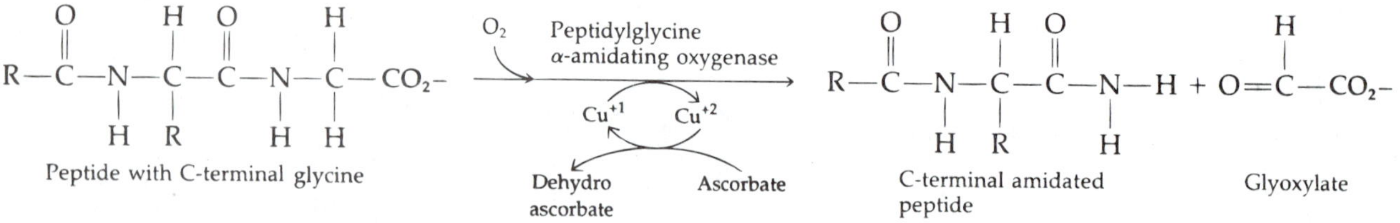

FIGURE 9.9 Amidation of peptides with C-terminal glycine requires vitamin C.

Vitamin C, tetrahydrobiopterin, and oxygen are also involved in the hydroxylation of tryptophan for the synthesis of the neurotransmitter serotonin (5-hydroxytryptamine) in the brain (Fig. 9.10). Tryptophan hydroxylase or mono-oxygenase catalyzes the first step in serotonin synthesis, whereby tryptophan is converted to 5-hydroxytryptophan in a tetrahydrobiopterin-dependent reaction; ascorbate may function in the regeneration of tetrahydrobiopterin from dihydro-biopterin. Subsequently 5-hydroxytryptophan is decarboxylated to generate serotonin.

Cholesterol Degradation for Bile Acid Synthesis Cholesterol 7-alpha-hydroxylase, found in the microsomes of the liver, is required for the initial step in the synthesis of bile acids from cholesterol. The hydroxylation of cholesterol's steroid nucleus by cholesterol 7-alpha-hydroxylase has been shown to be diminished in vitamin C-deficient guinea pigs [4,16]. Ascorbate 2-sulfate, a metabolite of vitamin C catabolism, may also act as a sulfating agent required for cholesterol catabolism [4,5].

Other Functions Many other diverse biochemical functions for vitamin C have been proposed. Experimental evidence supporting these functions varies considerably. Experimental results often conflict, and the mechanism by which ascorbate may be involved is generally unclear. Possible functions for vitamin C include roles in microsomal hydroxylation reactions of noncholesterol steroids and drugs [4,5]; regulation of cellular nucleotide concentrations [4,5]; roles in lipid metabolism [4,17,18], immune function, including complement synthesis [1,4,16,18]; prevention of oxidative destruction of other vitamins, such as vitamin A [4]; sulphation for proteoglycan synthesis [5,16]; and endocrine systems [19]. Vitamin C supplementation at 500 mg daily maintained reduced glutathione (GSH) blood concentrations and improved the antioxidant protection capacity of blood in adults [20]. GSH serves as a sulfhydryl buffer in cells, especially maintaining structural integrity of red blood cells.

Much attention has been directed toward the use of pharmacologic doses of vitamin C in treatment of both the common cold and cancer. The possible pharmacologic effects of vitamin C in the treatment of the common cold and other infectious diseases have been almost totally refuted by Briggs [21], who reviewed the literature (1936 to 1982) and investigated the effect of large doses of vitamin C on the incidence, severity, and duration of the common cold. Briggs concluded that high doses of ascorbate were only weakly prophylactic, if at all, and were of little or no use in the treatment of human infections. One gram of vitamin C per day had no more effect in protection against or in combatting the common cold than 50 mg per day. There were no significant differences between the groups for the number of colds, their severity, or their duration. Other reports conflict

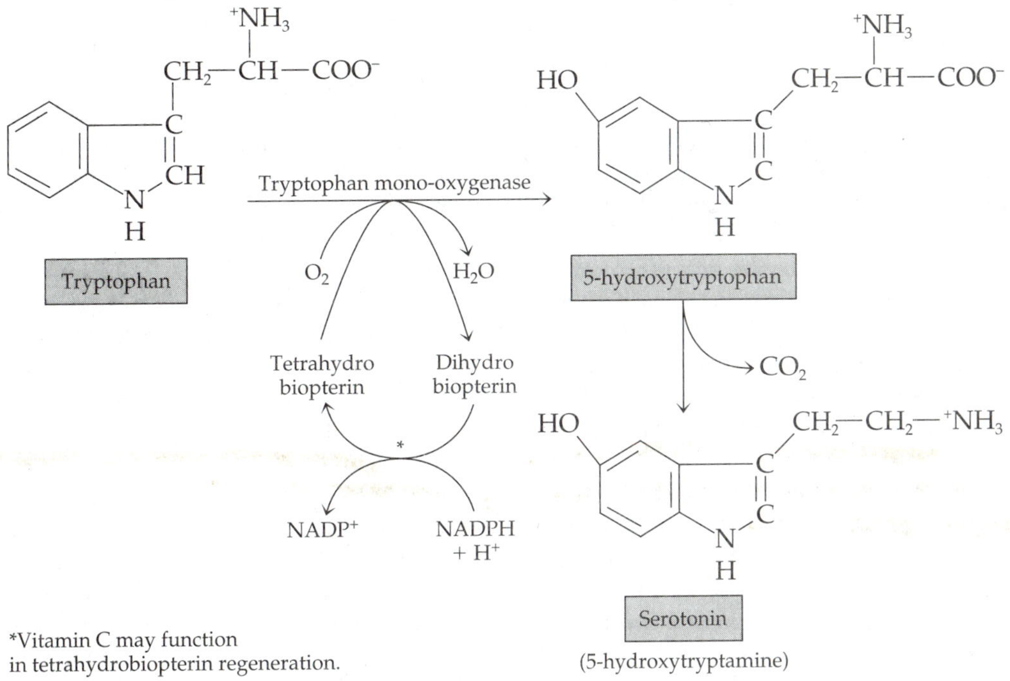

*Vitamin C may function
in tetrahydrobiopterin regeneration.

FIGURE 9.10 Serotonin synthesis.

those by Briggs [21], and suggest a considerable decrease in the duration of cold episodes and the severity of the symptoms [22]. Vitamin C is hypothesized to react with oxidized products released from white blood cell phagocytosis, which occurs at higher rates with infection than with no infection. The reaction of vitamin C with the oxidized products minimizes the inflammatory effects of the oxidized products [22], and thus the severity of the cold.

The possible effect of vitamin C in the prevention and treatment of cancer is controversial. Block [23,24] has reviewed epidemiologic studies of vitamin C and cancer and the mechanisms by which vitamin C may function to prevent cancer. Epidemiologic studies providing indirect evidence suggest strong associations between vitamin C status and cancers of the oral cavity, esophagus, and uterine cervix [4,23]. Possible relationships may exist between vitamin C and cancer of the larynx, bladder, and pancreas [4,23]. Other reviews [25] both support some and negate some of these associations. In clinical trials, whereas some researchers have shown that the survival time in cancer patients could be prolonged through massive doses of vitamin C, no such success has been demonstrated by others [4,23,24,26,27].

Possible mechanisms of ascorbate action against cancer development include a role in immunocompetence, an ability to act as a free radical scavenger or antioxidant, thereby preventing oxidative damage and an ability to detoxify carcinogens or to block carcinogenic processes [4,23,27]. The fact that vitamin C, when ingested with nitrates and/or nitrites, can prevent formation of carcinogenic nitrosamines or nitrosamides supports this latter theory and has led credence that the vitamin is somewhat protective against stomach and/or esophageal cancers [4,26,27]. Vitamin C is not unique in this regard; other reducing agents and some food components are also effective in preventing nitrosocarcinogens [27,28].

Further directions of research with respect to vitamin C as an antioxidant include its use in the prevention of cataracts and cardiovascular disease [25].

Interactions with Other Nutrients

The interaction between the mineral iron and vitamin C is related not only to the vitamin's effect on intestinal absorption of nonheme iron but also on the distribution of iron in the body. Specifically, ascorbate enhances the intestinal absorption of nonheme iron by either reducing iron to a ferrous (Fe^{+2}) form from a ferric (Fe^{+3}) form or by forming a soluble complex with the iron in the alkaline pH of the small intestine to thereby enhance iron's absorption. Excessive iron in the presence of vitamin C, however, can accelerate the oxidative catabolism of vitamin C, thus negating the enhancing effects of vitamin C on iron absorption. Incorporation of iron into ferritin, the storage form of iron, and stabilization of ferritin by ascorbate have also been demonstrated [13,29]. The effect of the vitamin in the distribution and storage of iron is uncertain. Ascorbic acid supplements can cause a change in the distribution of iron in patients suffering with iron overload [6,30], but not necessarily in other individuals [31]. Iron held in the reticuloendothelial cells of the spleen and liver may be mobilized in iron overload patients and then deposited in the parenchymal cells, posing a potential risk for liver damage [30].

In addition to its effects on iron, ascorbic acid may also increase the absorption and excretion of heavy metals, such as lead, from the body by forming chelates with the metals [18]. With respect to copper, vitamin C intakes of 1.5 g daily for about two months resulted in decreased serum copper and ceruloplasmin, a copper-containing protein with oxidase activity; however, despite the decrease, serum copper levels remained within normal range [32]. Dietary vitamin C intakes in excess of 600 mg daily have also been shown to decrease the oxidase activity of ceruloplasmin. Ascorbate may cause copper dissociation from ceruloplasmin or may influence the binding of copper to enzymes [26,33]. Human cells treated with vitamin C have exhibited enhanced copper uptake from ceruloplasmin [26]. Decreased intestinal absorption of copper by ascorbic acid has been observed in several animal species. A proposed mechanism of interaction for this effect suggested that vitamin C stimulated iron mobilization and the mobilized iron in turn inhibited copper absorption [33]. In addition, vitamin C may inhibit the binding of copper to metallothionein, a protein found in the intestinal cells and other body cells. The delayed binding has been proposed to inhibit copper transport across the intestinal cell [33].

Ascorbic acid also appears necessary for folate metabolism. Specifically, vitamin C is thought to be needed to maintain folate in a reduced state, as either tetrahydrofolate, the active form of the vitamin, or dihydrofolate.

Metabolism and Excretion

Vitamin C is typically oxidized to dehydroascorbate. This oxidized form of the vitamin is readily reduced by GSH (Fig. 9.3) or by niacin as nicotinamide adenine dinucleotide (NADH) or nicotinamide adenine dinucleotide phosphate (NADPH) to regenerate ascorbate (p. 228).

The postulated biochemical steps in the metabolism of ascorbic acid, which occurs primarily in the liver but to some extent in the kidneys, are given in Figure 9.4. To metabolize ascorbate, it is first oxidized to form dehy-

droascorbate. This process involves the removal of two electrons and two protons and is thought to occur following the formation of a free radical intermediate. Further oxidation (opening of the ring) of dehydroascorbate yields 2,3-diketogulonic acid, which possesses no vitamin C activity. Diketogulonate is cleaved by separate pathways (Fig. 9.4) into either oxalic acid and a four-carbon sugar threonic acid or into a variety of 5-carbon sugars (xylose, xylonate, and lyxonate). The 4- and 5-carbon sugars can be converted into cellular compounds or can be oxidized and excreted as CO_2 and water.

Vitamin C metabolites including dehydroascorbate, diketogulonate, oxalic acid, 2-O-methyl ascorbate, and 2-ketoascorbitol plus excess ascorbate are excreted in the urine. About 25% of vitamin C intake is excreted in the form of oxalic acid [8]. The kidneys can reduce dehydroascorbate to ascorbate and can conserve ascorbic acid and dehydroascorbate through reabsorption by the kidney tubules so long as the body pool of the vitamin is less than, or approximates, 1,500 mg [6,15]. Tissues are thought to be saturated with body pools between 1,500 and 3,000 mg [26]. The specific amount of vitamin C filtered and then reabsorbed by the kidneys depends on plasma vitamin C concentrations. Plasma ascorbate levels of about 0.8 to 1.4 mg/dL constitute the renal threshold whereby vitamin C in amounts in excess of this level will not be reabsorbed and will thus be excreted in the urine [4]. When the body pool of ascorbic acid is less than 1,500 mg, little or no ascorbic acid appears in the urine; only its metabolites are excreted. As the pool increases above 1,500 mg, the efficiency of kidney reabsorption of the vitamin decreases, and ascorbate along with its metabolites are excreted.

Recommended Dietary Allowances (RDA)

Because the need for vitamin C may change with physiologic status, determination of the actual requirement is difficult in species unable to synthesize it [1]. Multiple approaches to establish vitamin C needs by humans exist; which approach is best remains controversial, as does what is the optimal dietary vitamin C intake [15].

In the United States, the RDA for ascorbate for men has ranged from 75 mg/day in 1943 to 45 mg/day in 1974. The 1989 RDA [34] for vitamin C is 60 mg for adults and is based on maintenance of a body pool of 1,500 mg. This level represents the amount of the vitamin that could be held within the body tissues and fluids without loss via the kidneys and is the same level recommended in the 1980 edition of the RDA [34]. In the 1989 RDA, cigarette smokers for the first time were singled out for an increased vitamin C requirement; recommendations are 100 mg daily for cigarette smokers. Increased metabolic turnover of vitamin C was seen in smokers as compared with nonsmokers.

Recommendations from a 1980 to 1985 Committee on RDA have been published and are referred to as Recommended Dietary Intakes (RDI) [6]. The RDI for adult males and females for vitamin C are 40 mg and 30 mg, respectively [6]. The RDI for vitamin C is based on a body pool of 900 mg, a level believed by some investigators to exceed by 300 mg the amount needed by normal people under ordinary circumstances [6].

Deficiency—Scurvy

Vitamin C intakes of less than 10 mg daily may result in scurvy. Scurvy is typically manifested when the total body pool of vitamin C falls below about 300 mg [15]. Scurvy may be characterized by a multitude of signs and symptoms. Most notable signs and symptoms include bleeding gums, small skin discolorations due to ruptured blood vessels (petechiae), sub-lingual hemorrhages, easy bruising (ecchymoses and purpurae), impaired wound and fracture healing, joint pain (arthralgia), loose and decaying teeth, and hyperkeratosis of hair follicles. The four H's—*hemorrhagic* signs, *hyperkeratosis* of hair follicles, *hypochondriasis* (psychological manifestation), and *hematologic* abnormalities (associated with impaired iron absorption)—are often used as a mnemonic device for remembering scurvy signs [15].

Although scurvy is rare in the United States, low plasma vitamin C levels have been observed in the elderly, especially if institutionalized. People who have poor diets, especially if coupled with alcoholism or drug abuse, are likely to be deficient, as are people with diseases, such as diabetes mellitus and some cancers that increase the turnover rate of the vitamin.

Toxicity

More vitamin C is absorbed, and thus toxicity more likely, with ingestion of several large (<1 g) doses of the vitamin throughout the day than with one single dose. The greater absorption occurs because intestinal vitamin C absorption is saturable and dose dependent. Therefore, maximal absorption of vitamin C occurs more frequently with ingestion of several doses of vitamin C throughout the day versus one more massive dose (>1 g). Unabsorbed vitamin C in the intestinal tract may produce an osmotic diarrhea, a common side effect of ingestion of megadoses of vitamin C [2,4,9,26,35]. Many potentially harmful effects have been attributed to excessive intakes of ascorbic acid, but the frequency of recorded toxicity is quite low [6,35].

Because vitamin C is metabolized in the body to oxalate and because calcium oxalate is a common constituent of kidney stones (nephrolithiasis), ingestion of large doses of vitamin C has been purported as an etiologic factor in nephrolithiasis. Doses up to 10 g of vitamin C have been shown to increase the amount of oxalate excreted; the amount of oxalate excreted (typically <50 mg), however, usually remains within a normal and safe range [4,36,37]. Those people predisposed to calcium oxalate kidney stones should, however, avoid high doses of vitamin C [4,7,9,16,37]. Large doses of ascorbic acid (up to approximately 4 g) can also increase the amount of uric acid excreted in the urine through competitive inhibition of renal reabsorption of uric acid [6,16,38]. The resulting urine acidification along with the excessive amount of uric acid being excreted could cause precipitation of urate crystals and urate kidney stones [35]. The actual clinical importance of uricosuria (high uric acid in the urine) with regard to stone formation is unknown [14,35].

Because ascorbic acid increases nonheme iron absorption, chronic high doses of vitamin C may be unsafe for those people unable to regulate absorption of iron, including individuals with hemochromatosis, thalassemia, and sideroblastic anemia [24,35].

Excessive ascorbate excretion in the urine and feces can interfere with a variety of clinical laboratory tests. Vitamin C in the urine, for example, may act as a reductive agent and thus interfere with the diagnostic tests using redox chemistry [4]. False-negative tests for fecal occult blood may be generated and occult blood in the urine may not be detected. Tests for glucose in the urine can be rendered invalid [4,26,35].

The issue of systemic conditioning to high intakes of vitamin C is still in question. Because scurvylike symptoms have been reported in some individuals on abrupt withdrawal of large intakes of vitamin C, people are advised to gradually diminish the intake of vitamin C over a 2- to 4-week period [4].

Assessment of Nutriture

The measurement of blood, serum, or plasma levels of ascorbate is the most commonly used and practical procedure for determining vitamin C nutriture [4,7,35,39]. Blood, plasma, and serum vitamin C concentrations respond to changes in dietary vitamin C intakes, and are thus used to assess recent vitamin C intake. Plasma vitamin C levels are deemed superior to blood levels because the latter is less sensitive to vitamin C deficiency [4]. White blood cell content of the vitamin better reflects body stores, but this measurement is technically more difficult to perform. Following is a list of the serum levels of vitamin C considered to be deficient, marginal, and adequate [40]:

	Criteria of Status		
	Deficient	Marginal	Adequate
Vitamin C serum (mg/dL)			
<20 years male and female	<0.2	0.2–0.6	>0.6
>20 years male and female	<0.2	0.2–0.4	>0.4
Vitamin C WBC (mg/dL)	0–7	7–15	>15

References Cited for Vitamin C

1. Englard S, Seifter S. The biological functions of ascorbic acid. Ann Rev Nutr 1986;6:365–406.
2. Sauberlich HE. Bioavailability of vitamins. Prog Food Nutr Sci 1985;9:1–33.
3. Rose RC. Intestinal transport of vitamins. J Inherited Metab Dis 1985;8(suppl):13–16.
4. Jacob RA. Vitamin C. In: Shils ME, Olson JA, Shike M., eds. Modern nutrition in health and disease, 8th ed. Philadelphia: Lea and Febiger, 1994:432–448.
5. Basu TK, Schorah CJ. Vitamin C in health and disease. Westport, CT: AVI, 1982.
6. Olson A, Hodges RE. Recommended dietary intakes (RDI) of vitamin C in humans. Am J Clin Nutr 1987;45:693–703.
7. Sauberlich HE. Ascorbic acid. In: Brown ML., ed. Present knowledge in nutrition, 6th ed. Washington, DC: International Life Sciences Institute Nutrition Foundation, 1990:132–141.
8. Bender DA. Nutritional biochemistry of the vitamins. New York: Cambridge University Press, 1992:360–393.
9. Passmore R. How vitamin C deficiency injures the body. Nutr Today 1977;12:6–11,27–31.
10. Niki E. Action of ascorbic acid as a scavenger of active and stable oxygen radicals. Am J Clin Nutr 1991;54:1119S–1124S.
11. Frei B. Ascorbic acid protects lipids in human plasma and low density lipoprotein against oxidative damage. Am J Clin Nutr 1991;54:1113S–1118S.
12. Stadtman ER. Ascorbic acid and oxidative inactivation of proteins. Am J Clin Nutr 1991;54:1125S–1128S.
13. Aberts B, Bray D, Lewis J, et al. Molecular biology of the cell. New York: Garland, 1983:693–701.
14. Rebouche CJ. Ascorbic acid and carnitine biosynthesis. Am J Clin Nutr 1991;54:1147S–1152S.
15. Levine M. New concepts in the biology and biochemistry of ascorbic acid. N Engl J Med 1986;314:892–902.
16. Combs GF. The vitamins. San Diego, CA: Academic Press, 1992:223–249.
17. Gey KF, Moser UK, Jordan P, Stahelin HB, Eichholzer M, Ludin E. Increased risk of cardiovascular disease at suboptimal plasma concentrations of essential antioxidants: An epidemiological update with special attention to carotene and vitamin C. Am J Clin Nutr 1993;57(suppl.):787S–797S.
18. Moser U, Bendich A. Vitamin C. In: Machlin LJ, ed. Handbook of vitamins, 2nd ed. New York: Dekker, 1991:195–232.
19. Levine M, Morita K. Ascorbic acid in endocrine systems. Vitamins & Hormones 1985;42:2–64.
20. Johnston CS, Meyer CG, Srilakshmi JC. Vitamin C elevates red blood cell glutathione in healthy adults. Am J Clin Nutr 1993;58:103–105.
21. Briggs M. Vitamin C and infectious disease: A review of the literature and the results of a randomized, double-blind, prospective study over 8 years. In: Briggs MH, ed. Recent vitamin research. Boca Raton, FL: CRC Press, 1984:39–81.
22. Hemila H. Vitamin C and the common cold. Br J Nutr 1992;67: 3–16.
23. Block G, Menkes M. Ascorbic acid and cancer prevention. In: Moon TE, Micozzi MS, eds. Nutrition and cancer prevention. New York: Dekker, 1989:341–388.
24. Block G. Vitamin C and cancer prevention: The epidemiologic evidence. Am J Clin Nutr 1991;53:270S–282S.
25. Gershoff SN. Vitamin C (ascorbic acid): New roles, new requirements? Nutr Rev 1993:51;313–326.
26. Davies MB, Austin J, Partridge DA. Vitamin C. Its chemistry and biochemistry. Cambridge, England: Royal Society of Chemistry, 1991.
27. Carpenter MP. Roles of vitamins E and C in cancer. In: Laidlaw SA, Swendseid ME. Contemporary issues in clinical nutrition. New York: Wiley-Liss, 1991:61–90.
28. Bright-See E. Vitamin C and cancer prevention. Semin Oncol 1983;10:294–298.
29. Hoffman KE, Yanelli K, Bridges KR. Ascorbic acid and iron metabolism: Alterations in lysosomal function. Am J Clin Nutr 1991;54:1188S–1192S.
30. Nienhuis AW. Vitamin C and iron. N Engl J Med 1981;304: 170–171.
31. Cook JD, Watson SS, Simpson KM, Lipschitz DA, Skikne BS. The effect of high ascorbic acid supplementation on body iron stores. Blood 1984;64:721–726.
32. Finley EB, Cerklewski FL. Influence of ascorbic acid supplementation on copper status in young adult men. Am J Clin Nutr 1983;37:553–556.
33. Harris ED, Percival SS. A role of ascorbic acid in copper transport. Am J Clin Nutr 1991;54:1193S–1197S.
34. National Research Council. Recommended dietary allowances, 10th ed. Washington, DC: National Academy Press, 1989:115–124.
35. Alhadeff L, Gualtieri CT, Lipton M. Toxic effects of water-soluble vitamins. Nutr Rev 1984;42:33–40.
36. Tsao CS, Salimi SL. Effect of large intake of ascorbic acid on urinary and plasma oxalic acid levels. Internatl J Vit Nutr Res 1984;54:245–249.

37. Hughes C, Dutton S, Truswell AS. High intakes of ascorbic acid and urinary oxalate. J Human Nutr 1981;35:274–280.
38. Sutton JL, Basu TK, Dickerson JWT. Effect of large doses of ascorbic acid in man on some nitrogenous components of urine. Human Nutr Appl Nutr 1983;37A:136–140.
39. Jacob RA. Assessment of human vitamin C status. J Nutr 1990;120:1480–1485.
40. Simko MD, Cowell C, Gilbride JA. Nutrition assessment. Rockville, MD: Aspen, 1984:165–166.

The following discussion outlines the B-complex vitamins.

THIAMIN

Thiamin (vitamin B_1), the structural formula of which is shown in Figure 9.11, consists of a pyrimidine ring and a thiazole moiety (meaning one of two parts), which are linked by a methylene (CH_2) bridge.

Sources

Thiamin is found widely distributed in foods. Foods considered rich sources of thiamin are yeast, lean pork, legumes, and whole or enriched grain products. Organ meats and nuts are also relatively high in thiamin.

Digestion, Absorption, and Transport

In plants, thiamin exists in its free form, while in animal products over 95% of thiamin occurs in a phosphorylated form, primarily thiamin diphosphate (TDP), also called *thiamin pyrophosphate (TPP)* [1]. Intestinal phosphatases hydrolyze the phosphates from the thiamin prior to absorption.

The bioavailability of thiamin occurring naturally in foods is believed to be high [2]. Occasionally, however, antithiamin factors may be present in the diet. For example, thiaminases present in raw fish catalyze the cleavage of thiamin, thereby destroying its activity. These thiaminases are thermolabile, thus cooking of fish renders the enzymes inactive. Other antithiamin factors, such as tannic and caffeic acids, that are thermostable may be found in coffee, tea, betel nuts, and certain fruits and vegetables such as blueberries, black currants, brussels sprouts, and red cabbage [2]. Calcium, magnesium, and other divalent cations assist in the precipitation of thiamin by tannic acid. Thiamin destruction may be prevented by the presence of reducing compounds such as vitamin C and citric acid, among others.

Free thiamin, not phosphorylated thiamin, is absorbed from the intestine. Absorption of thiamin can be both active and passive, depending on the amount of the vitamin presented for absorption. At low physiologic concentrations, thiamin absorption is active and sodium dependent. Absorption occurs primarily in the upper jejunum, but can occur in the duodenum and ileum [2–5]. When intakes of thiamin are high, absorption is predominantly passive.

Thiamin absorption is typically high except in the case of ethanol ingestion [2]. Ethanol ingestion interferes with active transport of thiamin from the mucosal cell across the basolateral membrane, but not the brush border membrane [4].

Within the mucosal cells, thiamin may be phosphorylated (that is, converted into a phosphate ester). Thiamin transport across the basolateral membrane is sodium and energy dependent [1]. Thiamin appearing on the serosal side of the enterocyte is not initially bound to phosphates.

Thiamin in the blood is typically in the form of thiamin monophosphate (TMP) [6]. Thiamin may be

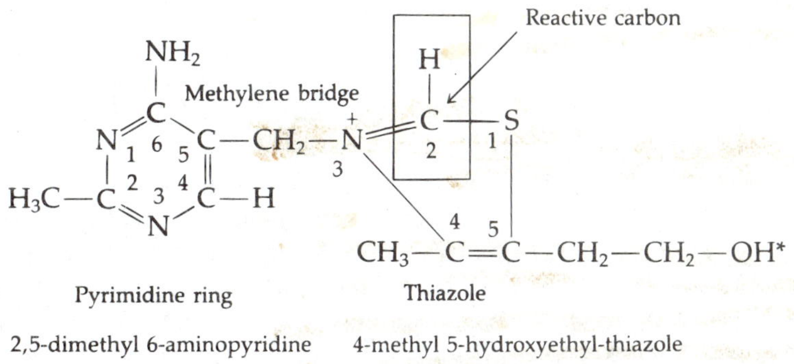

FIGURE 9.11 Structure of thiamin.

2,5-dimethyl 6-aminopyridine   4-methyl 5-hydroxyethyl-thiazole

*Diphosphate addition occurs here to form the active coenzyme thiamin diphosphate (TDP).

bound to albumin for plasma transport, and thiamin in excess of albumin's binding capacity is found free [4,6]. The majority (about 90%) of thiamin in the blood is present within the blood cells. Transport of thiamin into red blood cells is thought to occur by facilitated diffusion whereas transport into other tissues requires energy. Only free thiamin or TMP is thought to be able to cross cell membranes.

The human body contains approximately 30 mg of thiamin, with high concentrations found in the skeletal muscles, heart, liver, kidney, and brain. Approximately half of the body's thiamin is found distributed throughout the skeletal muscle. Most of the free thiamin is taken up by the liver and phosphorylated, although other tissues have the capacity to convert thiamin to its coenzyme phosphorylated form, thiamin diphosphate (TDP). Conversion of thiamin to TDP requires adenosine triphosphate (ATP) and thiamin pyrophosphokinase, an enzyme found in the liver, brain, and perhaps in other tissues as well [7]. About 80% of the total thiamin in the body exists as TDP [3].

Another form of thiamin, thiamin triphosphate (TTP) represents about 10% of total body thiamin and is synthesized by action of a TDP-ATP phosphoryl transferase that phosphorylates TDP [1,3,4]. The terminal phosphate on TTP may be hydrolyzed by thiamin triphosphatase to yield TDP. TTP, as well as TDP and TMP, can be found in small amounts in several tissues, including the brain, heart, liver, and kidney. TMP is thought to be derived from the catabolism of the terminal phosphate on TDP and is believed to be inactive [1].

Functions and Mechanisms of Action

At the cellular level, thiamin plays essential roles in (1) energy transformation; (2) synthesis of pentoses and NADPH (a coenzyme form of niacin, nicotinamide adenine dinucleotide phosphate in a reduced form); and (3) membrane and nerve conduction.

Energy Transformation TDP functions as a coenzyme necessary for the oxidative decarboxylation of both pyruvate and alpha-ketoglutarate. These reactions (Fig. 9.12) are instrumental in generating ATP. Inhibition of these decarboxylation reactions prevents synthesis of ATP and acetyl CoA needed for the synthesis of, for example, fatty acids, cholesterol and other important compounds, and results in the accumulation of pyruvate, lactate, and α-ketoglutarate in the blood.

The steps that occur in the oxidative decarboxylation of pyruvate are shown in Figure 9.13 and require a

multienzyme complex, pyruvate dehydrogenase complex, which is bound to the mitochondrial membrane. Three enzymes make up the complex: first, a TDP-dependent pyruvate decarboxylase, followed by a lipoic acid-dependent dihydrolipoyl transacetylase and finally a FAD-dependent dihydrolipoyl dehydrogenase. The roles of four vitamins—thiamin (TDP), riboflavin (FAD), niacin (NAD+), and pantothenic acid (CoA)—in this decarboxylation process can be identified in Figure 9.13. Although lipoic acid functions as a prosthetic group, it is not considered a vitamin. Lipoic acid is classified as a sulfur-containing fatty acid; uncertainty exists as to whether it is synthesized in the body or is obtained by diet. In the dehydrogenase reactions, lipoate functions similar to biotin at the end of the long flexible side chain of the enzyme; specifically it rotates from one active site to another site on the multisubunit enzyme. Lipoamide (Fig. 9.13) picks up the acetyl group from TDP to form acetyl lipoamide. The acetyl group is transferred from acetyl lipoamide to CoA with the formation of acetyl CoA and dihydrolipoamide. The dihydrolipoamide is then oxidized back to the original lipoamide.

The decarboxylation of α-ketoglutarate by the α-ketoglutarate dehydrogenase complex is similar to that for pyruvate. α-ketoglutarate dehydrogenase serves to decarboxylate α-ketoglutarate and forms succinyl CoA.

A key feature of TDP (Fig. 9.14) is that the carbon atom between the nitrogen and sulfur atoms in the thiazole ring is more acidic than most CH groups [3,8]. It ionizes (deprotonizes) to form a carbanion at carbon 2 of the thiazole ring. The carbanion is stabilized by the positively charged nitrogen in the thiazole ring [3,8]. The carbanion combines with the 2-carbonyl group of pyruvate (Fig. 9.14), α-ketoglutarate and other α-ketoacids to form a covalent bond [7,8].

Decarboxylation of the branched-chain α-ketoacids, which arise from the transamination of valine, isoleucine, and leucine, is an oxidative process that also requires thiamin as TDP. Failure to oxidize the α-ketoacids, α-ketoisocaproic, α-keto β-methyl valeric, and α-ketoisovaleric acids from leucine, isoleucine, and valine respectively, results in the accumulation of both the branched-chain amino acids and their α-ketoacids in blood and other body fluids. Such findings are characteristic of maple syrup urine disease (MSUD). MSUD results from a genetic (inborn error of metabolism) absence or insufficient activity of the branched-chain α-ketoacid dehydrogenase enzyme complex. People with MSUD must avoid meat, poultry, fish, and dairy products in order to limit intakes of leucine, isoleucine, and

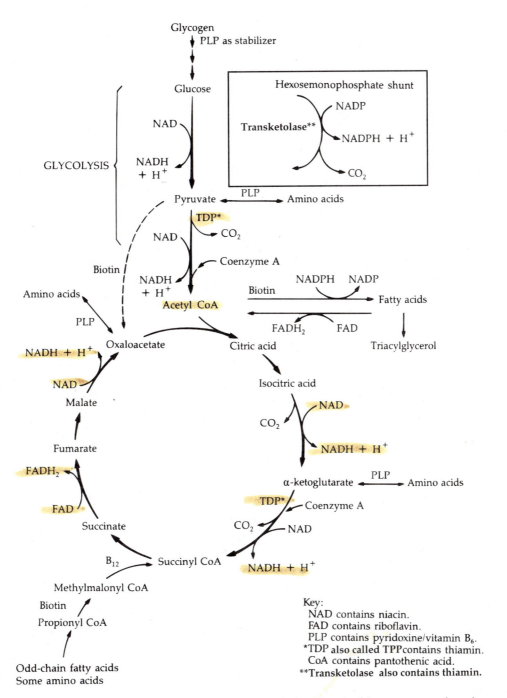

Glycogen
↓ PLP as stabilizer
↓↓
Glucose

Hexosemonophosphate shunt

Transketolase** ⟶ NADP
⟶ NADPH + H$^+$
⟶ CO_2

GLYCOLYSIS

NAD
NADH + H$^+$

Pyruvate ⟶ PLP ⟶ Amino acids

TDP*
NAD ⟶ CO_2
Coenzyme A

Biotin

NADH + H$^+$
Acetyl CoA

Biotin ⟶ NADPH NADP ⟶ Fatty acids
FADH$_2$ FAD
Triacylglycerol

Amino acids
PLP

NADH + H$^+$
NAD
Malate

Oxaloacetate Citric acid

Isocitric acid
NAD
CO_2
NADH + H$^+$

Fumarate

FADH$_2$
FAD
Succinate

α-ketoglutarate ⟶ PLP ⟶ Amino acids
TDP* ⟶ Coenzyme A
CO_2 ⟶ NAD
NADH + H$^+$

B$_{12}$ ⟶ Succinyl CoA

Methylmalonyl CoA
Biotin ↗
Propionyl CoA
↗
Odd-chain fatty acids
Some amino acids

Key:
NAD contains niacin.
FAD contains riboflavin.
PLP contains pyridoxine/vitamin B$_6$.
*TDP also called TPP contains thiamin.
CoA contains pantothenic acid.
**Transketolase also contains thiamin.

FIGURE 9.12 Various vitamin cofactors and their action sites in energy metabolism. The role of thiamin as TDP is shown by an asterisk(*).

valine. Medical foods devoid of these three amino acids provide the majority of nutrient intake.

Synthesis of NADPH and Pentoses TDP also functions as a loosely bound prosthetic group of transketolase, a key cytosolic enzyme in the hexose mono-

phosphate shunt. The hexose monophosphate shunt is the pathway in which sugars of varying chain lengths are interconverted. The shunt is essential for the generation of pentoses for nucleic acid synthesis and of NADPH, which is needed, for example, for fatty acid synthesis. TDP forms a carbanion (as in Fig. 9.14) that acts to

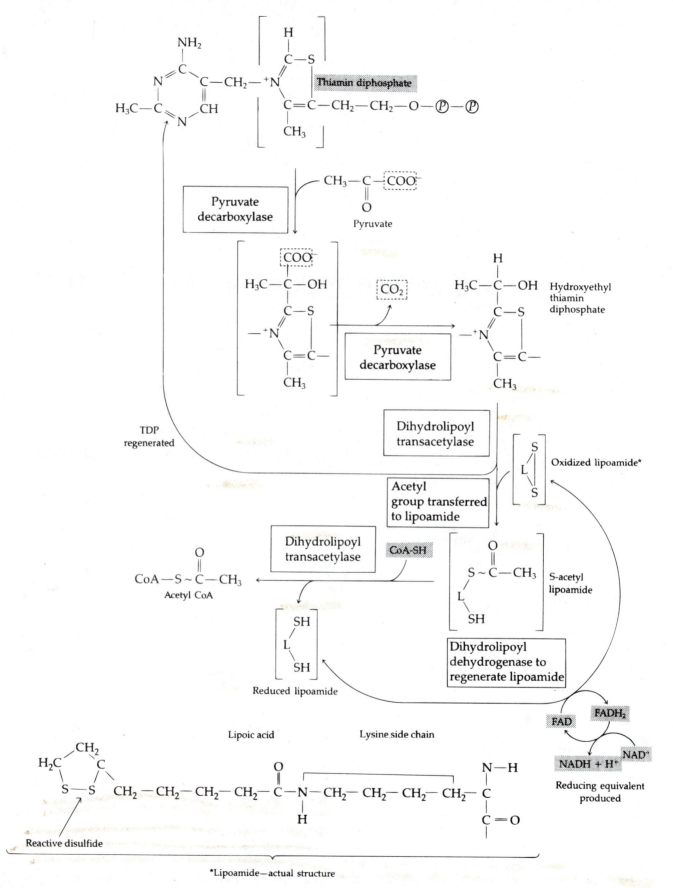

FIGURE 9.13 Oxidative decarboxylation of pyruvate by pyruvate dehydrogenase complex.

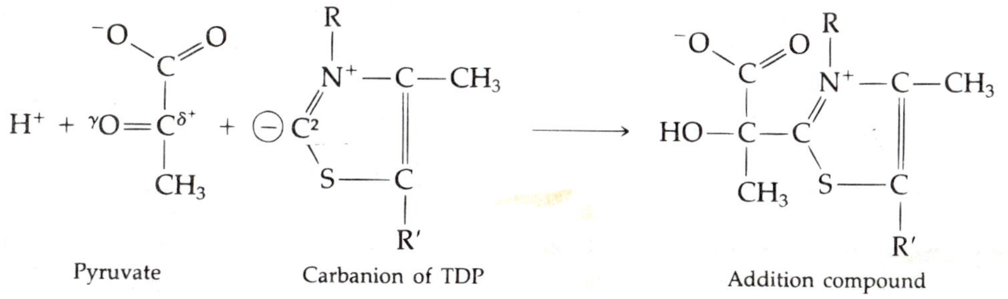

FIGURE 9.14 Combination of TDP carbanion with substrate pyruvate.

transfer an activated aldehyde from a donor ketose substrate to an acceptor. The acceptor in the hexose monophosphate shunt is xylulose. Transketolase hydrolyzes the carbon to carbon bond in xylose 5-P, sedoheptulose 7-P, and fructose 6-P (that is, ketoses) and transfers the two carbon fragment (carbons 1 and 2 of the ketoses) to an aldose receptor [8]. The transketolase-activated reaction that requires Mg^{+2} can be written as follows:

$$\text{xylulose 5-P + ribose 5-P} \xrightleftharpoons[\text{transketolase}]{}$$

$$\text{sedoheptulose 7-P + glyceraldehyde 3-P}$$

$$\text{xylulose 5-P + erythrose 4-P} \xrightleftharpoons[\text{transketolase}]{}$$

$$\text{glyceraldehyde 3-P + fructose 6-P}$$

Membrane and Nerve Conduction   Exactly how thiamin functions or in what form it functions in nerve membranes and in nerve conduction is unclear. However, it is believed that in the nervous system thiamin as either TDP or TTP exerts its action in some manner other than as a coenzyme. TDP and TTP are rapidly interconvertible; therefore, uncertainty exists about which is the neurophysiologically active form [9]. But evidence is emerging that TTP may be the form involved in nerve membrane function and nerve transmission [1,9].

Aberrations in nerve function may be due to a lack of energy; a decreased amount of acetylcholine, the synthesis of which requires TDP; or a reduced nerve impulse transmission. In the last instance it is postulated that thiamin, as TDP or TTP, may occupy a site on the nerve membrane. The site is either a sodium channel or is proximal to the channel. In this location thiamin could regulate nerve impulse transmission. Initiation of a nerve impulse could result in dephosphorylation of the thiamin ester, a reaction that somehow would allow sodium to cross the membrane freely, thereby permitting conduction of the nerve impulse [9].

Metabolism and Excretion

Thiamin in excess of tissue needs and storage capacity is metabolized for urinary excretion. When intake of the vitamin is adequate, the excretion products are almost equally divided between thiamin and its metabolites [4]. Free plasma thiamin is typically filtered by the kidney and excreted in the urine. Degradation of thiamin begins with the cleavage of the molecule into its pyrimidine and thiazole moieties; the two rings are then further metabolized. Over 40 metabolites from pyrimidine and thiazole catabolism have been identified [1,6].

Some thiamin appears to be catabolized at a fairly constant rate regardless of the level of thiamin intake [10]. The pathway for this degradation may not necessarily be related to physiological function [10]. These losses represent obligatory losses that must be met by dietary thiamin.

Recommended Dietary Allowances

Determination of the RDA for thiamin has been based on (1) relationship between varying levels of thiamin intake and occurrence of clinical signs of deficiency; (2) level of excretion of thiamin and/or its metabolites; and (3) degree of erythrocyte transketolase activity. Because of the importance of thiamin in energy metabolism, needed intake varies according to energy (caloric) intake. The RDA for adults is 0.5 mg/1,000 kcal; however, an intake of no less than 1 mg/day is advised [3,6,11].

Deficiency—Beriberi

Despite the known functional roles of thiamin at the cellular level, it has as yet been impossible to explain all the pathophysiologic manifestations in animals or humans that are associated with thiamin deficiency, beriberi. One of the first symptoms of thiamin deficiency is a loss of appetite (anorexia) and thus weight. As deficiency worsens, cardiovascular system involvement (such as hypertrophy and altered heart rate) and neurologic symptoms appear.

Three types of beriberi have been identified. Dry beriberi is found predominantly in older adults; it is thought to result from a chronic low thiamin intake especially if coupled with a high carbohydrate intake. Dry beriberi is characterized by muscle weakness and wasting especially in the lower extremities [1,6,8]. Wet beriberi results in more extensive cardiovascular system involvement than dry beriberi; right-side heart failure leads to respiratory involvement with edema [1,6]. Lastly, acute beriberi, seen mostly in infants, has been documented in countries such as Japan.

In the United States and in Western countries, thiamin deficiency associated with alcoholism is common and is referred to as Wernicke's encephalopathy or Wernicke-Korsakoff syndrome. This condition is characterized by mental confusion, loss of recent memory, ataxia, among other symptoms [1,6]. Alcoholics are particularly prone to thiamin deficiency because of (1) decreased intake of the vitamin due to decreased food consumption; (2) an increased requirement in the case of liver damage (decreased liver function impairs TDP formation and, consequently, vitamin use) and (3) decreased thiamin absorption is possible [6,11]. Elderly populations are also at risk for thiamin deficiency. People with diseases that impair absorption of the vitamin are also at greater risk of developing deficiency. Examples of conditions in which absorption is impaired include some cancers, biliary disease, and inflammatory bowel diseases. Folate and protein deficiencies that impair enterocyte turnover also diminish thiamin absorption. Excess glucose infusion intravenously and ingestion of diets that are made up primarily of refined, unenriched grain products necessitate increased thiamin intake. The enrichment of grain products that are not whole grain has helped to improve thiamin intakes in many populations of the United States.

Toxicity

There appears to be little danger of thiamin toxicity associated with oral intake of large amounts (500 mg daily for one month) of thiamin [11–13]. Excessive (100 times recommendations) thiamin, administered by the parenteral (intravenous or intramuscular) route, however, has been associated with headache, convulsions, cardiac arrythmia, anaphylactic shock, among other signs [8].

Pharmacologic levels of thiamin are used in the treatment of certain inborn errors of metabolism. One variant form of MSUD has been shown to respond to oral thiamin supplements (up to 500 mg daily). Other metabolic diseases that may respond to large doses of the vitamin are thiamin-responsive megaloblastic anemia and thiamin-responsive lactic acidosis. In the latter condition, large doses of thiamin can increase the activity of pyruvate dehydrogenase in the liver, thereby decreasing the level of lactic acid as more pyruvate is decarboxylated for entry into the Krebs cycle. How administration of the vitamin helps correct thiamin-responsive megaloblastic anemia has not been elucidated [14].

Assessment of Nutriture

Adequacy of thiamin nutriture is most accurately determined by measurement of erythrocyte transketolase activity in hemolyzed whole blood [15]. Transketolase, the thiamin-dependent enzyme of the hexose monophosphate shunt, increases activity with the addition of thiamin to the incubation medium. An increase in activity of more than 25% is indicative of thiamin deficiency.

	Thiamin Status		
	Deficient	Marginal	Adequate
Transketolase (effect of TDP)	> 25%	25 to 15%	<15%

References Cited for Thiamin

1. Gubler CJ. Thiamin. In: Machlin LJ., ed. Handbook of vitamins. 2nd ed. New York: Dekker, 1991:233–281.
2. Sauberlich HE. Bioavailability of vitamins. Prog Food Nutr Sci 1985;9:1–33.
3. Tanphaichitr V. Thiamin. In: Shils ME, Olson JA, Shike M., eds. Modern nutrition in health and disease. 8th ed. Philadelphia: Lea and Febiger, 1994:359–365.
4. Bender DA. Nutritional biochemistry of the vitamins. New York: Cambridge University Press, 1992:128–155.
5. Sauberlich HE. Vitamins—how much is for keeps? Nutr Today 1987;22:20–28.
6. Brown ML. Thiamin. In: Brown ML, ed. Present knowledge in nutrition, 6th ed. Washington, DC: The Nutrition Foundation, 1990:142–145.
7. Murray RK, Granner DK, Mayes PA, Rodwell VW. Harper's biochemistry, 23rd ed. Norwalk, CT: Appleton and Lange, 1993.
8. Combs GF. The vitamins. San Diego, CA: Academic Press, 1992:251–269.
9. Haas RH. Thiamin and the brain. Ann Rev Nutr 1988;8: 483–515.
10. Ariaey-Nejad MR, Balaghi M, Baker EM, Sauberlich HE. Thiamin metabolism in man. Am J Clin Nutr 1970;23: 764–778.
11. National Research Council. Recommended dietary allowances, 10th ed. Washington, DC: National Academy Press, 1989:125–132.

12. Council on Scientific Affairs, American Medical Association. Vitamin preparations as dietary supplements and as therapeutic agents. JAMA 1987;257:1929–1936.
13. Alhadeff L, Gualtieri CT, Lipton M. Toxic effects of water-soluble vitamins. Nutr Rev 1984;42:33–40.
14. Tanphaichiti V, Wood B. Thiamin. In: Olson RE, Broquist HP, Chichester CO, Darby WJ, Kolbye AC, Stalvey RM. Present knowledge in nutrition, 5th ed. Washington, DC: The Nutrition Foundation, 1984:273–284.
15. Simko MD, Cowell C, Gilbride JA. Nutrition assessment. Rockville, MD: Aspen, 1984.

RIBOFLAVIN

Riboflavin consists of flavin (isoalloxazine ring), to which is attached a ribitol (sugar alcohol) side chain. The structure of riboflavin along with its two coenzyme derivatives are given in Figure 9.15.

Sources

Riboflavin is found in a wide variety of foods. Milk and milk products such as cheeses are thought to contribute the majority of dietary riboflavin. Eggs, meat, and legumes also provide riboflavin in significant quantities to the diet. Fruits, vegetables, and cereal grains are minor contributors of dietary riboflavin.

The form of riboflavin in food varies. Free or protein-bound riboflavin is found in milk, eggs, and in enriched breads and cereals. In most other foods the vitamin occurs as one or the other of its coenzyme derivatives, FMN (flavin mononucleotide) or FAD (flavin adenine dinucleotide). Phosphorus-bound riboflavin is also found in some foods.

Digestion, Absorption, and Transport

Riboflavin attached noncovalently to proteins may be freed by the action of hydrochloric acid secreted within the stomach or by gastric and intestinal enzymatic hydrolysis of the protein. Riboflavin in foods as FAD, FMN, and riboflavin phosphate must also be freed prior to absorption. Within the intestinal lumen, FAD pyrophosphatase converts FAD to FMN; FMN is converted to free riboflavin by FMN phosphatase.

FAD $\xrightarrow{\text{FAD pyrophosphatase}}$ FMN $\xrightarrow{\text{FMN phosphatase}}$ riboflavin

Other intestinal phosphatases such as nucleotide diphosphatase and alkaline phosphatase may also hydrolyze bound riboflavin. A small amount (about 7%) of FAD is covalently bound to either of two amino acids, histidine or cysteine. For example, following consumption of foods containing succinate dehydrogenase or monoamine oxidase, these proteins are degraded; however, the riboflavin remains bound, typically to histidine or cysteine residues [1,2]. Absorption of the histidine- and cysteine-bound riboflavin does not usually occur; however, should absorption occur via amino acid transport systems, the complex is excreted unchanged in the urine [2].

Generally, animal sources of riboflavin are thought to be better absorbed than plant sources. Divalent metals such as copper, zinc, iron, and manganese have been shown to chelate riboflavin and FMN and inhibit riboflavin absorption [3].

Free riboflavin is absorbed via a saturable, sodium-dependent carrier mechanism primarily in the proximal small intestine. Riboflavin absorption has been shown to require ATP [4,5]. Absorption rate is proportional to dose until the rate levels off at approximately 25 mg [1,6]. Peak concentrations of the vitamin in the plasma correlate with intakes of 15 to 20 mg [2]. Absorption appears to be facilitated by bile salts [1,5].

On absorption into the mucosal cells, riboflavin is phosphorylated into FMN, a reaction catalyzed by flavokinase and requiring ATP (Fig. 9.15). At the serosal surface most of the FMN is probably dephosphorylated to riboflavin, which enters the portal system. The vitamin is carried to the liver, where it is converted to its coenzyme derivatives (Fig. 9.15).

Riboflavin, FMN, and FAD are transported in the plasma by a variety of proteins including albumin, fibrinogen, and globulins (principally immunoglobulins) [2,5,7]. Albumin appears to be the primary transport protein. Most of the flavins in the plasma are found as riboflavin rather than as one of its coenzyme forms. Of the free riboflavin, approximately 50% is bound via hydrogen bonds to albumin. The extent to which the flavins are bound to plasma proteins is not believed to be crucial in regulating tissue availability of the vitamin except that the proteins may decrease losses of the vitamin during glomerular filtration [7]. Regardless of the form in which the vitamin reaches the tissues, it is free riboflavin that traverses the cell membrane by a carrier-mediated process. Within the cell the vitamin can be converted to its coenzyme forms by flavokinase and FAD synthetase, both of which are widely distributed in tissues [8].

Although the affinity for binding riboflavin to plasma proteins is rather low, a high-affinity transport system for riboflavin coenzymes may exist in the brain. The tight binding of FAD to these transport proteins could help explain why the concentration of FAD in the brain does not decline appreciably even in a severe riboflavin deficiency [9].

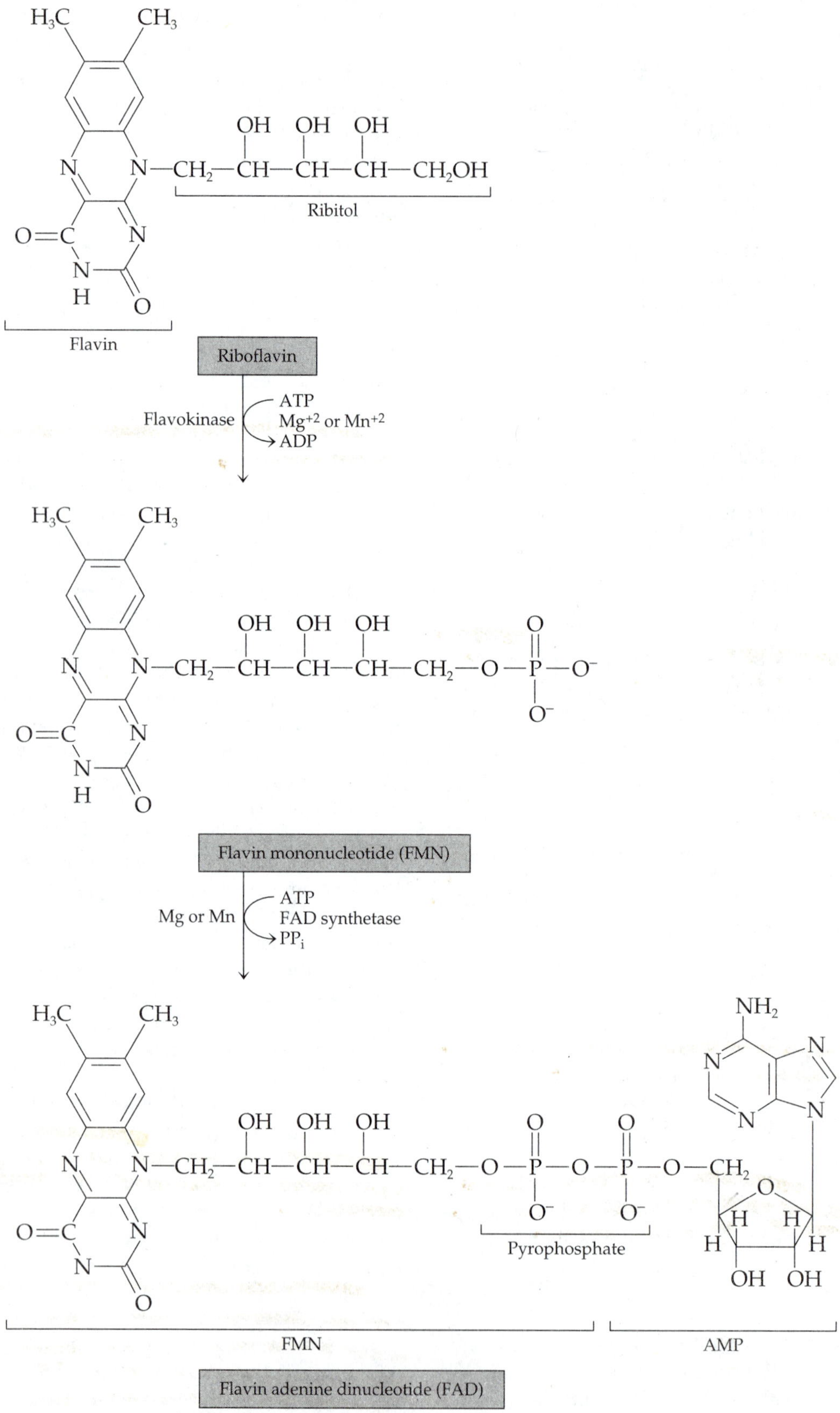

FIGURE 9.15 Structure of riboflavin and its coenzyme forms.

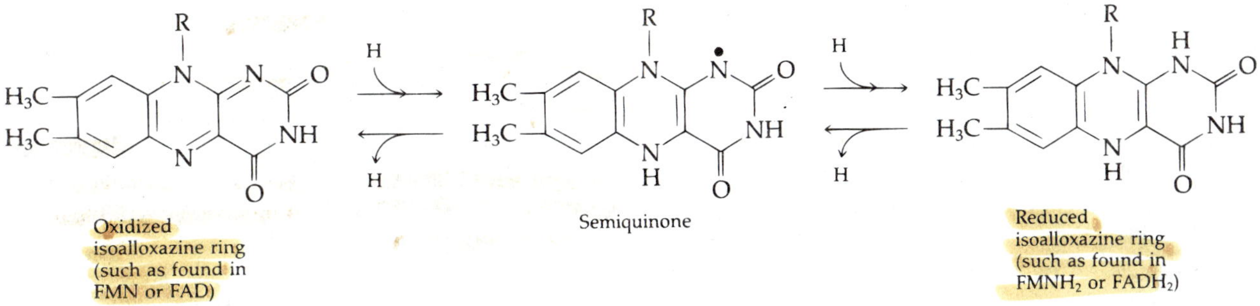

FIGURE 9.16 Oxidation and reduction of isoalloxazine ring.

Riboflavin is found in small quantities in a variety of tissues. The greatest concentrations of riboflavin are found in the liver, kidney, and heart. Intracellular phosphorylation of free riboflavin is necessary to prevent diffusion out of the tissue [2]. Most of the riboflavin in tissues is first converted to one of its coenzyme forms. Synthesis of FMN and FAD appear to be under hormonal regulation. Hormones shown to be particularly important in this regulation are ACTH, aldosterone, and the thyroid hormones, all of which accelerate the conversion of riboflavin into its coenzyme forms apparently by increasing the activity of flavokinase [1]. The coenzyme form of the vitamin is then bound to the apoenzyme. FMN and FAD function as prosthetic groups for enzymes involved in oxidation-reduction reactions. These enzymes are called *flavoproteins*.

Functions and Mechanisms of Actions

FMN and FAD function as cofactors for a wide variety of oxidative enzyme systems and remain bound to the enzymes during the oxidation-reduction reactions. Flavins can act as oxidizing agents because of their ability to accept a pair of hydrogen atoms. The isoalloxazine ring is reduced by two successive one-electron transfers with the intermediate formation of a semiquinone free radical, as shown in Figure 9.16. Reduction of the isoalloxazine ring yields the reduced forms of the flavoprotein, which can be found in $FMNH_2$ and $FADH_2$.

Flavoproteins exhibit a wide range of redox potentials and therefore can play a wide variety of roles in intermediary metabolism [8]. The role of flavoproteins in the electron transport chain is provided on p. 60–64. In the oxidative decarboxylation of pyruvate (Fig. 9.13) and α-ketoglutarate, FAD serves as intermediate electron carrier, with NADH being the final reduced product. Succinate dehydrogenase is an FAD flavoprotein that removes electrons from succinate to form fumarate, and forms $FADH_2$ from FAD (Fig. 9.12). The electrons

are then passed into the electron transport chain via coenzyme Q (Fig. 3.12, p. 64). In fatty acid oxidation, fatty acyl CoA dehydrogenase requires FAD. Sphinganine oxidase, in sphingosine synthesis, requires FAD.

As a coenzyme for an oxidase such as xanthine oxidase, FAD transfers electrons directly to oxygen with the formation of hydrogen peroxide. Xanthine oxidase, which contains both iron and molybdenum, is necessary for purine catabolism in the liver. The enzyme converts hypoxanthine to xanthine and then xanthine to uric acid (see Fig. 7.11). Similarly aldehyde oxidase using FAD converts aldehydes, such as pyridoxal (vitamin B6) to pyridoxic acid, an excretory product and retinal (vitamin A) to retinoic acid (Fig. 10.4) while also passing electrons to oxygen and generating hydrogen peroxide. Also in vitamin B6 metabolism (Fig. 9.38), pyridoxine phosphate oxidase—which converts pyridoxamine phosphate (PMP) and pyridoxine phosphate (PNP) to pyridoxal phosphate (PLP), the primary coenzyme form of vitamin B6—is dependent on FMN. Synthesis of an active form of folate, N^5 methyl THF, requires $FADH_2$ (Fig. 9.29).

In choline catabolism, several enzymes (such as choline dehydrogenase, dimethylglycine dehydrogenase, and monomethylglycine dehydrogenase) require FAD. Some neurotransmitters (such as dopamine) and other amines (tyramine and histamine) require FAD-dependent monoamine oxidase for metabolism.

Reduction of the oxidized form of glutathione (GSSG) to its reduced form (GSH) is also dependent on FAD-dependent glutathione reductase. This reaction forms the basis of one of the assays used to assess riboflavin status (see the section "Assessment of Nutriture").

Metabolism and Excretion

Riboflavin undergoes limited metabolism prior to excretion in the urine; primarily free riboflavin is found in the urine. Some of the riboflavin metabolites are thought to arise from tissue degradation of covalently bound flavins or are thought to be a reflection of bacterial action in the intestinal tract. It is believed that the metabolites formed in the intestinal tract can be absorbed and then excreted in the urine [10].

Riboflavin and riboflavin phosphate that are not bound to proteins in the plasma are filtered by the glomerulus. The phosphate is removed from the riboflavin prior to excretion of the riboflavin by the kidney [2]. Riboflavin bound to cysteine and histidine is also found in the urine if absorbed in such form from the gastrointestinal tract or if generated in body cells from the degradation of flavoenzymes such as succinate dehydrogenase and monoamine oxidase [1].

Urinary excretion of riboflavin may be noticeable a couple of hours following oral ingestion of the vitamin. Riboflavin is a fluorescent yellow compound. Thus, following riboflavin intake in a quantity such as 1.7 mg, similar to that found in a vitamin pill, a color change of the urine occurs whereby the urine will deepen in color from a typical light yellow to a brighter orangish yellow.

In addition to urine, free riboflavin may be secreted in the bile [2]. Small amounts of free riboflavin are found in the feces [5]. Fecal riboflavin metabolites are thought to arise from metabolism of riboflavin by intestinal flora [5].

Recommended Dietary Allowances

The level of riboflavin intake commensurate with adequate nutriture has been estimated through various studies: urinary excretion of riboflavin, relationship of dietary intake to clinical signs of deficiency, and the activity of erythrocyte glutathione reductase. The present RDA for riboflavin is given in mg per 1,000 kcal. The recommended allowance for people of all ages is 0.6 mg/1,000 kcal with a minimum intake of 1.2 mg for persons whose caloric intake may be less than 2,000 kcal. Through the years the recommended allowances for riboflavin have been calculated in relation to (1) protein requirement, (2) energy intake, and (3) metabolic body size. Because of the interdependence of these three variables, allowances calculated by the various methods have not differed significantly [11].

Deficiency

A deficiency of riboflavin rarely occurs in isolation; most often it is accompanied by other nutrient deficits [12]. No clear riboflavin deficiency disease has been characterized; however, clinical symptoms of deficiency after almost four months of inadequate intake include lesions on the outside of the lips (cheilosis) and corners of the mouth (angular stomatitis), inflammation of the tongue (glossitis), redness or bloody (hyperemia) and swollen (edema) mouth cavity, dermatitis, peripheral nerve dysfunction (neuropathy), among other signs. Severe deficiency of riboflavin may diminish the synthesis of the coenzyme form of vitamin B6 and niacin (NAD) synthesis from tryptophan.

Conditions and populations associated with increased need for riboflavin intake are many. Due to limited dietary intake, people with congenital heart disease, some cancers, and excess alcohol intake may develop deficiency. Riboflavin metabolism is altered with thyroid disease. Excretion of riboflavin is enhanced with diabetes mellitus, trauma, and stress. Women on oral contraceptives are also more likely to develop deficiency than women not taking these drugs.

Toxicity

Toxicity associated with large oral doses of riboflavin has not been reported, but neither can any benefit be ascribed to megadosing by the well-nourished individual [13].

Assessment of Nutriture

The most sensitive method for determining riboflavin nutriture is the measurement of the activity of erythrocyte glutathione reductase, an enzyme requiring FAD as a coenzyme. The method is based on the following reaction:

$$NADPH + H^+ + GSSG \xrightarrow{\text{glutathione reductase-FAD}} NADP^+ + 2\ GSH$$

Glutathione in its oxidized form is designated as GSSG and in its reduced form as GSH. In cases of a riboflavin deficiency or marginal riboflavin status, the activity of glutathione reductase is limited and less NADPH is used to reduce the oxidized glutathione. *In vitro* enzyme activity in terms of "activity coefficients" (AC) is determined both with and without the addition of FAD to the medium. When addition of FAD causes a marked stimulation of enzyme activity (AC >1.20), then riboflavin status is considered inadequate [14].

References Cited for Riboflavin

1. McCormick DB. Riboflavin. In: Shils ME, Olson JA, Shike M., eds. Modern nutrition in health and disease, 8th ed. Philadelphia: Lea and Febiger, 1994:366–375.
2. Bender DA. Nutritional biochemistry of the vitamins. New York: Cambridge University Press, 1992:156–183.

3. Cooperman JM, Lopez R. Riboflavin. In: Machlin LJ., ed. Handbook of vitamins, 2nd ed. New York: Dekker, 1991:283–310.

4. McCormick DB. Riboflavin. In: Brown ML, ed. Present knowledge in nutrition, 6th ed. Washington, DC: The Nutrition Foundation, 1990:146–154.

5. Combs GF. The vitamins. San Diego, CA: Academic Press, 1992:271–287.

6. Sauberlich HE. Vitamins—how much is for keeps? Nutr Today 1987;22:20–28.

7. White HB, Merrill AH. Riboflavin-binding proteins. Ann Rev Nutr 1988;8:279–299.

8. Merrill AH, Lambeth JD, Edmondson DE, et al. Formation and mode of flavoproteins. Ann Rev Nutr 1981;1:281–317.

9. Rivlin RS. Riboflavin. Nutrition Reviews' Present knowledge in nutrition, 5th ed. Washington, DC: The Nutrition Foundation, 1984:285–302.

10. Pike RL, Brown ML. Nutrition: An integrated approach, 3rd ed. New York: Wiley, 1984:92–97.

11. National Research Council. Recommended dietary allowances, 10th ed. Washington, DC: National Academy Press, 1989: 132–137.

12. McCormick DB. Riboflavin. In: Shils ME, Young VR, eds. Modern nutrition in diet and disease, 7th ed. Philadelphia: Lea and Febiger, 1988:362–369.

13. Council on Scientific Affairs, American Medical Association. Vitamin preparations as dietary supplements and as therapeutic agents. JAMA 1987;257:1929–1936.

14. Gibson RS. Principles of nutritional assessment. New York: Oxford University Press, 1990:425–444.

NIACIN

The term *niacin* is considered a generic term for *nicotinic acid* and *nicotinamide* (also called *niacinamide*) [1,2]. The vitamin activity of niacin is provided by both nicotinic acid and nicotinamide, the structural formulas of which are given in Figure 9.17.

Sources

The best sources of niacin include tuna, halibut, beef, chicken, turkey, pork, and other meats. In uncooked meats, niacin occurs as the nicotinamide nucleotides, including nicotinamide adenine dinucleotide (NAD) and nicotinamide adenine dinucleotide phosphate (NADP). In their oxidized forms, NAD and NADP possess a positive charge, and therefore may alternatively be written NAD^+ and $NADP^+$. Figure 9.17 shows the structures of these two nucleotides. NAD and NADP are thought to undergo hydrolysis following the slaughter of animals, thus meats provide niacin as free nicotinamide [3].

Cereal grains, seeds, and legumes also contain appreciable amounts of niacin. Niacin is also found in coffee and tea. In some foods, niacin may be bound covalently to complex carbohydrates and called *niacytin*, or bound to small peptides and called *niacinogens* [1–5]. Biologically unavailable niacin has been found primarily in corn, but also in wheat and a variety of cereal products [5]. Bound niacin is biologically unavailable, although chemical treatment with bases such as lime water can improve availability. Some niacin is also thought to be released from niacytin on exposure to gastric acid. At most, however, only about 10% of the niacin in maize is thought to be available for absorption [3].

In addition to dietary sources of niacin, NAD may be synthesized in the liver from the amino acid tryptophan. This biosynthetic pathway is depicted in Figure 9.18. Only about 3% of the tryptophan that is metabolized follows the pathway to NAD synthesis. It is estimated that 1 mg niacin (called *niacin equivalent* and abbreviated NE) can be expected from the ingestion of 60 mg dietary tryptophan. FAD and vitamin B_6 are required as coenzymes in several of the reactions involved in the conversion of tryptophan to NAD. Deficiency of vitamin B_6 can impair NAD synthesis. Moreover, synthesis will vary with different physiological states.

Digestion, Absorption, and Transport

NAD and NADP may be hydrolyzed within the intestinal tract by glycohydrolase to release free nicotinamide. Nicotinamide and nicotinic acid can be absorbed in the stomach, but are more readily absorbed in the small intestine [3–5]. Transport of niacin in the small intestine occurs primarily by a sodium-dependent, saturable system. Concentration of the vitamin in the lumen of the intestine, however, appears to determine its mode of absorption. At low concentrations niacin is absorbed via sodium-dependent, carrier-mediated, facilitated diffusion, while at high concentrations it is absorbed by passive diffusion [3–5].

Nicotinic acid is believed to be converted into nicotinamide in the mucosal cells. For this conversion to occur, nicotinic acid probably must first be incorporated into NAD and then released as the amide through NAD hydrolysis [2].

In the plasma, niacin is found primarily as nicotinamide, but nicotinic acid may also be found. Approximately 15 to 30% of nicotinic acid in the plasma is bound to plasma proteins [6]. Nicotinamide and nicotinic acid move across cell membranes by simple diffusion; however, nicotinic acid transport into the kidney

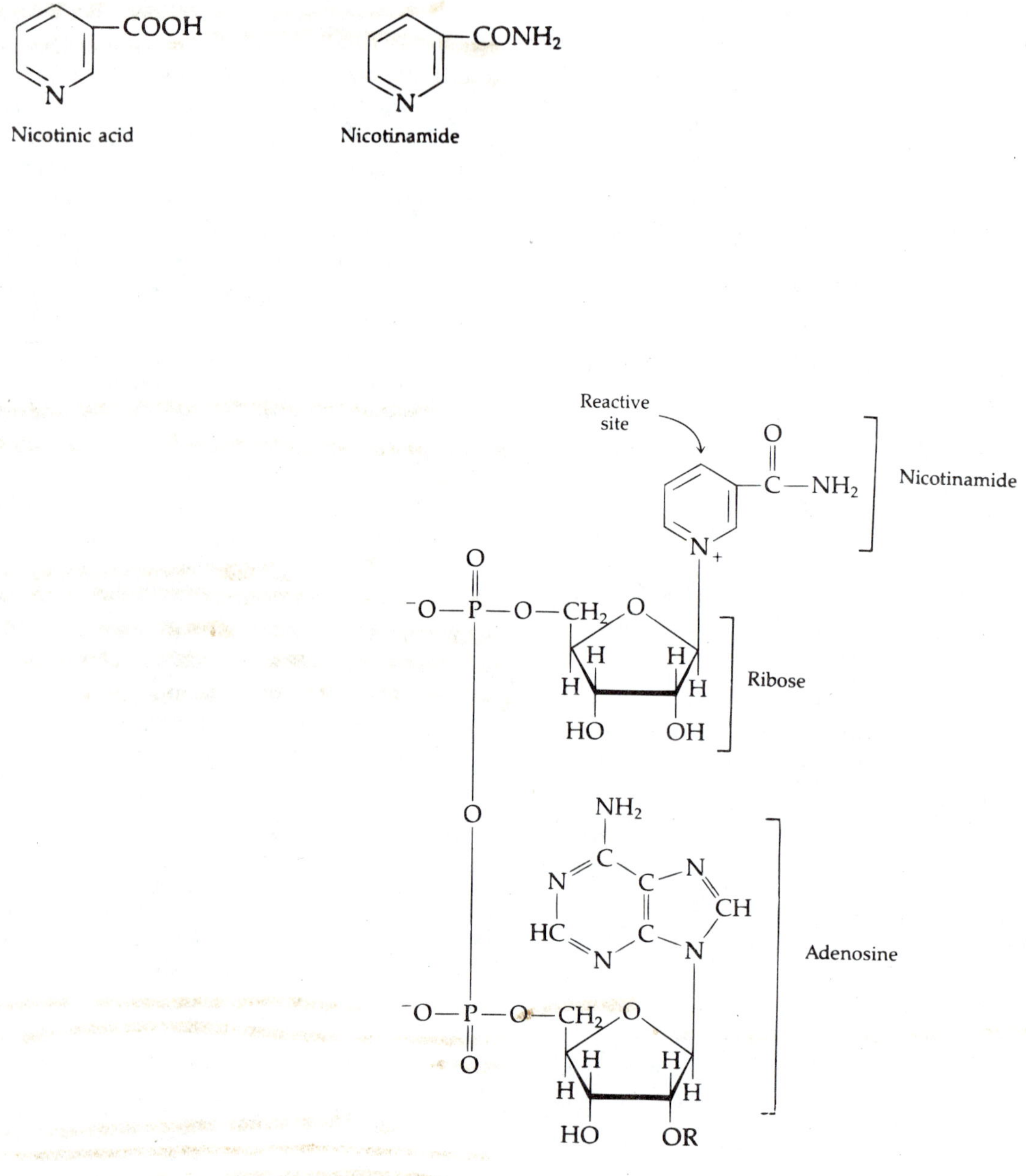

Nicotinic acid

Nicotinamide

R = H for NAD$^+$ nicotinamide adenine dinucleotide
R = PO$_3^{-2}$ for NADP$^+$ nicotinamide adenine dinucleotide phosphate

FIGURE 9.17   Structures of *nicotinic acid, nicotinamide,* NAD, and NADP.

tubules and red blood cells requires a sodium-dependent carrier system [1,7].

Nicotinamide serves as the primary precursor of NAD, which is synthesized in all tissues. In the liver, however, nicotinic acid also may be used to synthesize NAD. As NAD or NADP, the vitamin is trapped within the cell. Intracellular concentrations of NAD typically predominate over those of NADP. NAD may be degraded to yield nicotinamide.

Functions and Mechanisms of Action

Approximately 200 enzymes, primarily dehydrogenases, require NAD and NADP. Most of these enzymes func-

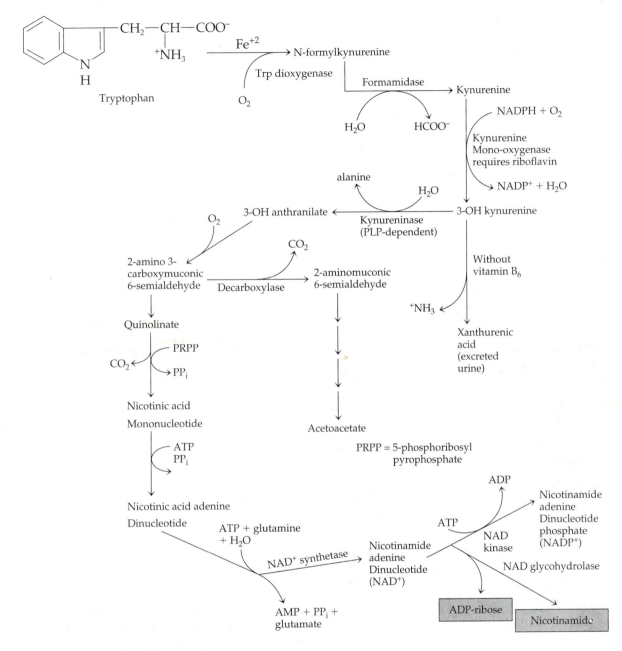

FIGURE 9.18 NAD+ synthesis from tryptophan.

tion reversibly [4]. Figure 9.19 demonstrates the oxidation reduction that may occur in the nicotinamide moiety of the coenzymes.

Although NAD and NADP are very similar and undergo reversible reduction in the same way, their functions are quite different in the cell. The major role of NADH, formed from NAD, is to transfer its electrons from metabolic intermediates through the electron transport chain (p. 60–64), thereby producing adenosine

triphosphate (ATP). NADPH, in contrast, acts as a reducing agent in many biosynthetic pathways such as fatty acid synthesis [1]. These coenzymes are not tightly bound to their apoenzymes and can easily transport hydrogen atoms from one part of the cell to another. Reactions in which they participate occur both in the mitochondria and the cytoplasm.

Oxidative reactions in which NAD participates and is reduced include glycolysis (p. 84), oxidative decar-

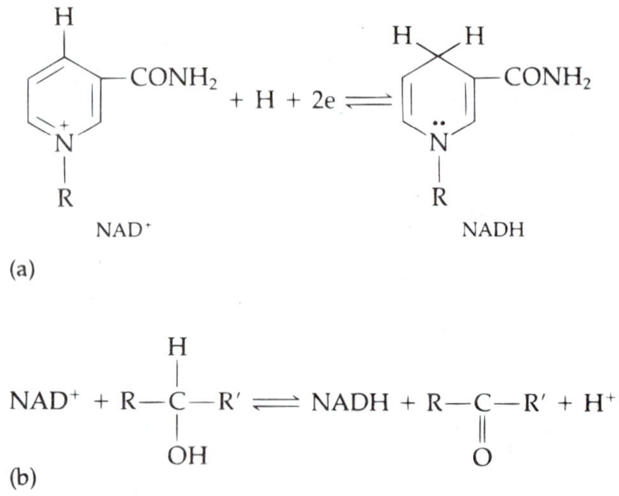

FIGURE 9.19 (a) The oxidation and reduction in the nicotinamide moiety; (b) NAD in dehydrogenation reactions. One H of the substrate goes to NAD.

boxylation of pyruvate (p. 90), oxidation of acetate via the Krebs cycle (p. 90), β-oxidation of fatty acids (p. 135), and oxidation of ethanol (p. 216). NAD is also required by aldehyde dehydrogenase for catabolism of vitamin B$_6$ as pyridoxal to its excretory product, pyridoxic acid.

NADP participates in the hexose monophosphate shunt (p. 87) and in the malate shuttle (p. 87) for transport of acetyl CoA out of the mitochondria. The resulting NADPH is used in a variety of reductive biosyntheses, including (1) fatty acid synthesis (p. 139); (2) cholesterol and steroid hormone synthesis; (3) oxidation of glutamate (p. 172); and (4) synthesis of deoxyribonucleotides (precursors of DNA). NADPH also may be used to reduce the oxidized form of vitamin C, dehydroascorbate. Enzymes such as glutathione reductase (p. 246), which functions to reduce glutathione from its oxidized state, also require NADPH. Conversion of folate to dihydrofolate (DHF) and tetrahydrofolate (THF) as well as synthesis of N^5 methyl THF and N^5 N^{10} methylene THF, active forms of folate require NADPH (Fig. 9.29).

Some nonredox functions of NAD have been discovered in recent years. First, in relation to protein synthesis, NAD acts as a donor of adenosine diphosphate ribose (ADP-ribose) (Fig. 9.18) for the posttranslational modification of proteins. The enzyme catalyzing the reaction is a polymerase that attaches ADP-ribose onto various chromosomal proteins. Proteins associated with chromosomes include both histone and nonhistone pro-

teins. It is the ADP-ribosyl moiety of the NAD that is posttranslationally attached by the polymerase to chromosomal proteins. In some cases, multiple ADP-ribosyl moieties may be attached to some of the proteins. This role of NAD suggests that niacin is involved in the regulation of a variety of cellular processes including growth and differentiation [1]. Secondly, niacin, along with chromium, is thought to be a component of glucose tolerance factor (GTF) that potentiates the action of insulin (Fig. 12.13). The exact function of niacin in the GTF is not clear.

Metabolism and Excretion

NAD, generated from nicotinamide or produced in the liver from tryptophan, and NADP can be degraded by glycohydrolase into nicotinamide and ADP-ribose (Fig. 9.18). The released nicotinamide is methylated and is then oxidized into a variety of products that are excreted in the urine. There is typically little excretion of nicotinic acid or nicotinamide since both compounds may be actively reabsorbed from glomerular filtrate.

The primary metabolites of nicotinamide are N′ methyl nicotinamide (representing about 20 to 30% of niacin) and N′ methyl-2-pyridone-5-carboxamide (representing about 40 to 60%). Nicotinic acid is metabolized to N′methylnicotinic acid. These metabolites may be used as a basis for assessing niacin status.

Recommended Dietary Allowances

Estimation of niacin requirements is complicated by the uncertain factor of the tryptophan-derived NAD. The efficiency of the conversion of tryptophan to the vitamin is affected by a variety of influences, including the amount of tryptophan and niacin ingested, protein and energy intake, and vitamin B$_6$ and riboflavin nutriture [8]. As previously mentioned, 60 mg tryptophan is thought to be equivalent to 1 mg niacin and is regarded as a niacin equivalent (NE) [8]. Thus, total niacin represents the sum of milligrams of both nicotinic acid and nicotinamide and 1/60 mg of tryptophan. The average U.S. diet usually contains at least 800 mg tryptophan a day [6].

Although recommendations are given in niacin equivalents, food composition tables report only preformed niacin. A rough estimate of niacin equivalents from a protein can be made by assuming that for every 1 g high-quality (complete) protein in the diet, 10 mg tryptophan are provided. For example, an intake of 60 g complete protein would provide 600 mg tryptophan.

Then since it takes 60 mg tryptophan to generate 1 mg niacin equivalent, about 10 niacin equivalents would be obtained from the 60 g protein. The calculations are shown here:

$$1 \text{ g complete, high-quality protein} = 10 \text{ mg tryptophan}$$

$$\frac{10 \text{ mg tryptophan}}{1 \text{ g protein}} \times 60 \text{ g protein} = 600 \text{ mg tryptophan}$$

$$600 \text{ mg tryptophan} \times \frac{1 \text{ mg niacin equivalent}}{60 \text{ mg tryptophan}} = 10 \text{ NE}$$

Information used in estimating niacin requirements has come from human depletion and repletion studies conducted in the 1950s. Requirements for adult subjects appear to range from 9.2 to 13.3 niacin equivalents per day.

Allowances for niacin are related to energy intake because of the involvement of NAD and NADP in the oxidation of energy-producing nutrients. The RDA for adults is 6.6 niacin equivalents per 1,000 kcal with an intake of not less than 13 niacin equivalents daily should caloric intake fall below 2,000 kcal per day.

Deficiency—Pellagra

Classical deficiency of niacin results in a condition known as pellagra. The four D's—*dermatitis, dementia, diarrhea,* and *death*—are often used as a mnemonic device for remembering signs of pellagra [7]. The dermatitis is similar to sunburn at first and appears on areas exposed to sun such as the face and neck, and on the extremities such as the back of the hands, wrists, elbow, knees, and feet. Neurologic manifestations include peripheral neuritis, paralysis of extremities, and dementia or delirium. Gastrointestinal manifestations include glossitis, cheilosis, stomatitis, nausea, vomiting, and diarrhea. If untreated, death occurs.

A niacin deficiency also can result from the use of the antituberculosis drug isoniazid. Isoniazid binds with PLP and thereby reduces PLP-dependent kynureninase activity required for niacin synthesis. Hartnup disease results in impaired tryptophan absorption, and thus decreases concentrations of the precursor tryptophan needed for niacin synthesis. Malabsorptive disorders (chronic diarrhea, inflammatory bowel diseases, some cancers) may impair niacin and tryptophan absorption and result in the increased likelihood of niacin deficiency. Individuals with poor nutrient intakes such as those who consume excessive amounts of alcohol are at risk for deficiency. In addition, people with stress, trauma, or prolonged fever may have increased needs for niacin.

Toxicity

Large doses of nicotinic acid (approximately 3 g/day, but given in divided doses such as 1 g three times a day) are used in the treatment of hypercholesterolemia (high blood cholesterol). These pharmacologic doses have been shown to significantly lower total serum cholesterol and low-density lipoproteins (LDLs) while causing an increase in high-density lipoproteins (HDLs) [4]. Although the mechanism of action is unclear, it is proposed that nicotinic acid decreases the levels of cAMP in the adipocytes, thereby decreasing lipase activity. Decreased lipase activity results in a decreased mobilization of fatty acids from the adipocytes and, therefore, a decreased substrate for synthesis of very low density lipoproteins (VLDLs) in the liver. Decreased production of VLDLs lowers triacylglycerol levels, because VLDLs contain relatively high amounts of triacylglycerols. Furthermore, with decreased VLDLs there is less synthesis of LDL and thus lower serum cholesterol levels. An increase in the HDL appears to be due to a decrease in their breakdown within the liver.

Despite the therapeutic benefits of nicotinic acid, many undesirable side effects are associated with its use as a drug. Some of these side effects include (1) release of histamine, which causes an uncomfortable flushing and which may be injurious to people with asthma and/or peptic ulcer disease; (2) possible injury to the liver, as indicated by elevated serum levels of enzymes of hepatic origin (such as transaminases and alkaline phosphatases) and by obstruction of normal bile flow from the liver to the small intestine; (3) competition of niacin with uric acid for excretion, thereby raising serum uric acid levels; (4) development of dermatologic problems such as itching; and (5) elevation of plasma glucose levels [9]. Gastrointestinal problems typically associated with intakes of large doses of nicotinic acid include heartburn and nausea with possible vomiting. Whether the beneficial effects of niacin in reducing blood lipids compensate for its possible toxic effects is a debatable question [9,10].

Nicotinamide in large doses does not exhibit toxic effects, but neither does it reduce blood lipids. Because of their stimulatory effects on the central nervous system (CNS), both nicotinic acid and nicotinamide have been tried during the past 25 years as therapeutic agents for some mental disorders. The current consensus among experts is that no improvement in brain function accrues from large doses of the vitamin [6,7].

Assessment of Nutriture

Status of niacin nutriture is assessed by measurement of urinary metabolites of nicotinamide. Although the best indication of status is the ratio of N'methyl-2-pyridone-5-carboxamide to N'methyl nicotinamide, the difficulty of measuring the pyridone compound prevents the ratio method from being the preferred one [6,11]. When, however, this particular method is used, a ratio < 1 is indicative of niacin deficiency.

A more commonly used method for assessing niacin nutriture is measurement of N'methyl nicotinamide (mg/g creatinine) during a period of four to five hours after a 50-mg test dose of nicotinamide. Guidelines are presented here [11]:

	Urinary N'methyl Nicotinamide (mg/g creatinine) Excretion		
	Deficient	Marginal	Adequate
All Ages	< 0.5	0.5–1.59	> 1.6

References Cited for Niacin

1. Swenseid ME, Jacob RA. Niacin. In: Shils ME, Olson JA, Shike M., eds., Modern nutrition in health and disease, 8th ed. Philadelphia: Lea and Febiger, 1994:376–382.
2. Jacob RA, Swendseid ME. Niacin. In: Brown ML, ed. Present knowledge in nutrition, 6th ed. Washington, DC: The Nutrition Foundation, 1990:163–169.
3. Bender DA. Nutritional biochemistry of the vitamins. New York: Cambridge University Press, 1992:184–222.
4. Henderson LM. Niacin. Ann Rev Nutr 1983;3:289–307.
5. Sauberlich HE. Bioavailability of vitamins. Prog Food Nutr Sci 1985;9:1–33.
6. van Eys J. Niacin. In: Machlin LJ, ed., Handbook of vitamins, 2nd ed. New York: Dekker, 1991:311–340.
7. Combs GF. The vitamins. San Diego, CA: Academic Press, 1992:289–309.
8. National Research Council. Recommended dietary allowances, 10th ed. Washington, DC: National Academy Press, 1989:137–142.
9. Alhadeff L, Gualtieri CT, Lipton M. Toxic effects of water-soluble vitamins. Nutr Rev 1984;42:33–40.
10. Council on Scientific Affairs, American Medical Association. Vitamin preparations as dietary supplements and as therapeutic agents. JAMA 1987;257:1929–1936.
11. Gibson RS. Principles of nutrition assessment. New York: Oxford University Press, 1990:437–444.

PANTOTHENIC ACID

Pantothenic acid or pantothenate, an amide, consists of β-alanine and pantoic acid joined together by a peptide bond. The structure of pantothenate is shown at the top of Figure 9.20 and as part of coenzyme A in Figure 9.21.

Sources

The Greek word *pantos* means everywhere, and the vitamin pantothenic acid, as its name implies, is found widely distributed in nature. Because this vitamin is present in virtually all plant and animal foods, a deficiency is quite unlikely. Meats, particularly liver; egg yolk; legumes; whole-grain cereals; mushrooms; broccoli; and avocados, among others, are good sources of the vitamin. Royal jelly from bees also provides large amounts of pantothenate.

Digestion, Absorption, and Transport

Most, about 85%, of the pantothenic acid in food occurs as a component of coenzyme A, or CoA (Fig. 9.21) [1]. During the digestive process, CoA is hydrolyzed to pantetheine and then to pantothenic acid. The free pantothenic acid is thought to be absorbed principally in the jejunum by passive diffusion [1,2], although animal studies suggest that when present in low concentrations, pantothenate may be absorbed by a sodium-dependent active process [3]. Approximately 40 to 61%, mean 50%, of the ingested pantothenic acid appears to be available for absorption [4,5]. Panthenol, an alcohol form of the vitamin used in multivitamins, may also be absorbed and converted to pantothenate. However, pantothenate absorption has been shown to decrease to about 10% when pantothenate ingestion approaches ten times recommended intakes in pill form.

From the intestinal cell, pantothenate enters into portal blood for transport to body cells. Although pantothenic acid is found in whole blood, plasma, serum, and red blood cells, most occurs as CoA within the red blood cells. Free pantothenic acid is found in serum and plasma, but higher concentrations are found in red blood cells [3]. Uptake of pantothenate by heart, muscle, and liver cells occurs by sodium-dependent active transport [1,2,6]. Central nervous system, adipose, and renal uptake of pantothenate is by facilitative diffusion [1,2]. Within cells, pantothenate may accumulate and is typically used to synthesize or resynthesize CoA. CoA is

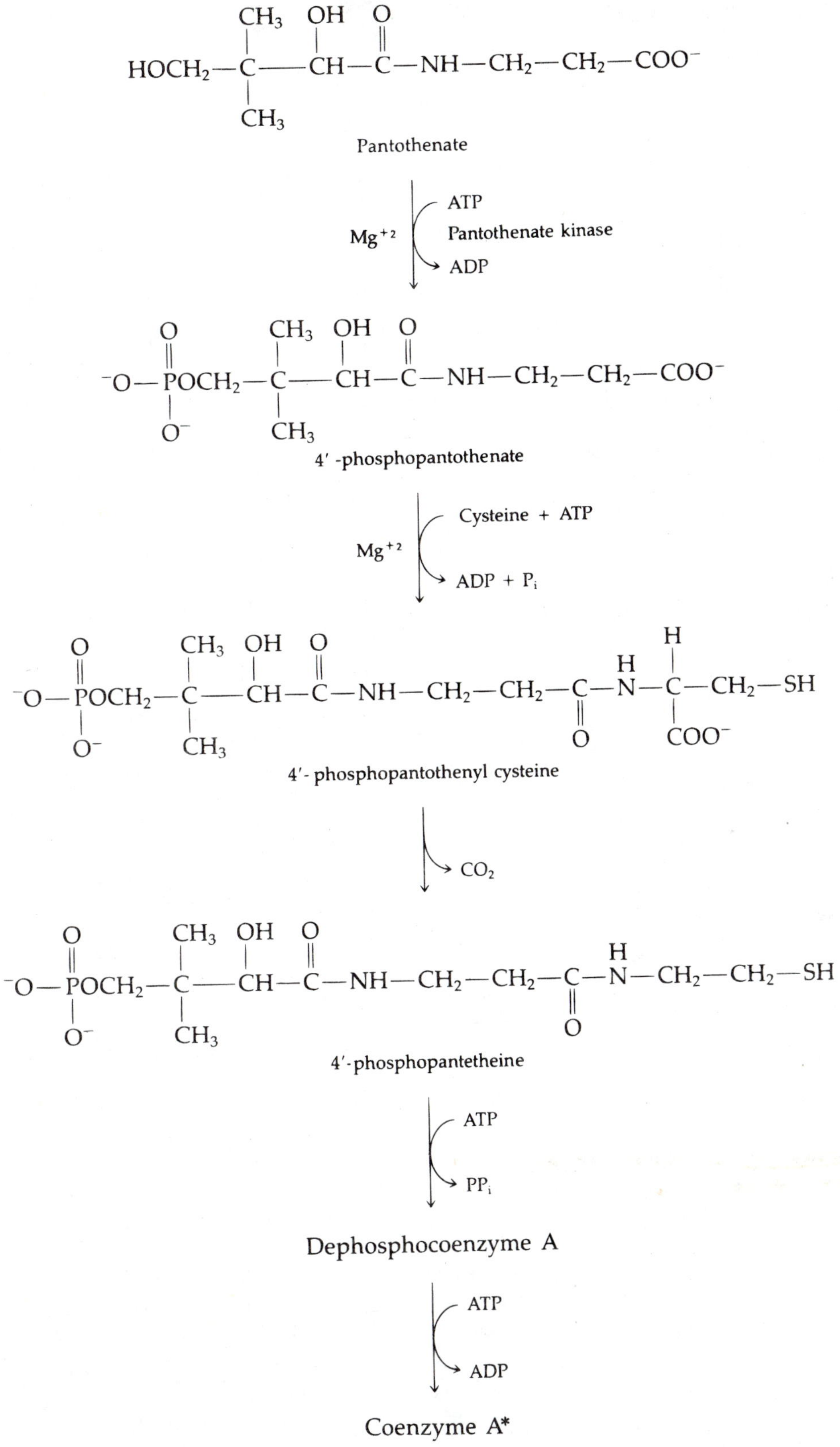

FIGURE 9.20 Synthesis of coenzyme A *(structure shown in Figure 9.21) from pantothenate.

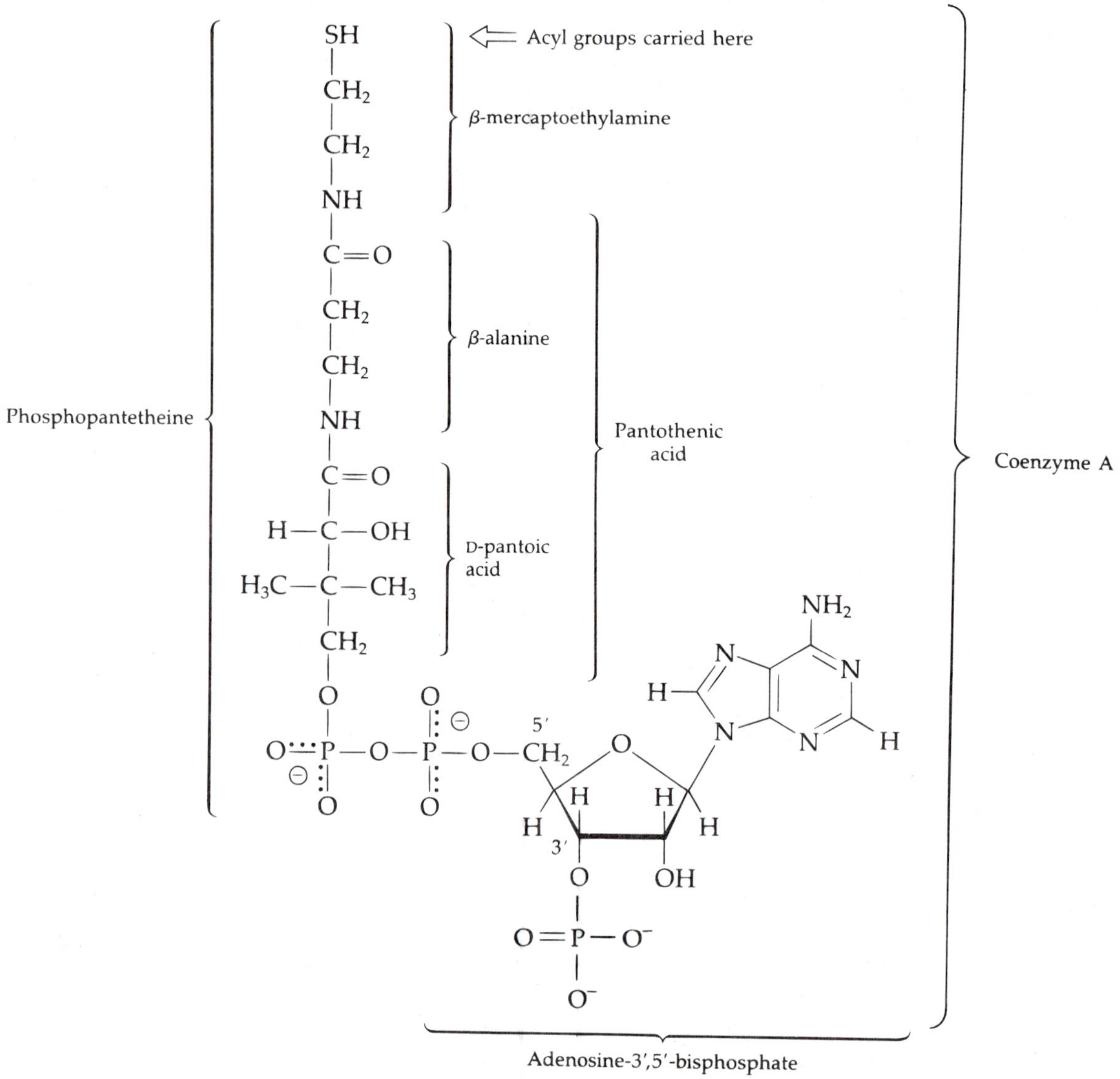

FIGURE 9.21   Structure of coenzyme A and identification of components.

found in the largest concentrations in the liver, adrenal gland, kidney, brain, and heart [6].

Functions and Mechanisms of Action

One of the primary functions of pantothenic acid relates to its role as a component of CoA, although 4'-phosphopantotheine, derived from CoA, may also function bound to a protein. The synthesis of CoA from pantothenate is depicted in Figure 9.20. The synthesis requires pantothenic acid, cysteine, and ATP. The synthesis of coenzyme A starts with the rate-limiting phosphorylation of pantothenic acid by pantothenate kinase and the formation of 4'-phosphopantothenate. ATP and Mg^{+2} are required for this reaction. Next in another ATP- and Mg^{+2}-requiring reaction, cysteine reacts with the 4'phosphopantothenate. A peptide bond is formed between the carboxyl group of the 4'-phosphopantothenate and the amino group of cysteine. Third, a carboxyl group from the cysteine moiety is removed to generate 4'-phosphopantotheine. An adenylation occurs whereby adenosine monophosphate (AMP) is added to the 4'-phosphopantotheine to form dephosphocoenzyme A. Lastly, phosphorylation with ATP of the 3'-hydroxyl group of the dephosphocoenzyme A produces CoA. Figure 9.21 gives the structure of coenzyme A, identifying its active site and its constituents. Synthesis of CoA is inhibited by acetyl CoA, malonyl CoA, and propionyl CoA as well as by other longer-chain acyl CoAs. CoA metabolism has been reviewed in depth by Robishaw and Neely [7].

As a component of CoA, pantothenic acid becomes essential for production of energy from carbohydrate,

$$\overset{O}{\underset{\parallel}{}}$$

fat, and protein. CoA can form thio esters ($-S-C-R$) with carboxylic acids and can transfer the acyl groups, typically 2–13 carbons, as needed for condensation and additional reactions. Examples of acids activated by CoA include acetic (2 carbons), malonic (3 carbons), propionic (3 carbons, found naturally in some fish, derived from the catabolism of both amino acids such as methionine, threonine, and isoleucine, and from the catabolism of odd-chain fatty acids), methylmalonic (4 carbons), and succinic (4 carbons, and found as an intermediate in the Krebs cycle as well as generated from the catabolism of amino acids such as methionine, threonine, isoleucine, and valine). Succinyl CoA is also necessary along with the amino acid glycine for the initial vitamin B_6-dependent step in heme synthesis (Figs. 9.42 and 12.5).

A crucial reaction in energy metabolism is the formation of acetyl CoA, which condenses with oxaloacetate to thereby introduce acetate for oxidation via the Krebs cycle (Fig. 9.12). Acetyl CoA, the common compound formed from the three energy-producing nutrients, holds the central position in the transformation of energy. Pantothenic acid, then, joins the other B vitamins thiamin, riboflavin, and niacin, in the oxidative decarboxylation of pyruvate (Fig. 9.12) and α-ketoglutarate. On the synthetic side of metabolism, condensation of acetyl CoA with activated CO_2 to form malonyl CoA is the first step in fatty acid synthesis (p. 139). Therefore pantothenic acid plays an important role in energy storage as well as energy release. Other synthetic reactions include the reaction of acetyl CoA and acetoacetyl CoA to form HMG CoA (Fig. 6.13), important in cholesterol synthesis and ketogenesis. Phospholipid and sphingomyelin production from phosphatidic acid and sphingosine respectively also use acyl CoA.

Another function of pantothenic acid is as the prosthetic group on acyl carrier protein (ACP). Figure 9.20 shows that 4'-phosphopantotheine is necessary as a prosthetic group for ACP. ACP acts as the acyl carrier in the synthesis of fatty acids and is a necessary component of the fatty acid synthase complex (p. 139). The sulfhydryl group in the 4'-phosphopantotheine and a sulfhydryl group in the protein are the active sites in the

ACP. These groups are located close to one another so that the acyl chain being synthesized can be transferred between the two of them.

Pantothenic acid is also involved in the modification of proteins. Specifically, the vitamin is involved in the protein acetylation process, which in turn affects protein functions. The donation of long-chain fatty acids or acetate by CoA to proteins occurs posttranslationally [8,9]. Acetylation of peptides may protect them from degradation and may determine activity, location, and function in the cell [8,9]. Acetylation of the N-terminal amino acids has been shown to affect resistance to ubiquitin-mediated proteolysis [8]. Other proteins that may undergo acetylation include microtubules of the cell's cytoskeleton, histones, and other DNA-binding proteins [8].

Another suggested role of pantothenic acid based on animal studies includes acceleration of the normal healing process following surgery [10]. The exact mechanism of the effect of pantothenate is unclear; however, an increase in cellular multiplication during the first postoperative period has been proposed [10].

Metabolism and Excretion

During metabolism, CoA is dephosphorylated and through a series of subsequent reactions generates pantothenate. Pantothenate is excreted as such primarily in the urine; no metabolites of the vitamin have been identified in humans. Fecal pantothenate excretion also occurs.

Urinary excretion of pantothenate is thought to reflect dietary intake. Whenever urinary excretion of pantothenate is < 1 mg/day, deficiency might be suspected. An excretion of < 1 mg/day is thought to correspond to an intake of < 4 mg daily [1].

Recommended Dietary Allowances

No recommended allowances have been formulated for the vitamin, but 4 to 7 mg/day have been stated as a safe and adequate range for children over age 11 and adults [11]. Intakes of about 4 to 6 mg daily are thought to be sufficient [1,11].

Deficiency

Pantothenate deficiency in humans has been reported in people with severe malnutrition [3]. Moreover, "Burning feet syndrome" characterized by abnormal skin sensations, exacerbated by warmth and diminished with cold, of the feet and lower legs has been reported and is thought to result from a pantothenic acid deficiency. The syndrome can be corrected with calcium pantothenate administration. Other symptoms of deficiency include vomiting, fatigue, and weakness. A metabolic inhibitor of pantothenate, omega methylpantothenate, has been used in studies to induce low pantothenate status in humans. Conditions and populations associated with increased need for intake include people with alcoholism, diabetes mellitus, and inflammatory bowel diseases. Increased excretion of the vitamin has been shown in people with diabetes mellitus. Absorption is likely to be impaired with inflammatory bowel diseases. Intake of the vitamin is typically low in people with excessive alcohol intake.

Toxicity

Pantothenate toxicity has not been reported to date in humans. Intakes of 100 mg panthothenate may increase niacin excretion [12]. Intakes of about 10 g pantothenate as calcium pantothenate daily for up to six weeks have resulted in no problems [1,6]. Intakes up to 20 g may cause mild intestinal distress and diarrhea [11].

Assessment of Nutriture

Plasma pantothenic acid concentrations < 100 μg/dL are thought to reflect low dietary pantothenate intakes [3]. Urinary pantothenate excretion of < 1 mg/day is considered to be low [1].

References Cited for Pantothenic Acid

1. Bender DA. Nutritional biochemistry of the vitamins. New York: Cambridge University Press, 1992:341–359.
2. Olson RE. Pantothenic acid. In: Brown ML, ed. Present knowledge in nutrition, 6th ed. Washington, DC: The Nutrition Foundation, 1990:208–211.
3. Fox HM. Pantothenic acid. In: Machlin LJ., ed., Handbook of vitamins, 2nd ed. New York: Dekker, 1991: 429–451.
4. Tarr JB, Tamura T, Stokstad ELR. Availability of vitamin B₆ and pantothenate in an average American diet in man. Am J Clin Nutr 1981;34:1328–1337.
5. Sauberlich HE. Bioavailability of vitamins. Prog Food Nutr Sci 1985;9:1–33.
6. Combs GF. The vitamins. San Diego, CA: Academic Press, 1992:345–356.
7. Robishaw JD, Neely JR. Coenzyme A metabolism. Am J Physiol 1985;248:E1–E9.
8. Plesofsky-Vig, N. Pantothenic Acid and Coenzyme A. In: Shils ME, Olson JA, Shike M., eds. Modern nutrition in health and disease, 8th ed. Philadelphia: Lea and Febiger, 1994:395–401.
9. Plesofsky-Vig N, Brambl R. Pantothenic acid and coenzyme A in cellular modification of proteins. Ann Rev Nutr 1988;8:461–482.
10. Aprahamian M, Dentinger A, Stock-Damge C, Kouassi JC, Grenier JF. Effects of supplemental pantothenic acid on wound healing: Experimental study in rabbit. Am J Clin Nutr 1985;41:578–589.
11. National Research Council. Recommended dietary allowances, 10th ed. Washington, DC: National Academy Press, 1989:169–173.
12. Clarke JF, Kies C. Niacin nutritional status of adolescent humans fed high dosage pantothenic acid supplements. Nutr Rep Internl 1985;31:1271–1279.

Additional Reference

Pike RL, Brown ML. Nutrition: An integrated approach, 3rd ed. New York: Wiley, 1984.

BIOTIN

Biotin was once referred to as vitamin H. Its structure consists of two rings, a ureido ring joined to a thiophene ring, with an additional valeric acid side chain (Fig. 9.22).

Sources

Biotin is found widely distributed in foods. Good food sources of the vitamin are liver, soybeans, and egg yolk. Cereals, legumes, and nuts also contain relative high amounts of biotin. Within many foods, biotin is found bound to protein or as *biocytin*, which is also called biotinyllysine (Fig. 9.23). Biotin is also produced by bacteria within the colon.

Avidin, a glycoprotein in raw egg whites, may irreversibly bind biotin in a noncovalent bond and prevent biotin absorption. Because avidin is heat labile (unstable with heat), ingestion of cooked egg whites does not compromise biotin absorption.

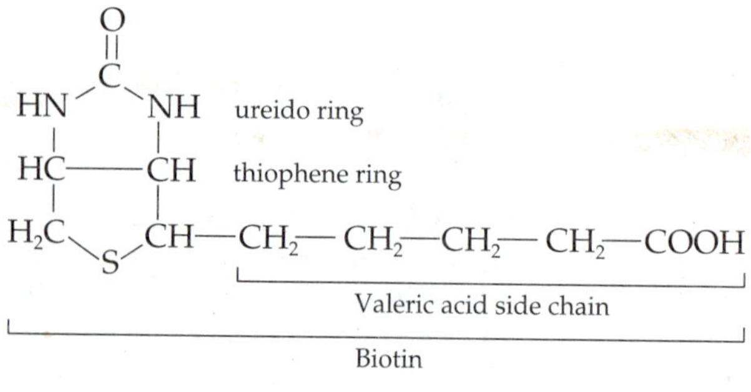

FIGURE 9.22 The structure of biotin.

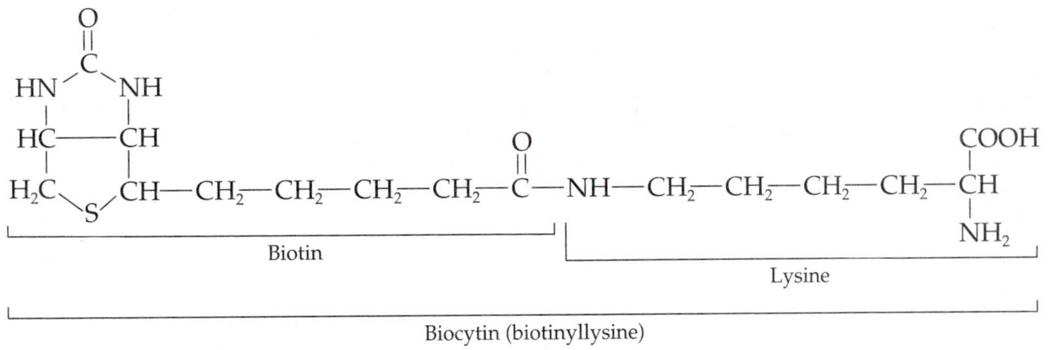

FIGURE 9.23 The structure of biocytin.

Digestion, Absorption, and Transport

Protein-bound biotin requires digestion by proteolytic enzymes prior to absorption. Proteolysis by proteases yields free biotin, biocytin, or biotinyl peptides. Biocytin and biotinyl peptides can be further hydrolyzed by biotinidase. Biotinidase, on the intestinal brush border or in pancreatic or intestinal juice, hydrolyzes the biocytin or biotinyl peptides to release free biotin, lysine, and possibly other amino acids from the peptides. Undigested biocytin may also be absorbed as such into the body and may be acted on by the biotinidase present in plasma, or other body tissues such as the liver, kidney, and adrenal glands. Any biocytin not metabolized by biotinidase is excreted in the urine [1]. Biotinidase is active over a wide pH range and is specific for the biotinyl moiety, hydrolyzing at amide or ester linkages [2]. Biotinidase deficiency due to an inborn error of metabolism has been documented in infants and children. Clinical features associated with the genetic disorder, as well as deficiency, include seizures, ataxia, skin rash, alopecia (hair loss), acidosis, among others [2]. The bioavailability of biotin contained in foods is highly variable, ranging from 100% in corn to near 0% in wheat.

Little is known about the mechanism of absorption of biotin in humans. Based on experimental studies in animals, it is proposed that most absorption of the vitamin occurs in the upper one-third to one-half of the small intestine. Absorption in the duodenum is thought to be greater than in the jejunum [3], which is thought to be greater than that in the ileum [4]. Absorption in the proximal and midtransverse colon occurs [4], but is small relative to biotin absorption in the small intestine [5]. Absorption in the small intestine is carrier mediated and thought to require sodium. Absorption may or may not require energy [4–6]: A small amount of biotin absorption may also occur by passive diffusion [5,6].

Both free biotin and protein-bound biotin are found in the plasma. Albumin and alpha- and beta-globulins bind biotin, as does a plasma biotinidase, which has two binding sites for biotin and is thought to arise from the liver [4,6]. Biotin is stored in small quantities in the muscle, liver, and brain. The rate and uptake of biotin by tissues is related to the need of the cells for the vitamin. When biotin enters the cells, its distribution corresponds to localization of the carboxylases, the enzymes requiring biotin as a coenzyme [7].

Functions and Mechanisms of Action

Biotin functions in cells covalently bound to enzymes. Biotin uptake into cells is by active transport. Within the cell, biotin reacts in a Mg^{+2}-requiring reaction with ATP to form biotinyl 5′-adenylate, or referred to as *activated biotin*. In subsequent reactions, holoenzyme (carboxylase) synthetase joins the biotinyl moiety with one of several apoenzymes to form a holoenzyme carboxylase with the release of AMP. Multiple carboxylase deficiencies due to inborn errors of metabolism of holoenzyme synthetase have been documented. Some of the genetic disorders benefit from biotin supplements (10 mg or more daily) and dietary amino acid restrictions to limit substrates for the missing or deficient enzymes.

Examples of biotin-dependent enzymes include acetyl CoA carboxylase, pyruvate carboxylase, propionyl CoA carboxylase, and β-methylcrotonyl CoA carboxylase. Table 9.2 lists the enzymes and their roles in metabolism. Knowles [8] has reviewed the mechanism of action of biotin-dependent enzymes.

The carboxylases are multisubunit enzymes to which biotin is attached by an amide linkage. The carboxyl terminus of biotin is linked to the epsilon amino group of a specified lysine residue in the apoenzyme. The chain connecting biotin and the apoenzyme is long and flexible, thereby allowing the biotin to move from one active site of the carboxylase to another. This long chain can be seen by examining the structure of biocytin (Fig. 9.23). In addition, Figure 9.24a depicts the

Table 9.2 Biotin-Dependent Enzymes

Enzyme	Role	Significance
1. Pyruvate carboxylase	Converts pyruvate to oxaloacetate	Replenishes oxaloacetate for Krebs cycle Necessary for gluconeogenesis
2. Acetyl CoA carboxylase	Forms malonyl CoA from acetate	Commits acetate units to fatty acid synthesis
3. Propionyl CoA carboxylase	Converts propionate to succinate	Provides mechanism for metabolism of some amino acids and odd-numbered chain fatty acids. Succinate formed enters Krebs cycle.
4. β-methylcrotonyl CoA carboxylase	Converts β-methyl-crotonyl CoA to β-methylglutaconyl CoA	Allows catabolism of leucine and certain isoprenoid compounds

attachment of biotin to the enzyme, emphasizing the long flexible chain and the amide linkage between the vitamin and the lysine residue of the enzyme. One active site on the apoenzyme generates the carboxybiotin enzyme, while the other transfers the activated carbon dioxide to a reactive carbon on the substrate. Figure 9.24b illustrates the formation of the CO_2 biotin enzyme complex and demonstrates the overall action of pyruvate carboxylase.

Pyruvate carboxylase is a particularly interesting and important enzyme because of its regulatory function. For its activation as shown in Figure 9.24b, this

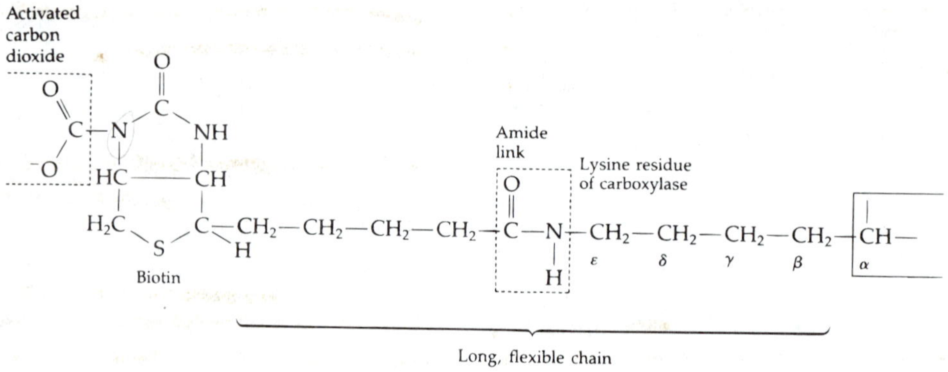

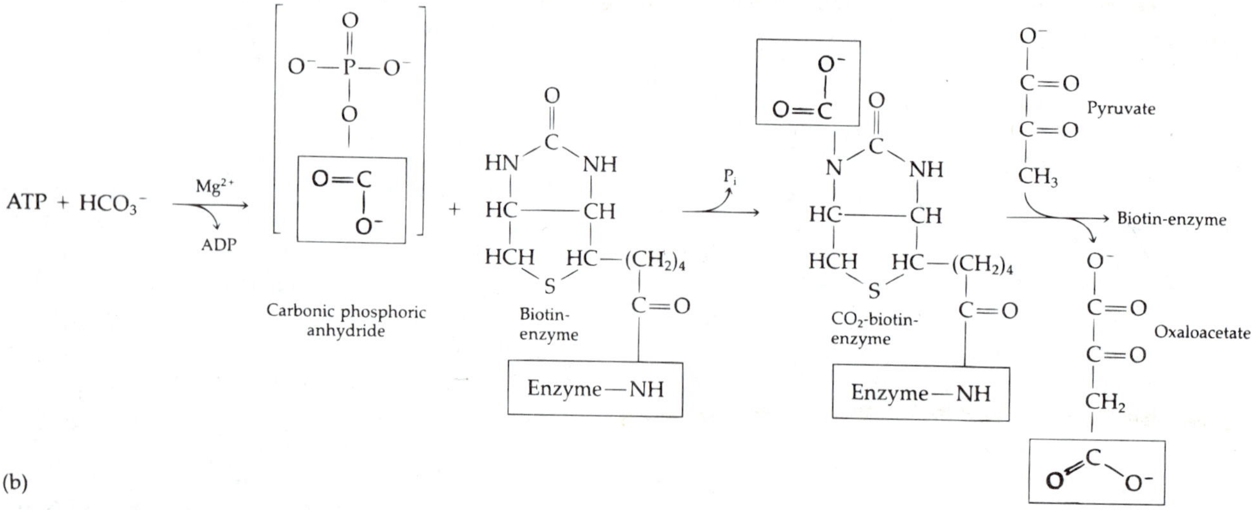

FIGURE 9.24 (a) Biotin: mobile carrier of activated CO_2; (b) conversion of pyruvate to oxaloacetate by biotin-dependent pyruvate carboxylase.

particular carboxylase requires the presence of acetyl CoA as well as ATP and Mg^{+2}. Acetyl CoA serves as an allosteric activator, and its presence indicates the need for increased amounts of oxaloacetate. Specifically, pyruvate carboxylase catalyzes the carboxylation of pyruvate to form oxaloacetate. If there is a surplus of ATP in the cell, the oxaloacetate is then used for gluconeogenesis. If, however, there is a deficiency of ATP, the oxaloacetate will enter the Krebs cycle on condensation with acetyl CoA (p. 90).

The importance of biotin in energy metabolism is further exemplified by its role in the initiation of fatty acid synthesis (p. 139); that is, the formation of malonyl CoA from acetyl CoA by the regulatory and rate-limiting enzyme acetyl CoA carboxylase. This enzyme is allosterically activated by citrate and isocitrate and inhibited by long-chain fatty acyl CoA derivatives. ATP and Mg^{+2} are required for the reaction.

Propionyl CoA carboxylase is important for the catabolism of isoleucine, threonine, and methionine, which each generate propionyl CoA. Propionyl CoA also arises from the catabolism of odd-number chain fatty acids found, for example, in some fish. Propionyl CoA carboxylase catalyzes the carboxylation of propionyl CoA to methylmalonyl CoA (Fig. 9.25). The reaction requires ATP and Mg^{+2}. Methylmalonyl CoA, after being acted on by racemase, generates succinyl CoA in a vitamin B12-dependent reaction (Fig. 9.25).

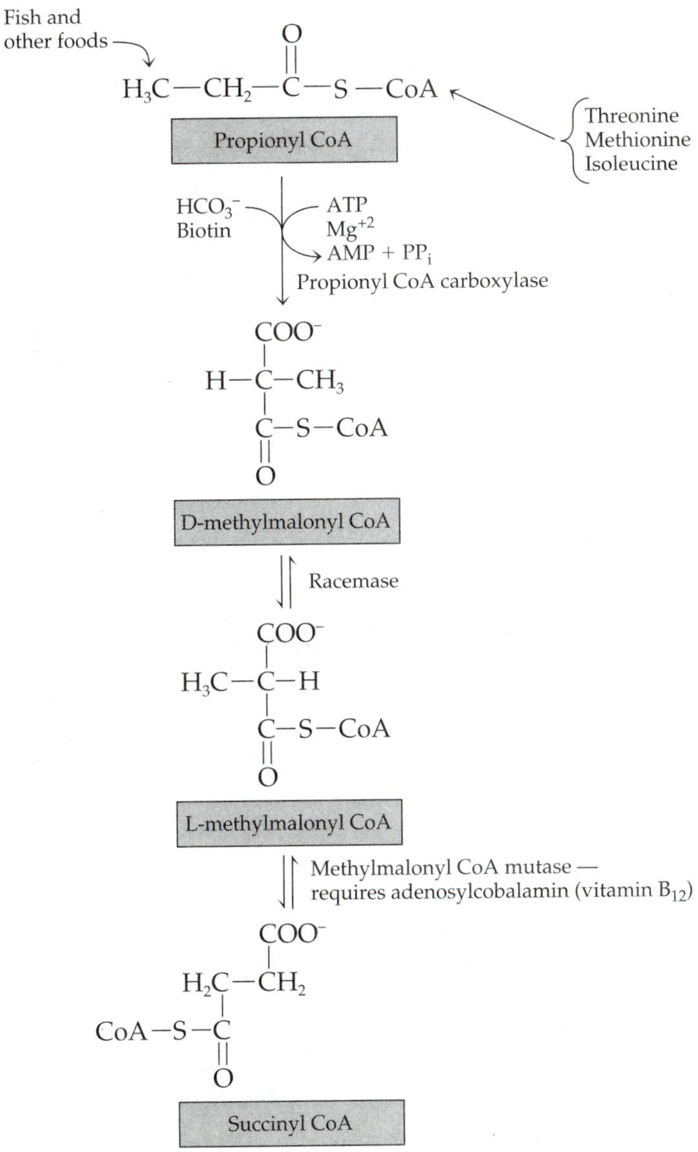

FIGURE 9.25 The oxidation of propionyl CoA and the role of biotin.

Beta-methylcrotonyl CoA carboxylase is important in the catabolism of the amino acid leucine. During leucine catabolism (Fig. 9.26), β-methylcrotonyl CoA is formed. This compound is carboxylated in an ATP-, Mg^{+2}-, and biotin-dependent reaction by β-methylcrotonyl CoA carboxylase to form β-methylglutaconyl CoA, which is further catabolized to generate acetoacetate and acetyl CoA.

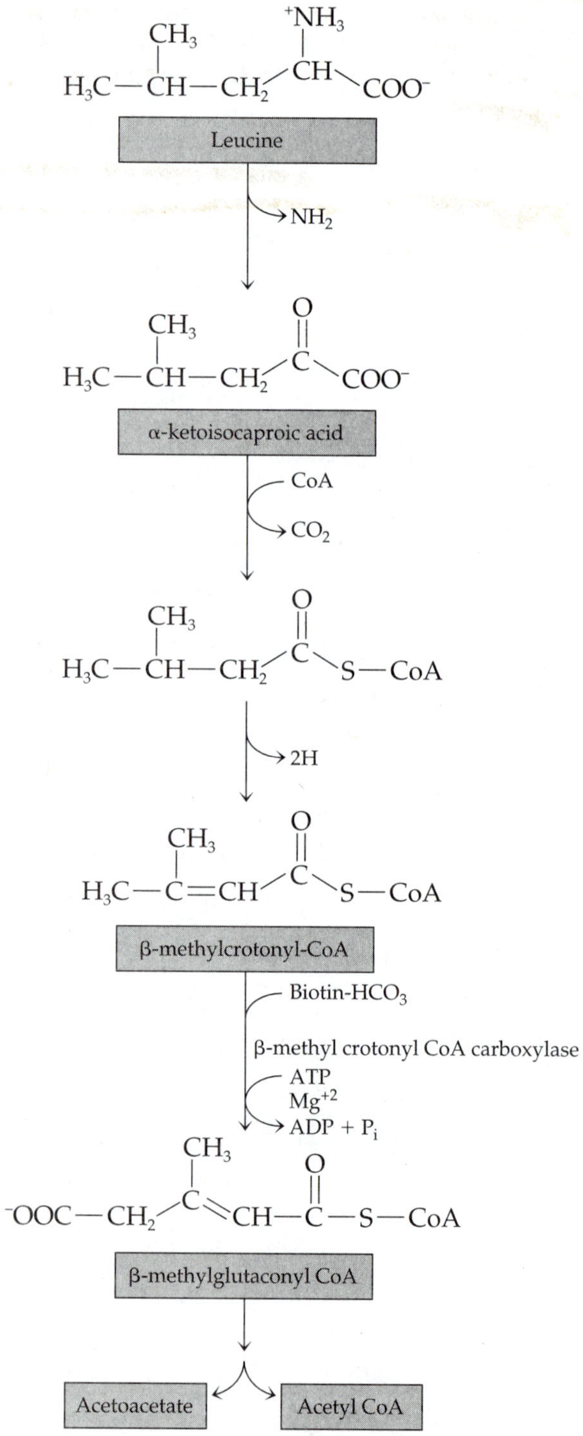

FIGURE 9.26 The role of biotin in leucine catabolism.

Metabolism and Excretion

Catabolism of the biotin holoenzymes or holocarboxylases by proteases yields biocytin. The biocytin is then degraded by biotinidase to yield free biotin. Some of this biotin is reused, and some is degraded. With respect to biotin catabolism (Fig. 9.27), the valerate side chain of biotin may be degraded by beta-oxidation to form bisnorbiotin. Little catabolism of the ring system of the vitamin occurs in humans [5,7]. Biotin is primarily excreted in the urine, as such, or as bisnorbiotin [9]. Small amounts of two other metabolites, biotin sulfoxide [9] and biotin sulfone (Fig. 9.27), may also be formed and excreted [4,5]. In addition, biocytin that has not been hydrolyzed by biotinidase may also be excreted in the urine [1].

Free biotin may be reabsorbed by the kidney, although saturation of the renal transport system results in urinary excretion [4]. Urinary biotin excretion ranges from <6 to 111 µg/day. United States diets supplying 28 to 42 µg biotin per day resulted in an urinary biotin excretion of 20 to 24 µg/day with no indication of inadequate status associated with this level of intake [10]. Adults ingesting 100 to 200 µg biotin daily excreted 18 to 46 µg biotin in the urine [7]. Unabsorbed biotin and biotin synthesized by intestinal bacteria are excreted in the feces. Excretion in the feces appears to be independent of dietary intake [5]. Urinary and fecal excretion of biotin are often greater than dietary intake presumably due to the intestine's contribution of biotin to the body. Urinary biotin excretion is typically less than dietary intake [3].

Recommended Dietary Allowances

Because of the uncertain contribution of intestinal synthesis to total biotin intake and the incomplete knowledge about the bioavailability of food biotin, a range of 30 to 100 µg/day is provisionally recommended for children 11 years or older and adults [10]. Based on the appearance of a biotin deficiency in studies of children with biotinidase deficiency not receiving supplements of free biotin, it has been concluded that intestinally synthesized biotin is not sufficient to maintain normal biotin status [3].

Deficiency

Biotin deficiency in humans is characterized by depression, hallucinations, muscle pain, localized paresthesia, anorexia, nausea, alopecia (hair loss), and scaly dermatitis. People ingesting raw eggs in excess amounts are likely to develop biotin deficiency due to impaired biotin absorption. Impaired biotin absorption may occur also with gastrointestinal disorders, such as inflammatory bowel disease and achlorhydria (lack of hydrochloric acid in gastric juices), or with people on anticonvulsant drug therapy. Excessive alcohol ingestion and sulfonamide therapy also increase the risk for deficiency.

Toxicity

Toxicity of biotin has not been reported. Biotin given in oral doses of 60 mg daily for over six months has not been shown to produce side effects.

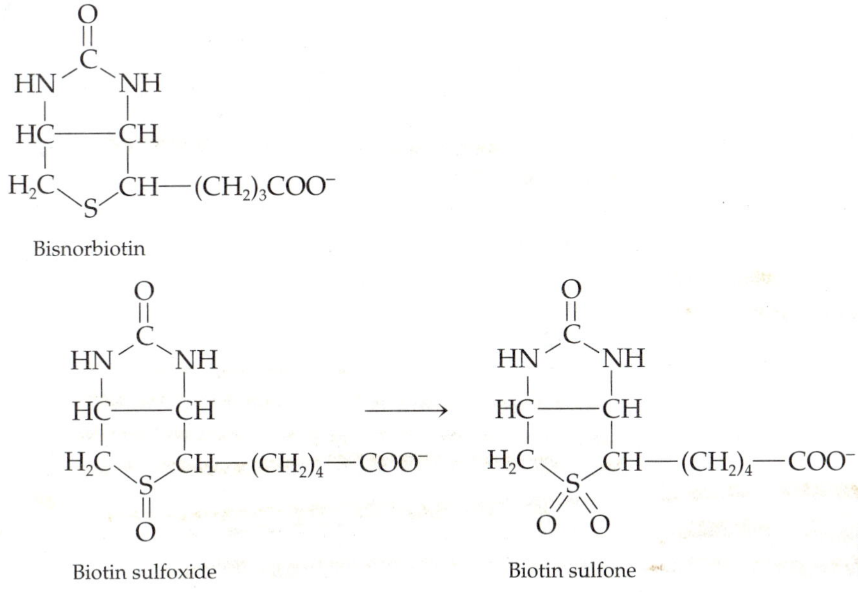

FIGURE 9.27 Selected metabolites from biotin degradation.

Assessment of Nutriture

Evaluation of biotin in blood, plasma, or serum as well as analysis in urine are most often used to assess biotin status. Plasma biotin concentrations below 1.02 nmol/L are thought to indicate deficiency [5]. Normal ranges for plasma biotin are 0.82 to 2.87 nmol/L [5]. Urinary biotin excretion is thought to reflect and has been used to assess biotin status [7,9]. Urinary biotin levels of <20 µg/day are thought to be inadequate.

References Cited for Biotin

1. Sauberlich HE. Vitamins—how much is for keeps? Nutr Today 1987;22:20–28.
2. Wolf B, Heard GS, McVoy JRS, Grier RE. Biotinidase deficiency. Ann NY Acad Sci 1985;447:252–262.
3. Bonjour JP. Biotin. In: Machlin LJ., ed., Handbook of vitamins, 2nd ed. New York: Dekker, 1991:393–427.
4. Bender DA. Nutritional biochemistry of the vitamins. New York: Cambridge University Press, 1992:318–340.
5. Dakshinamurti K. Biotin. In: Shils ME, Olson JA, Shike M., eds., Modern nutrition in health and disease, 8th ed. Philadelphia: Lea and Febiger, 1994:426–431.
6. Combs GF. The vitamins. San Diego, CA: Academic Press, 1992:329–343.
7. McCormick DB. Biotin. In: Shils ME, Young VR, eds., Modern nutrition in health and disease, 7th ed. Philadelphia: Lea and Febiger, 1988:436–439.
8. Knowles JR. The mechanism of biotin-dependent enzymes. Ann Rev Biochem 1989;58:195–221.
9. Mock DM, Lankford GL, Cazin J. Biotin and biotin analogs in human urine: Biotin accounts for only half of the total. J Nutr 1993;123:1844–1851.
10. National Research Council. Recommended dietary allowances, 10th ed. Washington, DC: National Academy Press, 1989:165–169.

FOLIC ACID

Folate and folacin are generic terms for compounds that have similar chemical structures and nutritional properties similar to those of folic acid, which is also called *pteroylglutamate* or *pteroylmonoglutamate* [1]. Folic acid is made up of three distinct parts, all of which must be present for vitamin activity. Figure 9.28 shows the structure of folic acid. As shown in Figure 9.28, pterin, also called *pteridine*, is conjugated to para-aminobenzoic acid (PABA) to form pteroic acid. The carboxy group of PABA is peptide bound to the alpha amino group of glutamate to form folic acid. Although mammals can synthesize all the component parts of the vitamin, they do not have the enzyme necessary for the coupling of the pterin molecule to PABA to form pteroic acid [2]. In the body, metabolically active folate has multiple glutamic acid residues attached.

Sources

Good food sources of folate include mushrooms, green vegetables such as spinach, brussels sprouts, broccoli, asparagus, turnip greens, among others, as well as legumes (especially lima beans), and liver. Raw foods are typically higher in folate than cooked foods due to folate losses incurred with cooking. Fruits and non-organ meats are typically poor sources of folate.

Folate in foods exists primarily in the form of pteroylpolyglutamates containing up to nine glutamate residues instead of the one glutamate as shown in Figure 9.28. The principal pteroylpolyglutamates in foods are N^5 methyl tetrahydrofolate (THF), N^{10} formyl THF [3], although over 150 different forms of folate have been reported [4,5].

Folate bioavailability in individual foods varies from as high as 96% in cooked lima beans to as low as 25% in romaine lettuce [4]. Moreover, reduced forms of pteroylpolyglutamates in foods are labile and easily oxidized. It is estimated that in food preparation or processing, 50 to 95% of the folates originally present can be lost [4,5]. The effect of thermal processing on folate bioavailability depends to a great extent on the form of folate present in food.

Availability of folate from food is also affected by inhibitory compounds known as *conjugase inhibitors*. The conjugase inhibitors prevent the digestion of folate, which is necessary for folate absorption [6].

Digestion, Absorption, and Transport

Before the polyglutamate forms of folate in foods can be absorbed, they must be hydrolyzed to the monoglutamate form. This hydrolysis is performed by the γ-glutamylcarboxypeptidases, also called *conjugases*. The group of conjugases exhibits separate activities in the human jejunal mucosa: one soluble and the other membrane bound and concentrated in the intestinal brush border [5,7]. The conjugases are also found in the pancreatic juice and bile. The brush border conjugase has been characterized; it is a zinc-dependent exopeptidase that stepwise cleaves the polyglutamate into monoglutamate. Zinc deficiency can impair conjugase activity and diminish digestion and thus absorption of folate [2,3]. In addition, chronic alcohol ingestion can diminish conjugase activity to impair folate absorption. Conjugase in-

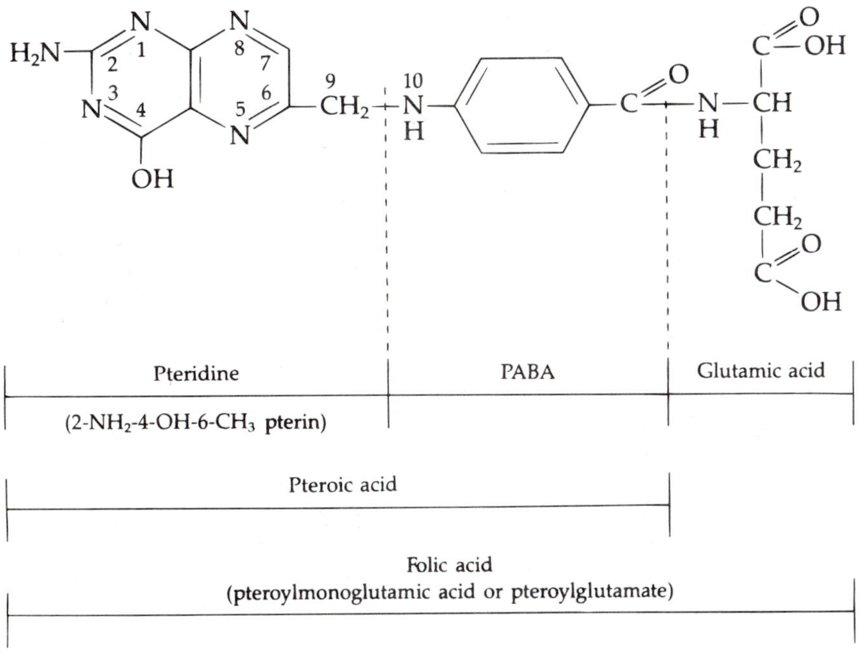

FIGURE 9.28 Structural formula of folic acid.

hibitors in foods such as legumes, lentils, cabbage, and oranges also prevent the digestion of polyglutamate forms of folate to the monoglutamate form. This digestion is necessary in order for folate to be absorbed [6].

The carrier system responsible for transporting folate across the cell membrane is believed to be saturable and pH, energy, and sodium dependent [3,4,7]. Folate-binding proteins (FBP) are found associated with the intestinal brush border and are believed to form a part of the transport system; the folate-binding proteins may be derived from the cellular membranes in which they serve transport functions [3,5,8]. Absorption is possible throughout the small intestine but is most efficient in the jejunum [2,6], where optimal transport occurs between a pH of 5 and 6 [6]. The folate in milk, however, appears to be absorbed more avidly in the ileum. Folate in milk is bound to a high-affinity folate-binding protein [2]. Diffusion may also account for 20 to 30% of folate absorption regardless of concentration [3]. Efficiency of folate absorption is estimated at 50% [3].

Within the intestinal cell, folate is typically reduced to THF and methylated to N^5 methyl THF or formylated. The reduction of various folate forms to THF occurs stepwise through action of NADPH-dependent dihydrofolate reductase (Fig. 9.29). Four additional hydrogens are added at positions 5, 6, 7, and 8. Most of the folate found in portal circulation is N^5 methyl THF, although dihydrofolate and formylated forms are also present.

Within the liver, about 33% of folate is present as THF, 37% of N^5 methyl THF, 23% as N^{10} formyl THF and 7% as N^5 formyl THF [2]. Bound to the N^5 methyl THF and N^{10} formyl THF are glutamates varying in length from typically 4 to 7. Dihydrofolate taken up by the liver is typically reduced and either conjugated for storage or converted to N^5 methyl THF [2]. Most of the N^5 methyl THF, along with N^{10} formyl THF, is secreted into the bile and then reabsorbed by way of enterohepatic circulation. This recirculation process may account for as much as 50% of the total folate that reaches peripheral tissues [7]. Intracellular folate-binding proteins in the liver have been identified and may serve a storage role [8].

In the blood folate is found as a monoglutamate. Almost two-thirds of the folate in blood plasma is bound to protein [7]; free folate accounts for the other one-third. Folate-binding proteins have been identified in plasma and within blood cells. Folate-binding protein binds folate with high affinity. Albumin and alpha-2 macroglobulin also bind folate, but with relatively low affinity. Monoglutamate forms of folate in the blood include THF, N^5 methyl THF, N^{10} formyl THF, among others [5].

Folate transport into tissue cells occurs by a carrier-mediated process that may or may not require ATP. Folate-binding proteins associated with renal and hepatic cell membranes have been identified [8]. Within cells, THF is converted into a polyglutamate form to become a functional coenzyme, accepting and transferring one-carbon fragments. Intracellular demethylation is

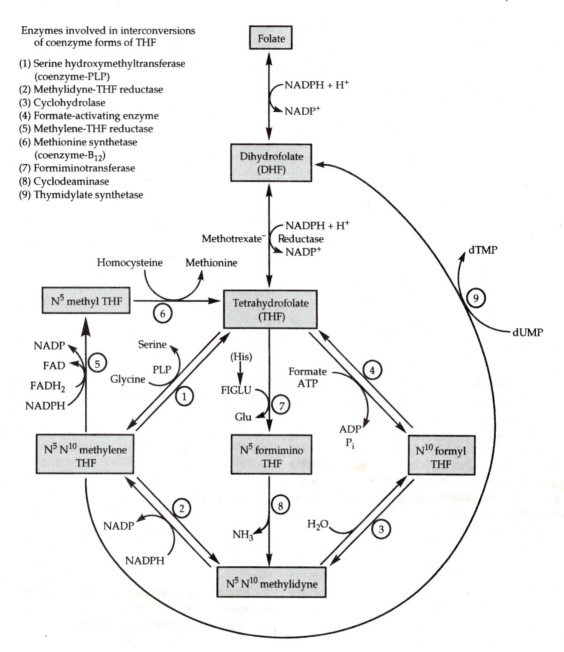

FIGURE 9.29 Interconversions of coenzyme forms of THF.

required, along with formation of polyglutamates by pteroylpolyglutamate synthetase (PPS). Five to seven glutamate residues are usually added to the monoglutamate in ATP requiring reactions. The glutamates are added to the vitamin by peptide bonds. Adding these glutamate residues not only allows the production of the various folate coenzyme forms but also traps the folate in the cell. For example, red blood cells accumulate considerable amounts of folate as polyglutamates. Total

body folate levels range from 5 to 10 mg, with the liver storing most of the vitamin [9].

Functions and Mechanisms of Action

Folic acid and subsequently dihydrofolate are both reduced by dihydrofolate reductase, a cytosolic enzyme, to generate THF (Fig. 9.29). THF accepts one-carbon groups from various degradative reactions in amino acid metabolism. These THF derivatives then serve as donors of one-carbon units in a variety of synthetic reactions. The one-carbon group accepted by THF is bonded to its N^5 or N^{10} atoms or to both (Fig. 9.29). The coenzyme forms are interconvertible, except that N^5 methyl THF cannot be converted back to N^5, N^{10} methylene (Fig. 9.29).

The five THF derivatives, which participate in a variety of reactions, are illustrated as follows. The first three derivatives represent the most oxidized forms of folate, while N^5 methyl THF is the most reduced form.

N^5 formyl THF $\qquad -C{\overset{\displaystyle O}{\|}}-H$

N^{10} formyl THF $\qquad -C{\overset{\displaystyle O}{\|}}-H$

N^5 formimino THF $\qquad -CH=NH$

N^5, N^{10} methylidyne/ methenyl THF $\qquad {>}CH$

N^5, N^{10} methylene THF $\qquad {>}CH_2$

N^5 methyl THF $\qquad -CH_3$

Amino Acid Metabolism Folate as N^5, N^{10} methylene THF is required for *serine* synthesis from *glycine*. N^5, N^{10} methylene THF contributes a hydroxy methyl group to glycine to produce serine. Vitamin B_6 as pyridoxal phosphate (PLP) is required for serine hydroxymethyltransferase activity.

$$\text{Glycine} \underset{N^5, N^{10} \text{ methylene THF} \quad THF}{\overset{\text{serine hydroxymethyltransferase}}{\rightleftharpoons}} \text{serine}$$

This reaction is reversible such that glycine may be synthesized from serine in a THF-dependent reaction. Serine represents a major source of one-carbon units used in folate reactions. Glycine degradation also requires THF.

$$\text{Glycine} \xrightarrow[\text{NAD}^+ \qquad \text{NADH} + H^+]{\text{THF} \quad N^5, N^{10} \text{ methylene THF}} CO_2 + NH_4^+$$

Methionine regeneration from homocysteine also involves folate as N^5 methyl THF. As shown in Figure 9.30, methionine adenosyl transferase catalyzed the conversion of methionine to S-adenosyl methionine (SAM) in an ATP-requiring reaction. S-adenosyl homocysteine (SAH) is generated from removal of a methyl group from SAM. Removal of the adenosyl group from SAH yields homocysteine. Remethylation of homocysteine to form methionine, requires N^5 methyl THF as a methyl donor and vitamin B_{12} in the form of methylcobalamin as a prosthetic group for homocysteine methyltransferase, also called *methionine synthetase*. Another homocysteine methyltransferase requiring betaine, which is formed from choline catabolism, and not requiring methylcobalamin, has also been demonstrated [2].

In order for homocysteine methyltransferase to transfer a methyl group from N^5 methyl THF to homocysteine, cobalamin must be tightly bound to the enzyme. Cobalamin, while bound to the apoenzyme, picks up the methyl group from N^5 methyl THF to generate methylcobalamin and THF. Methylcobalamin then serves as the methyl donor for converting homocysteine to methionine.

The roles of folate and vitamin B_{12} in the conversion of homocysteine to methionine have been receiving considerable attention since an association between elevated blood homocysteine concentrations and premature coronary artery disease as well as premature occlusive vascular disease and cerebral or peripheral vascular disease has been documented. Supplementation (folic acid, vitamin B_{12} and vitamin B_6) of healthy people with hyperhomocysteinemia (high blood homocysteine concentrations) for six weeks has been shown to normalize blood homocysteine concentrations, and thus, decrease a risk factor for heart disease [10].

Histidine Metabolism *Histidine* metabolism also requires THF (Fig. 9.31). Deamination of histidine generates urocanic acid, which can undergo further metabolism to yield formiminoglutamate (FIGLU). The formimino is removed from FIGLU with the help of formiminotransferase to generate *glutamic acid*; THF receives the formimino to yield N^5 formimino THF (Fig. 9.31). This reaction, FIGLU to glutamate, can be used as a basis for determination of folate deficiency whereby subjects are given an oral histidine load and FIGLU excretion is measured in the urine. FIGLU accumulates with folate deficiency, because if THF were available FIGLU would be converted into glutamate.

Purine and Pyrimidine Synthesis The involvement of THF derivatives in purine and pyrimidine synthesis (Figs. 7.9, 7.10) makes folate essential for cell division. Synthesis of cells with short life spans, such as enterocytes, are particularly dependent on adequate levels of folate.

In pyrimidine synthesis (Fig. 7.9, p. 168), thymidylate synthase uses N^5, N^{10} methylene THF to convert

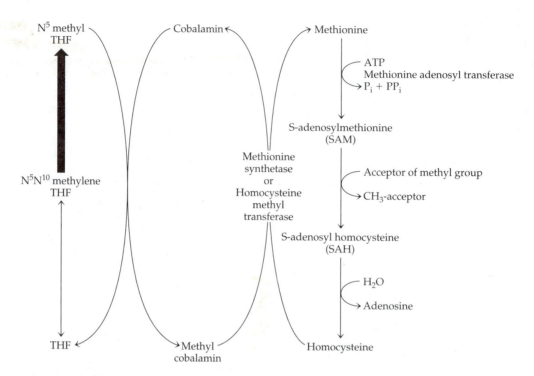

FIGURE 9.30 The resynthesis of methionine from homocysteine, showing the roles of folate and vitamin B_{12}.

dUMP to dTMP and dihydrofolate (DHF) (Fig. 9.29). dTMP is required for DNA synthesis. To regenerate N^5, N^{10} methylene THF, DHF is converted by dihydroreductase to THF in a reaction requiring NADPH. The THF is converted to N^5, N^{10} methenyl THF as serine is converted to glycine by serine hydroxymethyl transferase, a vitamin B_6-dependent reaction (Fig. 9.29). Both thymidylate synthetase and dihydrofolate reductase are active enzymes in cells undergoing cell division. Inhibitors of dihydrofolate reductase, such as the chemotherapeutic drug Methotrexate, which binds to the enzyme's active site, have been employed in the treatment of cancer to prevent synthesis of THF needed for actively dividing cancer cells.

Folate as N^{10} formyl THF is needed for purine ring formation (Fig. 7.10, p. 169). C8 of the purine atom involves the formylation of glycinamide ribotide (GAR) to form formylglycinamidine ribotide (FGAR). N^{10} formyl THF donates the formyl group in this reaction. Purine ring atom C2 is acquired by formylation of 5-aminoimidazole 4-carboxamide ribonucleotide (AICAR). N^{10} formyl THF formylates AICAR to generate 5-formaminoimidazole 4-carboxamide ribotide (FAICAR).

Interrelationships with Other Nutrients

Ascorbic acid, with its reducing capability, has been shown to protect folate from oxidative destruction. The relationship between folate and *zinc* remains unclear. Folate intakes of about 150 μg/day along with supplements containing 400 μg folate taken every other day have been shown to diminish zinc absorption, although dietary zinc intake averaged only 7.5 mg daily [11]. Rat studies suggest that in the presence of high concentrations of folate, folate and zinc form a complex in the intestinal lumen. This complex then inhibits zinc absorption. Zinc absorption after ingestion of 200 mg zinc sulfate was diminished in adults who had been receiving 350 μg oral folate daily [12]. Yet oral zinc (25 mg as zinc sulfate) when ingested with and without 10 mg folate, did not decrease serum zinc concentrations [13]. Thus, further research concerning interactions between folate and zinc are needed.

A synergistic relationship exists between folate and *vitamin B_{12}*, also called *cobalamin*; this relationship is sometimes called the *"methyl–folate trap"* whereby without vitamin B_{12} the methyl group from N^5 methyl THF can't be removed and is thus trapped. The following sequence of events leads to the methyl folate trap. Tracing the reactions shown in Figures 9.29 and 9.30 will be helpful. Serine donates single carbons through conversion to glycine and in the process THF is converted to N^5, N^{10} methylene THF. N^5, N^{10} methylene THF is readily reduced to N^5 methyl THF by a reductase (whose activity in inhibited by its end product, N^5 methyl THF, and by SAM). N^5 methyl THF is required

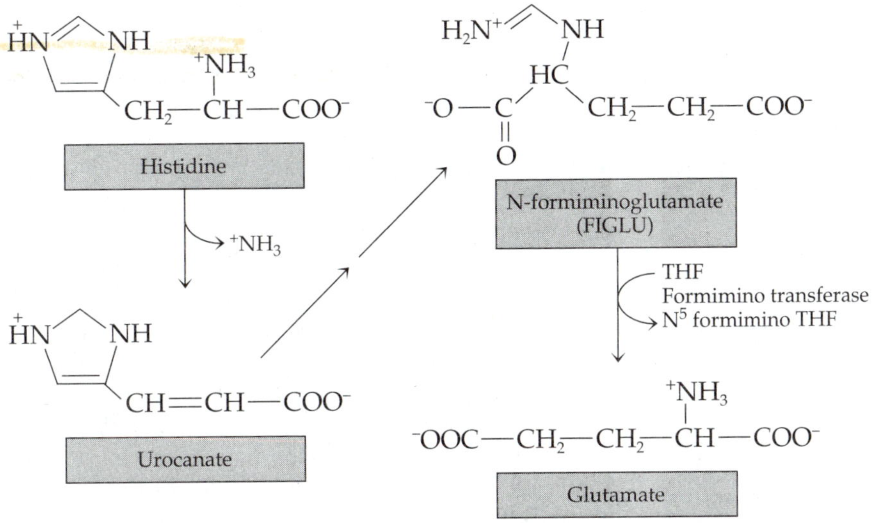

FIGURE 9.31 The role of folic acid in histidine catabolism.

for methionine synthesis from homocysteine. Methyl groups are transferred by the enzyme methionine synthetase from N^5 methyl THF to vitamin B_{12}. Adequate vitamin B_{12} must be present for the activity of methionine synthetase. The addition of the methyl group to cobalamin generates methylcobalamin, which serves as the methyl donor for converting homocysteine to methionine. Without cobalamin to accept the methyl group from N^5 methyl THF, the N^5 methyl THF accumulates, is trapped, and THF is not regenerated.

The THF, resulting from the synthesis of methionine, is important as a substrate for pteroylpolyglutamate synthetase, which adds the glutamate residues to the THF. The polyglutamate form of THF can now be used or converted into its various coenzyme forms. N^{10} formyl THF is needed for purine synthesis; $N^5 N^{10}$ methylene THF is needed for thymidylate synthesis, which in turn must be present for DNA synthesis. Thus, the synergism between folate and vitamin B_{12} is very important for support of rapidly proliferating cells.

Metabolism and Excretion

Under normal conditions, the body appears to hold on tenaciously to absorbed folate. Folate-binding proteins are present in the renal brush border and coupled with tubular reabsorption of folate in the kidney, very little folate is excreted in the urine.

Catabolism of folate occurs through the action of carboxypeptidase G. Two metabolites of folate are para-acetamidobenzoate and para-acetamidobenzoylglutamate, with the latter found in the greater amounts. The relative proportions of the various metabolites suggests that the principal route of catabolism occurs through oxidative cleavage of the folate molecule between positions 9 and 10 [6]. Acetylation of these compounds in the liver occurs prior to urinary excretion [6,9], although the excretion of folate metabolites is minimal.

Although much of the absorbed dietary folate is secreted by the liver into the bile, most of this folate is reabsorbed via enterohepatic recirculation and losses in the stool are minimal [7]. Folate from microbial origin may, however, appear in the feces in relatively high amounts.

Availability of folate to crucial tissues where rapid cell division is occurring appears to be carefully regulated when the supply of dietary folate is limited. The mechanisms of regulation are unclear, but regulation seems to occur through rate of synthesis of polyglutamates. The less metabolically active tissues return monoglutamates to the liver; the liver then redistributes the folate to the actively proliferating cells. How circulating folates are directed to specific tissues is uncertain, but one possibility is that folate-binding proteins and membrane-associated binding proteins could provide tissue-specific uptake [7].

Recommended Dietary Allowances

The minimal daily folate requirement is estimated at 50 μg based on intravenous administration, while 100 μg dietary folate is thought to prevent folate deficiency [1,6]. The 1989 RDA for folate is considerably lower than the amount recommended in the 1980 RDA. The 1989 RDA suggest approximately 3 μg/kg body wt/day for adults, with males and females needing 200 μg and 180 μg folate/day, respectively. This recommended amount is based on 50% folate bioavailability from foods and approximately 30% coefficient of variation. The RDI [14] suggest folate intakes similar to the 1989 RDA. Sauberlich et al. [15], however, suggest nonpregnant women need 200 to 250 μg folate/day to restore or maintain normal plasma folate concentrations. Bailey [16] has also suggested that the RDA for folate be re-evaluated.

The 1989 RDA for folate during pregnancy is more than double that for the nonpregnant female (400 μg versus 180 μg) to build or maintain maternal stores and to support the developing fetus. Additional recommendations by the Centers for Disease Control and Prevention [17] of 400 μg folate/day for women capable of becoming pregnant have been proposed because of the accumulating evidence that folate supplementation during periconceptional period of pregnancy may reduce the incidence of neural tube defects. Debates are ongoing concerning whether or not foods, and which foods, should be fortified with folate.

Deficiency—Megaloblastic, Macrocytic Anemia

Marginal folate deficiency is characterized initially by low plasma folate and hypersegmentation of polymorphonuclear leukocytes. Red blood cell folate concentrations diminish after about four months of low folate intake [18]. After approximately four to five months, bone marrow cells become megaloblastic and anemia occurs [18].

Megaloblastic anemia—the release into circulation of large immature erythrocytes—due to folate deficiency is relatively common in the United States. However, megaloblastic anemia also occurs due to a deficiency of vitamin B_{12}. The anemia results from decreased DNA synthesis and failure of the cells to divide properly, coupled with the continued formation of RNA. The quantity of RNA becomes greater than normal, leading to excess production of other cytoplasmic constituents, including hemoglobin. The result is immature, enlarged cells often containing excessive hemoglobin.

A review of the formation and maturation of erythrocytes is given in Figure 9.32, and may help better illustrate the effects of a folate and vitamin B_{12} deficiency. Briefly, the proerythroblast develops from stem cells in bone marrow under the stimulation of hypoxia (low blood oxygen) via erythropoietin (a hormone produced in the kidney). In the proerythroblast, active DNA and RNA synthesis occur and cell division begins. Cells resulting from first division are termed *basophilic erythroblasts* because they stain with basic dyes due to the many organelles present within the cell. During this stage, hemoglobin synthesis begins. The next generation of cells consists of the polychromatophil erythroblasts in which hemoglobin synthesis intensifies. The concentration of hemoglobin influences DNA synthesis and cell division. Cell division usually continues into the orthochromatic stage. The orthochromatic erythrocytes are characterized by continued hemoglobin synthesis, discontinuation of DNA synthesis, a slowing of RNA synthesis, and migration of the nucleus to the cell wall in preparation for extrusion. The cell now becomes the reticulocyte in which hemoglobin synthesis continues up to a concentration of approximately 34%. Once this concentration is reached, the ribosomes disappear, and the cells pass into blood capillaries by squeezing through pores of the membrane. In about two to three days, when the rest of the cell organelles have disappeared, reticulocytes become erythrocytes. The erythrocyte, or mature red blood cell, is all cytoplasm packed with hemoglobin. Glycolysis and hexose monophosphate shunt are the only metabolic pathways occurring in the erythrocyte. A deficiency of folate and/or vitamin B_{12} interferes with normal cell division. Large, malformed, and sometimes nucleated, red blood cells result.

Folate deficiency is also suspected in the development (initiation) of cancer. Folate deficiency in cells and tissues is thought to increase the potential for neoplastic changes in normal cells during the early stages of cancer [18, 19].

Some conditions and populations associated with increased need for folate intake include the elderly and people with excessive alcohol ingestion, achlorhydria, inflammatory bowel diseases, malignancies, oral contraceptive users, as well as pregnant and lactating women. Folate deficiency has been observed in people treated with diphenylhydantoin or phenytoin, anticonvulsants used in the treatment of epilepsy. Folate and phenytoin inhibit the cellular uptake of one another in the gastrointestinal tract and possibly in the brain [1,20]. However, although folate supplements of 5 to 30 mg/day corrected the hematological signs associated with the folate deficiency, seizure activity increased in some patients [6]. Other drugs, such as cholestyramine, used to treat high cholesterol concentrations, and sulfasalazine, used to treat inflammatory bowel diseases, have also been shown to interact with folate to create potential folate deficiency. Malabsorption of folate occurs with inflammatory bowel diseases and excessive alcohol ingestion.

Toxicity

Folate supplements in amounts greater than 0.4 mg daily are considered to be pharmacologic doses [6]. Some reports suggest no adverse effects of folate supplements,

Genesis of RBC

Proerythroblast

Basophil
erythroblast

Polychromatophil
erythroblast

Orthochromatic
erythroblast

Reticulocyte

Erythrocytes

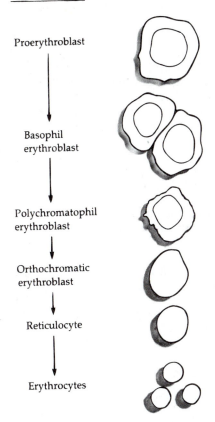

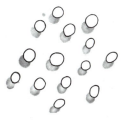

Microcytic,
hypochromic anemia

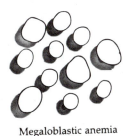

Megaloblastic anemia

FIGURE 9.32 Genesis and maturation of the red blood cell; red blood cells characteristic of microcytic and megaloblastic anemias.

400 mg/day for 5 months, 10 mg for 4 months, or 10 mg/day for 5 years, in adults [1,6]. Toxicity of oral folic acid in moderate doses is reportedly virtually nonexistent [21]. Other studies, however, indicate that folate intakes up to 15 mg daily are toxic in some individuals. Problems include insomnia, malaise, irritability, diminished zinc status, and gastrointestinal problems [20,22]. In addition, folate supplementation can mask a vitamin B_{12} deficiency. Folate supplements alleviate the megaloblastic anemia due to a vitamin B_{12} deficiency, while the neurologic damage due to a vitamin B_{12} deficiency progresses undetected.

Assessment of Nutriture

Folate status is most often assessed through measurement of folate levels in the plasma, serum, or red blood cells [6]. Serum or plasma folate levels reflect recent dietary intake, thus true deficiency must be interpreted through repeated measures of serum or plasma folate. Red blood cell folate levels, more reflective of folate status than serum folate, represent vitamin status at the time the red blood cell was synthesized [1,14,23]. Red

blood cell folate may indicate liver folate stores. A low red blood cell folate may, however, occur with a vitamin B_{12} deficiency [23].

	Folate Status		
	Deficient	Marginal	Adequate
Serum folate (ng/mL)	<3	3–6	>6
Red blood cell folate (ng/mL)	<140	140–160	>160

The deoxyuridine suppression test, another method to assess folate status, measures the availability of folate for *de novo* thymidine synthesis. In this test, the activity of thymidylate synthetase is measured in cultured lymphocytes or bone marrow cells. The reaction catalyzed by thymidylate synthetase is dependent on folate and indirectly on vitamin B_{12}; therefore the change in activity elicited by the addition of one or the other vitamin allows identification of the deficiency. In case of a deficiency of both vitamin B_{12} and folate, normalization of enzyme activity would be possible only after the addition of both vitamins.

Deoxyuridine suppression test (thymidylate synthetase activity)[24]

	Deficiency		
	B_{12}	Folate	Folate and B_{12}
Add B_{12}	Normalized	Abnormal	Abnormal
Add folate	Abnormal	Normalized	Abnormal
Add B_{12} and folate	Normalized	Normalized	Normalized

Source: Simko MD, Cowell C, Gilbride JA. Nutrition Assessment. Rockville, MD: Aspen Publishers, 1984. Reprinted with permission of Aspen Publishers, Inc.

N-formiminoglutamate (FIGLU) excretion may also be used to measure folate nutriture, because folate as THF must be available for the formimino group to be removed from FIGLU, and glutamate to be formed (see Fig. 9.31). FIGLU excretion is measured in a six-hour urine collection after ingestion of 2 to 5 g oral L-histidine. Normal FIGLU excretion is about 5 to 20 mg, whereas with folate deficiency FIGLU excretion is five to ten times above normal. A deficiency of vitamin B_{12}, however, will also cause an elevated FIGLU excretion.

References Cited for Folic Acid

1. National Research Council. Recommended dietary allowances, 10th ed. Washington, DC: National Academy Press, 1989;150–158.
2. Bender DA. Nutritional biochemistry of the vitamins. New York: Cambridge University Press, 1992:269–317.
3. Coombs GF. The vitamins. San Diego, CA: Academic Press, 1992:357–376.
4. Sauberlich HE. Bioavailability of vitamins. Prog Food Nutr Sci 1985;9:1–33.
5. Sauberlich HE. Vitamins—how much is for keeps? Nutr Today 1987;22:20–28.
6. Brody T. Folic acid. In: Machlin LJ., ed. Handbook of vitamins, 2nd ed. New York: Dekker, 1991:453–489.
7. Steinberg SE. Mechanisms of folate homeostasis. Am J Physiol 1984;246:G319–324.
8. Wagner C. Cellular folate binding proteins; function and significance. Ann Rev Nutr 1982;2:229–248.
9. Herbert V, Das KC. Folic acid and vitamin B_{12}. In: Shils ME, Olson JA, Shike M., eds. Modern nutrition in health and disease, 8th ed. Philadelphia: Lea and Febiger, 1994:402–425.
10. Ubbink JB. Vitamin B_{12}, vitamin B_6, and folate nutritional status in men with hyperhomocysteinemia. Am J Clin Nutr 1993;57:47–53.
11. Milne DB, Canfield WK, Mahalko JR, Sandstead HH. Effect of oral folic acid supplements on zinc, copper, and iron absorption and excretion. Am J Clin Nutr 1984;39:535–539.
12. Simmer K, Iles CA, James C, Thompson RPH. Are iron-folate supplements harmful? Am J Clin Nutr 1987;45:122–125.
13. Keating JN, Wada L, Stokstad ELR, King JC. Folic acid: Effect on zinc absorption in humans and in the rat. Am J Clin Nutr 1987;46:835–839.
14. Herbert V. Recommended dietary intakes (RDI) of folate in humans. Am J Clin Nutr 1987;45:661–670.
15. Sauberlich HE, Kretsch MJ, Skala JH, Johnson HL, Taylor PC. Folate requirement and metabolism in nonpregnant women. Am J Clin Nutr 1987;46:1016–1028.
16. Bailey LB. Evaluation of a new recommended dietary allowance for folate. J Am Diet Assoc 1992;92:463–468,471.
17. Centers for Disease Control and Prevention. Recommendations for the use of folic acid to reduce the number of cases of spina bifida and other neural tube defects. MMWSR 1992;41:1–7.
18. Hine RJ. Folic acid: Contemporary clinical perspective. Persp Appl Nutr 1993;1:3–14.
19. Folate, alcohol, methionine, and colon cancer risk: Is there a unifying theme? Nutr Rev 1994; 52:18–20.
20. Alhadeff LC, Gualtieri CT, Lipton M. Toxic effects of water-soluble vitamins. Nutr Rev 1984;42:33–40.
21. Krumdieck CL. Folic Acid. In: Brown ML, ed., Present knowledge in nutrition, 6th ed. Washington, DC: The Nutrition Foundation, 1990:179–188.
22. Zimmerman MB, Shane B. Supplemental folic acid. Am J Clin Nutr 1993;58:127–128.
23. Bailey LB. Folate status assessment. J Nutr 1990;120:1508–1511.
24. Simko MD, Cowell C, Gilbride JA. Nutrition assessment. Rockville, MD: Aspen, 1984.

Additional References

Herbert V. The 1986 Herman Award Lecture. Nutrition science as a continually unfolding story: The folate and vitamin B_{12} paradigm. Am J Clin Nutr 1987;46:387–402.
Shane B, Stokstad ELR. Vitamin B_{12}-folate interrelationships. Ann Rev Nutr 1985;5:115–141.

VITAMIN B_{12} (COBALAMINS)

Vitamin B_{12} is considered a generic term for a group of compounds called *corrinoids* because of their corrin nucleus. The corrin is a macrocyclic ring made of four reduced pyrrole rings linked together. The corrin of vitamin B_{12} has an atom of cobalt in the center of it to which is attached, at almost right angles, a nucleotide, 5,6-dimethylbenzimidazole. Also attached to the cobalt atom in vitamin B_{12} is one of the following:

Group Attached	Resulting Compound
—CN	Cyanocobalamin
—OH	Hydroxocobalamin
—H₂O	Aquocobalamin
—NO₂	Nitritocobalamin
5'-deoxyadenosyl	5'-deoxyadenosylcobalamin
—CH₃	Methylcobalamin

Cyanocobalamin is shown in Figure 9.33. Only two cobalamins, 5'-deoxyadenosylcobalamin (subsequently called *adenosylcobalamin*) and methylcobalamin, are active as coenzymes. The human body has the biochemical ability to convert most of the other cobalamins into an active coenzyme form of the vitamin.

Sources

The only dietary sources of vitamin B_{12} for humans are from animal products, which have derived their cobalamins from micro-organisms. All naturally occurring vitamin B_{12} is produced by micro-organisms. Any vitamin B_{12} found in plant foods could probably be traced to contamination with micro-organisms contained in manure or, in the case of legumes, to the presence of nitrogen-fixing bacteria in the plant root nodules [1]. Contaminated hands taking foods to the mouth may also provide vitamin B_{12}.

The best sources of the cobalamins are meat and meat products, poultry, fish, shellfish (especially clams and oysters), and eggs (especially the yolk); the cobalamins in these products are predominantly adenosyl- and hydroxocobalamin. Milk and milk products such as cheese and yogurt contain less of the vitamin, mainly as methyl- and hydroxocobalamins [2,3]. Cyanocobalamin may be found in a few foods as well as tobacco; it is also the form, along with hydroxocobalamin [4] that is commercially available in, for example, vitamin preparations. Within the body, cyanocobalamin is converted to aquo- or hydroxocobalamin.

Bioavailability of vitamin B_{12} may be impaired by vitamin C. Vitamin C in doses of 500 mg or more, taken with meals or up to one hour after a meal, may diminish vitamin B_{12} availability from food or destroy the vitamin [5–7].

Digestion, Absorption, and Transport

The digestion and absorption of vitamin B_{12} is believed to proceed according to the scheme depicted in Figure 9.34. Ingested cobalamins must first be released

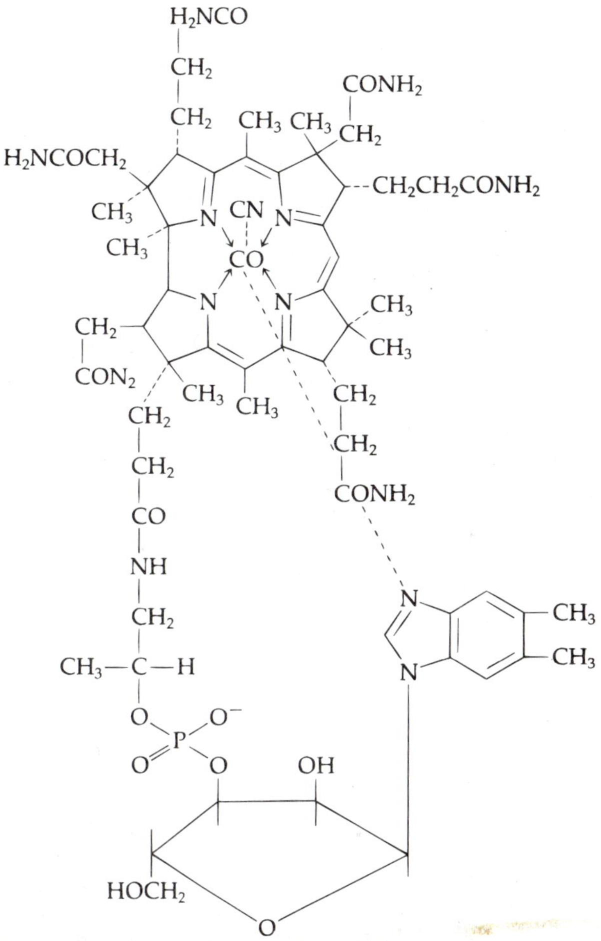

FIGURE 9.33 Structural formula of vitamin B_{12} (cyanocobalamin).

from the polypeptides to which they are linked in foods. This release usually occurs through the action of the gastric proteolytic enzyme pepsin in the stomach.

Once released from foods, vitamin B_{12} absorption involves contact with two proteins, intrinsic factor (IF) and R proteins. IF is a glycoprotein synthesized by the gastric parietal cells. Although it is made and released in the stomach, IF functions in the small intestine. R proteins, known collectively as *cobalophilins* or *haptocorrins* (HC), are found in most body fluids, including saliva and gastric juice [1,6,8,9]. R proteins have a high affinity for cobalamins. Free cobalamin released from food combines with R protein; the complex moves from the stomach into the small intestine. Within the duodenum, the R protein is hydrolyzed by pancreatic proteases, and free cobalamin is released. A pancreatic insufficiency could interfere with the release of cobalamin from the R protein and reduce the amount of the vitamin available for

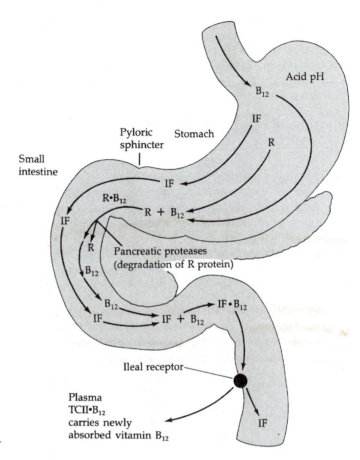

FIGURE 9.34 Vitamin B_{12} absorption.

absorption. R proteins may also serve to protect vitamin B_{12} from bacterial use [7,10].

In the proximal small intestine, IF, which escapes the catabolic action of the proteases, binds the cobalamin, any of the forms, once released from the R proteins. The cobalamin-IF complex travels to the ileum, where receptor sites for vitamin B_{12} are present. Absorption of the vitamin occurs throughout the entire ileum, especially the distal third [1,8].

The cobalamin absorption process is complex and poorly understood. It is known that calcium is needed for absorption to occur, and presently the belief is that calcium has some sort of specific action on the receptor site [6]. Whether cellular uptake of IF occurs with the vitamin is unclear.

Absorption of vitamin B_{12} is slow; after attachment of the IF-cobalamin complex to the receptor, there is a delay of three to four hours before the cobalamin appears in circulation. Peak levels of the vitamin in the blood may not be reached for 8 to 12 hours after ingestion [4].

When pharmacologic doses of vitamin B_{12} are ingested, passive diffusion can account for much of the absorption throughout the intestinal tract. However, passive diffusion can account for only about 1% and up to 3% of the total absorption of the vitamin when it is being obtained from ordinary dietary sources [7,10]. Absorption rate of the vitamin decreases with increased intake. At low levels of intake (0.1 µg), absorption averages 80%, while at higher intakes the absorption rate drops to 3% [4].

Enterohepatic circulation is very important in vitamin B_{12} nutriture, accounting in part for the long biological half-life of cobalamin. When enterohepatic circulation is effective, much of the cobalamin in the bile and in other intestinal secretions can be reabsorbed. Malabsorption syndromes not only cause a decrease in absorption of ingested cobalamin but also interfere with enterohepatic circulation, thereby increasing the amount of vitamin B_{12} required to meet body needs.

Following intestinal absorption, cobalamins bind to one of three transcobalamins (TC), designated as TCI, TCII, or TCIII in the blood. It is not known whether attachment to TC occurs within the enterocyte or at the serosal surface. The transcobalamins also are considered R proteins. The exact functions of TCI and TCIII are unknown. TCIII may function in the delivery of cobalamin from peripheral tissues back to the liver [8]. About 90% of vitamin B_{12} is bound to TCI, which may function as a circulating storage form of the vitamin [8].

TCII is the main protein that carries, in a one-to-one ratio, newly absorbed cobalamin to the tissues (Fig. 9.34). TCII is important for normal cobalamin metabolism and is thought to be synthesized in the liver [11]. In the blood, methylcobalamin comprises about 60 to 80%, and adenosylcobalamin may account for up to 20% of total plasma cobalamin. Other forms of cobalamin in the blood include cyanocobalamin and hydroxocobalamin.

TCII also assists uptake of the vitamin by tissues; all tissues appear to have receptors for TCII. Cobalamin, along with TC, are taken up by endocytosis. Within the lysosome, TCII is degraded and hydroxocobalamin is released. This form of the vitamin may undergo cytosolic methylation to generate methylcobalamin or may undergo reduction and subsequent reaction with ATP in the mitochondria to yield adenosylcobalamin [1].

Vitamin B_{12}, unlike other water-soluble vitamins, can be stored and retained in the body for long periods of time, years. The vitamin is stored mainly in the liver; however, small amounts are also found in the muscle, bone, kidneys, heart, brain, and spleen. Adenosylcobalamin is the primary storage form of the vitamin in the liver, and possibly in other organs; however, hydroxocobalamin and methylcobalamin are also stored to a lesser extent [4]. Haptocorrin represents the circulating storage form of vitamin B_{12} that is in equilibrium with body stores of the vitamin. Hepatocytes have receptors for the uptake of both haptocorrin and for TCII.

Functions and Mechanisms of Action

Three enzymatic reactions requiring vitamin B_{12} have been recognized in humans; one of these reactions requires methylcobalamin, while the other two must have adenosylcobalamin. Adenosyl- and methylcobalamin are formed by a complex reaction sequence resulting in the production of a carbon–cobalt bond between the cobalt nucleus of the vitamin and either the methyl or 5′-deoxyadenosyl ligand.

The reaction requiring methylcobalamin as a coenzyme is the conversion of homocysteine into methionine (see Figs. 9.29 and 9.30). This reaction occurs in the cytoplasm of the cell. To form the methylcobalamin needed in methionine synthesis, cobalamin, bound to the methionine synthetase (homocysteine methyl transferase) apoenzyme, picks up the methyl group from N^5 methyl THF and transfers it to homocysteine, thereby

producing methionine and free THF. THF can then be converted into any of its coenzyme forms. This reaction explains in large part the synergism between folate and vitamin B_{12}. Since the formation of N^5 methyl THF is irreversible, a vitamin B_{12} deficiency traps body folate in the methyl form. This is known as the folate methyl trap hypothesis (see p. 266).

Nitrous oxide has been shown to inhibit the activity of methionine synthetase; it reacts with cobalamin, converting the cobalt from a +1 to a +3 oxidation state. Vitamin B_{12}, to function as methylcobalamin coenzyme, must contain cobalt present in its reduced state, +1 [1,12]. Individuals who are vitamin B_{12} deficient may exhibit deterioration of nervous system function following nitrous oxide anesthesia [13].

Two reactions require adenosylcobalamin (Figs. 9.35 and 9.36). These reactions are catalyzed by mutases and occur in the mitochondria. First, adenosylcobalamin is needed for methylmalonyl CoA mutase, which converts L-methylmalonyl CoA to succinyl CoA (Fig. 9.35). L-methylmalonyl CoA is generated from propionyl CoA. Propionyl CoA, which arises from the oxidation of methionine, isoleucine, threonine, and odd-chain fatty acids, is converted into D-methylmalonyl CoA in an ATP-, Mg^{+2}-, and biotin-dependent reaction (Fig. 9.35). L-methylmalonyl CoA is made from the D form through the action of racemase. Methylmalonyl CoA mutase requires adenosylcobalamin to convert L-methylmalonyl CoA to succinyl CoA, the Krebs cycle intermediate (Fig. 9.35). With a deficiency of vitamin B_{12}, mutase activity is impaired, and methylmalonyl CoA and methylmalonic acid, formed from hydrolysis of methylmalonyl CoA, accumulate in body fluids. Genetic defects in methylmalonyl CoA mutase and adenosylcobalamin synthesis have also been demonstrated and result in the accumulation of methylmalonyl CoA and methylmalonic acid.

Leucine aminomutase also requires adenosylcobalamin (Fig. 9.36). This enzyme isomerizes L-leucine and beta-leucine. Beta-leucine generated from intestinal bacteria may be converted to L-leucine within the body [8]. Alternately, beta leucine generated from L-leucine may undergo subsequent transamination in a vitamin B_6 (PLP)-dependent reaction and provide an alternate pathway for leucine catabolism.

Metabolism and Excretion

Very little evidence exists to support any extensive degradation of cobalamin. Whole-body turnover of vitamin B_{12} is approximately 0.1%/day and loss of the vitamin is due primarily to fecal excretion, not catabolism

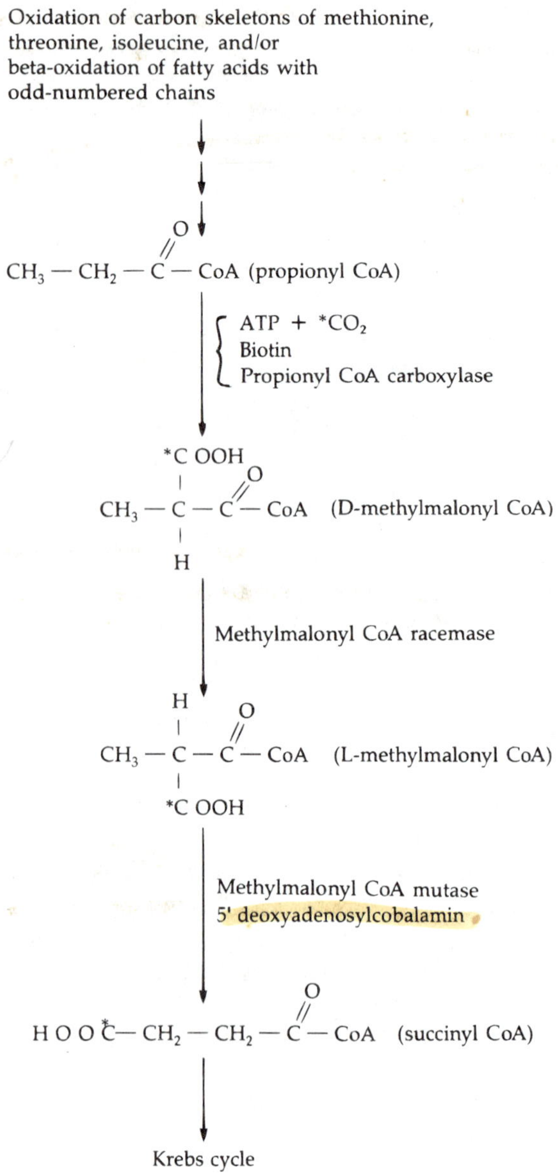

Oxidation of carbon skeletons of methionine, threonine, isoleucine, and/or beta-oxidation of fatty acids with odd-numbered chains

$$CH_3 - CH_2 - \overset{\overset{O}{\|}}{C} - CoA \quad \text{(propionyl CoA)}$$

$$\left\{ \begin{array}{l} ATP + {}^*CO_2 \\ Biotin \\ Propionyl\ CoA\ carboxylase \end{array} \right.$$

$$CH_3 - \overset{\overset{*C\ OOH}{|}}{\underset{|}{C}} - \overset{\overset{O}{\|}}{C} - CoA \quad \text{(D-methylmalonyl CoA)}$$
$$H$$

Methylmalonyl CoA racemase

$$CH_3 - \overset{\overset{H}{|}}{\underset{|}{C}} - \overset{\overset{O}{\|}}{C} - CoA \quad \text{(L-methylmalonyl CoA)}$$
$${}^*C\ OOH$$

Methylmalonyl CoA mutase
5' deoxyadenosylcobalamin

$$HOO{}^*\overset{}{C} - CH_2 - CH_2 - \overset{\overset{O}{\|}}{C} - CoA \quad \text{(succinyl CoA)}$$

Krebs cycle

FIGURE 9.35 Role of vitamin B_{12} in oxidation of odd-numbered chain fatty acids and selected amino acids.

[11]. Little urinary excretion of vitamin B_{12} occurs. Most of cobalamin excretion occurs via the bile, although 65 to 75% of the cobalamin, up to 5 μg/day, secreted into the gastrointestinal tract is reabsorbed in the ileum.

Recommended Dietary Allowance

The RDA for vitamin B_{12} is based on the amount of the vitamin necessary to initiate a hematologic response in strict vegetarians as well as in patients with pernicious

anemia. Because patients with pernicious anemia lack IF and are unable to reabsorb the vitamin excreted in the bile or consumed in the diet, their need for exogenous vitamin B_{12} is greater than in normal people. These patients need injections of as much as 1 μg daily for a satisfactory hematologic response, while an intake of 0.65 μg was sufficient to elicit response in vitamin B_{12}-deficient vegetarians [2,11].

Measuring with accuracy the vitamin B_{12} body pool size and determining what amount of the vitamin constitutes an ideal pool have not been accomplished. Nevertheless, studies of vitamin B_{12} nutriture and turnover rate in healthy subjects have led to the belief that 1 μg/day can be expected to sustain normal people [2,11]. The 1980 RDA for vitamin B_{12} was set at 3 μg/day and allowed maintenance of an upper-limit body pool size [14]. The 1980 to 1985 RDA Committee formulated a RDI of 2 μg/day for vitamin B_{12}. This lower level was chosen because no proven advantage has been associated with maintenance of a higher-than-normal body pool size [2,11]. Two micrograms daily was also chosen for the 1989 RDA for vitamin B_{12} [2].

Deficiency—Megaloblastic, Macrocytic Anemia

Inadequate absorption of the vitamin rather than inadequate dietary intake is responsible for more than 95% of the vitamin B_{12} deficiency seen in the United States. Although a strict vegetarian diet can produce a deficiency of the vitamin, clinical symptoms may not appear for up to 20 to 30 years on such a diet [6]. An exception would be the infant and/or very young child maintained on unfortified foods of plant origin; vitamin B_{12}-fortified tofu provides an excellent source of the vitamin.

Vitamin B_{12} deficiency occurs in stages. Initially, serum concentrations diminish as indicated by low holotranscobalamin II. Secondly, cell concentrations of the vitamin diminish. Thirdly, biochemical deficiency occurs, as evidenced by decreased DNA synthesis, and by elevated homocysteine and methylmalonic acid concentrations in the serum. Finally, anemia occurs [15].

The megaloblastic anemia associated with a vitamin B_{12} deficiency is detailed under folic acid deficiency (p. 268) since deficiencies of both vitamins result in megaloblastic anemia. In fact, the megaloblastic anemia due to a vitamin B_{12} deficiency can be corrected with large doses of folate [16]. The neuropathy, characterized by demyelination of nerves, caused by a lack of vitamin B_{12} is not responsive to folate therapy, however. The cause of the neuropathy may be related to the availability of methionine [6,17]. The neuropathy can be ame-

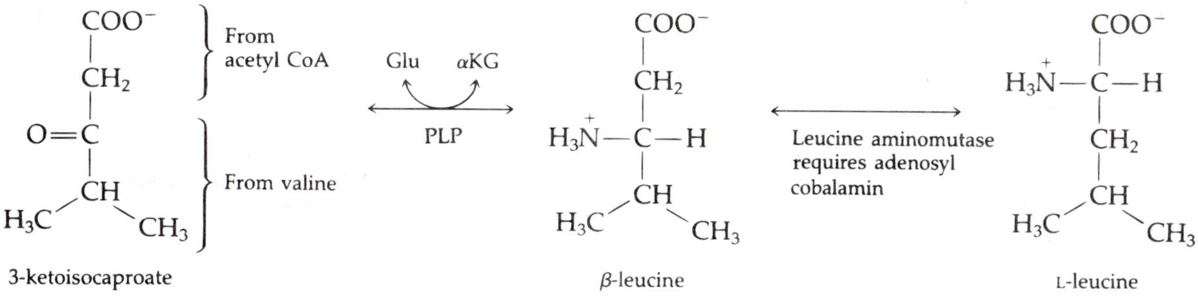

FIGURE 9.36 Isomerization of leucine by a vitamin B_{12}- dependent enzyme.

liorated through increased exogenous methionine or an accelerated production of methionine from homocysteine, a reaction that requires vitamin B_{12}. An inadequate amount of methionine caused by a deficiency of vitamin B_{12} decreases the availability of S-adenosylmethionine (SAM). SAM is required for methylation reactions, essential to the myelin maintenance and thus neural function. SAM deficiency in the nervous system (that is, cerebrospinal fluid) has been suggested in the pathogenesis of cobalamin neuropathy [16]. In addition, plasma vitamin B_{12} concentrations have been reported to be inversely associated with plasma homocysteine concentrations [18,19]. Elevated plasma homocysteine concentrations are thought to play a role in early onset (≤ 50 years) coronary heart disease, and may be lowered with vitamin B_{12} and/or folate supplements [18].

Population groups in which a vitamin B_{12} deficiency is most often encountered are the elderly, alcoholics, and gastrectomy patients. In all these groups, absorption is usually impaired. Conditions and populations associated with increased need for intake include those with a lack of IF secretion (gastrectomy and destruction of gastric mucosa), those with decreased absorptive surface (blind loop syndrome associated with intestinal surgery, ileal resection, celiac and tropical sprue, ileitis, Zollinger-Ellison syndrome), and those who may ingest a diet low in vitamin B_{12} (strict vegetarians). In addition, people with parasitic infections such as tapeworms may develop a vitamin B_{12} deficiency due to use of the vitamin by the parasite and consequent limited availability to the infected person.

Toxicity

Although no clear toxicity from massive doses of vitamin B_{12} has ever been recorded, neither has there been noted any benefit from an excessive intake of the vitamin by nondeficient people [2].

Assessment of Nutriture

Serum B_{12} concentrations are commonly used to assess nutriture.

	Vitamin B_{12} Status	
	Deficient	Adequate
Serum B_{12} (pg/mL)	< 100	> 100

Red blood cell vitamin B_{12} concentrations can also be used, but are less specific, decreasing with both cobalamin and folate deficiencies. Other tests used to assess vitamin B_{12} nutriture are found under "Assessment of Nutriture" in the folate section (p. 269).

The Schilling test may be used to determine problems of vitamin B_{12} absorption (that is, IF insufficiency). The test involves oral administration of radioactive vitamin B_{12}. Urinary excretion of the vitamin is measured. Below-normal urinary excretion of the vitamin suggests impaired absorption. Elevated concentrations of methylmalonic acid in the urine are also used to detect cobalamin deficiency.

References Cited for Vitamin B_{12}

1. Seatharam B, Alpers DH. Absorption and transport of cobalamin (vitamin B-12). Ann Rev Nutr 1982;2: 343–369.
2. National Research Council. Recommended dietary allowances, 10th ed. Washington, DC: National Academy Press, 1989;158–165.
3. Sandberg DP, Begley JA, Hall CA. The content, binding and forms of vitamin B_{12} in milk. Am J Clin Nutr 1981;34:1717–1724.
4. Ellenbogen L, Cooper BA. Vitamin B_{12}. In: Machlin LJ., ed. Handbook of vitamins, 2nd ed. New York: Dekker, 1991:491–536.

5. Herbert V. Vitamin B$_{12}$. In: Brown ML, ed. Present knowledge in nutrition, 6th ed. Washington, DC: The Nutrition Foundation, 1990:170–178.

6. Davis RE. Clinical chemistry of vitamin B$_{12}$. Adv Clin Chem 1984;24:163–216.

7. Sauberlich HE. Bioavailability of vitamins. Prog Food Nutr Sci 1985;9:1–33.

8. Bender DA. Nutritional biochemistry of the vitamins. New York: Cambridge University Press, 1992:269–317.

9. Herbert V. Recommended dietary intakes (RDI) of vitamin B-12 in humans. Am J Clin Nutr 1987;45:671–678.

10. Sauberlich HE. Vitamins—how much is for keeps? Nutr Today 1987;22:20–28.

11. Herbert V, Das KC. Folic acid and vitamin B$_{12}$. In: Shils ME, Olson JA, Shike M., eds. Modern nutrition in health and disease, 8th ed. Philadelphia: Lea and Febiger, 1994:402–425.

12. Metz J. Cobalamin deficiency and the pathogenesis of nervous system disease. Ann Rev Nutr 1992;12:59–79.

13. Flippo TS, Holder WD. Neurologic degeneration associated with nitrous oxide anesthesia in patients with vitamin B$_{12}$ deficiency. Archives Surg 1993;128:1391–1395.

14. National Research Council. Recommended dietary allowances, 9th ed. Washington, DC: National Academy of Sciences, 1980;113–120.

15. Herbert V. Staging of vitamin B-12 (cobalamin) status in vegetarians. Am J Clin Nutr 1994;59(suppl):1213S–1222S.

16. Council on Scientific Affairs, American Medical Association. Vitamin preparations as dietary supplements and as therapeutic agents. JAMA 1987;257:1929–1936.

17. Metz J. Pathogenesis of cobalamin neuropathy: Deficiency of nervous system S-adenosylmethionine. Nutr Rev 1993;51:12–15.

18. Pancharuniti N, Lewis CA, Sauberlich HE, Perkins LL, Go RCP, Alvarez JO, Masaluso M, Acton RT, Copeland RB, Cousins AL, Gore TB, Cornwell PE, Roseman JM. Plasma homocyst(e)ine, folate, and vitamin B-12 concentrations and risk for early-onset coronary artery disease. Am J Clin Nutr 1994;59:940–948.

19. Mansoor MA, Ueland PM, Svardal AM. Redox status and protein binding of plasma homocysteine and other aminothiols in patients with hyperhomocysteinemia due to cobalamin deficiency. Am J Clin Nutr 1994;59: 631–635.

Additional References

Herbert V. The 1986 Herman Award Lecture. Nutrition science as a continually unfolding story: The folate and vitamin B$_{12}$ paradigm. Am J Clin Nutr 1987;46:387–402.

Shane B, Stokstad ELR. Vitamin B$_{12}$-folate interrelationships. Ann Rev Nutr 1985;5:115–141.

Coombs GF. The vitamins. San Diego, CA: Academic Press, 1992:377–392.

VITAMIN B$_6$

Vitamin B$_6$ exists as several vitamers, the structural formulas of which are given in Figure 9.37. These vitamers are interchangeable and comparably active (Fig. 9.38). Pyridoxine represents the alcohol form, pyridoxal the aldehyde form, and pyridoxamine the amine form. Each has a 5'-phosphate derivative.

Sources

All vitamers are found in food. Pyridoxine, the most stable of the compounds, is found almost exclusively in plant foods. Very small amounts, if any, of pyridoxal and pyridoxamine or its phosphorylated form are present in plant foods. Excellent sources of vitamin B$_6$ in commonly consumed foods are bananas, navy beans, and walnuts. The other vitamers, primarily pyridoxal phosphate and pyridoxamine phosphate, are found in animal products, with sirloin steak, salmon, and the light meat of chicken being rich sources [1,2].

In some plants, vitamin B$_6$ is found in a conjugated form, pyridoxine beta-glucoside. Mammalian glycosidase is not thought to be able to free the pyridoxine from the glucoside. Thus, unless hydrolyzed by glucosidase from intestinal flora, this form of the vitamin is not well utilized [2].

The bioavailability of vitamin B$_6$ from different food sources is also influenced by the extent and type of processing to which the foods are subjected. Much of the vitamin originally present in foods can be lost through processing, including, for example, heating, canning, milling of wheat, sterilization, and freezing [1–3].

Digestion, Absorption, and Transport

For absorption of vitamin B$_6$ to occur, the phosphorylated vitamers must be dephosphorylated. Alkaline phosphatase, found at the intestinal brush border, or other intestinal phosphatases hydrolyze the phosphate to yield either pyridoxine (PN), pyridoxal (PL), and pyridoxamine (PM).

Absorption of PL, PN, and PM occurs primarily in the jejunum by passive diffusion. At physiologic intakes, the vitamin is absorbed rapidly in its free form; however, when the phosphorylated vitamers are ingested in high concentrations, some of these compounds may be absorbed per se [3]. Absorption of pyridoxine glucosides may also occur by passive diffusion; however, the complex will be excreted unchanged in the urine [4]. Overall absorption of vitamin B$_6$ furnished by the average U.S. diet ranges from 71 to 82%.

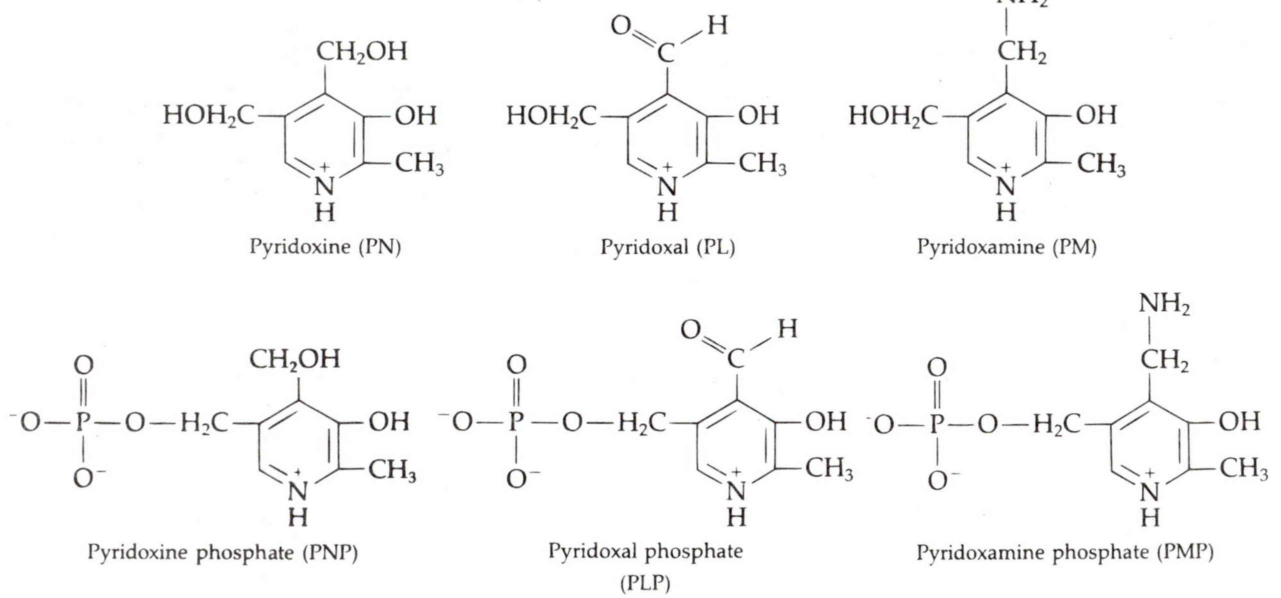

FIGURE 9.37 Vitamin B$_6$ structures.

Within the intestinal cell, PN may be converted into pyridoxine phosphate (PNP) by the action of pyridoxine kinase using ATP. PL is typically converted to pyridoxal phosphate (PLP) also through the action of kinase and ATP. PNP may be converted to PLP through the action of pyridoxine phosphate oxidase, which requires riboflavin as FMN.

PLP is the main form (about 60% of the total) of the vitamin found in the blood; it does not cross cell membranes without hydrolysis to PL by extracellular alkaline phosphatase [4]. Other forms of the vitamin, especially PL (comprising about 14% of blood vitamin B$_6$ content) also may be present in the blood. PL may be found in both red blood cells and in plasma. In the erythrocytes, PL binds to the alpha chain of hemoglobin and PLP binds to the beta chain [5]. In the plasma, both PLP and PL are bound to albumin during transport. Plasma PLP, however, is very tightly bound to albumin and probably is unavailable for use by the tissues. Another 15% of the vitamin circulates as PM, which also can be used after tissue uptake.

The liver is the main organ that takes up by passive diffusion the newly absorbed vitamin B$_6$. The liver stores about 5 to 10% of the vitamin [6]. Unphosphorylated forms of the vitamin are typically phosphorylated within the cytoplasm of the hepatocyte (liver cell) as shown in Figure 9.38. PN and PMP are then generally converted to PLP. Figure 9.38 depicts the interconversion of the B$_6$ vitamers, a process that occurs mainly in the liver. From the liver, PLP and PL are released for transport to extrahepatic tissues.

Extrahepatic tissues, especially muscles, possess the majority (75 to 80% [6]) of PLP. Only PL is taken up by these tissues and, thus, PLP in blood must be hydrolyzed before cellular uptake. Within the cell, PL is phosphorylated by pyridoxine kinase. Pyridoxine kinase is found in almost all tissues, and phosphorylation traps the vitamin in the cells. Most tissues, however, lack sufficient PNP/PMP oxidase, which converts PNP and PMP into the coenzyme form of the vitamin, PLP. PNP/PMP oxidase is found mainly in the liver and intestine, but also in the kidney, brain, and red blood cell, although the activity in the latter cells is low [4]. PNP/PMP oxidase, crucial to activity of vitamin B$_6$, is a flavin mononucleotide (FMN)-dependent enzyme. Thus, normal vitamin B$_6$ metabolism is closely interrelated with riboflavin.

Functions and Mechanisms of Action

The coenzyme form of vitamin B$_6$ is associated with a vast number of enzymes, the majority of which are involved in amino acid metabolism. PLP, through the formation of a Schiff base (the product formed by an amino group and an aldehyde), labilizes all of the bonds around the α-carbon of the amino acid. The specific bond that

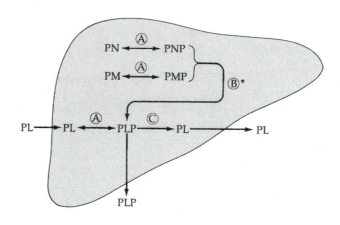

FIGURE 9.38 Vitamin B$_6$ metabolism in the liver. *Oxidase is found mainly in the liver and enterocytes.

Enzymes
(A) Kinase—ATP dependent
(B) PMP and PNP oxidase*—FMN dependent
(C) Phosphatase

is broken is determined by the catalytic groups of the particular enzyme to which PLP is attached. The covalent bonds of an α-amino acid that can be made labile by its binding to specific PLP-containing enzymes are given in Figure 9.39.

Reactions catalyzed by PLP include transamination (which can also be catalyzed by PMP), decarboxylation, transulfhydration and desulfhydration, cleavage, synthesis, and racemization. Glycogen metabolism and the action of steroid hormones also appear to involve vitamin B$_6$.

Transamination Of particular importance are the transamination reactions in which PMP as well as PLP can serve as a coenzyme. The most common aminotransferases for which PLP (or PMP) is a coenzyme are glutamate oxaloacetate transaminase (GOT) (also called aspartic amino transferase (AST)) and glutamate pyruvate transaminase (GPT) (also called alanine aminotransferase (ALT)) (Fig. 7.13). Figure 9.40a and b show the two phases of transamination and demonstrate how PLP forms a Schiff base. In the first phase, the corresponding alpha keto acid of the amino acid is produced along with PMP. In the second phase, the transamination cycle is completed as a new alpha keto acid substrate receives the amino group from the PMP. The corresponding amino acid is generated, along with regeneration of PLP.

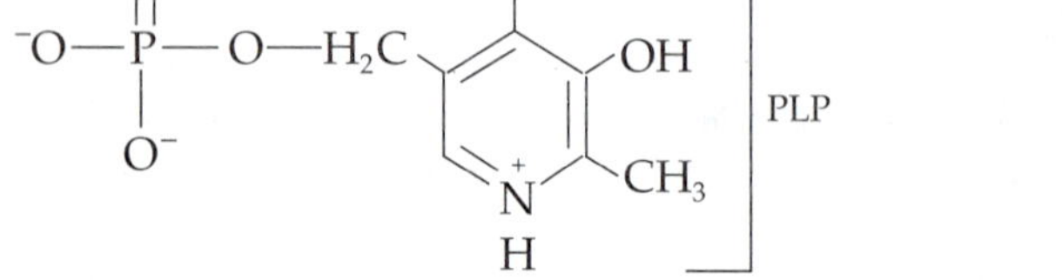

Decarboxylation Common decarboxylation reactions include the formation of γ-aminobutyric acid (GABA) from glutamate (Fig. 7.26) and the production of serotonin from 5-hydroxytryptophan (Fig. 7.24).

Transulfhydration and Desulfhydration PLP is required for transulfhydration reactions in which cysteine is synthesized from methionine (Fig. 9.41). Both cystathionine synthase and cystathionine lyase require PLP. Cysteine undergoes desulfhydration followed by transamination to generate pyruvate.

Cleavage An example of a cleavage reaction in which PLP is required is the removal of the hydroxymethyl group from serine. In this reaction PLP is the coenzyme for a transferase that transfers the hydroxy-

FIGURE 9.39 The covalent bonds of an alpha amino acid that can be made labile by its binding to PLP-containing enzymes.

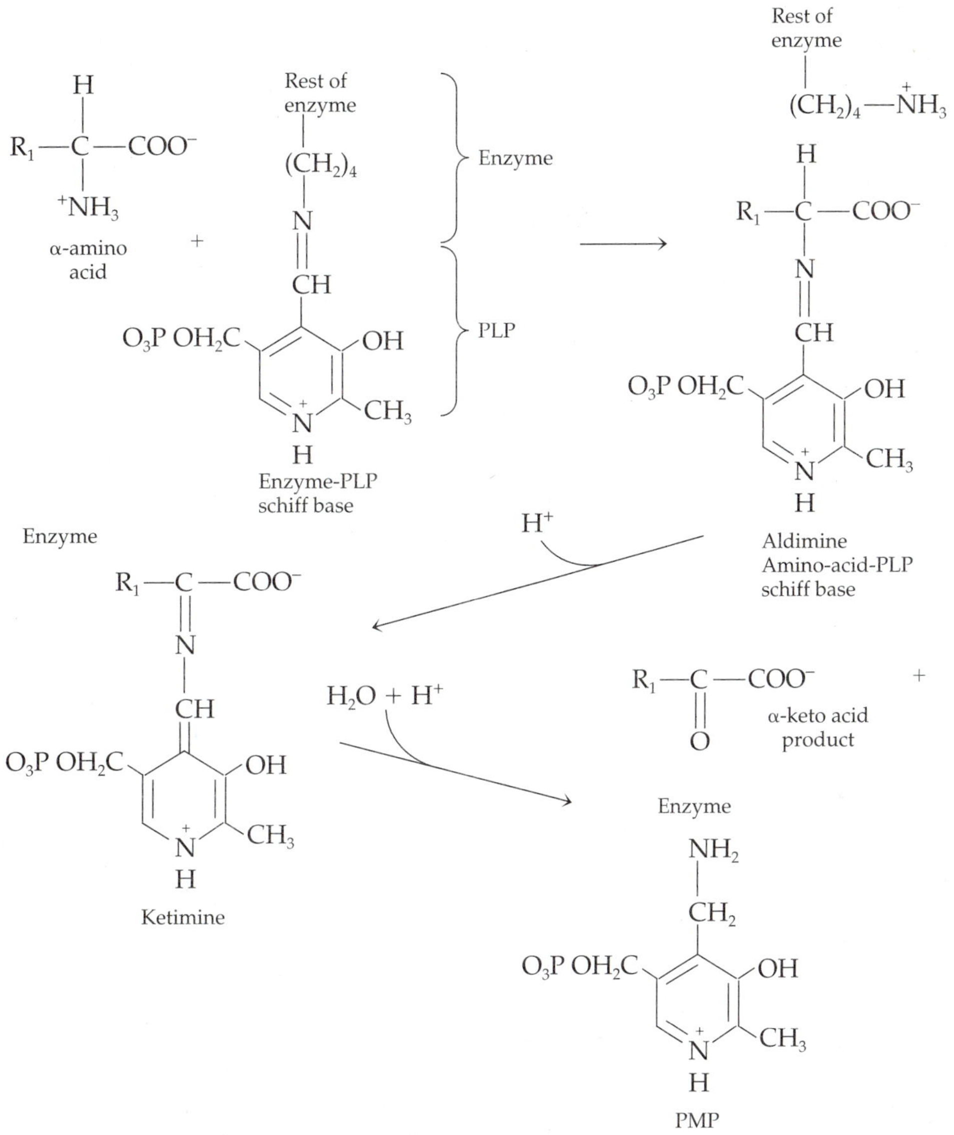

FIGURE 9.40 (a) The role of vitamin B_6 in transamination, Phase 1.

methyl group of serine to tetrahydrofolate (THF) so that glycine is formed (p. 264, Fig. 9.29; 265).

Racemization PLP is required by racemases that catalyze the interconversion of D- and L- amino acids. Although such reactions are more prevalent in bacterial metabolism, some occur in humans.

Synthesis Vitamin B_6 is also necessary in the synthesis of heme. PLP is required for delta-aminolevulinic acid synthetase, which catalyzes the condensation of glycine with succinyl CoA to form δ-aminolevulinic acid (ALA) in the mitochondria of the cell (Fig. 9.42). ALA moves into the cytosol of the cell, where it is used to synthesize porphobilinogen (PBG), the parent pyrrole compound in porphyrin synthesis. Through a series of reactions, PBG is converted into protoporphyrin IX. Protoporphyrin IX with the addition of Fe^{+2} by ferrocheletase forms heme. Heme synthesis is shown in Figure 12.5.

Niacin (NAD) synthesis from tryptophan also requires an important PLP-dependent reaction. Specifi-

(b)

FIGURE 9.40 continued (b) The role of vitamin B$_6$ in transamination, Phase 2.

cally, kynureninase required for the conversion of 3-hydroxykynurenine to 3-hydroxyanthranilate requires vitamin B$_6$ as a coenzyme (Fig. 9.18).

Other compounds synthesized in the body in vitamin B$_6$-dependent reactions include histamine from the amino acid histidine, carnitine, a nitrogen-containing compound (p. 230), and compounds, such as taurine and dopamine, with neuromodulatory functions.

Glycogen Catabolism The function of PLP in glycogen degradation is poorly understood. Glycogen is catabolized by glycogen phosphorylase to form glucose 1-PO$_4$ (p. 83); vitamin B$_6$ is required for glycogen phos-

phorylase activity. The mechanism of action of the coenzyme appears to be different from that exerted with other enzymes. The phosphate of the coenzyme is believed to be involved as a proton shuttle or buffer to stabilize the compound and permit covalent bonding of the phosphate to form glucose 1-PO$_4$ [4]. Most of vitamin B$_6$ found in muscle is present as PLP, which is in turn bound to glycogen phosphorylase [7].

Steroid Hormone Action Vitamin B$_6$ as PLP has been shown to react with lysine residues in steroid hormone receptor proteins to prevent or interfere with hormone binding. These receptor proteins mediate nuclear

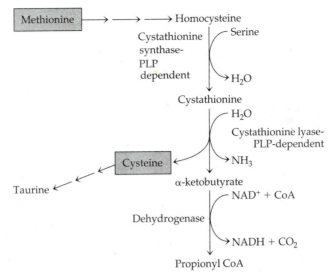

FIGURE 9.41 Cysteine synthesis from methionine requires vitamin B_6.

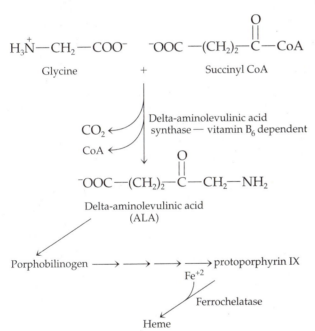

FIGURE 9.42 Synthesis of delta-aminolevulinic acid by vitamin B_6-dependent delta-aminolevulinic acid synthase.

uptake of the steroid hormone and the interaction of the nucleoproteins with the DNA [6]. PLP has also been shown to bind to receptors on steroids [5]. Thus, vitamin B_6 appears to be able to diminish the actions of steroids. Diminishing the action of, for example, glucocorticoid hormones can in turn influence metabolism of protein, carbohydrate, and lipid.

Metabolism and Excretion

The intracellular level of PLP is believed to be controlled by enzymatic hydrolysis. The suggested mech-

anism for control lies primarily with the concentration of the PLP-binding proteins in the cells. When these proteins are saturated, then the newly synthesized PLP will be hydrolyzed by intracellular phosphatase. Another possibility for regulating PLP formed in the cell is product inhibition of PNP/PMP oxidase, operative primarily in the liver and intestinal cells (Fig. 9.38) [3].

Pyridoxic acid (PIC) is the major excretory product resulting from the oxidation of PL by either NAD-dependent aldehyde dehydrogenase, found in all tissues, or by FAD-dependent aldehyde oxidases found in the liver and kidneys. The amount of PIC excreted is thought to be more indicative of recent vitamin intake than of vitamin stores because newly formed PLP is not freely exchangeable with endogenous PLP [3]. Newly formed PLP is instead quickly converted to PL and PIC and is released into the plasma.

The form in which the vitamin is ingested appears to influence the percentage of intake that is excreted as PIC. When large doses (100 mg) of the vitamin were given as PL, PM, or PN, 90% of the PL and PM appeared in the urine as PIC within 36 hours. In contrast, only 70% of the PN was excreted as PIC; much of the PN was excreted as such in the urine within two hours. It appears that when PN is administered at high levels, the kidney tubules reduce plasma content of the vitamer by secreting some of it into the urine [8].

Recommended Dietary Allowances

Adequate intake of vitamin B_6 has been estimated through depletion and repletion studies. The requirement for vitamin B_6 has been found to be related to the level of protein intake [9]. Therefore, in formulating the

RDA, consideration was given to the average protein intake among the United States population. Given the assumption that 126 g protein daily represents the upper limit of a customary intake by adult males, the RDA for vitamin B_6 for this population group is set at 2.0 mg daily. Because women are expected to consume a little less protein (upper limit 100 g daily), the RDA for vitamin B_6 for this group is reduced to 1.6 mg daily [10]. An intake of 0.016 mg vitamin B_6/1 g protein is considered sufficient to meet the needs of adults under normal conditions [10].

Deficiency

Vitamin B_6 deficiency is relative rare in the United States. In the 1950s, deficiency occurred in infants due to severe heat treatment of infant milk. The heat processing resulted in a reaction between the PLP and the epsilon amino group of lysine in the milk proteins to form pyridoxyl-lysine, which possesses little vitamin activity. Signs of vitamin B_6 deficiency [11] include sleepiness, fatigue, cheilosis, glossitis, stomatitis in adults, and abnormal EEGs, seizures, and convulsions in infants. A hypochromic, microcytic anemia may also result from a vitamin B_6 deficiency due to impaired heme synthesis. Deficiency also alters calcium and magnesium metabolism [12] and impairs niacin synthesis from tryptophan [7].

Groups particularly at risk for vitamin B_6 deficiency are (1) breastfed infants born with low plasma vitamin B_6 levels; (2) the elderly, who have a poor intake of the vitamin and may also have accelerated hydrolysis of PLP and oxidation of PL to PIC; (3) people who consume excessive amounts of alcohol (alcohol can impair conversion of PN and PM to PLP, and the presence of acetaldehyde formed from ethanol metabolism may enhance hydrolysis of PLP to PL with subsequent formation of PIC in blood) [1,2]; (4) renal patients on maintenance dialysis, which causes an abnormal loss of the vitamin; and (5) people on a variety of drug therapies that inhibit activity of the vitamin, primary among which are those employing isoniazid, penicillamine, corticosteroids, and/or anticonvulsants. Pregnant women exhibit increased xanthurenic acid excretion with a tryptophan load, but it is uncertain whether this is an indication of a vitamin insufficiency or is a normal physiologic condition [8–10]. Other conditions and populations with possible increased needs for the vitamin include those with hyperthyroidism, high protein intake, liver disease, or stress.

Toxicity

Pharmacologic doses of vitamin B_6 have been advocated for the prevention or treatment of a variety of disease states including atherosclerotic heart disease, carpal tunnel syndrome, premenstrual syndrome, depression, muscular fatigue, paresthesia, and autism [7,13]. Although some beneficial results from megadoses of the vitamin have been noted in selected individuals, indiscriminate use of the vitamin is not without risk. Adults chronically ingesting 2 to 6 g pyridoxine per day have been reported to suffer from sensory and peripheral neuropathy. Some symptoms include unsteady gait, numbness of the feet and hands, impaired tendon reflexes, and paresthesia [7,14]. Excessive amounts of pyridoxine appear to cause degeneration of dorsal root ganglia in the spinal cord, loss of myelination, and degeneration of sensory fibers in peripheral nerves [4,13–15]. The minimal dosage at which toxicity occurs is not clear [7].

Assessment of Nutriture

A commonly used index of vitamin B_6 nutriture is a functional test measuring xanthurenic acid excretion following tryptophan loading (100 mg tryptophan/kg body weight). Abnormally high xanthurenic acid (>25 mg in 6 hours) excretion is found in vitamin B_6 deficiency because 3-hydroxykynurenine, an intermediate in tryptophan metabolism, cannot lose its alanine moiety and be converted to 3-hydroxyanthranilate, as should occur (Fig. 9.18). Instead, 3-hydroxykynurenine becomes xanthurenic acid. Interpretation of this test is sometimes difficult due to factors other than vitamin B_6 in tryptophan metabolism. Acceptable xanthurenic acid excretion following the tryptophan load is <25 mg per 6 hours.

Plasma PLP assays are being used more frequently to assess vitamin B_6 nutriture, although intakes of both the vitamin and protein among other factors will affect plasma concentrations of PLP. Plasma PLP concentrations in excess of 30 nmol/L are thought to suggest adequate vitamin status [16].

Estimates of urinary vitamin B_6 and pyridoxic acid have also been used to assess status of vitamin B_6. Urinary vitamin B_6 excretion measured over several 24-hour urine collections for a period of 1 to 3 weeks is recommended to more accurately assess vitamin B_6. Urinary vitamin B_6 excretion in comparison to creatinine excretion is also used such that urinary levels of <20 μg/g creatinine suggests B_6 deficiency, while excretion >20 μg/g creatinine suggests acceptable vitamin B_6 status. Urinary pyridoxic acid excretion is considered to be a short-term indicator of vitamin B_6 status [16].

Measurement of erythrocyte transaminase activity before and after vitamin B_6 addition are also useful in determining vitamin B_6 nutriture; however, due to a variety of limitations with the assays, these tests are better used as an adjunct to other tests. Erythrocyte transaminase index examines activity of erythrocyte glutamic oxaloacetic transaminase (EGOT) (also called *aspartic amino transferase*, or EAST) after the addition of vitamin B_6. This assay and the assay discussed next are thought to represent long-term vitamin status. Deficient vitamin B_6 status is suggested by activity of >1.8 following the addition of the vitamin [16]. Similarly, if activity of erythrocyte glutamic pyruvic transaminase (EGPT) (also called *alanine aminotransferase*, or EALT) increases >1.25, then B_6 deficiency is suggested while activity of <1.25 indicates adequate status [16,17].

References Cited for Vitamin B_6

1. Sauberlich HE. Bioavailability of vitamins. Prog Food Nutr Sci 1985;9:1–33.
2. Sauberlich HE. Vitamins—how much is for keeps? Nutr Today 1987;22:20–28.
3. Ink SL, Henderson LM. Vitamin B_6 metabolism. Ann Rev Nutr 1984;4:455–470.
4. Bender DA. Nutritional biochemistry of the vitamins. New York: Cambridge University Press, 1992:223–268.
5. Leklem JE. Vitamin B_6. In: Shils ME, Olson JA, Shike M., eds. Modern nutrition in health and disease, 8th ed. Philadelphia: Lea and Febiger, 1994:383–394.
6. Allgood VE, Cidlowski JA. Novel role for vitamin B_6 in steroid hormone action: A link between nutrition and the endocrine system. J Nutr Biochem 1991;2:523–534.
7. Leklem JE. Vitamin B_6. In: Machlin LJ, ed. Handbook of Vitamins, 2nd ed. New York: Dekker, 1991:341–392.
8. Henderson LM. Vitamin B_6. In: Olson RE, Chairman, Broquist HP, Chichester CO, Darby WJ, Kolbye AC, Jr, Stalvey RM, eds. Present knowledge in nutrition, 5th ed. Washington, DC: The Nutrition Foundation, 1984:303–317.
9. Committee on Dietary Allowances, Food and Nutrition Board. Human vitamin B_6 requirements. Washington, DC: National Academy of Sciences, 1978.
10. National Research Council. Recommended dietary allowances, 10th ed. Washington, DC: National Academy Press, 1989;142–150.
11. Coombs GF. The vitamins. San Diego, CA: Academic Press, 1992:311–328.
12. Turlund JR, Betschart AA, Liebman M, Kretsch MJ, Sauberlich HE. Vitamin B_6 depletion followed by repletion with animal or plant source diets and calcium and magnesium metabolism in young women. Am J Clin Nutr 1992;56:905–910.
13. Alhadeff L, Gualtieri CT, Lipton M. Toxic effects of water-soluble vitamins. Nutr Rev 1984;42:33–40.
14. Council on Scientific Affairs, American Medical Association. Vitamin preparations as dietary supplements and as therapeutic agents. JAMA 1987; 257:1929–1936.
15. Sensory neuropathy from megadoses of pyridoxine. Nutr Rev 1984;42:49–51.
16. Leklem JE. Vitamin B_6: A status report. J Nutr 1990;120:1503–1507.
17. Simko MD, Cowell C, Gilbride JA. Nutrition assessment. Rockville, MD: Aspen, 1984.

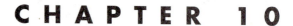

CHAPTER 10

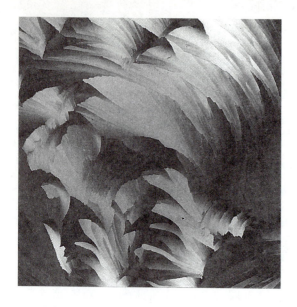

THE FAT-SOLUBLE VITAMINS

Vitamin A

Vitamin D

Vitamin E

Vitamin K

For each vitamin, the following subtopics will be discussed:
> Sources
> Digestion (when applicable), Absorption, and Transport
> Functions and Mechanisms of Action
> Interactions with Other Nutrients (when applicable)
> Metabolism and Excretion
> Recommended Dietary Allowance
> Deficiency
> Toxicity
> Assessment of Nutriture

Perspective: **The Antioxidant Nutrients**

Photo: Photomicrograph of crystallized beta-carotene

This chapter addresses each of the four fat-soluble vitamins, A, D, E, and K. The reader is referred to Chapter 9 for an overview of vitamins and information pertaining to the water-soluble vitamins. The absorption and transport of the fat-soluble vitamins, in contrast to that of the water-soluble vitamins, are closely associated with the absorption and transport of lipids. As with dietary lipids, optimal fat-soluble vitamin absorption requires the presence of bile salts. Similarly, the transport of the fat-soluble vitamins in the body occurs initially by chylomicrons. Moreover, the fat-soluble vitamins are stored in body lipids, although the amount stored varies widely among the four fat-soluble vitamins. Table 10.1 provides an overview of the discovery, functions, deficiency syndrome, foods sources, and the Recommended Dietary Allowance (RDA) of each of the fat-soluble vitamins. Appendix A provides the 1989 RDA for all nutrients and for all age groups.

VITAMIN A

The term *vitamin A* or *preformed vitamin A* is used to refer to retinol (an alcohol) and retinal (the aldehyde form). Retinoic acid is a metabolite of retinal. The term *provitamin A* refers to beta-carotene and other carotenoids that can be converted into retinol.

Sources

Free (all-trans) retinol (Fig. 10.1a) is not generally found in foods, but is present as precursor fatty acid esters, among which the most commonly occurring is retinyl palmitate (Fig. 10.1b). Retinyl esters are found in selected foods of animal origin, primarily egg yolks, butter, whole milk products, liver, and fish liver oils. In pharmaceutical preparations, retinyl acetate is commonly used.

284

TABLE 10.1 The Fat-Soluble Vitamins: Discovery, Function, Deficiency Syndrome, Food Sources, and Recommended Dietary Allowance (RDA)

Vitamin	Discovery	Biochemical or Physiologic Function	Deficiency Syndrome or Symptoms	Good Sources in Rank Order	RDA[a]
Vitamin A (retinol, retinal, retinoic acid) Provitamins: carotenoids, particularly beta-carotene	McCollum (1916)	Synthesis of rhodopsin and other light receptor pigments; unknown metabolites involved in growth and differentiation of epithelia, nervous, bone tissue and immune function	*Children:* poor dark adaptation, xerosis, keratomalacia, growth failure *Adults:* night blindness, xeroderma	Beef liver, sweet potato, carrots, spinach, butternut squash, dandelion greens	1000 μg RE 800 μg RE
Vitamin D Provitamins: ergosterol 7-dehydrocholesterol Vitamin D_2 (ergocalciferol) Vitamin D_3 (cholecalciferol)	McCollum (1922)	Regulator of bone mineral metabolism, primarily calcium	*Children:* rickets *Adults:* osteomalacia	Synthesized in skin exposed to ultraviolet light; fortified milk is the only constantly reliable good source	10 μg[b] 5 μg
Vitamin E tocopherols tocotrienols	Evans and Bishop (1922)	Antioxidant	*Infants:* anemia *Children and Adults:* neuropathy and myopathy	Vegetable seed oils are major source; widely distributed in foods	10 mgαTE 8 mgαTE
Vitamin K phylloquinones menaquinones menadione	Dam (1935)	Activates blood-clotting factors II, VII, IX, X by γ-carboxylating glutamic acid residues; carboxylates bone and kidney proteins	*Children:* hemorrhagic disease of newborns *Adults:* defective blood clotting	Synthesized by intestinal bacteria; green leafy vegetables, soy beans, beef liver	70 μg[c] 60 μg[c]

[a]Adults, aged 19–50 years, males and females.
[b]10 μg aged 19–24 years, both genders, then 5 μg aged 25–50 years, both genders.
[c]For males and females respectively, aged 19–24 years, then increases to 80 μg and 65 μg for males and females, respectively, aged 25–50 years.

Other dietary components providing vitamin A activity are carotenoids, which possess at least one unsubstituted β-ionone ring. Carotenoids, the red, orange, and yellow pigments synthesized by a wide variety of plants, are many in number (over 400), but only about 10% of these pigments have vitamin A activity. The pigment with the greatest vitamin A activity is β-carotene (Fig. 10.1c); two other commonly occurring carotenoids with vitamin A activity are α- and γ-carotene (Fig. 10.1d and e). Alpha- and γ-carotene activity as compared with that of β-carotene ranges from 50 to 54% and 42 to 50%, respectively [1]. These nutritionally active carotenoids are found in a variety of fruits and vegetables. Yellow and orange (brightly colored) vegetables provide significant amounts of carotenoids. All green vegetables contain some β-carotene equivalents, although the pigment cannot be seen because it is masked by chlorophyll.

Digestion, Absorption, and Transport

Carotenes and retinyl esters in foods are often complexed with protein from which they must be released.

Hydrolysis from protein occurs by the action of pepsin in the stomach and other proteolytic enzymes in the proximal small intestine. Hydrolysis of retinyl and carotenoid esters by various esterases occurs at the same time triacylglycerols, phospholipids, and cholesteryl esters are being hydrolyzed by pancreatic enzymes. Pancreatic lipase, cholesterol ester hydrolase, as well as esterases from the intestinal brush border are thought to be responsible for de-esterification [2–5].

The released carotenoids and retinols in the small intestine are solubilized into micellar solutions along with the other fat-soluble food components. The micellar solutions containing the vitamin A diffuse through the glycoprotein layer surrounding the microvilli of the duodenum and jejunum and into the enterocyte. Approximately 70 to 90% of retinol from the diet is absorbed [6,7]. β-Carotene absorption ranges from about 20 to 50% [7,8], but carotenoid absorption may be as low as 5% [3,4]. Carotenoid absorption decreases as carotenoid intake increases. Figure 10.2 depicts the absorption of vitamin A and carotenoids.

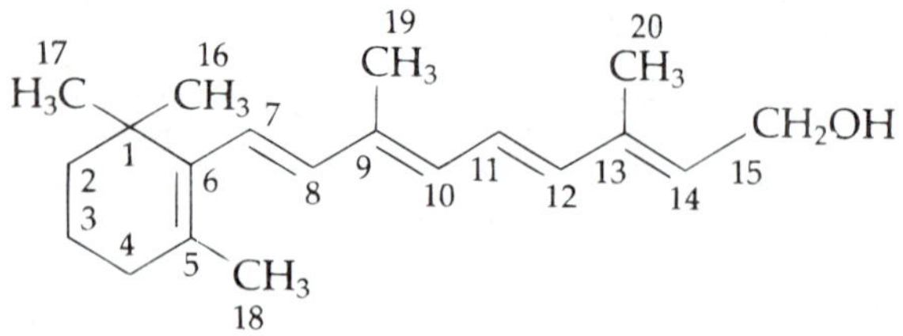

(a) All-trans-retinol

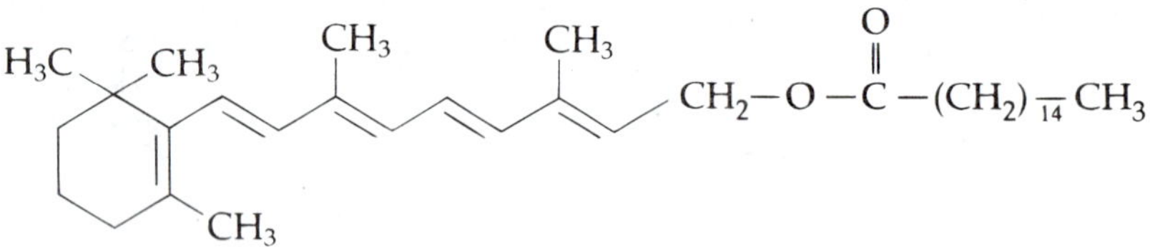

(b) Retinyl palmitate

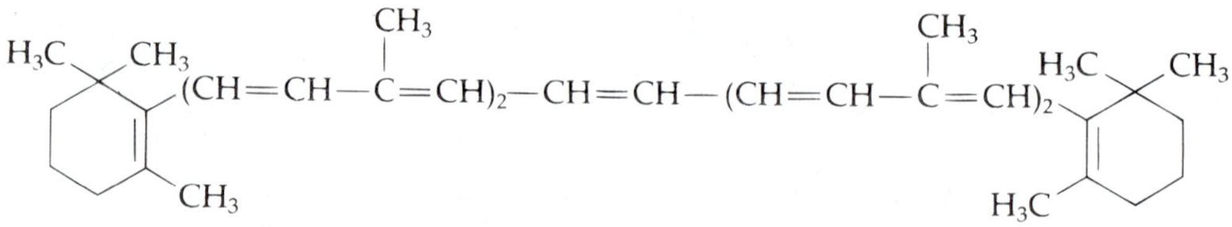

(c) β-carotene

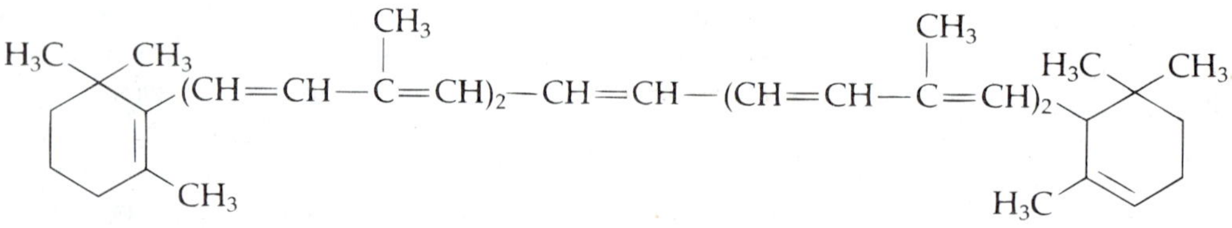

(d) α-carotene

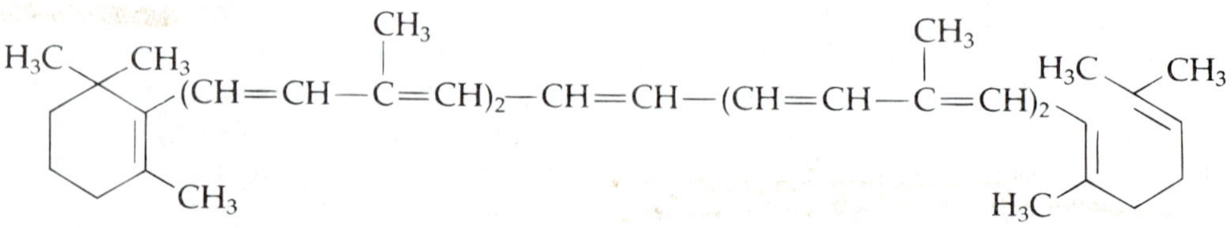

(e) γ-carotene

FIGURE 10.1 Selected forms of vitamin A and carotenoids.

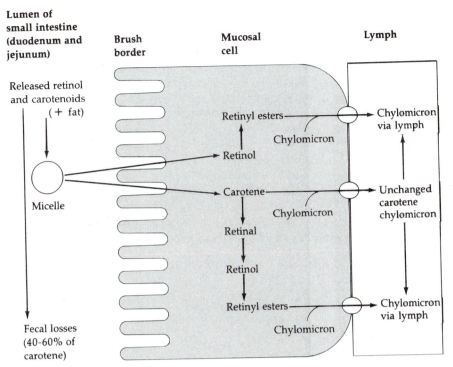

FIGURE 10.2 Absorption of vitamin A.

Within the intestinal mucosal cell (and to a very small extent the liver), β-carotene 15,15′-dioxygenase can convert β-carotene into retinal (Fig. 10.3). Retinal, formed from β-carotene, can subsequently be converted to retinol by retinal reductase, a NADH/NADPH-dependent enzyme. β-Carotene theoretically can produce 2 mol of retinol, but *in vivo* this does not occur because activity of β-carotene 15,15′-dioxygenase is relatively low. Thus, some (up to 30%) β-carotene may leave the intestine without oxidation. It is estimated that 6 μg β-carotene are required to produce the vitamin A activity of 1 μg retinol. See Table 10.2 for factors used for the interconversion of units of vitamin A and carotenoids.

Although the retinal is interconvertible with retinol, some of the retinal may be irreversibly oxidized into retinoic acid (Fig. 10.4) within the intestinal cell. Retinoic acid, in contrast to retinol, is picked up by the portal vein, and transported in the plasma bound tightly to albumin.

Retinol, formed from the oxidation of carotenoids, follows the same metabolic pathways of re-esterification in the intestinal cell as retinol originating from dietary retinyl esters. One of two metabolic pathways may be followed for retinol re-esterification in the enterocyte. The primary pathway involves cellular retinol-binding protein (CRBP) II, whose synthesis may depend on retinoic acid [3,4]. CRBP II binds both retinol and reti-

nal and is present in the cytoplasm of epithelial cells of the small intestine [2]. CRBP II directs the reduction of retinal and subsequent esterification [9]. CRBP II-bound retinol is esterified by lecithin retinol acyl transferase (LRAT) to form mainly retinyl palmitate, but also

TABLE 10.2 Factors Used in Interconversion of Vitamin A Units and Carotenoids

1 retinol equivalent (RE)
= 1 μg all-trans retinol
= 6 μg all-trans β-carotene
= 12 μg other provitamin A carotenoids
= 3.33 IU_a (i.e., the IU of vitamin A)
= 10 IU_c (i.e., the IU of provitamin A carotenoids)
1 international unit of preformed vitamin A (1 IU_a = 0.3 μg of all-trans retinol, and
1 IU_a
= 0.3 RE
= 3 IU_c
= 1.8 μg all-trans β-carotene
= 3.6 μg other provitamin A carotenoids
1 IU of provitamin A carotenoids (1 IU_c) = 0.6 μg of all-trans β-carotene, and
1 IU_c
= 0.1 RE
= 0.33 IU_a
= 0.1 μg all-trans retinol
= 1.2 μg other provitamin A carotenoids

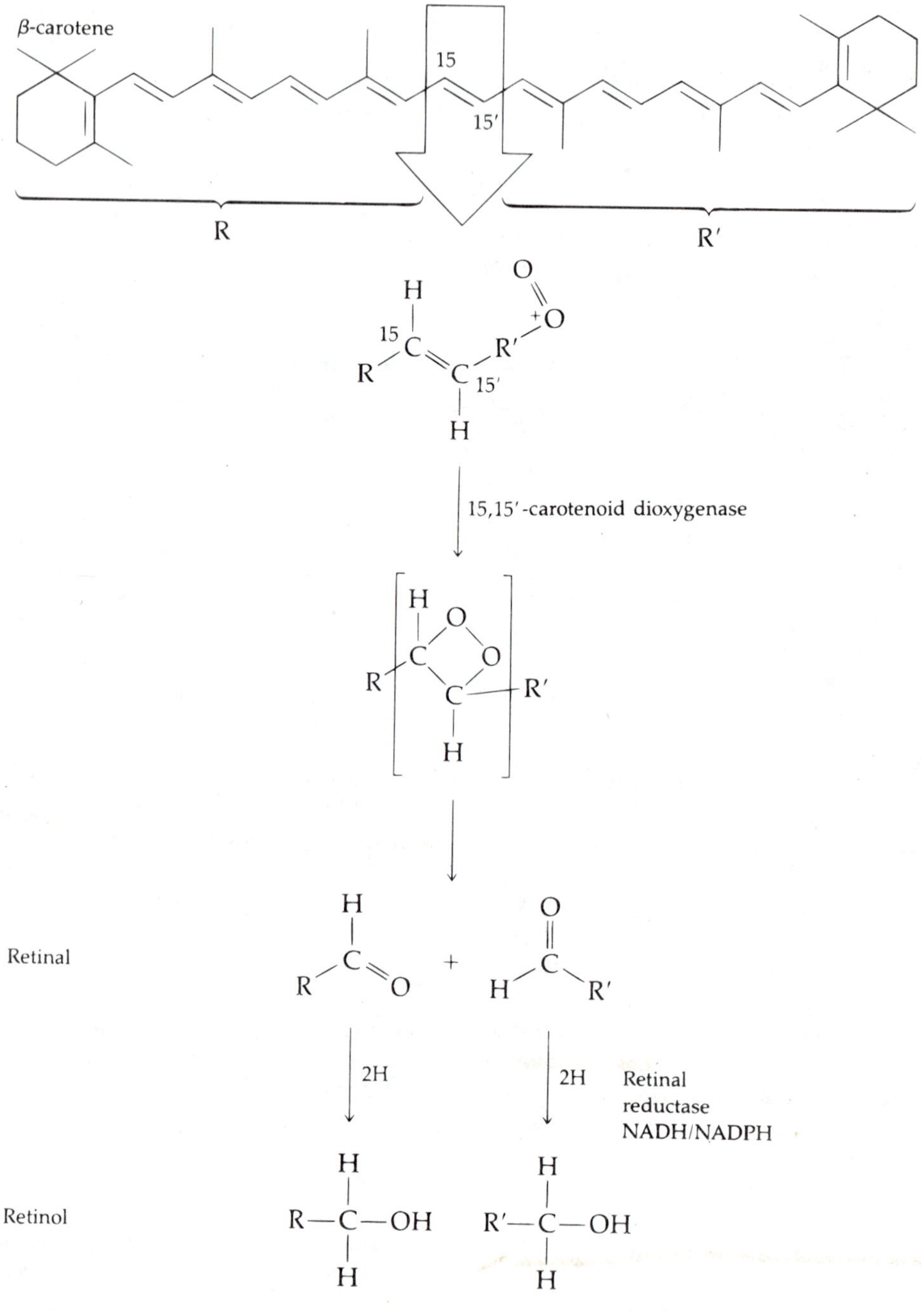

β-carotene

$$15$$

$$15'$$

R   R′

15,15′-carotenoid dioxygenase

Retinal

2H   2H   Retinal
reductase
NADH/NADPH

Retinol

FIGURE 10.3 Cleavage of carotene to retinal and its reduction to retinol.

retinyl stearate and retinyl oleate, among others. The minor second pathway for re-esterification involves binding of retinol to a cellular protein that is non-specific, with subsequent re-esterification by acyl CoA retinol acyl transferase (ARAT) [2,10]. ARAT may serve to esterify retinol when large doses of the vitamin are ingested [11]. The newly formed retinyl esters, along with a small amount of unesterified retinol, and any carotenoids that have been absorbed unchanged, are incorporated into chylomicrons containing cholesterol esters, phospholipid, triacylglycerols, and apoproteins; these chylomicrons are then carried first into the lymphatic system and then into general circulation.

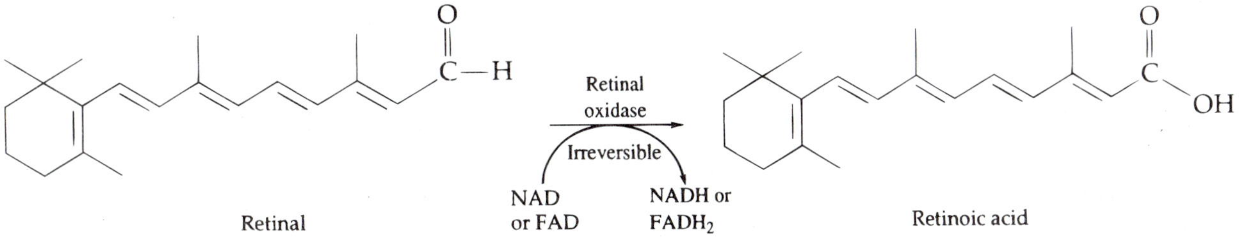

FIGURE 10.4 The irreversible oxidation of retinal to retinoic acid.

Chylomicrons deliver retinyl esters, some unesterified retinol, and carotenoids to many extrahepatic tissues such as bone marrow, blood cells, spleen, adipose tissue, muscle, lungs, and kidneys. Chylomicron remnants deliver retinyl esters and a portion of the carotenoids not taken up by peripheral tissue to the liver.

Carotenoids reaching the liver can follow three routes: (1) a small portion may be cleaved to form retinol; (2) some may be incorporated into the very low density lipoproteins (VLDLs) synthesized in the liver, and then be released as part of VLDLs for circulation to various tissues of the body; and (3) some can be stored in the liver. Excess carotenoids not stored in the liver will be deposited in body lipids. Serum carotene levels are reflective of recent intake, and not body stores.

The handling of retinyl esters reaching the liver is shown in Figure 10.5; however, most cells of the body are able to metabolize retinol generated from the retinyl esters through a number of metabolic pathways. Hydrolysis of the retinyl esters occurs following their uptake by the hepatic parenchymal cells. Within the cell, retinol binds with a cellular retinol-binding protein (CRBP). CRBPs have been found in many body cells, especially the intestine (CBRP II), the liver, and the kidney. CRBP is thought to function both to help control concentrations of free retinol within the cell cytoplasm and thus prevent its oxidation, and to direct the vitamin through a series of protein-protein interactions to specific enzymes of metabolism [9,12,13]. Enzymatic metabolism of retinol includes possible esterification by enzymes such as LRAT or ARAT, oxidation of retinol to retinal by NAD(P)H-dependent retinol dehydrogenase, phosphorylation of retinol to retinyl phosphate using ATP, and hydrolysis of membrane-associated retinyl esters [10,13]. CRBP may also assist in the transfer of retinal from the microsomal retinol dehydrogenase to the cytosolic retinal dehydrogenase [12].

Retinol not metabolized or transported from the liver may be stored following re-esterification. Some storage of retinol occurs in the parenchymal cells, but about 80 to 95% of the retinol is stored in special peri-sinusoidal cells called *stellate cells*. Vitamin A is stored in these stellate cells along with lipid droplets [14,15]. When liver stores of vitamin A are adequate, the stellate cells will store recently ingested vitamin A as retinyl esters (primarily retinyl palmitate, but also as retinyl stearate, oleate, and linoleate). For a given person, plasma vitamin A levels remain quite constant over a wide range of dietary intakes and liver stores. Only after the hepatic stellate cells can accept no more retinol for storage does hypervitaminosis A occur.

Retinol mobilization from the liver and delivery to target tissues are dependent on the synthesis and secretion of retinol-binding protein (RBP) by the parenchymal cells (Fig. 10.6). Each mole of retinol released by a hydrolase from its ester storage form combines with 1 mole of RBP to form holo-RBP. In the plasma, the holo-RBP also interacts with a molecule of transthyretin (TTR), a protein formerly known as *prealbumin* that also binds to one thyroxine (T_4) per tetramer. The retinol-RBP-TTR complex circulates in the plasma (Fig. 10.6); it is not filtered by the glomerulus. Some tissues that take up retinol from the RBP-TTR complex include adipose, skeletal muscle, kidney, white blood cells, and bone marrow [3,4]. There is extensive recycling of retinol (in rats 7 to 13 times prior to degradation) among plasma, extrahepatic tissues, and the liver, with both the parenchymal and stellate cells of the liver taking up retinol directly from its complexed form in the plasma [3,4,11].

Entry of the retinol into target cells (Fig. 10.6) is believed to involve slow release from RBP with subsequent association with the target cell [16]. It may also be mediated by specific cell surface receptors that recognize the RBP and internalize the retinol, but not the RBP [16]. The apo-RBP that remains after retinol release can no longer bind to TTR, and this apo-RBP is typically catabolized by the kidney.

In contrast to retinol, which is mobilized from the liver for transport to other tissues, retinoic acid is thought to be produced in small amounts by individual cells. Whether or not central production of retinoic acid

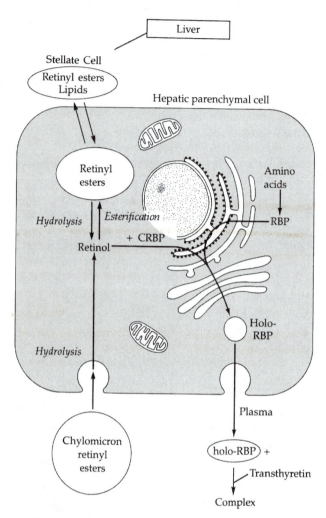

FIGURE 10.5 Diagram summarizing the metabolism of vitamin A and RBP in the liver.

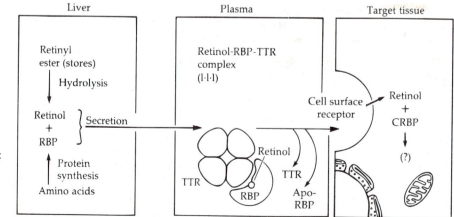

FIGURE 10.6 Schematic summary of processes involved in vitamin A mobilization from the liver, transport in plasma, and delivery and uptake into target cell.

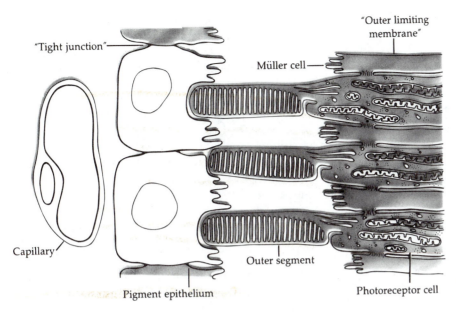

"Tight junction"

"Outer limiting membrane"

Müller cell

Capillary

Outer segment

Pigment epithelium

Photoreceptor cell

FIGURE 10.7 The photoreceptor cell and its restrictive boundaries.

occurs by the intestine or liver for transport to other tissues is unclear. Plasma retinoic acid concentrations are, however, typically low. Within the cell cytoplasm, retinoic acid binds to cellular retinoic acid-binding proteins (CRABPs). CRABPs are thought to function in a capacity similar to that described for CRBPs. Both CRBPs and CRABPs are often found in the same tissues; however, their relative distribution in the tissues differs [17]. CRABP, like CRBP, functions to help control concentrations of free retinoic acid within the cell and thus prevent its catabolism, and to direct the usage of retinoic acid intracellularly.

Functions and Mechanisms of Action

Vitamin A is recognized as being essential for vision, and for systemic functions including cellular differentiation, growth, reproduction, bone development, and the immune system.

Visual Cycle Retinol transported to the retina via the RBP-TTR complex appears to move into the pigment epithelium of photoreceptor rod cells. The photoreceptor cell is shown in Figures 10.7 and 10.8. The movement of retinol into the outer rod segments, where the visual cycle occurs, involves at least two proteins specific to the retina, cellular retinal-binding protein (CRALBP), and interstitial or interphotoreceptor retinol-binding protein (IRBP) [14]. In addition, CRBP and CRABP are also found in the retina [14].

Within the retina, retinol may be converted into a retinyl ester and stored. The retinyl ester is hydrolyzed as needed to release retinol, which is oxidized in the rod cells by an NAD-activated dehydrogenase to generate all trans retinal. This reaction occurs in the rod outer segments. The all-trans retinal produced is equilibrated with its 11-cis isomer either spontaneously or by an isomerase. The 11-cis retinal binds as a protonated Schiff base to a lysine amino acid residue in the protein opsin (Fig. 10.9) to produce the compound rhodopsin. Rhodopsin is embedded in disks, located in the rod's outer segment, which is enclosed within a restricted compartment of the retina created by tight junctions between cells (Figs. 10.7 and 10.8) [18]. The cells on the blood side are one layer thick and form the pigment epithelium. The "outer limiting membrane" is formed on the vitreal side of the photoreceptor cells by specific junctions between the photoreceptor cells and the retinal glial cells of Müller (Fig. 10.7) [18]. Despite the barriers around the photoreceptor cells, vitamin A moves into and within the cells so that rhodopsin can be generated. CRBP and CRALBP are believed to assist in vitamin A transport through the pigment epithelium, while IRBP is required for transport of the various forms of vitamin A between the cell types [18,19]. Specifically, IRBP, a glycolipoprotein, resides within the retinal interphotoreceptor space that lies between the pigment epithelium and the photoreceptor cells. IRBP transports two molecules of retinol between the tissues [19].

Rod cells with rhodopsin detect small amounts of light, thus they are important for night vision. When a quantum of light (hv) hits the rhodopsin (Fig. 10.10), rhodopsin breaks down in a series of reactions. The term *bleaching* is often used because a loss of color

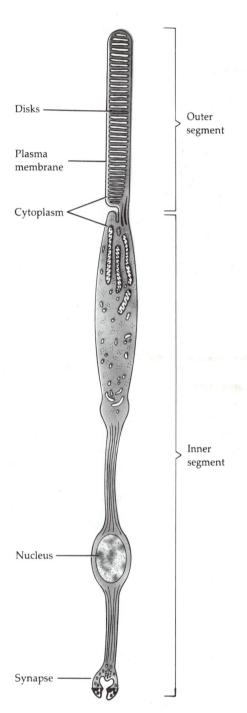

FIGURE 10.8 A photoreceptor (rod) cell, emphasizing its disks, and the location site of rhodopsin.

occurs as the rhodopsin splits. During the degradation of rhodopsin, all-trans retinal is generated. These processes also lead to an electrical signal to the optic nerve. A transmitter is required for carrying through the cell to the plasma membrane the message that light

has hit the rhodopsin. Two possible candidates for the role of transmitter are calcium and cyclic GMP. Whatever the transmitter, the result is that the sodium channels in the plasma membrane are blocked, and the rod cell hyperpolarizes.

Recovery of the rod's dark current and thus vision in dim light is believed to be made possible by the phosphorylation of opsin. With this phosphorylation, the cascade of light-activated enzymes is terminated. The all-trans retinal formed as a result of light must be converted back to 11-cis retinal; the exact steps involved and the location of the reaction (outer segment versus pigment epithelium) are unclear. The visual cycle is, however, completed when all-trans retinal is converted back to 11-cis retinal and bound once again to rhodopsin.

Cellular Differentiation Retinoic acid acts as a hormone to affect gene expression and thus control cell development. Retinoic acid may also act to diminish degradation of retinol by affecting CRBP II synthesis. Retinoic acid or 9-cis retinoic acid (generated from 9-cis retinol) are transported to the nucleus bound to CRABP. Within the nucleus, retinoic acid and 9-cis retinoic acid bind to one or more of three retinoic acid receptors (RAR) or to one or more of three retinoid X receptors (RXR), respectively. Binding of retinoic acid or 9-cis retinoic acid to RAR or RXR, respectively, permits interaction with specific nucleotide sequences of nuclear DNA to regulate gene transcription, with the potential to affect a wide variety of body proteins and thus body processes (Fig. 10.11).

Only a few of the vast number of processes affected by the binding of retinoic acid (or 9-cis retinoic acid) to nuclear receptors are unknown. Retinoic acid is thought to act as a morphogen in embryonic developments [19]. Nuclear retinoic acid receptors appear in different cells during different times of development. Thus, retinoic acid may serve to signal morphogenesis [17].

Retinoic acid is needed by epithelial cells found in such places as the lungs, trachea, skin, and gastrointestinal tract, among others. Retinoic acid helps to maintain both the normal structure and the functions of the epithelial cells [13]. For example, retinoic acid directs the differentiation of keratinocytes (immature skin cells) into mature epidermal cells. Retinoic acid appears to have more specific effects on cellular differentiation than 9-cis retinoic acid [17]. Retinoic acid is thought to act as a signal to "switch on" the genes for keratin proteins [13]. Vitamin A also appears to direct the synthesis of keratins, with genes for smaller (versus larger) keratin molecules transcribed and translated in the presence of vitamin A [16,20]. Vitamin A, *in vitro*, directs differen-

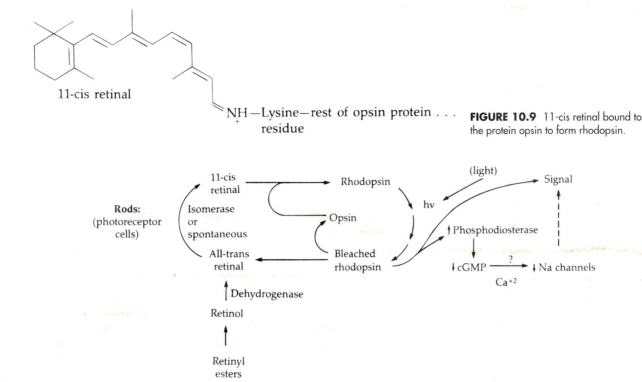

FIGURE 10.9 11-cis retinal bound to the protein opsin to form rhodopsin.

FIGURE 10.10 The visual cycle.

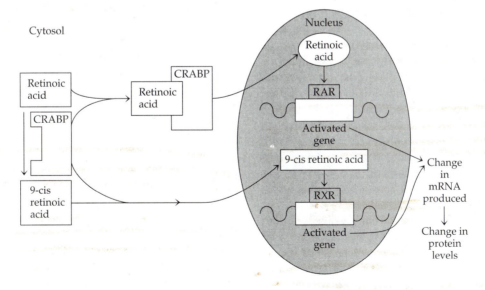

FIGURE 10.11 Hypothesized mode of action for retinoic acid.

tiation of squamous epithelial keratinizing cells into mucus-secreting cells [20].

Growth Vitamin A deficiency has long been characterized in animals by impaired growth that can be stimulated with replacement by either retinol or retinoic acid. Specifically, vitamin A has been shown to stimulate the growth of epithelial cells. Cell growth is stimulated, in part, by growth factors that bind to specific receptors on cell surfaces. Retinoic acid appears to increase the number of specific receptors for growth factors [20]. The mechanism by which vitamin A affects growth is unclear; however, the vitamin may act by increasing the synthesis of cell surface components such as glycoproteins (see next section). Retinyl β-glucuronide, formed in a variety of tissues from retinol and UDP-GA, has been shown to actively support growth and differentiation [10]. Retinoyl β-glucuronide has also been shown to improve acne lesions in patients [21].

Cell Surface Functions—Glycoproteins One cell surface function of vitamin A is thought to be mediated through glycoproteins, principal cell surface constituents involved in, for example, cell communication, cell recognition, cell adhesion, and cell aggregation. Vitamin A is thought to play a role in the synthesis of glycoproteins. The possible mode of action involves the formation of retinyl phosphate, formed from the conjugation of retinol and ATP (Fig. 10.12). Retinyl phosphate can be converted into retinyl phosphomannose (also called *mannosyl retinylphosphate*) in the presence of GDP-mannose. Retinyl phosphomannose can in turn transfer the mannose to a glycoprotein acceptor. The glycoprotein receptor, on receipt of the mannose, becomes a mannosylated glycoprotein [10]. Such changes in the glycan portion of the glycoprotein in turn can greatly affect differentiation of cells or tissues through their effects on cell communication, recognition, adhesion, and cell aggregation.

Retinoic acid has also been shown to affect cell membranes by increasing the number of junctions between cells (called *gap junctions*). These junctions are important for cell to cell communication and for cell adhesion. Vitamin A and retinoic acid can modify cell surfaces, possibly again through increasing glycoprotein synthesis at the gene level or by improving attachment of glycoproteins to cell surfaces to induce cell adhesion [20].

Other Functions Vitamin A, as retinol but not retinoic acid, is essential for *reproductive processes* in both males and females, although the mechanism(s) of its action(s) are unclear at present. *Bone development and maintenance* also requires vitamin A. Vitamin A is necessary for bone metabolism through involvement with osteoblasts and osteoclasts. Although the mechanism of action is unclear, vitamin A deficiency results in excessive deposition of bone by osteoblasts and reduced osteoclasts. Several aspects of *immune system function* also appear to be influenced by vitamin A. Depletion studies suggest that vitamin A appears to be needed for T-

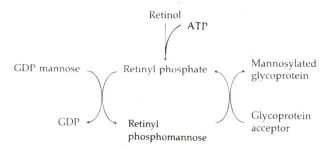

FIGURE 10.12 The role of vitamin A in the mannosylation of glycoproteins.

lymphocyte function and for antibody response to viral, parasitic, and bacterial infections [22]. Natural killer cell activity and phagocytosis are also impaired with vitamin A deficiency [17,22].

Beta-carotene, lycopene (a carotenoid, red in color and found in tomatoes, for example), and other carotenoids are thought to function as *antioxidants*, because they possess the ability to react with and quench free-radical reactions in membrane systems, or possibly in solution. Quenching is a process by which electronically excited molecules, such as singlet molecular oxygen (generated from lipid peroxidation of membranes, enzymatic or photochemical reactions) are inactivated [23]. Singlet oxygen, like free radicals, can damage cellular components unless removed. Carotenoids, like β-carotene or lycopene, can react with singlet oxygen. The singlet oxygen transfers its excitation energy and returns to the ground state, while the carotenoid receiving the energy enters an excited state. Quenching is attributed to the conjugated double-bond systems within the carotenoids. In addition, β-carotene has the ability to react directly with peroxyl radicals (O_2^{2-}) involved in lipid peroxidation.

With respect to atherosclerosis, oxidation of cholesterol in low-density lipoproteins (LDLs) increases the likelihood of monocyte uptake of the oxidized LDL cholesterol and deposition of the lipids as fatty streaks in blood vessels [24]. Once deposited within the vessels, the monocytes differentiate into macrophages and, when filled with cholesterol, become foam cells. Although postulated to protect human cells from reactive oxygen species that may induce oxidation and lead to atherosclerosis and cancer, the actual mechanism(s) by which carotenoids, such as lycopene, lutein, α-carotene, among others, prevent the oxidation of LDL and other cell membranes is unclear [25,26]. Nevertheless, many studies suggest that β-carotene and other carotenoids can protect LDL from oxidation, although α-tocopherol (vitamin E) appears to be more effective than β-carotene [27].

Interrelationships with Other Nutrients

Vitamin A interacts with both vitamins E and K. Cleavage of β-carotene into retinal requires *vitamin* E. Vitamin E is probably necessary to protect the substrate and the product from oxidation; however, large doses (ten times the RDA) of vitamin E may inhibit β-carotene absorption or conversion to retinol in the intestine [1,6]. Excess vitamin A appears to interfere with vitamin K absorption.

Protein status also influences vitamin A status and transport. The activity of the enzyme carotenoid dioxygenase that cleaves β-carotene is depressed by inadequate protein intake. Overall vitamin A metabolism is closely related to protein status because transport and use of the vitamin depend on several vitamin A-binding proteins synthesized in the body.

A *zinc* deficiency interferes with vitamin A metabolism. Its effect appears to operate at two levels. First, a general reduction in growth accompanied by decreased food intake and a reduction in the synthesis of plasma proteins, particularly RBP, which is made in the liver. Thus, with zinc deficiency, plasma retinol concentrations decrease, and liver retinol concentrations increase. Secondly, with zinc deficiency there is a decreased hepatic mobilization of retinol from its storage as retinyl esters. The activity of the enzyme retinyl ester hydrolase, which releases the vitamin from its storage form, may be inhibited by the lack of zinc or possibly by vitamin E [15]. In peripheral tissue, alcohol dehydrogenase, which converts retinol into retinal, is also dependent on zinc.

Iron status is also interrelated with vitamin A. Vitamin A deficiency may result in microcytic anemia. Vitamin A supplementation in turn corrects the anemia with observed increases in indices of iron status [15]. Vitamin A may be directly acting on iron metabolism or storage, or may be affecting differentiation of the red blood cell [15,17].

Metabolism and Excretion

Retinol conversion to retinal is reversible, but the oxidation of retinal to retinoic acid is irreversible. Retinoic acid does not accumulate in the liver or any other tissues in appreciable amounts [28].

The major pathway of retinoic acid catabolism is oxidation to 4-hydroxy (OH) retinoic acid in a NADPH-dependent reaction (Fig. 10.13). This compound is subsequently converted to 4-oxoretinoic acid in an NAD-requiring reaction. The latter compound is further oxidized to a variety of metabolites for excretion.

The oxidized products of vitamin A that contain intact chains are conjugated to glucuronide (Fig. 10.13) and excreted primarily via the bile into the feces. About 70% of the vitamin A metabolites is excreted in the feces. Some of the polar products, however, can be absorbed and returned to the liver via enterohepatic circulation. This recycling mechanism helps conserve the body's supply of vitamin A. Urinary excretion of vitamin A metabolites accounts for about 30% of vitamin A excretion [7] while a small amount is expired by the lungs as CO_2 [15,17].

Carotenoids, newly absorbed and not stored or converted to retinal or retinol, may be metabolized into a variety of compounds depending on the individual carotenoid. Carotenoid metabolites are excreted into the bile [21].

Recommended Dietary Allowances

The 1989 recommended dietary allowances (RDA) [7] for vitamin A are 800 μg RE for adult women and 1,000 μg (1 mg) RE for adult men; these recommendations do not differ from those published in 1980 [29].

Recommendations for adequate intake of vitamin A have been based on the amounts needed to correct night blindness among vitamin A-deficient subjects, and to raise plasma vitamin A levels to a normal level in depleted subjects. In addition, estimates of vitamin need have been based on amounts of the vitamin needed to maintain a given body pool size in well-nourished subjects. A concentration of 20 μg retinol/g liver was used to represent a satisfactory total body reserve [6]. With this latter approach, the recommended level for vitamin A intake was reduced to 700 RE for adult men and 600 RE for adult women; however, the recommendations (referred to as *recommended dietary intakes*, or RDI) of the committee were never officially accepted [6]. Studies of vitamin A utilization rates in adult men, although few in number, generated wide variations in vitamin A utilization. The minimum requirement was determined as 600 μg retinol; however, neither liver stores nor plasma retinol concentrations are optimal at this level. A comparison of the 1987 RDI and 1989 RDA for vitamin A in different population groups is given in Table 10.3.

Deficiency

Vitamin A deficiency is less common in the United States than in developing countries, where inadequate

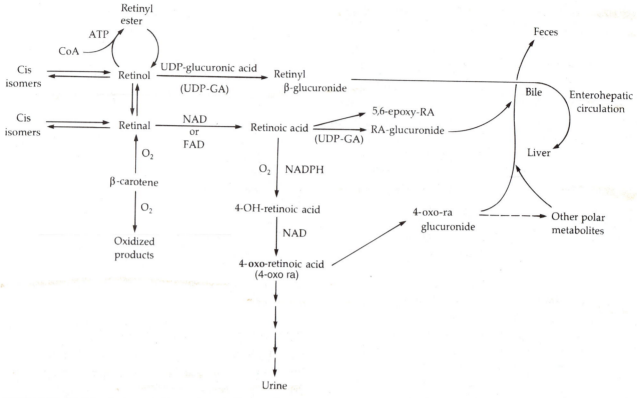

FIGURE 10.13 Vitamin A metabolism and metabolite excretion.

TABLE 10.3 Comparison of 1987 RDIs and 1989 RDAs for Vitamin A in Different Population Groups

Population Groups	RDI (μg)	RDA (μg)
Infants, 0–24 mo	375	375–400
Children, 2–6 yr	400	400–500
Children, 6–9 yr	500	500–700
Males, 10–11 yr	600	700–1,000
Males, 12–70+ yr	700	1,000
Females, 10–70+ yr	600	700–800
Pregnancy, 6–9 mo	+200	800
Lactation, 0–5 mo	+400	1,300
Lactation, 6+ mo	+320	1,200

Note: Population groups are divided differently in various recommendations.

intake is fairly common in children under 5 years of age. Increased mortality is associated with both clinically evident vitamin A deficiency in children as well as with children with inadequate vitamin A stores but no clinical signs of deficiency [30]. Selected signs and symptoms of deficiency include anorexia, retarded growth, increased susceptibility to infections, obstruction and enlargement of hair follicles, and keratinization of epithelial (mucous) cells of the skin with (thus) failure of normal differentiation [10,17]. Night blindness results from impaired production of rhodopsin in the outer segments of the rods. Xerophthalmia occurs with vitamin A deficiency and is characterized by abnormalities of the conjunctiva and cornea of the eye. Conjunctival changes include the disappearance of goblet cells in the conjunctiva, epithelial cells become enlarged and keratinized, and Bitot's spots appear overlying the keratinized epithelia. The Bitot's spots are white accumulations of sloughed cells thought to result from decreased retinol and glycoproteins in tear fluid as well as slower diffusion of retinol from plasma to the epithelial layer [15,17]. Keratomalacia may occur if the changes in the cornea become severe and irreversible (such as with corneal perforation and loss of aqueous humor).

Conditions and populations associated with increased need for vitamin A include those with malabsorptive disorders such as those with steatorrhea, pancreatic, liver, or gallbladder diseases. People with chronic nephritis, acute protein deficiency, intestinal parasites, or acute infections may also become vitamin A deficient. Measles infections in developing countries are associated with high mortality. Measles is thought to depress vitamin A status, which may be already low in children from developing countries. Vitamin A supplements are recommended by WHO and UNICEF for children with measles and living in a country with measles fatality rates of 1% or greater [22]. Serious infections increase urinary vitamin A excretion [31].

Toxicity

That toxicity can result from an excessive intake of vitamin A has been brought to the public's attention in recent years by the teratogenic effects of 13-cis retinoic acid (Acutane), which is used extensively in the treatment of acne. Use of this compound by women in the early months of their pregnancy has resulted in a number of birth defects among the infants born to these women [15,17].

In adults, a chronic intake of vitamin A in amounts ten times greater than the RDA (10 mg RE) can result in hypervitaminosis, manifested by a variety of maladies (anorexia, dry, itchy and desquamating skin, alopecia and coarsening of the hair, ataxia, headache, bone and muscle pain, conjunctivitis, among others). Most manifestations of toxicity appear to subside gradually once excessive intake of the vitamin is discontinued.

When vitamin A intake is in excess, serum retinol levels may rise above 200 μg/dL (normal is 45 to 65 μg/dL). Retinol is no longer transported exclusively by RBP but can be carried to the tissues by plasma lipoproteins. It has been suggested that when retinol is presented to the cell membranes in a form other than in a RBP complex, the released retinol produces potentially toxic effects [16].

Beta-carotene ingestion by adults in amounts as high as 180 mg daily appears to pose no serious side effects. Hypercarotenosis can however cause a yellow discoloration of the skin occurring especially in the fat pads or fatty areas of the palms of the hands and soles of the feet. The condition usually disappears following removal of the carotenoids from the diet.

Assessment of Nutriture

Vitamin A status may be assessed in a variety of ways including clinical assessment for Bitot's spots, measurements of dark adaptation threshold, and electrophysiological measurements including electroretinograms to measure the level of rhodopsin and its rate of regeneration [32].

The conjunctival impression cytology (CIC) method measures the reduction in goblet cells and the derangement of epithelia on the conjunctiva of the eye, which occurs with impaired vitamin A status [33].

Plasma retinol concentrations are frequently measured as a biochemical indicator of vitamin A status.

Plasma retinol levels reflect status best if the individual has exhausted their stores of the vitamin, as with deficiency, or if their stores are filled to capacity, as with toxicity.

Measurement of changes in plasma retinol concentrations before and 5 hours after oral administration of retinyl esters (450–1000 μg) in oils, a process referred to as *Relative Dose Response (RDR)*, is also done to assess vitamin A status.

$$RDR\ (\%) = \frac{\text{plasma retinol at 5 hr} - \text{initial plasma retinol}}{\text{plasma retinol concentration at 5 hr}} \times 100$$

Criteria for RDR and plasma vitamin A status are as follow [7,17,32]:

	Vitamin A Status			
	Deficient	Marginal	Acceptable	Better
Plasma vitamin A (μg/dL)	<10	10–20	>20	>30
RDR (%)	>50	50–20	<20	

References Cited for Vitamin A

1. Erdman JW, Poor CL, Dietz JM. Factors affecting the bioavailability of vitamin A, carotenoids, and vitamin E. Food Tech 1988;42:214–221.
2. Ong DE. Retinoid metabolism during intestinal absorption. J Nutr 1993;123:351–355.
3. Blomhoff R, Green MH, Norum KR. Vitamin A: Physiological and biochemical processing. Ann Rev Nutr 1992;12:37–57.
4. Norum KR, Blomhoff R. McCollum Award Lecture, 1992: Vitamin A absorption, transport, cellular uptake, and storage. Am J Clin Nutr 1992;56:735–744.
5. Rigtrup KM, McEwen LR, Said HM, Ong DE. Retinyl ester hydrolytic activity associated with human intestinal brush border membranes. Am J Clin Nutr 1994;60:111–116.
6. Olson JA. Recommended dietary intakes (RDI) of vitamin A in humans. Am J Clin Nutr 1987;45:704–716.
7. National Research Council. Recommended dietary allowances, 10th ed. Washington, DC: National Academy Press, 1989:78–92.
8. Bender DA. Nutritional biochemistry of the vitamins. New York: Cambridge University Press, 1992:19–50.
9. Ong DE. Cellular transport and metabolism of vitamin A: Roles of the cellular retinoid-binding proteins. Nutr Rev 1994;52: S24–S31.
10. Combs GF. The vitamins. New York: Academic Press, 1992:119–150.
11. Blomhoff R. Transport and metabolism of vitamin A. Nutr Rev 1994;52: S13–S23.

12. Napoli JL. Biosynthesis and metabolism of retinoic acid: Roles of CRBP and CRABP in retinoic acid: roles of CRBP and CRABP in retinoic acid homeostasis. J Nutr 1993;123:362–366.
13. Ross AC, Ternus ME. Vitamin A as a hormone: Recent advances in understanding the actions of retinol, retinoic acid, and beta carotene. J Am Diet Assoc 1993;93:1285–1290.
14. Ross AC. Overview of retinoid metabolism. J Nutr 1993;123:346–350.
15. Olson JA. Vitamin A. In: Machlin LJ. Handbook of Vitamins, 2nd ed. New York: Dekker, 1991:1–57.
16. Creek KE, St. Hilaire P, Hodam JR. A comparison of the uptake, metabolism and biologic effects of retinol delivered to human keratinocytes either free or bound to serum retinol-binding protein. J Nutr 1993;123:356–361.
17. Olson JA. Vitamin A. In: Shils ME, Olson JA, Shike M, eds. Modern nutrition in health and disease, 8th ed. Philadelphia: Lea and Febiger, 1994:287–307.
18. Ong DE. Vitamin A-binding proteins. Nutr Rev 1985;43:225–232.
19. Wolf G. The intracellular vitamin A-binding proteins: An overview of their functions. Nutr Rev 1991;49:1–12.
20. Wolf G. Multiple functions of vitamin A. Physiol Rev 1984;64: 873–937.
21. Olson JA. 1992 Atwater Lecture: The irresistible fascination of carotenoids and vitamin A. Am J Clin Nutr 1993;57:833–839.
22. Ross AC. Vitamin A and protective immunity. Nutr Today 1992;27 (July–Aug):18–26.
23. Mascio PD, Murphy ME, Sies H. Antioxidant defense systems: The role of carotenoids, tocopherols, and thiols. Am J Clin Nutr 1991;53:194S–200S.
24. Luc G, Fruchart J-C. Oxidation of lipoproteins and atherosclerosis. Am J Clin Nutr 1991;53:206S–209S.
25. Prince MR, Frisoli JK. Beta-carotene accumulation in serum and skin. Am J Clin Nutr 1993;57:175–181.
26. Krinsky NI. Actions of carotenoids in biological systems. Ann Rev Nutr 1993;13:561–587.
27. Abbey M, Nestel PJ, Baghurst PA. Antioxidant vitamins and low-density-lipoprotein oxidation. Am J Clin Nutr 1993;58:525–532.
28. Goodman DS. Vitamin A and retinoids in health and disease. N Engl J Med 1984;310:1023–1031.
29. National Research Council. Recommended dietary allowances, 9th ed. Washington, DC: National Academy of Sciences, 1980:55–60.
30. Olson JA. Hypovitaminosis A: Contemporary scientific issues. J Nutr 1994;124:1461S–1466S.
31. Stephensen CB, Alvarez JO, Kohatsu J, Hardmeier R, Kennedy JI, Gammon RB. Vitamin A is excreted in the urine during acute infection. Am J Clin Nutr 1994;60:388–392.
32. Underwood BA. Methods for assesment of vitamin A status. J Nutr 1990;120:1459–1463.
33. Olson JA. Needs and sources of carotenoids and vitamin A. Nutr Rev 1994;52:S67–S73.

VITAMIN D

Through the years vitamin D has been associated with skeletal growth and strong bones. This association arose because early in the twentieth century it was shown that rickets, a childhood disease characterized by improper development of bones, could be prevented by a fat-soluble factor D in the diet or by body exposure to ultraviolet light. The emphasis was placed on the dietary factor; therefore, any compound with curative action on rickets was designated as *vitamin D*.

Sources

Dietary vitamin D is provided primarily by foods of animal origin especially eggs, liver, butter, fatty fish, and foods such as milk and margarine that are fortified with the vitamin. Table 10.4 provides information on major food sources of the vitamin. Dietary vitamin D is a stable compound not prone to cooking, storage, or processing losses [1].

In plants a commonly occurring steroid, ergosterol, can be activated by irradiation to ergocalciferol (also called *vitamin D₂* or *ercalciol*)(Fig. 10.14), the antirachitic compound most commonly sold commercially. No ergosterol occurs in animals, but another steroid, 5,7-cholestradienol, commonly called *7-dehydrocholesterol*, is found in animals and humans. 7-dehydrocholesterol is synthesized in the sebaceous glands of the skin, secreted onto the surface, and reabsorbed into the various layers of the skin. This steroid appears to be uniformly distributed throughout the epidermis and dermis. During exposure to sunlight, some of the epidermal cutaneous

TABLE 10.4 Major food sources of Vitamin D

Food	Vitamin D content (µg/100g)
Nonfortified	
Butter	0.8
Milk—winter	0.03
Milk—summer	0.13
Cheese	0.2–0.3
Liver	0.1–0.2
Herring	22
Canned pilchards	8
Tuna	6
Sardines	7.5
Fortified	
Milk	1.0
Margarine	11.0

Source: Adapted from Lawson, Eric. Vitamin D. In: Diplock AT, ed. *Fat Soluble Vitamins.* Lancaster, PA: Technomic, 1985;135.

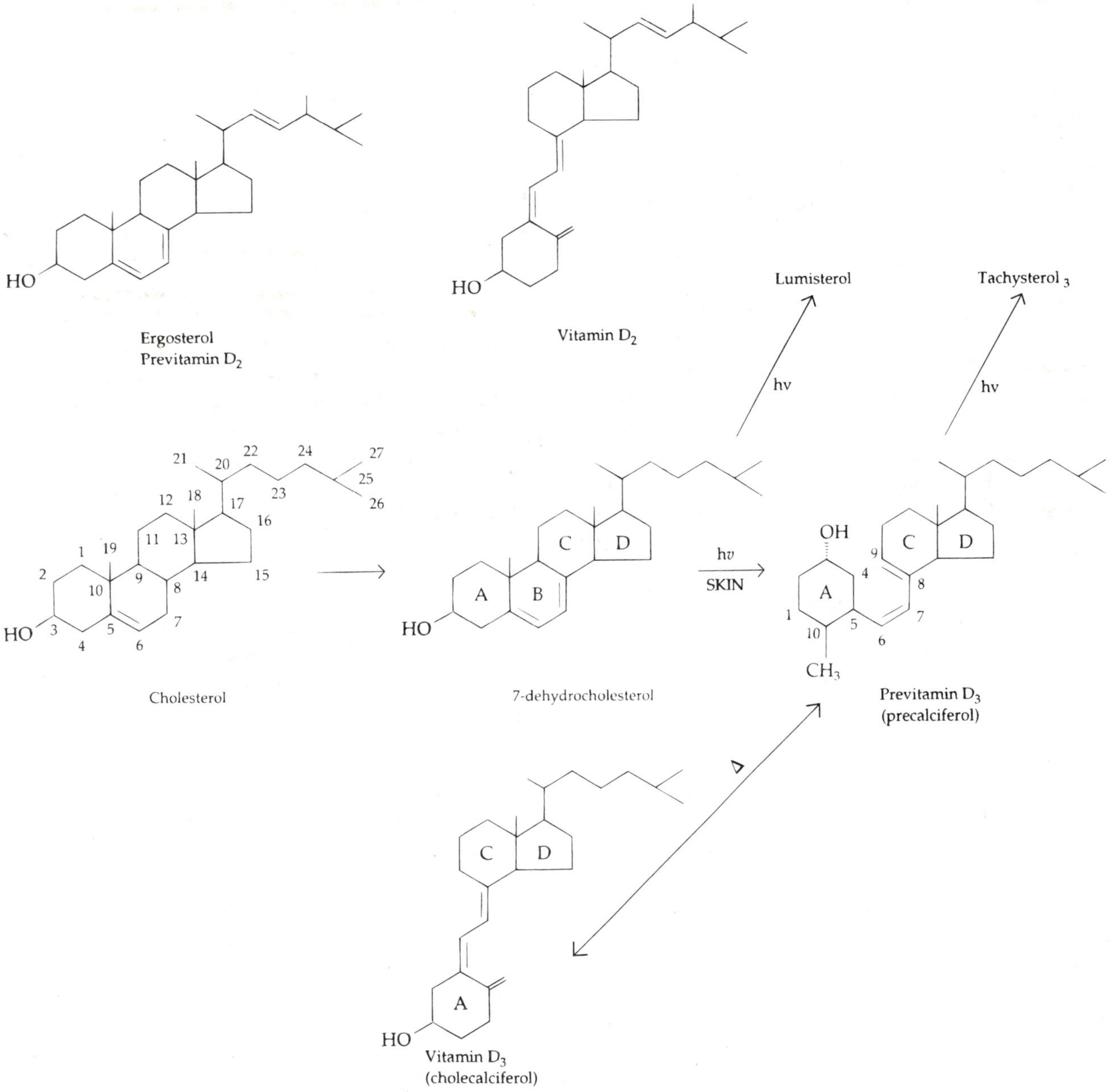

FIGURE 10.14 Production of vitamin D_3 in skin via previtamin D_3.

reservoir of 7-dehydrocholesterol is converted to previtamin D_3 (also called *precalciferol*) (Fig. 10.14). Lumisterol is also produced from 7-dehydrocholesterol in the presence of ultraviolet light; tachysterol is generated by further irradiation of previtamin D_3 [2,3]. Much of the previtamin D_3 is thermally isomerized within two to three days into vitamin D_3, also called *cholecalciferol* or *calciol*. Cholecalciferol diffuses from the skin into the blood with transport in the blood occurring by a transport α-2 globulin vitamin D-binding protein (DBP)

(also called *transcalciferin*) that is synthesized in the liver [2,3]. Neither lumisterol, tachysterol, nor previtamin D_3 has much affinity for the DBP. Therefore, rather than entering the blood, they are sloughed off during turnover of the skin [4].

Absorption and Transport

Vitamin D from the diet is absorbed from a micelle, in association with fat and with the aid of bile salts, by passive diffusion into the intestinal cell. About 50% of dietary vitamin D is absorbed. Although the rate of absorption is most rapid in the duodenum, the largest amount of vitamin D is absorbed in the distal small intestine.

Within the intestinal cell, vitamin D is incorporated primarily into chylomicrons. These chylomicrons enter the lymphatic system with subsequent entry into the blood. Chylomicrons transport about 40% of the cholecalciferol in the blood, although some vitamin D may be transferred from the chylomicron to DBP for delivery to extrahepatic tissues. Chylomicron remnants deliver the vitamin to the liver.

Cholecalciferol, which slowly diffuses from the skin into the blood, is picked up for transport by DBP. About 60% of plasma cholecalciferol is bound to DBP for transport. The vitamin D bound to DBP travels to the liver; however, much of the vitamin is deposited in muscle and adipose tissue prior to hepatic uptake [5]. Thus, the difference in the transport mechanism for cholecalciferol formed in the skin and that absorbed from the digestive tract impacts on the distribution of the vitamin in the body.

Cholecalciferol reaching the liver either by way of chylomicron remnants or by DBP is hydroxylated at carbon 25 to form 25-OH D_3 (also called *calcidiol*) (Fig. 10.15). The efficiency of the liver 25-hydroxylase in converting cholecalciferol into 25-OH D_3 appears related to vitamin D status. The NADPH-dependent enzyme is more efficient during periods of vitamin D deprivation than when normal amounts of the cholecalciferol are available. The relative activity of the enzyme in various organs including lung, intestine, and kidney [2], and the distribution of activity may be species dependent [2]. 25-hydroxylase is poorly regulated, thus blood levels of 25-OH D_3 are thought to represent vitamin D status [6].

Most of the 25-OH D_3 synthesized in the liver is secreted into the blood, and transported by DBP. Because little 25-OH D_3 remains in the liver and very little of this metabolite is taken up by the extrahepatic tissues, the blood is the largest single pool (storage site) of 25-OH D_3, which has a half-life of about three weeks [7,8]. When the 25-OH D_3 pool has been depleted during vitamin D deprivation, maintenance of vitamin D activity is made possible for variable time periods through the release of cholecalciferol from its skin reservoir and from other sites in muscle and adipose tissues [9].

Following hydroxylation in the liver, 25-OH D_3 bound to DBP is released into the blood and taken up by the kidney. In the kidney, a second hydroxylation of 25-OH D_3 occurs at the 1 position, resulting in $1,25\text{-}$

$(OH)_2 D_3$ (also called *calcitriol*) which is considered the active vitamin. Calcitriol is formed (Fig. 10.15) in the kidney tubules through the action of another NADPH-dependent enzyme, 25-OH D_3 1 α-hydroxylase (1-hydroxylase), a mitochondrial mixed-function oxidase. This enzyme is also present in macrophages and some cancer cells. Calcitriol in the blood has a half-life of about 4 to 6 hours.

The activity of 1-hydroxylase is influenced by a variety of factors. Parathyroid hormone (PTH) and low plasma calcium concentrations stimulate 1-hydroxylase activity. In contrast, dietary phosphorus intake impairs calcitriol production by 1-hydroxylase. A high intake of phosphorus causes a decrease in serum $1,25\text{-}(OH)_2 D_3$, whereas a low phosphorus intake stimulates production of calcitriol [10]. When sufficient amounts of calcitriol are present, the activity of 1-hydroxylase in the kidney is decreased significantly, and the activity of another enzyme, 24-hydroxylase, is increased in the kidney, and possibly other tissues such as cartilage and the intestine. $24,25\text{-}(OH)_2 D_3$ is formed from 24-hydroxylation of 25-OH D_3 (Fig. 10.15), and may be involved in bone mineralization, or may represent a step in the degradation of the vitamin [11]. Production of $24,25\text{-}(OH)_2 D_3$ appears to increase during periods of adequate vitamin D status and calcium homeostasis.

Functions and Mechanisms of Action

Calcitriol, $1,25\text{-}(OH)_2 D_3$, is considered the active form of vitamin D and functions like a steroid hormone. Initially the target tissues of the vitamin were believed to be limited to the intestine, bone, and kidney. The presence of specific receptors for the hormone in many other tissues, however, supports the present belief that calcitriol acts in a wide variety of tissues, including the heart, brain, and stomach [7,11]. Vitamin D receptors have a much greater affinity for the calcitriol metabolite of the vitamin than for any of the others. The reverse, however, is true for DBP. DBP transports calcitriol more loosely bound than the other metabolites. Consequently, on reaching its target tissues, the hormone is easily released from the DBP and is quickly bound by its receptor.

Calcitriol plays a role in the parathyroid hormone (PTH)-directed homeostasis of blood calcium concentrations, which impacts several tissues including the intestine, bone, and kidney (Fig. 10.16). Hypocalcemia stimulates secretion of PTH from the parathyroid gland. The PTH, in turn, stimulates 1-hydroxylase in the kidney such that 25-OH D_3 is converted to calcitriol. Calcitriol then acts alone or with PTH on its target tis-

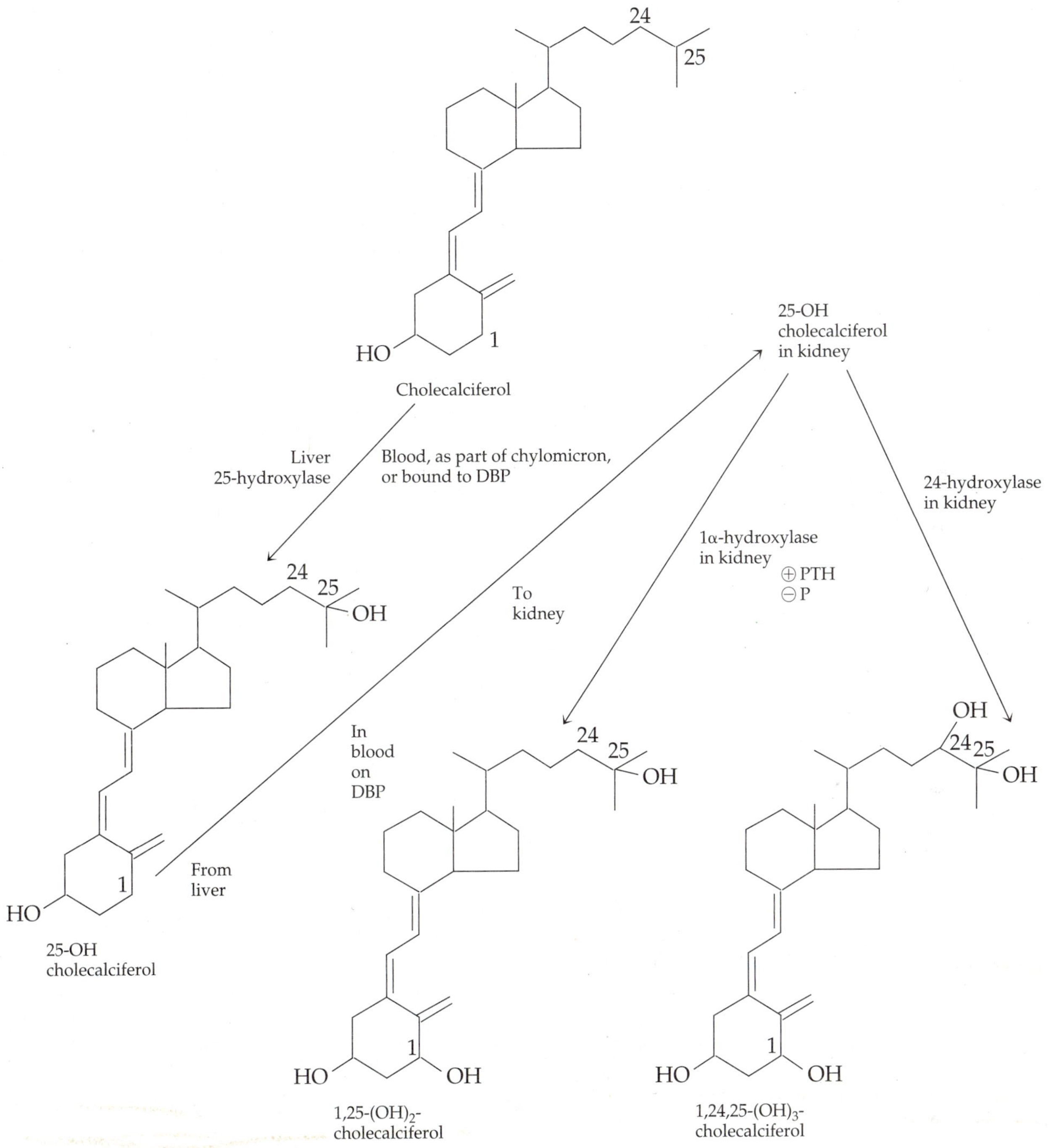

FIGURE 10.15 Hydroxylation of vitamin D.

sues, causing serum calcium and phosphorus concentrations to rise.

Calcitriol and the Intestine A more thoroughly investigated target tissue of calcitriol is the intestine (Fig. 10.17). The primary function of calcitriol in the intestine is increased absorption of calcium and phosphorus. In this function the vitamin is believed to act as a steroid hormone. Calcitriol interacts with high-affinity receptors in the enterocyte and is carried to the nucleus, where it interacts with specific genes encoding for proteins involved in calcium transport [11]. As the result of this interaction, a selective DNA transcription occurs that results in biosynthesis of new messenger RNA

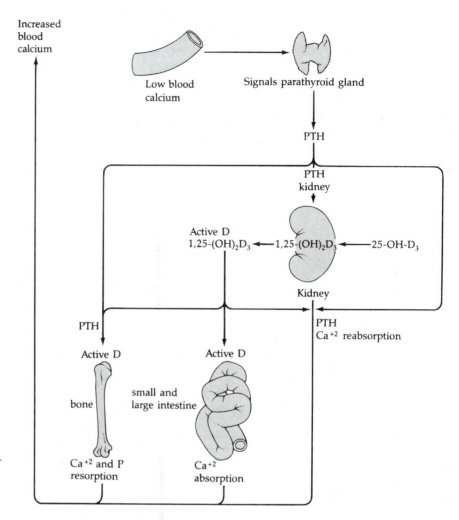

FIGURE 10.16 1,25-(OH)₂ D₃ synthesis and actions. Sites are shown where 1,25-(OH)₂ D₃ and PTH act to increase plasma calcium concentration.

(mRNA) molecules. These mRNA molecules are then translated on the endoplasmic reticulum into selected proteins. These proteins act at the brush border, in the cytoplasm, and/or at the basolateral membrane of the intestinal cells to promote calcium absorption. With respect to calcium, calcitriol is thought to induce changes in brush border composition and topology to increase calcium absorption. Calbindin, a calcium-binding protein in the intestinal mucosa, has been shown to be synthesized in response to the action of calcitriol. Although the amount of this calcium-binding protein is positively correlated with calcium absorption and transport, its exact role in the process is not yet defined. Final extrusion of calcium from the intestinal cell and into the blood requires another transport system. One system is a Ca^{+2}-Mg^{+2} ATPase with magnesium entering the cell as calcium exits, and ATP supplying the energy. This system is thought to be present and active mainly in the duodenum [4]. In the jejunum and ileum, a sodium–calcium exchange system is thought to exist whereby three Na⁺

are exchanged for one Ca^{+2} [4,6]. With respect to phosphorus, calcitriol is thought to increase the activity of brush border alkaline phosphatase, which hydrolyzes phosphate ester bonds allowing phosphorus absorption. Calcitriol is also thought to modulate the number of carriers available for sodium-dependent phosphorus absorption at the brush border membrane [4].

Calcitriol and the Kidney Calcitriol appears to be involved in the parathyroid hormone stimulation of calcium and phosphorus reabsorption in the distal renal tubule (Fig. 10.16) [6]. Although more research is needed to clarify the actions of calcitriol in the kidney, vitamin D is thought to have more effect on increasing phosphorus reabsorption than on calcium reabsorption in the kidney [4].

Calcitriol and the Bone With respect to bone, PTH, alone or with calcitriol, directs the mobilization of

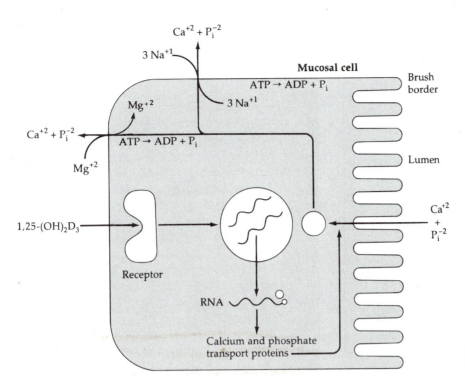

$$Ca^{+2} + P_i^{-2}$$

$3\,Na^{+1}$

Mucosal cell

Brush border

$ATP \rightarrow ADP + P_i$

$3\,Na^{+1}$

Mg^{+2}

$Ca^{+2} + P_i^{-2}$

$ATP \rightarrow ADP + P_i$

Mg^{+2}

Lumen

$1,25\text{-}(OH)_2D_3$

Ca^{+2}
$+$
P_i^{-2}

Receptor

RNA

Calcium and phosphate transport proteins

FIGURE 10.17 The actions of vitamin D on the intestinal absorption of calcium.

calcium and phosphorus from bone to help achieve a normal blood calcium concentration (Fig. 10.16). This process may be mediated by calcitriol-induced cell differentiation of hemopoietic cells to osteoclasts. Osteoclasts in turn mediate bone resorption. Alternately, the process may be mediated by calcitriol-induced increases in osteoclast activity [10].

Should blood calcium levels begin to rise above normal concentrations, calcitonin (a hormone produced by endocrine cells located in the connective tissue of the thyroid gland) is released and promotes the deposition (mineralization) of calcium and phosphorus in bones. Calcitriol or the metabolite $24,25\text{-}(OH)_2 D_3$ may also be involved in bone mineralization and suppression of PTH [12,13]. Elevated serum calcitriol and elevated ionized serum calcium in turn cause a decrease in PTH production through feedback loops. The long feedback loop is an indirect one due to the inhibitory effect of elevated ionized serum calcium on PTH secretion. The short feedback loop is direct; the calcitriol decreases the transcription of the gene for preparathyroid hormone, presumably by interacting with the vitamin D receptor in the parathyroid tissue and influencing the regulatory region of the PTH gene [10].

Modeling and remodeling of bone may also involve calcitriol. Calcitriol appears important in the synthesis of a prominent noncollagenous protein, osteocalcin, found in bone. Vitamin D stimulates osteoblasts to syn-

thesize osteocalcin, a γ-carboxyglutamate vitamin K-dependent protein found in bone matrix and dentine. Osteocalcin (also discussed on p. 317) is associated with new bone formation and when found in circulation is thought to be a sensitive marker of vitamin D action and bone disease.

Calcitriol and Cell Differentiation, Proliferation, and Growth Calcitriol also appears to trigger differentiation of stem cells to osteoclasts, which mediate bone resorption and release of calcium into blood [14]. This stimulation is believed due to an increase in the number of osteoclasts, derived from hematopoietic cells, and suggests a role for the vitamin in cellular differentiation (long-term effect) [10]. In addition, stimulation is due to increased activity of the osteoclasts (short-term effect) whereby calcitriol induces the release of osteoblast-derived resorption factors that stimulate osteoclast activity [10].

Further evidence supports a role for calcitriol in cell proliferation, differentiation, and growth. For example, calcitriol has been shown to inhibit cancer cell proliferation and growth, and stimulate skin epidermal cell differentiation, while preventing proliferation. These functions of the vitamin have been applied in vitamin D treatment of psoriasis (a disorder in which there is proliferation of the keratinocytes and a failure to differenti-

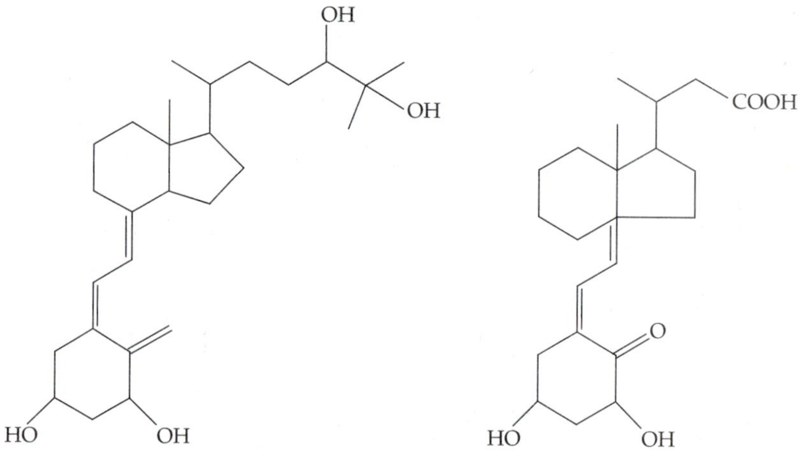

FIGURE 10.18 Some metabolites of vitamin D catabolism.

1,24,25-(OH)₃
Vitamin D₃

Calcitroic acid

ate rapidly) [2,10,11,13–15]. Calcitriol has also been shown to increase receptor sites for epidermal growth factor and to transform growth factors on the bone cells from rats [16].

Interaction with Other Nutrients

Discussion of vitamin D metabolism is impossible without noting the interrelationships existing among this vitamin or hormone and calcium, phosphorus, and vitamin K. The relationships with calcium and phosphorus are shown in Figures 10.16 and 10.17, and are discussed in the text corresponding to each figure. Interaction of calcitriol and vitamin K is provided on page 317. Also speculated is a decrease in vitamin D absorption as a result of *iron* deficiency [17].

Metabolism and Excretion

Calcitriol hydroxylation at carbon 24 generates the metabolite 1,24,25-(OH)₃ D₃ (Fig. 10.18), which may be further oxidized to 1,25-(OH)₂ 24-oxo D₃. Subsequent reactions, including side-chain cleavage, yield calcitroic acid (Fig. 10.18), a major excretory product that is excreted into the bile [11]. Other vitamin D metabolites are also formed after hydroxylation and oxidation. These other vitamin D metabolites may be conjugated and then excreted primarily in the bile. Less than 5% of the metabolites are excreted in the urine.

Recommended Dietary Allowance

Although the exact requirement for vitamin D has not been elucidated, the recommended intake for infants over 6 months of age, children, and adolescents is 10 μg or 400 IU daily. One IU is defined as the activity contained in 0.025 μg of cholecalciferol [9].

Recommended allowances for vitamin D decrease with the cessation of growth. The RDA for adults over 24 years of age is 5 μg (200 IU) daily; this amount of the vitamin is thought to be obtainable by exposure to sunlight. In the continental United States about 1.5 IU vitamin D/cm²/hour during the winter, and about 6 IU/cm²/hour during the summer can be synthesized in the skin [12]. Alternately, it takes about 10 minutes of summer sun on the face and hands to produce 10 μg (400 IU) of cholecalciferol [13]. A vitamin D supplement may be necessary for the elderly, particularly those who drink little milk and are partially or totally housebound.

Deficiency—Rickets and Osteomalacia

In infants and children, vitamin D deficiency results in rickets. Rickets is characterized by failure of bone to mineralize. In vitamin D-deficient infants, epiphyseal cartilage continues to grow and enlarge without replacement by bone matrix and minerals. Long bones of the legs bow, and knees knock as weight-bearing activity such as walking begins. The spine becomes curved, and pelvic and thoracic deformities occur.

In adults, deprivation of vitamin D leads to impaired calcium—and possibly phosphorus—absorption. Serum calcium homeostasis occurs in part through the action of PTH, which may remain elevated for prolonged time periods. With a marginal phosphorus intake and an insufficiency of vitamin D, an adequate serum phosphorus level may also be impossible to maintain, thereby further jeopardizing bone mineralization. Without sufficient serum calcium and phosphorus, the mineralization of bones under the direction of calcitonin cannot occur.

Thus, in vitamin D-deficient adults, as bone turnover occurs, the bone matrix is preserved, but remineralization is impaired. The bone matrix becomes progressively demineralized, resulting in bone pain and osteomalacia (soft bone).

Natural exposure to sunlight maintains adequate vitamin D nutrition for most of the world's population [3]. However, certain diseases, conditions, and populations may be at risk for vitamin D deficiency. Impaired vitamin D absorption may occur in disorders in which there is fat malabsorption, such as tropical sprue and Crohn's disease. Disorders affecting the parathyroid, liver, and/or kidney will impair the synthesis of active form of the vitamin. People with insufficient sun exposure may be at risk for vitamin D deficiency. People on anticonvulsant drug therapy may develop an impaired response to vitamin D, and exhibit problems with calcium metabolism. Infants may be at risk for deficiency because human milk is low in vitamin D and infant's exposure to sunlight typically is minimal. In addition, aging may reduce synthesis of cholecalciferol in the skin and may reduce the activity of 1-hydroxylase in response to PTH.

Toxicity

Although excessive exposure to sunlight may be the primary risk factor in development of skin cancer, it poses no risk of toxicity through overproduction of endogenous cholecalciferol. Extensive whole-body irradiation with ultraviolet light will generally raise the level of circulating 25-OH D_3 to 40 to 80 ng/mL; levels above 150 ng/ml are associated with possible toxicity [7]. Photochemistry regulates the cutaneous production of vitamin D_3, thus protecting people excessively exposed to sunlight from vitamin D intoxication [3].

Excessive dietary ingestion of vitamin D causes a much greater increase in 25-OH D_3 levels because exogenous vitamin D is absorbed and incorporated into chylomicrons, the remnants of which deliver the vitamin to the liver. Here the vitamin is hydroxylated in position 25 and released to the blood. Although the efficiency of 25-hydroxylase is decreased when the vitamin is in abundance, an excessive amount of the metabolite can still be produced with oversupplementation.

Exogenous vitamin D is the most likely of all vitamins to cause overt toxic reactions when the RDA is chronically exceeded [18]. Small multiples of the RDA ingested on a continuous basis can be toxic [18]. In the 1950s, an epidemic of "idiopathic hypercalcemia" among English infants was traced to an intake of vitamin D between 2,000 to 3,000 IU per day. Symptoms of toxicity in the infants included anorexia, nausea, vomiting, hypertension, renal insufficiency, and failure to thrive [18].

For adults the lowest safe intake of vitamin D is unclear. Intakes of as little as 2,000 IU per day of vitamin D (or five times the RDA) may pose a risk for adults if this level of intake is prolonged [19]. Some authorities suggest that intakes should not exceed 1,200 IU [20]. Dosages of 10,000 IU/day for several months have resulted in hypercalcemia—with possible calcification of soft tissues (calcinosis) such as the kidney, heart, lungs, and blood vessels—hyperphosphatemia, hypertension, anorexia, nausea, weakness, polyuria, polydypsia, azotemia, nephrolithiasis, renal failure, and in some cases, death [18].

Assessment of Nutriture

No ready method of measuring vitamin D status exists. Elevations in plasma alkaline phosphatase released from osteoclasts have been used to detect preclinical rickets [8,14]. The plasma concentration of 25-OH D_3 is thought to provide an index of vitamin D status. Normal plasma concentration of 25-OH D_3 ranges from 8 to 60 ng/mL [7] (with an average between 25 to 30 ng/mL) [9]. A level less than 10 ng/mL is regarded as an indicator for vitamin D therapy and levels above 150 ng/mL are associated with possible toxicity [7]. However, because cholecalciferol can be stored in extrahepatic tissues such as fat and muscles, measurement of serum 25-OH D_3 will not fully reflect pools of the vitamin [5]. Osteocalcin released into circulation is thought to represent a measure of vitamin D action, but is not always present in the blood in detectable quantities even if the individual has adequate vitamin D status.

References Cited for Vitamin D

1. Sauberlich HE. Vitamins—how much is for keeps? Nutr Today 1987;22:20–28.
2. Henry HL, Norman AW. Vitamin D: Metabolism and biological actions. Ann Rev Nutr 1984;4:493–520.
3. Webb AR, Holick MF. The role of sunlight in cutaneous production of vitamin D_3. Ann Rev Nutr 1988;8:375–399.
4. Lawson E. Vitamin D. In: Diplock AT, ed. Fat soluble vitamins. Lancaster, PA: Technomic, 1985:76–153.
5. Fraser DR. Vitamin D. In: Olson RE, Broquist HP, Chichester CO, Darby WJ, Kolbye AC Jr, Stalvey RM, eds. Nutrition reviews' present knowledge in nutrition, 5th ed. Washington, DC: The Nutrition Foundation, 1984:209–225.
6. Combs GF. The vitamins. New York: Academic Press, 1992:151–178.

7. Holick MF. The use and interpretation of assays for vitamin D and its metabolites. J Nutr 1990;120:1464–1469.
8. Bender DA. Nutritional biochemistry of the vitamins. New York: Cambridge University Press, 1992:51–86.
9. National Research Council. Recommended dietary allowances, 10th ed. Washington, DC: National Academy Press, 1989:92–98.
10. Reichel H, Koeffler HP, Norman AW. The role of the vitamin D endocrine system in health and disease. N Engl J Med 1989;320: 980–991.
11. Haussler MR. Vitamin D receptors: Nature and function. Ann Rev Nutr 1986;6:527–562.
12. Collins ED, Norman AW. Vitamin D. In: Machlin LJ. Handbook of vitamins, 2nd ed. New York: Dekker, 1991:59–98.
13. DeLuca HD. Vitamin D: 1993. Nutrition Today 1993;28(Nov–Dec):6–11.
14. Holick MF. Vitamin D. In: Shils ME, Olson JA, Shike M, eds. Modern nutrition in health and disease, 8th ed. Philadelphia: Lea and Febiger, 1994:308–325.
15. Vitamin D: New perspectives. Lancet 1987;1:1122–1123.
16. 1,25-dihydroxyvitamin D_3 affects growth factors in bone cells. Nutr Rev 1988;46:265–266.
17. Heldenberg D, Tenenbaum G, Weisman Y. Effect of iron on serum 25-hydroxyvitamin D and 24,25-dihydroxyvitamin D concentrations. Am J Clin Nutr 1992;56: 533–536.
18. Council on Scientific Affairs, American Medical Association. Vitamin preparations as dietary supplements and as therapeutic agents. JAMA 1987;257:1929–1936.
19. Marshall CW. Vitamins and minerals: help or harm? Philadelphia: Stickley, 1983.
20. National Institutes of Health Consensus Development Panel. Osteoporosis. JAMA 1984;252:799–802.

VITAMIN E

Vitamin E includes eight compounds (vitamers) synthesized by plants [1,2]. These compounds fall into two classes: the tocols, which have saturated side chains, and the tocotrienols (also called *trienols*), which have unsaturated side chains. Each class is comprised of four vitamers that differ in the number and location of methyl groups on the chromanol (chroman) ring. Vitamers in both classes are designated as alpha, beta, gamma, or delta, and possess characteristic biological activity [2]. Another compound, all-rac α-tocopheryl acetate, with vitamin E activity is used in fortification of foods [1].

Figure 10.19 gives the basic structure of the compounds with vitamin E activity and defines the biological activity of each. Vitamin E activity is greatest in α-tocopherol, followed by beta, which is greater than gamma and delta. Of the tocotrienols, only the alpha vitamer has significant activity; α-tocotrienol has an activity slightly less than β-tocopherol (0.4 versus 0.3, respectively) [1].

Sources

Vitamin E is widely distributed in foods. Plant foods, especially oils from plants, provide the primary source of vitamin E in the diet. The leaves and other green (chloroplast) portions of plants contain mostly α-tocopherol with small amounts of γ-tocopherol. Gamma-, delta-, and beta-tocopherols are found mainly in nonchloroplast regions of plants. In contrast to the tocopherols, the tocotrienols are found in the bran and germ sections of some plants, thus wheat germ oil represents a significant source of tocotrienols [4]. In foods of animal origin, vitamin E, primarily α-tocopherol, is found concentrated in fatty tissues of the animal [5]; however, in comparison to plants, animal products represent an inferior source of vitamin E. Fish oils, for example, are low in tocopherols [1].

Table 10.5 lists the approximate α-tocopherol equivalents found in commonly consumed foods; 1 α-tocopherol equivalent has the vitamin E activity of 1 mg α-tocopherol. However, the tocopherol content of foods quoted are only approximate. Methodology used for the analyses, as well as processing and storage affect the vitamin E content of foods [6,7]. The level of vitamin E best correlates with the level of polyunsaturated fat in the food. Most vitamin E in foods is found as α-tocopherol. However, with the increased consumption of oils from, for example, soybeans, the γ-tocopherol content, and to a lesser extent the δ-tocopherol content, of the U.S. diet is increasing relative to α-tocopherol [3].

Digestion, Absorption, and Transport

While the tocopherols are found free in foods, the tocotrienols are found esterified and must be hydrolyzed prior to absorption. Pancreatic esterase and/or duodenal mucosal esterase are thought to function in the lumen or at the brush border of the intestine to hydrolyze tocotrienol for absorption [2,4,8].

Absorption of vitamin E as free alcohols occurs primarily in the jejunum by nonsaturable, passive (requiring no carrier) diffusion [4,5,8]. Both bile salts and pancreatic juice are needed for micelle formation allowing the vitamin to diffuse through the unstirred water layer and the enterocyte membrane. Simultaneous digestion and absorption of dietary lipids, including medium-chain triacylglycerols, with vitamin E improves absorption of vitamin E [9]. A specific factor not associated with general fat absorption may also be required for

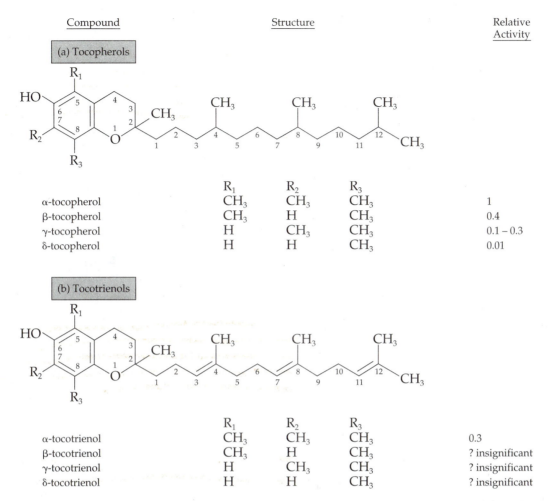

Compound	R₁	R₂	R₃	Relative Activity

(a) Tocopherols

	R_1	R_2	R_3	
α-tocopherol	CH₃	CH₃	CH₃	1
β-tocopherol	CH₃	H	CH₃	0.4
γ-tocopherol	H	CH₃	CH₃	0.1 – 0.3
δ-tocopherol	H	H	CH₃	0.01

(b) Tocotrienols

	R_1	R_2	R_3	
α-tocotrienol	CH₃	CH₃	CH₃	0.3
β-tocotrienol	CH₃	H	CH₃	? insignificant
γ-tocotrienol	H	CH₃	CH₃	? insignificant
δ-tocotrienol	H	H	CH₃	? insignificant

FIGURE 10.19 Structure and activity of natural tocopherols and tocotrienols. *(Diplock AT. Vitamin E. In: Diplock AT., ed. Fat soluble vitamins. Lancaster, PA: Technomic, 1984:156.)*

absorption of vitamin E as suggested by studies in vitamin E-deficient patients who have no problems absorbing fat [10].

The absorption of vitamin E varies from about 20 to 50% [4] and possibly as high as 80% [3,8]. As vitamin intake increases, vitamin E absorption decreases whereby absorption of pharmacologic doses, 200 mg, of vitamin E is less than 10% [1].

Absorbed tocopherol is incorporated into chylomicrons in the enterocyte and is transported through the lymph into circulation. The tocopherol in the chylomicrons equilibrates with the other plasma lipoproteins, including the high-density lipoproteins (HDLs) and low-density lipoproteins (LDLs) and interchanges with erythrocytes [3,11]. Tocopherol found in erythrocytes appears to be largely localized in the cell membrane [6,7]. Plasma tocopherol has been shown to be highly correlated with total plasma lipids.

Tocopherol is distributed to the tissues primarily by the low-density lipoproteins. Uptake of vitamin E into cells can occur (a) as LDL receptor-mediated uptake occurs [8,12], or (b) through lipoprotein lipase-mediated hydrolysis of chylomicrons and very low density lipoproteins (VLDLs) [4], and (c) possibly by other mechanisms [8]. Within the cell cytoplasm as well as other parts of the cells, vitamin E appears to bind to specific proteins, tocopherol-binding proteins, for transport [2,4]. The precise intracellular distribution of tocopherol is controversial, but most agree that the vitamin is primarily located in cell membranes, such as the plasma, mitochondrial, and microsomal membranes [1,2,8]. As described by Machlin [2], the vitamin is likely to be oriented with the chromanol "head" group toward the surface of the membrane near the phosphate region of the phospholipid, and with the hydrophobic phytyl "tail" buried within the hydrocarbon region.

TABLE 10.5 Approximate Vitamin E Content of Foods as α-Tocopherol Equivalents

Food	mg/100 g
Oils	
Wheat germ	156.9
Corn	15–20
Cottonseed	40–50
Peanut	15–20
Safflower	25–40
Soybean	10–17
Sunflower	49–50
Margarine	10–15
Vegetable shortening	10–15
Peanuts	7–10
Whole wheat	0.2–1
Vegetables	0.1–1
Fruits	0.1–0.3
Meat, fish	0.2–0.6
Eggs	0.5

Source: Adapted from Bieri JG. Sources and consumption of antioxidants in the diet. J Am Oil Chem Soc 1984;61:1917–1918; and Farrell PM. Vitamin E. In: Shils M, Young V, eds. Modern nutrition in health and disease, 7th ed. Philadelphia: Lea and Febiger, 1988: 340–354.

There is no single storage organ for vitamin E. The largest amount of the vitamin is concentrated in an unesterified form in the adipose tissue, with smaller amounts in liver, lung, heart, muscle, adrenal glands, and brain. The concentration of vitamin E in adipose tissues increases linearly with dosage of vitamin E, whereas the other tissues maintain a constant concentration or increase only at a very slow rate [1,11]. In times of low intake, withdrawal of tocopherol occurs slowly from adipose (thus it is not readily available), whereas withdrawal from the liver and plasma is rapid [7]. Depletion of vitamin E stored in the heart and muscle occurs at an intermediate rate [2].

Functions and Mechanisms of Actions

The principal function of vitamin E is the maintenance of membrane integrity in body cells. Some investigators believe that vitamin E may also provide physical stability to membranes [7]. The mechanism by which vitamin E functions to protect the membranes from destruction is through its ability to prevent the oxidation (peroxidation) of unsaturated fatty acids contained in the phospholipids of the cellular membranes. The phospholipids of the mitochondrial membrane and endoplasmic reticulum contain more unsaturated fatty acids than the plasma membrane. These membranes, therefore, are at greater risk for oxidation with a vitamin E deficiency

than is the membrane surrounding the cell [7]. Cell membranes are, however, still vulnerable to oxidation. Tissues with cell membranes especially susceptible to oxidation include the lungs, brain, and erythrocytes. Erythrocyte membranes, for example, are high in polyunsaturated fatty acids, and are exposed to high concentrations of oxygen. Because vitamin E prevents oxidation, it is referred to as an *antioxidant*.

Generation of Free Radicals Reduction of oxygen occurs as a normal process in the body. For example, reduction of oxygen takes place in the microsomal terminal oxidase system or cytochrome P_{450}. Reduction of molecular oxygen to water also occurs as part of the respiratory chain (electron transport, p. 59) occurring in the cell mitochondria. Intermediate metabolites, formed during these and other normal cellular processes (such as phagocytosis of foreign substances by macrophages and neutrophils), can be potentially damaging to cells. During the reduction of molecular oxygen to water, molecular oxygen may gain an electron; for example, one that has left the electron transport chain at an odd point. This reaction causes the generation of a free radical known as *superoxide radical*, O_2^-.

$$O_2 \xrightarrow{e^-} O_2^- \quad \text{(superoxide radical)}$$

Free radicals, as defined by Diplock [13], are atoms or molecules that have one or more unpaired electron(s); the imbalance in electrons results in most cases in the high reactivity of the free radicals.

A superoxide radical, once formed, can gain another electron, again from electron transport, from the cytochrome P_{450} system, or from an organic compound in the vicinity, to generate a peroxy anion.

$$O_2^- \xrightarrow{e^-} O_2^{2-} \quad \text{(peroxy anion)}$$

The peroxy anion can react with hydrogen ions in solution to form peroxide, also called *hydrogen peroxide*.

$$O_2^{2-} \xrightarrow{H^+} HO_2^- \xrightarrow{H^+} H_2O_2 \quad \text{(peroxide)}$$

Peroxides are also formed with normal cellular metabolism such as with phagocytosis.

Once formed, peroxides and superoxide radicals need to be removed from the cell. Without removal, superoxide radicals and hydrogen peroxide can react with iron to generate a more highly reactive free hydroxy radical, OH^-.

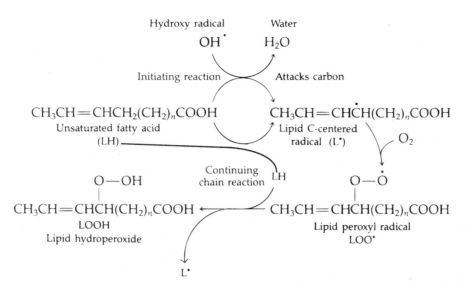

Hydroxy radical   Water

$$OH \cdot \qquad H_2O$$

Initiating reaction   Attacks carbon

$$CH_3CH = CHCH_2(CH_2)_nCOOH \qquad CH_3CH = CH\overset{\cdot}{C}H(CH_2)_nCOOH$$

Unsaturated fatty acid
(LH)

Lipid C-centered
radical (L·) O_2

Continuing
chain reaction   LH

$$\begin{array}{cc} O{-}OH & O{-}\overset{\cdot}{O} \\ | & | \\ CH_3CH{=}CHCH(CH_2)_nCOOH & CH_3CH{=}CHCH(CH_2)_nCOOH \end{array}$$

LOOH
Lipid hydroperoxide

Lipid peroxyl radical
LOO·

L·

FIGURE 10.20 The initiating and chain reactions caused by hydroxy free radical attack on an unsaturated fatty acid.

$$O_2^- + Fe^{+3} \longrightarrow O_2 + Fe^{+2}$$

Peroxide can react with the ferrous iron, or possibly copper, to generate hydroxide ions (OH^-) and free hydroxy radicals ($OH\cdot$).

$$Fe^{+2} + H_2O_2 \longrightarrow Fe^{+3} + OH^- + OH\cdot$$

Hydrogen peroxide also can react with an electron and hydrogen to generate a free hydroxy radical.

$$H_2O_2 \xrightarrow{\; e^- \; H^+ \;} H_2O + OH\cdot$$

Free Radicals, PUFA, and Vitamin E Free hydroxy radicals ($OH\cdot$) are very highly reactive, rapidly taking electrons from the surroundings. Often the electron taken by the reactive free hydroxy radical is from nearby organic molecules. If the organic molecule is a polyunsaturated fatty acid (PUFA) present in phospholipid portion of the cell membrane, damage to the membrane occurs. Membrane lipid oxidation is thought to represent a primary event in oxidative cellular damage [14]. The reaction between organic lipid compounds (LH) and free hydroxy radicals leads to the formation of a lipid carbon-centered radical (L·) and water, as shown below and in Figure 10.20.

$$LH + OH\cdot \longrightarrow L\cdot + H_2O$$

Organic lipid compounds can also react with molecular oxygen to generate lipid carbon-centered radicals and $HO_2\cdot$, perhydroxy radical.

$$LH + O_2 \longrightarrow L\cdot + HO_2\cdot$$

Lipid carbon-centered radicals can, in turn, react with molecular oxygen to form lipid peroxyl radicals, LOO·, shown as follows and in Figure 10.20.

$$L\cdot + O_2 \longrightarrow LOO\cdot \text{ (also written } LO_2\cdot\text{)}$$

Lipid peroxyl radicals can also be generated from reactions between Fe^{+3} and LOOH (lipid hydroperoxide), thus necessitating the removal of LOOH from the environment (see p. 322 for how this is done).

Once formed, lipid peroxy radicals can abstract a hydrogen atom from other organic compounds like PUFA to generate a chain reaction with the L·. This reaction is shown as follows and in Figure 10.20:

$$LOO\cdot + LH \longrightarrow L\cdot + LOOH$$

Chain reactions involving L· must be terminated to minimize cellular damage. Prevention of damage from oxygen radicals depends on a complex protective system of which vitamin E is a part.

Vitamin E located in the membranes can break the chain of radical attack by reacting with the peroxyl radical (LOO·) and preventing further abstraction of hydrogen (H) from the fatty acids. Thus, vitamin E terminates chain-propagation reactions. Vitamin E is less effective, however, in terminating peroxidation initiated by Fe^{+2}, which generates free hydroxy radicals, $OH\cdot$.

Vitamin E (EH, reduced state), because of the reactivity of the phenolic hydrogen on its carbon 6 hydroxyl group and the ability of the chromanol ring system to stabilize an unpaired electron [4], can provide a hydrogen for the reduction of the lipid peroxy radical.

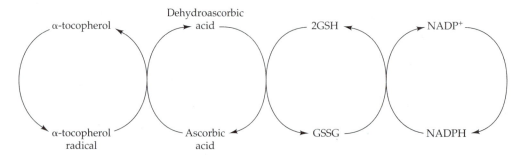

FIGURE 10.21 The regeneration of vitamin E.

$$LOO \cdot + EH \longrightarrow LOOH + E \cdot$$

E· represents oxidized vitamin E. The process is sometimes referred to as "free-radical scavenging."

The oxidized vitamin E (E·) must be regenerated. The regeneration is thought to require vitamin C, reduced glutathione, and NADPH (Fig. 10.21).

Vitamin E is only one line of defense against oxidative tissue damage. Other parts of the protective system are enzymes that require a variety of trace or microminerals (iron, selenium, zinc, copper, and manganese) for their activation; therefore, an interrelationship exists between vitamin E and these minerals involved in antioxidant activities. The relationship between vitamin E and these other nutrients with antioxidant functions is reviewed in the "Perspective" section at the end of this chapter.

Clinical trials with vitamin E suggest that the vitamin may decrease susceptibility of LDL to oxidation by free radicals [15–18]. These findings have implications in preventing atherosclerosis, which is thought to begin with the accumulation of lipid-laden foam cells in the arterial intima. Macrophages, which develop into foam cells, are thought to more readily take up oxidized LDL versus nonoxidized LDL. With continued accumulation, fatty streaks develop and represent the initial steps in atherosclerosis. Oxidized LDL may also (1) reduce macrophage motility in the arterial intima, (2) increase monocyte accumulation in endothelial cells, and (3) increase cytotoxicity of endothelial cells to contribute to atherogenicity [17,18]. Evidence of high intakes of vitamin E associated with a lower risk of coronary heart disease has been demonstrated in men [18] and women [17].

In addition, vitamin E supplementation appears to be beneficial to people with non–insulin-dependent diabetes mellitus who are experiencing poor metabolic control and microangiopathy [19]. Vitamin E supplementation (900 mg α-tocopherol) by non–insulin-dependent diabetics improved metabolic control [19].

Plasma GSH-to-GSSG ratio increased, and was thought to perhaps improve plasma membrane structure and its related activities required for glucose transport and/or metabolism (and thus metabolic control) [19].

Oxygen and oxyradicals are also thought to contribute to the development of cataracts. Vitamin E is being tested for prevention and treatment of cataracts [20,21].

Vitamin E may also be useful in the treatment of iron toxicity, which leads typically to lipid peroxidation through production of free radicals and excessive damage to organs especially the liver. Vitamin E may help to protect against the iron-induced cellular damage [22].

Interrelationships with Other Nutrients

Because the function of vitamin E in the body is closely tied to that of glutathione peroxidase as discussed in the "Perspective" section at the end of this chapter, an interrelationship exists between vitamin E and *selenium*. Selenium functions as an integral part of glutathione peroxidase that converts a lipid peroxide into a lipid alcohol. To a lesser extent, interrelationships also exist between vitamin E and *sulfur-containing amino acids* (S-aa). Cysteine, an S-aa generated from another S-aa, methionine, is necessary for synthesis of glutathione, which serves as the reducing agent in the glutathione peroxidase reaction. Superoxide dismutase (SOD) activity to remove superoxide radicals requires *zinc, manganese*, and *copper*.

High intakes of vitamin E can interfere with the functions of the other fat-soluble vitamins [4,11]. At dosages exceeding 1 g/day, vitamin E has been shown to be antagonistic to the action of *vitamin K* and to enhance the effect of oral coumarin anticoagulant drugs [2,22]. Vitamin E or its quinone (α-tocopheryl quinone) may block the oxidation of vitamin K (p. 316) and may affect prothrombin formation [11,22]. Vitamin E may also impact vitamin K absorption [2]. Problems with bone mineralization involving *vitamin D* have been reported in animals given high doses of vitamin E [4].

Another relationship is that between vitamin E and *vitamin A*. In a vitamin A deficiency, vitamin E is able to lower the rate at which vitamin A is depleted from the liver. Although the mechanism of this interaction is controversial, it appears to be unrelated to the prevention of lipid peroxidation [7]. Cleavage of β-carotene into retinal also requires vitamin E. Vitamin E is probably necessary to protect the substrate and product from oxidation; however, large doses (ten times the RDA) of vitamin E may inhibit β-carotene absorption or conversion to retinol in the intestine [5,23].

The relationship between vitamin E and dietary *PUFA* is particularly strong because requirement for the vitamin increases or decreases as the dietary intake of PUFA rises or falls. Some investigators believe that the dietary level of PUFA needs to be specified for a minimal vitamin E requirement to be determined [6,7,24].

Metabolism and Excretion

The metabolic fate of vitamin E in humans is largely unknown. Alpha-tocopherol, in a nonpolar solvent, is oxidized to a tocopheroxy radical, which can be reduced back to active vitamin E [7]. However, in polar solvents such as water this tocopheroxy radical is not formed [7]. In polar solvents the chromanol ring of α-tocopherol appears to be irreversibly oxidized into tocopheryl quinone [7]. Metastable tocopheroxide is formed as an intermediary product in this oxidation reaction, and it is speculated that tocopheroxide may be the primary tissue oxidation product of vitamin E [7].

The major route of α-tocopherol excretion is via the feces. Fecal tocopherol arises from vitamin E that was not absorbed, from secretion of the vitamin from enterocytes back into the intestinal lumen, from desquamation of intestinal epithelial cells, and from secretion into the bile [7]. Vitamin E excreted in bile exists as a presently unidentified metabolite conjugated with glucuronic acid [7].

Two water-soluble metabolites (α-tocopheronic acid and α-tocopheronolactone) resulting from the oxidation of the side chain of α-tocopherol can be conjugated to glucuronic acid and excreted in the urine [4]. Normally these metabolites represent no more than 1% of the α-tocopherol intake [2,4,9]. However, with high α-tocopherol intake, urinary excretion of the vitamin appears to rise [7].

Another possible excretion (or secretion) route for α-tocopherol is the skin, as suggested by the presence of large amounts of radioactivity in dermal tissue following intravenous injection of ^3H-α-tocopherol [4,7].

Recommended Dietary Allowances

The RDA for vitamin E is 8 mg α-tocopherol equivalents for the adult female and 10 mg for the adult male [6]. Diets of adults in the United States providing 2,000 to 3,000 kcal supplied 7 to 11 mg α-tocopherol equivalents, as well as met the RDA for other nutrients [3,6,11,24].

The adequacy of the RDA will vary if PUFA content deviates significantly from that which is customary [24]. Concern that increased intakes of PUFA will necessitate larger amounts of vitamin E in the diet is tempered by the notation that most foods, but not all, high in PUFA are also high in vitamin E, but not necessarily α-tocopherol [24]. Horwitt [26] believes that the need for vitamin E may be related more to changes in depot fat that occur with a prolonged, high intake of PUFA than to current PUFA intake.

Deficiency

Although determining a precise requirement for vitamin E has proved difficult, a deficiency in humans is quite rare. Usually the population groups exhibiting deficiency symptoms include premature, low-birthweight infants, people with abetalipoproteinemia, and people with malabsorption syndromes. Abetalipoproteinemia, a rare genetic disease, may result in vitamin E deficiency due to lack of apolipoprotein B, necessary for chylomicrons, VLDL, and LDL [7,8]. Malabsorption of fat is common in a variety of disorders including cystic fibrosis (characterized by pancreatic lipase deficiency), and various disorders of the hepatobiliary system, particularly chronic cholestasis characterized by decreased production of bile.

Some of the symptoms of vitamin E deficiency include retinal degeneration, ceroid pigment accumulation, hemolytic anemia, muscle weakness, degenerative neurologic problems, cerebellar ataxia, loss of vibratory sense, incoordination of limbs, among others [8,10]. Exactly how vitamin E deficiency is related to the neuromuscular degeneration is unknown. A likely explanation is the lack of antioxidant protection in neural and muscle tissues. In a deficiency of vitamin E, free radicals can cause an oxidant injury to the PUFA-rich membranes of these tissues [8].

Toxicity

Vitamin E appears to be one of the least toxic of the vitamins [4]. Although a few adverse symptoms from large oral doses of vitamin E have been reported, vitamin intakes of 400 to 800 mg α-tocopherol equivalents have been taken for months to years without apparent harm [6,27]. At higher doses (800 mg to 3.2 g), there have been occasional reports of muscle weakness, fatigue, double vision, and more predominant symptoms of gastrointestinal distress including nausea, diarrhea, and flatulence [4,11,22,27]. High intakes of vitamin E can interfere with the functions of the other fat-soluble vitamins [4,11], as discussed in the section on interrelationships with other nutrients.

Although oral supplementation appears harmless for most people and even beneficial for others, it is not wise to conclude that chronic ingestion of large amounts of vitamin E is without risk. The toxicity noted in premature infants given parenteral vitamin E suggests that an upper limit of safety may exist [1].

Assessment of Nutriture

No truly accurate evaluation of vitamin E status exists. Normal levels of total tocopherol range from 0.8 to 1.2 mg/dL serum in adults with values less than 0.5 mg/dL indicative of deficiency [1,4,6]. Because of the linear relationship between serum vitamin E concentrations and total serum lipids, serum vitamin E concentrations may not accurately reflect vitamin E status during hyper- or hypolipoproteinemia conditions [1,2,11,28]. To correct for serum lipid concentrations, the ratio of serum vitamin E (mg) to total serum lipids (g) is recommended by some [28]. A ratio greater than 0.6 mg/g for a child under 12 years and greater than 0.8 mg/g for older children and adults is considered normal [1,2,28].

A crude estimation of vitamin E status can be obtained from an erythrocyte hemolysis test that compares the amount of hemoglobin released by red cells during dilute hydrogen peroxide versus distilled water incubations. The result is expressed as a percentage whereby > 20% indicates a deficiency [2]. Variables other than vitamin E status, however, can affect *in vitro* hemolysis [1].

Two functional tests, which assess oxidative changes in lipids, may be used to assess vitamin E status. Both tests are related to the peroxidation of PUFA. The erythrocyte malondialdehyde test is done *in vitro* whereby peroxidation of PUFA of erythrocytes exposed to hydrogen peroxide is determined through measurement of generated malondialdehyde [28]. Malondialdehyde can be determined by a reaction with thiobarbituric acid [7]. The breath pentane test is done *in vivo*. Peroxidation of PUFA (such as linoleic acid) occurring in the body is determined by measuring the exhaled hydrocarbon gas

pentane [9]. Negative correlations between breath pentane levels and plasma vitamin E have been reported [28].

References Cited for Vitamin E

1. Farrell PM, Roberts RJ. Vitamin E. In: Shils ME, Olson JA, Shike M, eds. Modern nutrition in health and disease, 8th ed. Philadelphia: Lea and Febiger, 1994:326–341.
2. Machlin LJ. Vitamin E. In: Machlin LJ. Handbook of vitamins, 2nd ed. New York: Dekker, 1991:99–144.
3. Bieri JG. Vitamin E. In: Brown ML, ed. Present knowledge in nutrition. Washington, DC: International Life Sciences Institute Nutrition Foundation, 1990:117–121.
4. Combs GF. The vitamins. New York: Academic Press, 1992:179–203.
5. Erdman JW, Poor CL, Dietz JM. Factors affecting the bioavailability of vitamin A, carotenoids and vitamin E. Food Tech 1988;42:214–221.
6. National Research Council. Recommended dietary allowances, 10th ed. Washington, DC: National Academy Press, 1989:99–107.
7. Diplock AT. Vitamin E. In: Diplock AT, ed. Fat-soluble vitamins. Lancaster, PA: Technomic, 1984:154–224.
8. Sokol RJ. Vitamin E deficiency and neurologic disease. Ann Rev Nutr 1988;8:351–373.
9. Bender DA. Nutritional biochemistry of the vitamins. New York: Cambridge University Press, 1992:87–105.
10. Anon. Vitamin E deficiency without fat malabsorption. Nutr Rev 1988;46:189–194.
11. Bieri JG, Corash L, Hubbard VS. Medical uses of vitamin E. N Engl J Med 1983;308:1063–1071.
12. Traber MG, Kayden HJ. Vitamin E is delivered to cells via the high-affinity receptor for low-density lipoprotein. Am J Clin Nutr 1984;40:747–751.
13. Diplock AT. Antioxidant nutrients and disease prevention: An overview. Am J Clin Nutr 1991;53:189S–193S.
14. Niki E, Yamamota Y, Komuro E, Sato K. Membrane damage due to lipid oxidation. Am J Clin Nutr 1991;53:201S–205S.
15. Jialal I, Grundy SM. Effect of dietary supplementation with alpha tocopherol on the oxidative modification of low density lipoprotein. J Lipid Res 1992;33:899–906.
16. Esterbauer H, Dieber-Rotheneder M, Striegl G, Waeg G. Role of vitamin E in preventing the oxidation of low-density lipoprotein. Am J Clin Nutr 1991;53:314S–321S.
17. Stampfer MJ, Hennekens CH, Manson JE, Colditz GA, Rosner B, Willett WC. Vitamin E consumption and the risk of coronary disease in women. N Eng J Med 1993;328:1444–1449.
18. Rimm EB, Stampfer MJ, Ascherio A, Giovannucci E, Colditz GA, Willett WC. Vitamin E consumption and the risk of coronary heart disease in men. N Eng J Med 1993;328:1450–1456.
19. Paolisso G, D'Amore A, Giugliano D, Ceriello A, Varricchio M, D'Onofrio F. Pharmacologic doses of vitamin E improve insulin action in healthy subjects and non-insulin

dependent diabetic patients. Am J Clin Nutr 1993;57: 650–656.

20. Varma SD. Scientific basis for medical therapy of cataracts by antioxidants. Am J Clin Nutr 1991;53: 335S–345S.

21. Robertson JM, Donner AP, Trevithick JR. A possible role for vitamins C and E in cataract prevention. Am J Clin Nutr 1991; 53:346S–351S.

22. Bendich A, Machlin LJ. Safety of oral intake of vitamin E. Am J Clin Nutr 1988;48:612–619.

23. Olson JA. Recommended dietary intakes (RDI) of vitamin A in humans. Am J Clin Nutr 1987;45:704–716.

24. Lehmann J, Martin HL, Lashley EL, Marshall MW, Judd JT. Vitamin E in foods from high and low linoleic acid diets. J Am Diet Assoc 1986;86:1208–1216.

25. Omara FO, Blakley BR. Vitamin E is protective against iron toxicity and iron-induced hepatic vitamin E depletion in mice. J Nutr 1993;123:1649–1655.

26. Horwitt MK. Interpretations of requirements for thiamin, riboflavin, niacin-tryptophan, and vitamin E plus comments on balance studies and vitamin B-6. Am J Clin Nutr 1986;44:973–985.

27. Council on Scientific Affairs, American Medical Association. Vitamin preparations as dietary supplements and as therapeutic agents. JAMA 1987;257:1929–1936.

28. Gibson RS. Principles of nutritional assessment. New York: Oxford Press, 1990:397–404.

VITAMIN K

Several compounds possess vitamin K activity; these compounds all have a 2-methyl 1,4-naphthoquinone ring [1]. The naturally occurring forms of vitamin K are phylloquinone (K$_1$ or 2-methyl 3-phytyl 1,4-naphthoquinone), isolated from plants, and menaquinones (K$_2$) synthesized by bacteria. Most of the menaquinones contain six to ten isoprenoid units attached at carbon 3. Menadione (K$_3$) is not found naturally but is a common synthetic form of vitamin K that must be alkylated for activity. This alkylation can be accomplished rapidly by tissue enzymes. Figure 10.22 depicts menadione, phylloquinone, and one of the menaquinones, specifically menaquinone 7, which has 7 isoprenoic units and was originally isolated from putrefied fish meal [1].

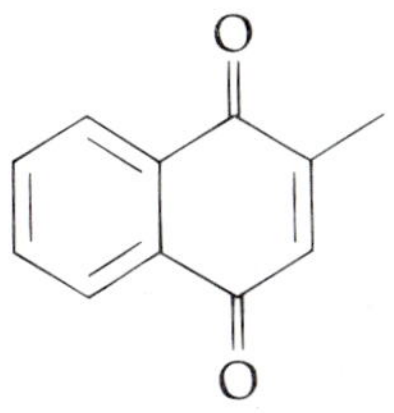

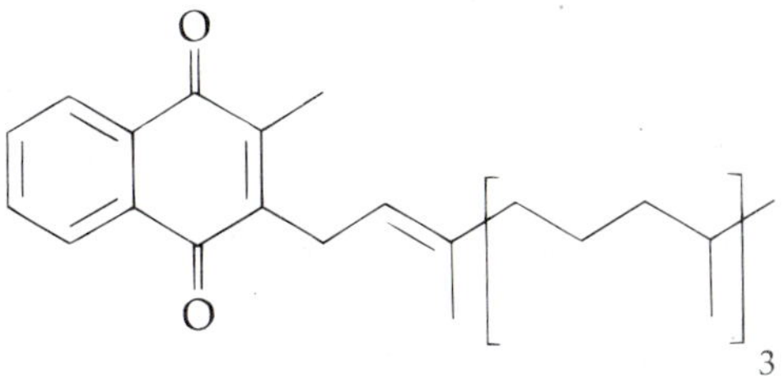

Sources

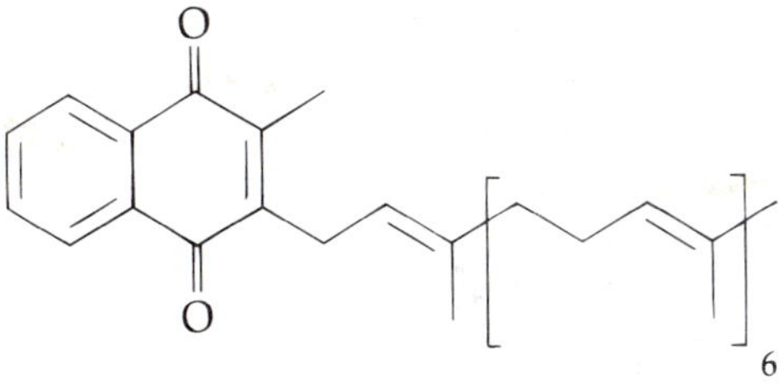

Dietary vitamin K is provided as phylloquinone in plant foods and as a mixture of menaquinones in animal products. The approximate vitamin K content of various foods is given in Table 10.6; the precise content of the vitamin in foods is unknown [1–3].

It is evident from Table 10.6 that dietary vitamin K is provided primarily by plant foods, especially spinach,

FIGURE 10.22 Biologically active forms of vitamin K.

broccoli, kale, brussels sprouts, cabbage, lettuce, among others [1,2], and therefore most of the vitamin consumed is phylloquinone. Smaller amounts of the vitamin are found in cereals, fruits, dairy products, and meats.

Bacteria in the gastrointestinal tract, especially the colon, also provide a source of menaquinones for humans.

Absorption and Transport

Phylloquinone is absorbed from the small intestine, particularly from the jejunum, by a saturable, energy-dependent process [2,4]. Menaquinones and synthetic menadione, in contrast, appear to be absorbed from the distal small intestine and colon by passive diffusion [1,4]. Menaquinones synthesized by bacteria in the lower digestive tract can also be absorbed by passive diffusion in the colon; however, the ability to absorb the bacterially produced vitamin varies from human to human [1].

TABLE 10.6 Vitamin K Content of Various Common Foods

Vitamin K, μg/100g			
<10	10–50	50–100	> 100
Fluid milk	Cheese	Beef liver	Broccoli
Skeletal meats	Butter	Cauliflower	Cabbage
Whole corn	Liver (most)	Watercress	Spinach
Whole wheat	Eggs	Asparagus	Lettuce
Bread	Corn oil		Brussels sprouts
Potatoes	Sunflower oil		Green tea (dry)
Carrots	Oats		Turnip greens
Tomatoes	Green beans		
Oranges	Peas		
Peaches	Coffee (dry)		
Apple sauce			

Source: Table 4.4 from chapter 4 by John W. Suttie of *Fat Soluble Vitamins,* edited by A. T. Diplock, published by Heinemann Professional Publishing Ltd., 1985, 22 Bedford Square, London WCIB 3HH. Reprinted with permission.

Absorption of vitamin K is enhanced by the presence of both bile salts and pancreatic juice [1]. Absorption varies from 40 to 80% of dietary vitamin K [3–5]; those with impaired fat absorption may absorb as little as 20 to 30% of the ingested vitamin [1].

Within the intestinal cell, vitamin K is incorporated into the chylomicron that enters the lymphatic and then the circulatory system for transport to tissues. Chylomicron remnants deliver vitamin K to the liver, although vitamin K has a relatively short hepatic duration, thereby suggesting very little long-term hepatic storage of the vitamin. In the liver, menadione is alkylated, and then, along with phylloquinone and menaquinone, is incorporated into very low density lipoproteins (VLDLs) and ultimately carried to extrahepatic tissues in low-density lipoproteins (LDLs) [5]. Extrahepatic tissues that store vitamin K in high quantities include the adrenal glands, lungs, bone marrow, kidneys, and lymph nodes [1,2,4]. The body pool size of vitamin K, estimated at 50 to 100 μg, is quite low for a fat-soluble vitamin, and smaller than that for vitamin B_{12} [5]. Turnover of vitamin K is rapid, approximately once every 2.5 hours [5].

Functions and Mechanisms of Action

Vitamin K is necessary for the posttranslational carboxylation of specific glutamic acid residues to form γ-carboxyglutamate (Fig. 10.24) on 4 of 13 factors required for the normal coagulation of blood. The 4 vitamin K-dependent factors include factors II (prothrombin), VII, IX, and X.

Overview of Blood Clotting In order for blood to clot, fibrinogen, a soluble protein, must be converted into fibrin, an insoluble fiber network. Thrombin cat-alyzes the proteolysis of fibrinogen to yield fibrin. Fibrin molecules aggregate to form a polymer, which then undergoes cross-linking by fibrin-stabilizing factor (activated by thrombin or factor XIII) to form an insoluble clot and stop bleeding (hemorrhage).

Thrombin, however, circulates in the blood as prothrombin, an inactive enzyme (zymogen). Two pathways, extrinsic and intrinsic (Fig. 10.23), can be used to generate prothrombin and thus thrombin for blood clotting. In the intrinsic pathway, the coagulation process is initiated by the adsorption of factor XII onto a substance such as collagen. Once XII is activated (XII_a), it proceeds to cleave XI to generate an active compound XI_a, which in turn cleaves IX. Factor IX is vitamin K dependent, thus once carboxylated it binds calcium, and, with phospholipids made from aggregated platelets, converts X to X_a, which is also vitamin K dependent. X_a in turn can hydrolyze prothrombin (factor II) into thrombin (II_a), which completes the conversion of fibrinogen to fibrin for clot formation. In the extrinsic pathway (which functions for example with tissue injury), compounds such as tissue thromboplastin activate VII. VII_a is vitamin K dependent, and through a similar cascade of reactions as described for the intrinsic pathway results in the synthesis of thrombin from prothrombin (Fig. 10.23).

The Role of Vitamin K in Carboxylation of Glutamic Acid Residues Four factors, II (prothrombin), VII, IX, and X, require vitamin K; prothrombin will be used as a model to describe the carboxylation process. Prothrombin requires vitamin K for the carboxylation of 10 to 12 glutamic acid residues residing in its N-terminal. This glutamic acid portion once carboxylated forms γ-carboxyglutamic acid (Gla). The carboxylation is required for the protein to become functional. The en-

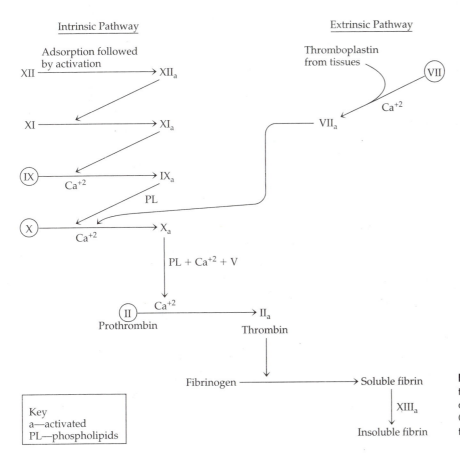

Intrinsic Pathway

Extrinsic Pathway

FIGURE 10.23 The activation of prothrombin and the roles of vitamin K-dependent clotting factors. Circled factors require vitamin K for their formation.

zyme responsible for the γ-carboxylation is referred to as vitamin K-dependent γ-glutamyl carboxylase and is found associated with the rough endoplasmic reticulum (RER), primarily in the liver, where the hemostatic factors are synthesized [5], but also in the RER of other tissues such as lung, spleen, kidney, thyroid, pancreas, cartilage, bone, and skin [4]. The widespread occurrence of γ-glutamyl carboxylase suggests that the need for carboxylated proteins that can bind calcium is much broader than just the regulation of blood coagulation.

Figure 10.24 illustrates the conversion of a specific polypeptide glutamic acid residue into Gla through the action of carboxylase and its vitamin K coenzyme. Gla residues function to bind calcium. The calcium then mediates the binding of Gla proteins to negatively charged phospholipid surfaces [6,7]. This adsorption of specific proteins on phospholipid surfaces is essential in hemostasis.

The participation of vitamin K in the carboxylation of proteins is a cyclic process (Fig. 10.25) often referred to as the *vitamin K cycle*. For the cycle to begin, vitamin K is needed in the reduced form, vitamin KH$_2$. Vitamin K, however, is present in the body generally in its oxidized quinone form due to the presence of oxygen in the

blood. Reduction of vitamin K quinone to the active dihydroxy or hydroquinone (KH$_2$) form can be accomplished by quinone reductases that require either dithiol (indicated by RSH—HSR) or NAD(P)H. The dithiol-dependent quinone reductase appears to be the main physiologic pathway for generating vitamin KH$_2$ from the quinone. Once KH$_2$ is present, along with oxygen and carbon dioxide as the carboxyl precursor, carboxylase can carboxylate the glutamic acid residues on the protein. The carboxylation of glutamic acid is believed to be coupled with the formation of the vitamin K 2,3-epoxide, as illustrated in Figure 10.25. No adenosine triphosphate (ATP) is required for the reaction. The reaction is probably accomplished by the free energy produced through the oxidation of vitamin KH$_2$ to 2,3-epoxide, whereby vitamin K provides reducing equivalents [3–5]. As the cycle continues, vitamin K 2,3-epoxide is subsequently converted to vitamin K quinone by an epoxide reductase. The quinone is then converted back to the dihydroxy vitamin K (KH$_2$) by one of the two quinone reductases, requiring either NAD(P)H or 2 RSH (Figure 10.25) as previously described.

Coumarin and warfarin are anticoagulants that antagonize the action of vitamin K. Oral anticoagulants

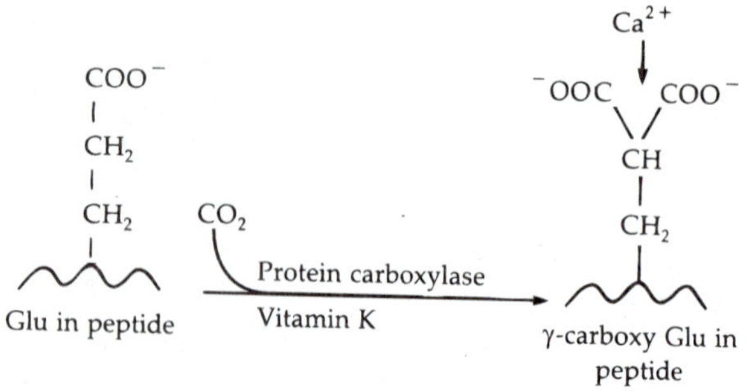

FIGURE 10.24 Production of gamma-carboxyglutamic acid (Gla) via vitamin K-dependent carboxylation.

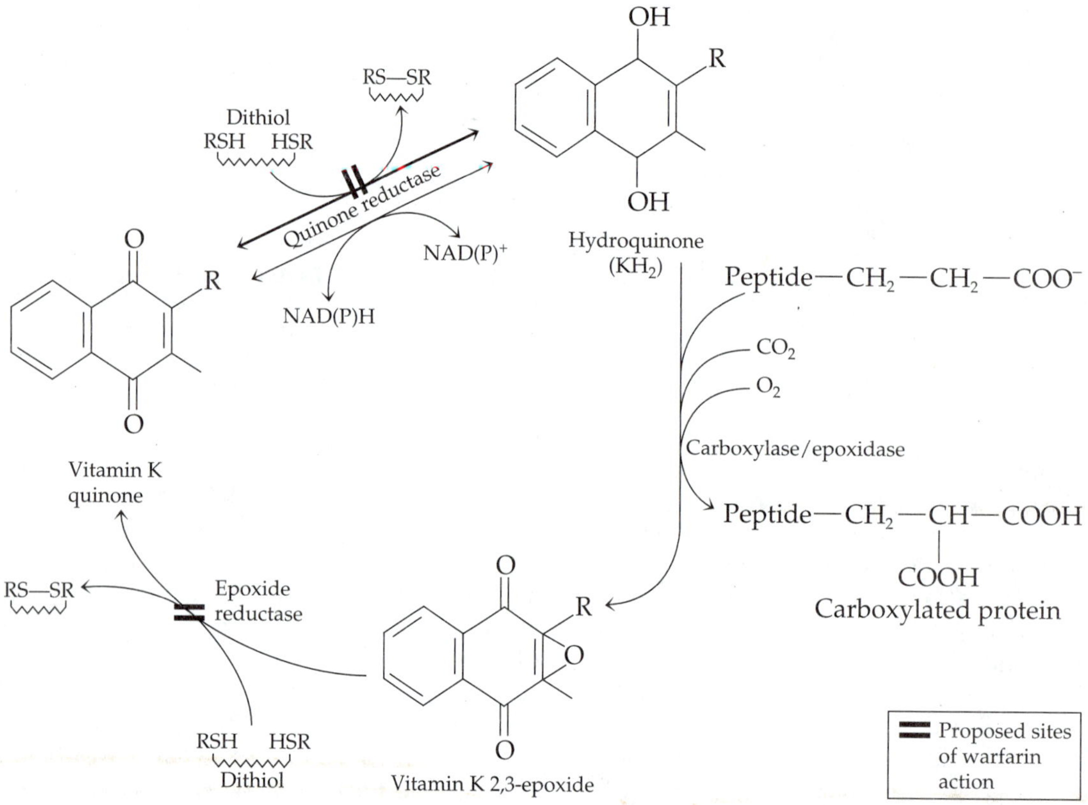

FIGURE 10.25 The vitamin K cycle.

regulate the hepatic biosynthesis of vitamin K-dependent blood-clotting factors. Warfarin, for example, interferes with the dithiol-catalyzed quinone reductase necessary for reducing the oxidized vitamin K to the KH_2 form. Warfarin may also act on the epoxide reductase also preventing KH_2 regeneration [5]. The NAD(P)H quinone reductase, however, is relatively insensitive to warfarin [4,5]. Ingestion of diets high in vitamin K, as obtained from ingestion of about a pound of broccoli daily, can lead to warfarin resistance [8].

Four other proteins, C, S, Z, and M, have also been identified as being vitamin K dependent. Although the functions of proteins Z and M are unknown, proteins C and S mediate, in part, the blood-clotting process. Protein C, a protease, inhibits coagulation, and with protein S, promotes fibrolysis and clot lysis [4,6]. Protein M appears to promote thrombin synthesis from prothrombin; however, further research is needed [5].

Two vitamin K-dependent proteins identified in skeletal tissues include bone Gla protein (BGP, also

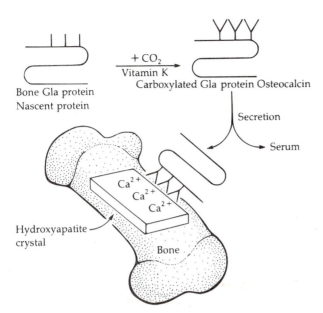

FIGURE 10.26 Schematic outline of the probable relationship between bone Gla protein secretion by osteoblasts and its accumulation in bone or serum. *(Price PA. Role of vitamin K-dependent proteins in bone metabolism. "Reproduced, with permission, from the Annual Review of Nutrition, volume 8:574, 1988, © 1988 by Annual Review, Inc.)*

called *osteocalcin*), and matrix Gla protein (MGP). Figure 10.26 illustrates osteocalcin synthesis. Osteocalcin, secreted by osteoblasts, is found in bone and dentine. On carboxylation involving vitamin K, the Gla residues facilitate the binding of calcium ions [9]. Osteocalcin appears to inhibit hydroxyapatite formation necessary for bone mineralization; however, further research is necessary [10,11]. Long-term vitamin K deficiency in animals results in cessation of longitudinal growth and bone crystallization problems [2]. MGP is found in bone, dentine, and cartilage and is associated with the organic matrix. Both osteocalcin and MGP are thought to promote mobilization of bone calcium [10,11]. Moreover (p. 303), their synthesis appears to be stimulated by 1,25-(OH)$_2$ D$_3$ [10,11]. Although BGP and MGP are better characterized than kidney Gla protein (KGP), which has been identified in the cortex of the kidney, further research to delineate the roles of these Gla proteins is necessary.

Interrelationships with Other Nutrients

The fat-soluble *vitamins A and E* are known to antagonize vitamin K. Excess vitamin A appears to interfere with vitamin K absorption. The antagonistic effect of alpha-tocopherol on vitamin K, however, has yet to be elucidated, but is thought to affect either absorption, function and/or metabolism [5,12]. Vitamin E or its quinone (alpha-tocopheryl quinone) may block the regeneration of the reduced form of vitamin K and/or may affect prothrombin formation by another manner [13,14]. Vitamin E may also impact vitamin K absorption [2].

A possible interrelationship between vitamins K and D is suggested based on their relationship to the mineral calcium. Vitamin D functions impact calcium metabolism, and vitamin K-dependent proteins bind calcium. Two sites of action of 1,25-OH$_2$ D$_3$ are the bone and kidney, and in both these tissues vitamin K-dependent calcium-binding proteins have been identified. 1,25-OH$_2$ D$_3$ is thought to regulate, in part, production of BGP, MGP, and KGP [10,11]. Further research is needed to better characterize the interrelationships.

Metabolism and Excretion

Phylloquinone, degraded much more slowly than menaquinone, is typically converted to 2,3-epoxide (vitamin K cycle, Fig. 10.25) and then to 3-hydroxyquinone. Several other metabolites are generated. These metabolites of phylloquinone are excreted primarily as glucuronides in the urine and feces via the bile [1]. Little is known about the metabolism and excretion of menaquinone.

Menadione is rapidly metabolized to menadiol, which then reacts with phosphate, sulfate, or glucuronide. Menadiol phosphate and menadiol sulfate are excreted both in the bile, and thus ultimately feces, and in the urine; menadiol glucuronides are excreted mostly in the feces via the bile [4,6].

Recommended Dietary Allowances

The 1989 RDA contain for the first time recommendations for vitamin K intakes in definitive values [15]. The RDA for a 79-kg adult male is 80 µg/day and for a 63-kg adult female, 65 µg/day [15]. In the past,

TABLE 10.7 Comparison of 1987 RDIs, 1980 and 1989 RDAs of Vitamin K in Various Population Groups[a]

Population Groups	RDI (1987) (µg)	RDA (1980) (µg)	RDA (1989) (µg)
Infants, 0–12 mo	10	10–20	5–10
Children, 1–3 yr	15	15–30	15
Children, 4–6 yr	20	20–40	20
Children, 7–10 yr	25	30–60	30
Adolescents, 11–14 yr	30	50–100	45
Adolescents, 15–18 yr	35	50–100	55–65
Adult males, 19–70+ yr	45	70–140	70–80
Adult females, 19–70+ yr	35	70–140	60–65
Pregnancy	+10	—	65
Lactation	+20	—	65
[Lactation (2nd 6 mo)]	—	—	62

[a]Population groups are divided differently in the various recommendations.

a range of in-takes has been suggested based on the assumption that the amount of vitamin K supplied by intestinal bacteria could vary from zero to as much as 50% of requirement [16]. Bacterial synthesis of menaquinones appears, however, insufficient to meet vitamin requirements when the intake of subjects is limited to approximately 50 µg per day [15]. Based on these studies and on the response of people with depressed levels of vitamin K to intravenously administered doses of the vitamin [15], a dietary intake of about 1 µg/kg body wt/day appears sufficient to maintain normal clotting time in adults. Requirements for vitamin K appear to range from 0.4 µg/kg/day to 1.0 µg/kg/day [1,2,6].

The Recommended Dietary Intakes (RDIs) suggested by the 1980–1985 Committee on RDA were lower than either the 1980 or 1989 RDA (Table 10.6) [3]. In his article justifying the RDI for vitamin K, Olson [3] explains the decrease in the amount of vitamin K for adolescents and adults by citing studies that show 0.15 µg vitamin K/kg body weight per day is sufficient to maintain vitamin K-dependent clotting factors and clotting times in the normal range even when subjects are being given large doses of antibiotics.

Deficiency

A deficiency of vitamin K is unlikely in healthy adults. A normal diet contains from 300 to 500 µg vitamin K per day and therefore supplies at least three times the amount of vitamin K recommended [5]. The population groups that appear most at risk for a vitamin K deficiency are newborn infants and people who have been injured, have renal insufficiency, and/or are being treated chronically with antibiotics [3]. The newborn infant is particularly at risk because its food is limited to milk, which is

low in vitamin K, and because its intestinal tract is not yet populated by vitamin K-synthesizing bacteria. Supplementation with vitamin K is considered advisable for all newborns; currently it is recommended that 0.5 to 1 mg phylloquinone be injected intramuscularly into infants very shortly after birth [3]. Those people on prolonged sulfa and antibiotic drug therapy are at risk due to destruction of gastrointestinal bacteria that manufacture the vitamin and contribute a source of vitamin K. Other conditions and populations associated with increased need for intake include those with malabsorptive disorders: biliary fistula, obstructive jaundice, steatorrhea or chronic diarrhea, intestinal bypass surgery, chronic pancreatitis, and liver disease.

Toxicity

Natural forms of vitamin K such as phylloquinone, even when supplemented in large amounts, have caused no symptoms of toxicity [3,11]. However, because of its unsubstituted carbon 3 (Fig. 10.22) the synthetic product menadione can combine with sulfhydryl groups such as those in glutathione, resulting in glutathione oxidation and excretion [7]. Ultimately there is oxidation of membrane phospholipids. Toxic effects reported in infants supplemented with menadione include hemolytic anemia, hyperbilirubinemia, and severe jaundice [4,11,14].

Assessment of Nutriture

Measurement of prothrombin time, the time required for a fibrin clot to form, is often used to identify potential defects in vitamin K-dependent or other blood-clotting proteins. A normal prothrombin time is considered to be between 11 and 13 seconds, while times greater than 25 seconds are associated with major bleeding [16]. In addition, maintenance of plasma prothrombin concentrations in the normal range (80 to 120 µg/mL) [3] suggests adequate vitamin K status.

Vitamin K status can also be assessed by the measurements of both plasma prothrombin and des γ-carboxyglutamyl prothrombin. Because human vitamin K deficiency results in the secretion of partially carboxylated prothrombin molecules (des γ-carboxyglutamyl prothrombin) into the plasma, measurement of the ratio of des γ-carboxyglutamyl prothrombin to prothrombin appears to be a useful indicator of alterations in vitamin K sufficiency [1,3]. The 24-hour urine excretion of γ-carboxyglutamic acid along with plasma vitamin K concentrations have also been used to assess vitamin K status [18].

References Cited for Vitamin K

1. Suttie JW. Vitamin K. In: Diplock AT, ed. Fat soluble vitamins. Lancaster, PA: Technomic, 1985:225–311.
2. Suttie JW. Vitamin K. In: Machlin LJ. Handbook of vitamins, 2nd ed. New York: Dekker, 1991:145–194.
3. Olson, JA. Recommended dietary intakes (RDI) of vitamin K in humans. Am J Clin Nutr 1987;45:687–692.
4. Combs GF. The vitamins. New York: Academic Press, 1992:205–222.
5. Olson RE. The function and metabolism of vitamin K. Ann Rev Nutr 1984;4:281–337.
6. Bender DA. Nutritional biochemistry of the vitamins. New York: Cambridge University Press, 1992:106–127.
7. Esmon CT. Cell mediated events that control blood coagulation and vascular injury. Ann Rev Cell Biol 1993;9:1–26.
8. Kempin SJ. Warfarin resistance caused by broccoli. N Eng J Med 1983;308:1229–1230.
9. Saupe J, Shearer MJ, Kohlmeier M. Phylloquinone transport and its influence on gamma-carboxyglutamate residues of osteocalcin in patients on maintenance hemodialysis. Am J Clin Nutr 1993;58:204–208.
10. Price PA. Role of vitamin-K dependent proteins in bone metabolism. Ann Rev Nutr 1988;8:565–583.
11. The function of the vitamin K-dependent proteins, bone Gla protein (BGP) and kidney Gla protein (KGP). Nutr Rev 1984;42:230–233.
12. Council on Scientific Affairs, American Medical Association. Vitamin preparations as dietary supplements and as therapeutic agents. JAMA 1987;257:1929–1936.
13. Bieri JG, Corash L, Hubbard VS. Medical uses of vitamin E. N Engl J Med 1983;308:1063–1071.
14. Bendich A, Machlin LJ. Safety of oral intake of vitamin E. Am J Clin Nutr 1988;48:612–619.
15. National Research Council. Recommended dietary allowances. 10th ed. Washington, DC: National Academy Press, 1989:107–114.
16. National Research Council. Recommended dietary allowances, 9th ed. Washington, DC: National Academy of Sciences, 1980:69–71.
17. Simko M, Cowell C, Gilbride JA. Nutrition assessment. Rockville, MD: Aspen, 1984.
18. Sadowski JA, Bacon DS, Hood S et al. The applications of methods used for the evaluation of vitamin K nutritional status in human and animal studies. In: Suttie JW, ed. Current advances in vitamin K research. New York: Elsevier, 1988: 453–463.

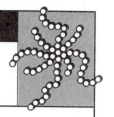

PERSPECTIVE

The Antioxidant Nutrients

DNA, proteins, and polyunsaturated fatty acids (PUFA) found in the body may be attacked by free radicals. Attack of DNA, proteins (especially those with free sulfhydryl groups), and polyunsaturated fatty acids by free radicals has been implicated in the etiologies of diseases including atherosclerosis and cancer, among others.

Free radicals, as defined by Diplock [1], are atoms or molecules that have one or more unpaired electron(s). Electrons in atoms reside in orbitals. The imbalance in electrons in the orbitals results in most cases in the high reactivity of the free radicals. Some examples of free radicals and reactive oxygen species include O_2^- (superoxide radical), O_2^{2-} (peroxyl radical), H_2O_2 (hydrogen peroxide), $OH^.$ (hydroxy free radicals), $L^.$ (lipid carbon-centered radical), $HO_2^.$ (perhydroxy or hydroperoxyl radical), and $LOO^.$ (lipid peroxyl radical). Once formed, free radicals attack membranes and tissues. For example, aqueous peroxyl radicals may induce oxidation of low-density lipoproteins, and oxidation and hemolysis of red blood cell membranes among others [2,3]. The formation of free radicals in the cell and the destruction of free radicals by antioxidant nutrients will be discussed in this "Perspective" section.

Superoxide radicals (O_2^-) are generated during several cellular processes. For example, molecular oxygen may gain an electron leaked from the electron transport chain to form a superoxide radical.

$$O_2 \xrightarrow{e^-} O_2^-$$

Superoxide radicals are also formed from activated phagocytic cells such as macrophages and neutrophils. In fact, the production of the superoxide radical is important for the destruction of some bacterial strains. In addition, superoxide radicals generated by neutrophils heighten the inflammatory response by acting as a chemoattractant for other neutrophils.

However, with excessive production and without removal, superoxide radicals can damage tissues. Damage may be extensive in the presence of metals such as iron. Superoxide radicals can react with free ferric iron to generate ferrous iron and molecular oxygen.

$$O_2^- + Fe^{+3} \longrightarrow O_2 + Fe^{+2}$$

Ferrous iron can react with hydrogen peroxide to form an extremely reactive free hydroxy radical ($OH^.$). Hydrogen peroxide and free hydroxy radicals are discussed further in the next several paragraphs.

$$Fe^{+2} + H_2O_2 \longrightarrow Fe^{+3} + OH^- + OH^. \text{ (Fenton reaction)}$$

Normally, however, iron, as well as copper, are not found free and available within the body; the minerals are typically (non-pathological condition) bound, as an antioxidant defense, to transport or storage proteins. It is thought that superoxide radicals may be able to mobilize iron, or copper, which then may be available to catalyze reactions resulting in the formation of the more reactive free hydroxy radical.

Superoxide radicals can generate other free radicals. For example, they can react with available electrons to form a peroxy radical (O_2^{2-}), which can subsequently react with hydrogen ions to form another destructive compound, hydrogen peroxide.

$$O_2^- \xrightarrow{e^-} O_2^{2-} \xrightarrow{H^+} HO_2^- \xrightarrow{H^+} H_2O_2$$

Hydrogen peroxide can react with an electron and hydrogen to generate a very reactive free hydroxy radical.

$$H_2O_2 \xrightarrow{e^- \ H^+} H_2O + OH^.$$

Concentrations of hydrogen peroxide as well as superoxide radicals need to be controlled in the body to prevent cellular destruction. Ascorbic acid (AH^-) acts as an antioxidant in aqueous solutions by reacting with the superoxide radical and hydrogen ion (H^+) to form semidehydroascorbate radical (A^-) and hydrogen peroxide (H_2O_2).

$$AH^- + O_2^- + H^+ \longrightarrow A^- + H_2O_2$$

Uric acid also may act as a reducing agent (antioxidant in aqueous solutions). Uric acid may scavenge various free radicals including $OH^.$. Superoxide dismutase (SOD) also reacts with O_2^-. SOD is found both in the cytosol and in the mitochondria. SOD activity in the cytosol requires Zn^{+2} and Cu^{+2}; while SOD in the mitochondria needs Mn^{+2} for activation. Deficiencies of these minerals can reduce the activity of this important enzyme.

PERSPECTIVE (continued)

Cytosol

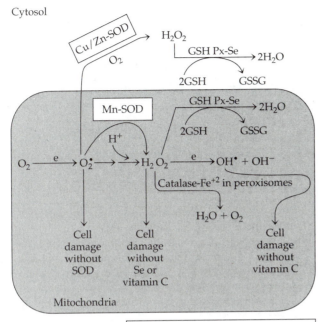

Key: SOD—superoxide dismutase
GSH Px—glutathione peroxidase

FIGURE 1 The interaction between the microminerals zinc, copper, manganese, iron, and selenium to prevent cell damage.

$$O_2^- + O_2^- + 2H^+ \xrightarrow{\text{superoxide dismutase (SOD)}} H_2O_2 + O_2$$

If more superoxide radicals are produced than can be handled by SOD, hydrogen peroxide and singlet oxygen ($^1O_2$) (both damaging to cells) may be generated. Singlet oxygen is discussed further on page 323.

As mentioned previously, hydrogen peroxides (H_2O_2) also damage cells. This compound is formed in cells from several reactions including, for example, (1) superoxide radicals reacting with an electron and $2H^+$, (2) ascorbate reacting with superoxide radicals and H^+, and (3) activated neutrophils. Because hydrogen peroxide can damage cells, it, like superoxide radicals, must be removed.

Ascorbate, just as it reacted with superoxide radicals, also can react with hydrogen peroxide to produce water and dehydroascorbate (DHAA).

$$AH^- + H_2O_2 + H^+ \longrightarrow 2 H_2O + DHAA$$

The accumulation of H_2O_2 also is prevented by two enzymes: (1) catalase, a heme Fe^{+2}-containing enzyme located primarily in peroxisomes, but to a small extent in the mitochondria, and (2) glutathione peroxidase, a selenium-requiring enzyme located in both the mito-

chondria and cytoplasm. In addition to requiring four selenium atoms, glutathione peroxidase uses two glutathione molecules (a tripeptide composed of glycine, cysteine, and glutamic acid) present in the reduced state (GSH). Glutathione, as well as cysteine, lipoic acid, and methionine are thiols (R-SH). Thiols may act in aqueous and lipid environments as an antioxidant. Glutathione serves as a substrate for various enzymes including glutathione peroxidase, and during the reaction, GSH becomes oxidized (GSSG). Each of the two glutathione molecules gives up a hydrogen from its sulfhydryl group (SH). A radical center is formed on the sulfur atom until two such radicals join to form a disulfide bond. Both catalase and glutathione peroxidase can react with H_2O_2 as follows:

$$2 H_2O_2 \xrightarrow{\text{catalase-Fe}^{+2}} 2 H_2O + O_2$$

$$H_2O_2 + 2GSH \xrightarrow{\substack{\text{glutathione} \\ \text{peroxidase-Se}}} 2 H_2O + GSSG$$

Glutathione peroxidase, because of its dual (mitochondrial and cytosolic) locations in the cell, is thought to be more active in the removal of hydrogen peroxide than catalase. Figure 1 shows the complex interaction between the antioxidant minerals—zinc, copper, manganese, iron, and selenium.

Again, the removal of hydrogen peroxide and the prevention of its reaction with free ferrous iron, or possibly copper, are important to prevent the generation of free hydroxy radicals (OH·).

$$Fe^{+2} \text{ or } Cu^{+1} + H_2O_2 \longrightarrow Fe^{+3} \text{ or } Cu^{+2} + OH· + OH^-$$

In addition, removal of hydrogen peroxide is needed to prevent its reacting with another electron and hydrogen ion to also form a free hydroxy radical (p. 320).

Free hydroxy radicals (OH·) are extremely reactive, rapidly taking electrons from the surroundings. According to Diplock [1], OH· is a severe threat to living systems. Often the electron taken by the reactive free hydroxy radical is from nearby organic molecules such as enzymes or other proteins, polyunsaturated fatty acids, and DNA. Hydroxy radical-induced changes in purine and pyrimidine bases in DNA may lead to mutations or breakages, which, if not repaired, may result, for example, in cancer [4]. If the organic molecule is a polyunsaturated fatty acid present in the phospholipid portion of the cell membranes, damage to the membrane and thus the cell occurs [5]. Vitamin C (AH⁻), however, can react with the hydroxy radical to produce water and semidehydroascorbate radical.

$$AH^- + OH· \longrightarrow H_2O + A^-$$

Frei [3] reported that ascorbate can effectively react, in aqueous solutions such as blood, with oxidants prior to their initiation of oxidative damage to lipids such as those within lipoproteins or membranes.

Removal of free hydroxy radicals is important to ensure membrane integrity. Organic lipid compounds (LH) can react with (1) free hydroxy radicals to form a lipid carbon-centered radical (L·) and water

$$(1) \quad LH + OH· \longrightarrow L· + H_2O$$

or (2) molecular oxygen to form a lipid carbon-centered radical and perhydroxy radical (HO₂·). This is sometimes referred to as initiation.

$$(2) \quad LH + O_2 \longrightarrow L· + HO_2·$$

Lipid carbon-centered radicals, in turn, can react with molecular oxygen to form lipid peroxyl radicals, LOO·.

$$L· + O_2 \longrightarrow LOO· \text{ (also written } LO_2·)$$

Once formed, lipid peroxy radicals can abstract a hydrogen atom from other organic compounds such as polyunsaturated fatty acids to generate a chain reaction (propagation) with the L·.

$$LOO· + LH \longrightarrow L· + LOOH$$

Lipid peroxyl radicals can also be generated from reactions between iron and LOOH (lipid hydroperoxide or peroxidized fatty acids),

$$LOOH + Fe^{+2} \longrightarrow LO· + OH^- + Fe^{+3}$$

$$LOOH + Fe^{+3} \longrightarrow LOO· + H^+ + Fe^{+2}$$

thus necessitating the removal of LO·, LOO·, and LOOH from the environment, and the removal of L·, which can initiate a chain reaction to destroy the cell. Sequestration of iron by transport and storage proteins is also essential for protection against free radical generation. Without the removal of these lipid free radicals, alterations in membrane integrity, potential, and fluidity may occur, with possible membrane rupture and cell death.

Vitamin E located in the membranes can break the chain of radical attack by reacting with the lipid peroxyl radical (LOO·) and preventing further abstraction of hydrogen (H) from the fatty acids. Vitamin E (EH) provides a hydrogen for the reduction of the lipid peroxyl radical.

$$LOO· + EH \longrightarrow LOOH + E·$$

Thus, vitamin E terminates chain-propagation reactions, but generates LOOH.

Destruction of peroxidized fatty acids (LOOH, also called *lipid hydroperoxides*) is also necessary. Peroxidized fatty acids, generated in the hydrophobic region of the cell membranes from the action of vitamin E, are polar compounds. Phospholipase A₂ may cleave the peroxidized fatty acid from the phospholipid in the membrane to allow migration. The polar peroxidized fatty acids can then destroy the normal architecture of the cell in migration from the nonpolar region of generation.

Peroxidized fatty acid destruction can be accomplished by the action of glutathione peroxidase. Glutathione peroxidase can react with peroxidized free fatty acids and convert them into hydroxyfatty acids, LOH.

$$2LOOH + 2GSH \xrightarrow{\text{glutathione peroxidase-Se}} 2LOH + H_2O + GSSG$$

Regeneration of reduced glutathione, as well as vitamins C and E is important to the cellular defense against free radicals. The regeneration of vitamin E is thought initially to require the migration of the vitamin to the membrane surface, followed by the actions of ascorbate (AH⁻), reduced glutathione, and NADPH. First, ascorbate is used to regenerate alpha-tocopherol and in the process forms dehydroascorbate (DHAA).

P E R S P E C T I V E   (continued)

Tocopherol radical + AH$^-$ $\longrightarrow$ tocopherol + DHAA

Ascorbate is regenerated from dehydroascorbate by glutathione.

$$DHAA + 2GSH \longrightarrow AH^- + GSSG + H^+$$

NADPH then regenerates GSH from GSSG.

$$NADPH + GSSG \longrightarrow NADP + 2GSH$$

Regeneration of ascorbic acid (AH$^-$) from semide-hydroascorbate radical (A$^-$) can also be accomplished by the following reactions [6]. Again, niacin and glutathione in its reduced form (GSH) may be involved.

$$2A^- \longrightarrow AH^- + DHAA$$

$$2A^- + 2GSH \longrightarrow 2AH^- + GSSG$$

$$2A^- + NADH + H^+ \longrightarrow 2AH^- + NAD^+$$

Beta-carotene, lycopene, and other carotenoids also function as antioxidants because they possess the ability to react with and quench free-radical reactions either in solution or in membrane systems. Quenching is a process by which electronically excited molecules, such as singlet molecular oxygen ($'O_2$) generated from lipid peroxidation of membranes, enzymatic or photochemical reactions (shown as follows), are inactivated [7].

$$O_2 \xrightarrow{\text{hv}} {'O_2}$$

In singlet oxygen, the peripheral electron in the oxygen structure is excited to an orbital above that which it normally occupies [1]. Singlet oxygen, like free radicals, can damage cells and tissues. The ability of carotenoids such as beta-carotene and lycopene to quench singlet oxygen is attributed to the conjugated double-bond systems within the carotenoids. The carotenoids can absorb energy without chemical change to return the "excited" $'O_2$ to its ground state [1]. Lycopene appears to be more effective than β-carotene in quenching singlet oxygen [1]. Carotenoids can also act to break chain reactions by LOO$\cdot$; however, these reactions only occur with low oxygen concentrations ($_pO_2$).

Results from studies comparing the effectiveness of the antioxidant nutrients differ because of the numerous experimental designs and conditions. However, studies clearly show the important role of the antioxidant nutrients with implications for prevention of disease. An increased risk of ischemic heart disease has been shown with low plasma concentrations of antioxidants, primarily vitamin E, but to lesser extents, in rank order, carotene = ascorbate > vitamin A [8].

Oral supplementation of α-tocopherol (but not β-carotene) rendered low-density lipoproteins less susceptible to oxidation *in vitro* and is linked to a lower risk of coronary heart disease in men and women [9–11]. However, in the presence of pro-oxidants such as ferrous iron, vitamin E's ability to prevent oxidation is diminished [7].

Prevention of endothelial cell injury and the oxidization of low-density lipoproteins appear to be important in preventing atherosclerosis. Injury to endothelial cells enhances monocyte attachment to the cells, migration through the endothelium to the intima, and differentiation of the monocytes into macrophages. Macrophages scavenge oxidized low-density lipoproteins and take up the lipoprotein through a receptor-mediated process. With lipid accumulation, foam cells form and create over time fatty streaks and plaque in the intima of the blood vessel. Clinical trials with vitamin E suggest that the vitamin may decrease susceptibility of low-density lipoproteins to oxidation by free radicals [9–13].

Risks for some types of cancer have been strongly correlated with low intakes or low nutritional status of many of the antioxidants, especially vitamins A and C, carotenoids, and selenium [14].

Recovery of tissue following ischemia–reoxygenation injuries also appears to benefit from the inclusion of antioxidants. Tissues deprived of oxygen, such as the heart during a myocardial infarction, need oxygen restoration to prevent or minimize tissue damage. However, restoration of oxygen results in free radical production within the damaged tissue, and thus in additional tissue damage. Three possible reasons [15–17] for the free radical production observed in ischemic tissue include (1) activation of neutrophils by compounds released by the damaged tissues and the neutrophil's subsequent generation of hydrogen peroxide and superoxide radicals. Second, with injury there may be disruption of the respiratory chain with more electrons leaked to oxygen for superoxide radical formation. Third, for tissues such as the intestine and possibly endothelial cells of blood vessels, the presence of xanthine oxidase or the conversion of xanthine dehydrogenase into xanthine oxidase may result in free radical formation [4,15–17]. During ischemia, xanthine dehydrogenase is converted into xanthine oxidase due to changes in thiol groups and/or proteolysis [15,16]. Following reoxygenation of the ischemic tissue, xanthine oxidase acts on hypoxanthine (generated from ATP or adenosine degradation).

$$Hypoxanthine + 2O_2 + H_2O \xrightarrow{\text{xanthine oxidase}} xanthine + 2O_2^- + 2H^+$$

P E R S P E C T I V E (continued)

The production of free radicals such as the superoxide radical by xanthine oxidase can further damage injured tissue [15–17]. And if iron or other metals like copper have been released from bound proteins, subsequent reactions of these metals with the free radicals, superoxide radicals, and hydrogen peroxide, can lead to the formation of more highly reactive free hydroxy radicals. Improved tissue recovery has been demonstrated with inclusion of antioxidant nutrients and enzymes as part of oxygen restoration following tissue ischemia.

As studies continue to document the roles of the antioxidant nutrients, scientists and other health professionals are re-evaluating the Recommended Dietary Allowances and the concept of prevention of vitamin and mineral deficiency diseases. Perhaps new guidelines defining optimal levels of nutrients to prevent diseases such as heart disease and cancer will emerge.

References Cited for Perspective

1. Diplock AT. Antioxidant nutrients and disease prevention: An overview. Am J Clin Nutr 1991;53:189S–193S.
2. Niki E. Action of ascorbic acid as a scavenger of active and stable oxygen radicals. Am J Clin Nutr 1991;54:1119S–1124S.
3. Frei B. Ascorbic acid protects lipids in human plasma and low density lipoprotein against oxidative damage. Am J Clin Nutr 1991;54:1113S–1118S.
4. Halliwell B, Evans PJ, Kaur H, Aruoma OI. Free radicals, tissue injury, and human disease: A potential for therapeutic use of antioxidants? In: Kinney JM and Tuck HN, eds. Organ metabolism and nutrition: Ideas for future critical care. New York: Raven Press, 1994:425–445.
5. Niki E, Yamamota Y, Komuro E, Sato K. Membrane damage due to lipid oxidation. Am J Clin Nutr 1991;53:201S–205S.
6. Stadtman ER. Ascorbic acid and oxidative inactivation of proteins. Am J Clin Nutr 1991;54:1125S–1128S.
7. Mascio PD, Murphy ME, Sies H. Antioxidant defense systems: The role of carotenoids, tocopherols, and thiols. Am J Clin Nutr 1991;53:194S–200S.
8. Gey KF, Moser UK, Jordan P, Sahelin HB, Eichholzer M, Ludin E. Increased risk of cardiovascular disease at suboptimal plasma concentrations of essential antioxidants: an epidemiological update with special attention to carotene and vitamin C. Am J Clin Nutr 1993;57(suppl):787S–797S.
9. Stampfer MJ, Hennekens CH, Manson JE, Colditz GA, Rosner B, Willett WC. Vitamin E consumption and the risk of coronary disease in women. N Eng J Med 1993;328:1444–1449.
10. Rimm EB, Stampfer MJ, Ascherio A, Giovannucci E, Colditz GA, Willett WC. Vitamin E consumption and the risk of coronary heart disease in men. N Eng J Med 1993;328:1450–1456.
11. Abbey M, Nestel PJ, Baghurst PA. Antioxidant vitamins and low-density-lipoprotein oxidation. Am J Clin Nutr 1993;58:525–532.
12. Jialal I, Grundy SM. Effect of dietary supplementation with alpha tocopherol on the oxidative modification of low density lipoprotein. J Lipid Res 1992;33:899–906.
13. Esterbauer H, Dieber-Rotheneder M, Striegl G, Waeg G. Role of vitamin E in preventing the oxidation of low-density lipoprotein. Am J Clin Nutr 1991;53:314S–321S.
14. Weisburger JH. Nutritional approach to cancer prevention with emphasis on vitamins, antioxidants, and carotenoids. Am J Clin Nutr 1991;53:226S–237S.
15. Halliwell B, Gutteridge HMC. Free radicals in biology and medicine. Oxford: Clarendon Press, 1989.
16. McCord JM. Free radicals and myocardial ischemia: Overview and outlook. Free Radical Biol Med 1988;4:9–14.
17. Baker GL, Corry RJ, Autor AP. Oxygen free radical induced damage in kidneys subjected to warm ischemia and reperfusion. Ann Surgery 1985;202:628–641.

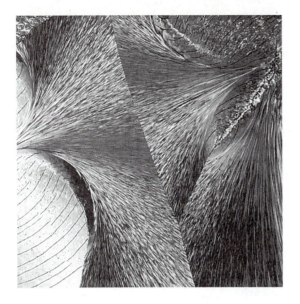

MACROMINERALS

Photo: Photomicrograph of crystallized calcium phosphate

The importance of minerals in normal nutrition and metabolism cannot be overstated, despite the fact that they constitute only about 4% of total body weight. Their functions are many and varied. They provide the medium essential for normal cellular activity, determine the osmotic properties of body fluids, impart hardness to bones and teeth, and function as obligatory cofactors in metalloprotein activity.

Historically, the knowledge that minerals are required in normal nutrition evolved from knowledge of the mineral composition of body tissues and fluids. This knowledge has expanded greatly as a result of accumulating improvements in analytic techniques for quantification of minerals.

Macrominerals (Table 11.1), also referred to as *major minerals* or *macronutrient elements*, are distinguished from the microminerals (Chapter 12) by their occurrence in the body. Using this as a criterion, various definitions of a macromineral have been expressed, such as the requirement that it constitute at least 0.01% of total body weight or that it occur in a minimum quantity of 5 g in a 60-kg human body. Unfortunately, however, these values are clearly not equivalent, a discrepancy that in itself indicates the desirability for a less ambiguous, standard definition such as required in amounts greater than 100 mg per day. Because of their importance in the maintenance of electrolyte balance in body fluids, the macrominerals sodium, chlorine, and potassium also are discussed in Chapter 13. Although sulfur is found in the body and is considered a macromineral, because the body does not use it alone as a nutrient, the mineral is not discussed as a subsection of this chapter. Sulfur is found in the body associated structurally with vitamins such as thiamin and biotin, and as part of the sulfur-containing amino acids methionine, cysteine, and taurine. Thus, sulfur is commonly found within proteins, especially those found in skin, hair, and nails.

Table 11.1 Macrominerals—Functions, Deficiency Symptoms, and Recommended Dietary Allowances (RDA)

Mineral	Selected Physiological Functions	Selected Enzyme Cofactors	Deficiency Symptoms	Food Sources in Rank Order	RDA[a]
Calcium	Structural component of bones and teeth, role in intracellular and hormonal secretion regulation, muscle contraction, blood clotting, and activation of some enzyme systems	Adenylate, cyclase, kinases (see Table 11.2)	Rickets, osteomalacia, osteoporosis, scurvy, tetany, parathyroid hyperplasia, stunted growth, laryngospasm	Milk, milk products, sardines, clams, osyters, turnip greens, mustard greens, broccoli, legumes, dried fruits	1,200 mg 19–24 years, then 800 mg
Chloride	Functions as a major anion; maintains pH balance, enzyme activation, component of gastric hydrochloric acid		Noted in infants: loss of appetite, failure to thrive, muscle weakness, lethargy, severe hypokalemia, metabolic acidosis	Table salt, seafood, milk, meat, eggs	
Magnesium	Component of bones; role in nerve impulse transmission, protein synthesis, enzyme activation (in glycolysis and many ATP-dependent reactions)	Involved in hydrolysis and transfer of phosphate groups by phosphokinase; important in numerous ATP-dependent enzyme reactions	Depression, muscle weakness, tetany, abnormal behavior, convulsions, depressed serum levels, growth failure	Nuts, legumes, cereal grains, soybeans, parsnips, chocolate, blackstrap molasses, corn, peas, carrots, seafood, brown rice, parsley, lima beans, spinach	350 mg males, 280 mg females
Phosphorus	Structural component of bone, teeth, cell membranes, phospholipids, nucleic acids, nucleotide coenzymes, ATP-ADP phosphate energy-transferring system in cells; participates in regulation of pH and osmotic pressure of intracellular fluids	Activates many enzymes in phosphorylation and dephosphorylation	Neuromuscular, skeletal, hematologic, and renal manifestations; rickets, osteomalacia, anorexia	Meat, poultry, fish, eggs, milk, milk products, nuts, legumes, cereals, grains, chocolate	1,200 mg 19–24 years, then 800 mg
Potassium	Functions as an electrolyte; role in water, electrolyte and pH balances, cell membrane transfer	Pyruvate kinase, Na^+/K^+-ATPase	Muscular weakness, mental apathy; cardiac arrhythmias, paralysis, bone fragility, adrenal hypertrophy, decreased growth rate, weight loss	Avocado, banana, dried fruits, orange, peach, potatoes, dried beans, tomato, wheat bran, dairy products, eggs	
Sodium	Functions as an electrolyte; role in water, pH, and electrolyte regulation, nerve transmission, muscle contraction	Na^+/K^+-ATPase	Anorexia, nausea, muscle atrophy, poor growth, weight loss	Table salt, meat, seafood, cheese, milk, bread, vegetables (abundant in most foods except fruits)	
Sulfur	Component of sulfur-containing amino acids, thiamin, biotin, lipoic acid		Unknown	Protein foods (meat, poultry, fish, eggs, milk, cheese, legumes, nuts)	

Note: Abbreviations: ATP, adenosine triphosphate; ADP, adenosine diphosphate.
[a]For adults.

CALCIUM

Calcium (Ca) is the most abundant divalent cation of the human body, averaging about 1.5% of total body weight [1]. Bones and teeth contain about 99% of the calcium. The other 1% of the body's calcium is distributed in both intracellular and extracellular fluids.

Sources

The best food sources of calcium are listed in Table 11.1 and include milk, cheese, ice cream, yogurt, tofu, salmon, sardines (with bones), clams, oysters, turnip greens, mustard greens, broccoli, kale, legumes, and dried fruits. Meats, grains, and nuts tend to be poor sources of calcium.

Digestion, Absorption, and Transport

Calcium is present in foods, and dietary supplements, as relatively insoluble salts. Because calcium is absorbed only in its ionized (Ca^{+2}) form, it must first be released from the salts. Calcium is solubilized from most calcium salts in about one hour at a mildly acidic pH. Solubilization, however, does not necessarily ensure better absorption, because within the more alkaline pH of the small intestine, calcium may complex with minerals or other selected dietary constituents [2]. Formation of these complexes in the small intestine may limit calcium bioavailability.

Ingestion of food or lactose along with the calcium source appears to improve overall calcium absorption [3]. In infants, the effects of lactose on calcium diffusion, especially in the ileum, are thought to be more pronounced than in the adult [3]. Other sugars, and protein, also seem to have the same positive effect on calcium absorption [4,5].

Fiber as well as phytate may decrease calcium absorption and retention. Nonfermentable fibers such as cellulose or those found in wheat bran can increase the bulk of intestinal contents and decrease transit time, thus decreasing the time available for calcium absorption to occur. Nonfermentable or slowly fermentable fibers such as some of the hemicelluloses stimulate proliferation of microbes, which in turn bind minerals such as calcium and make them unavailable for absorption. Phytate (myoinositol hexaphosphate) is found in some of the same plant foods in which fiber is found; for example, legumes, nuts and cereals. Phytates appear to bind calcium and decrease its availability. A phytate-to-calcium molar ratio greater than 0.2 has been suggested to increase the risk of calcium deficiency [6]. Calcium retention was depressed in young men after switching from white bread to whole-wheat bread providing 2 g phytate and 40 g fiber per day [7].

Calcium absorption in the intestine may also be inhibited by the presence of oxalate, which chelates the calcium and increases fecal excretion of the complex. Oxalate is found in a variety of vegetables (such as spinach, beets, celery, eggplant, greens, okra, and squash), fruits (such as straw-, black-, blue-, and gooseberries, and currents), nuts (pecans, peanuts), and beverages (tea, Ovaltine, cocoa), among other foods.

Magnesium and calcium, both divalent cations, appear to compete with each other for intestinal absorption whenever an excess of either is present in the gastrointestinal tract. A dietary calcium-to-phosphorus ratio of 1:1 is recommended by the Food and Nutrition Board [4]; however, diets high in phosphorus relative to calcium (in amounts suggested by the RDA) in humans have not been shown to impair calcium balance [1]. Absorption of calcium from low-calcium diets (230 mg) that include zinc supplements is also thought to be impaired [8]. The effect of calcium supplements on iron absorption is discussed in the section "Interactions with Other Nutrients."

Unabsorbed dietary fatty acids found in significant quantities associated with steatorrhea (> 7 g fecal fat/day) [9] can interfere with calcium absorption through the formation of insoluble calcium soaps (calcium–fatty acid complexes) in the lumen of the small intestine. These calcium soaps cannot be absorbed and are excreted in the feces.

Calcium absorption from calcium supplements varies depending on the calcium salt. Calcium (250 mg) absorption was 39% ± 3% from calcium carbonate, 32% ± 4% from calcium acetate, 32% ± 4% from calcium lactate, 27% ± 3% from calcium gluconate, and 30% ± 3% from calcium citrate [2]. Other studies suggest that calcium absorption from chelated forms of calcium such as calcium citrate, calcium citrate-malate, and calcium gluconate is better than that from calcium carbonate [10,11]. Calcium carbonate is widely used as a calcium supplement; it is relatively inexpensive and contains 40% calcium by weight. Calcium carbonate from fossilized oyster shell or dolomite, however, may be contaminated with aluminum and lead [11]. Bone meal preparations also contain lead [11]. Ingestion of these products as a calcium source should be avoided, because excessive intakes of these toxic metals may occur [11].

Two transport processes are responsible for the absorption of calcium, which occurs along the length of the small intestine, especially the ileum, where food remains for the longest time [3]. One of the transport processes, operative primarily in the duodenum and proximal jejunum, is saturable, requires energy, involves a calcium-binding protein (CBP or calbindin), and is regulated by calcitriol [1,25-$(OH)_2$ D_3]. For calcium to be absorbed by this process, three sequential steps, all regulated by vitamin D, must occur. These steps include entry at the brush border, intracellular movement, and, finally, extrusion at the basolateral membrane [12]. When available calcium is insufficient for body needs, absorption by the saturable mechanism accelerates. This acceleration is due to the action of calcitriol, which is produced in response to an increase in parathyroid hormone (PTH) secretion caused by a reduction in plasma levels of ionized calcium. Calcitriol-induced calcium absorption involves changes in membrane lipid composition and topology and the synthesis of a CBP. The extrusion of calcium from the enterocyte into the extracellular fluid requires ATP and a vitamin D-regulated Ca^{+2}-Mg^{+2} ATPase, an enzyme that hydrolyzes ATP and releases energy for pumping Ca^{+2} out of the cell, as Mg^{+2} moves in. Sodium is also exchanged for Ca^{+2} in the extrusion process in the basolateral membrane (Fig. 10.17) [3,13]. With age, however, the vitamin D-regulated absorption of calcium becomes impaired by decreased efficiency in the calcitriol production in response to PTH [14]. Estrogen deficiency at menopause also decreases vitamin D-mediated calcium absorption.

The other process for calcium absorption occurs throughout the small intestine, is nonsaturable, passive, and appears to be paracellular (that is, absorbed between cells rather than through them) [3]. The amount of calcium absorbed via the nonsaturable, paracellular mechanism depends on the supply of calcium in the intestinal lumen. Increased absorption via this mechanism becomes possible when there is an increased intake of the mineral.

The large intestine also appears to play a role in calcium absorption. Bacteria in the colon may release calcium bound to some fermentable fibers such as pectins. Up to 4% (or about 8 mg) of dietary calcium is absorbed by the colon per day; this amount may be higher in people who are absorbing less calcium in the small intestine [3].

Although calcium absorption varies among people because of the several factors just discussed, absorption in adults averages about 30% with a 200-mg calcium intake; other studies report calcium absorption in the range 20 to 50% [3,4,15]. Recker [16] reported 21 to 26% absorption of calcium from whole, chocolate, and imitation milk; yogurt; cheese; and calcium carbonate supplying 250 mg calcium. Sheikh [2] reported an average of 31% absorption of calcium from milk providing 250 mg calcium. As calcium intakes increase, absorption decreases. For example, with an intake of 800 mg calcium by adults about 15% is absorbed [4].

The efficiency of calcium absorption also is affected by physiologic states. Children, for example, absorb up to 75% of dietary calcium in contrast with adults, who average about 30% absorption [4]. In addition, pregnancy and lactation increase dietary calcium absorption.

Calcium is transported in the blood in three forms. Some calcium (about 40%) is bound to proteins, mainly albumin. Some calcium (about 10%) is complexed with sulfate, phosphate, or citrate. Lastly, about 50% of calcium is found free in the blood.

Functions

Mineralization Approximately 99% of total body calcium is found in bones and teeth. About 60 to 66% of the weight of bones is due to minerals (present mainly as hydroxyapatite and calcium phosphate) with the remaining 34 to 40% bone weight due to water and protein [1,17]. Proteins in bone include collagen, osteonectin, osteopontin, BGP (bone Gla protein or osteocalcin), and MGP (matrix Gla protein). The latter two proteins are dependent on vitamin K for carboxylation of their glutamic acid residues, and function in calcium binding. Calcium facilitates interactions between proteins or between proteins and phospholipids in cell membranes. Osteonectin is a phosphoprotein that binds both calcium and collagen [18].

Bone may be divided into two types, cortical and trabecular (Fig. 11.1). Most bones possess an outer layer of cortical bone that surrounds trabecular bone. Some bones also contain a cavity for bone marrow. Cortical bone is compact or dense, represents about 75% of total bone in the body, and consists of layers of mineralized collagen; it is found mainly in long bones of the limbs. Trabecular bone has a spongy appearance, represents about 25% of bone in the body, and is found in relatively high concentrations in the axial skeleton (vertebrae and pelvic region). Trabecular bone is more active metabolically, with a high turnover rate, and thus is more rapidly depleted of calcium with calcium deficiency than cortical bone [3].

Bone is constantly being made and resorbed, a process that is lifelong, and involves several types of bone cells. Osteoblasts, one of the bone cell types, secrete collagen to form a matrix. This matrix forms around the osteoblasts and with time becomes calcified. Osteoblast activity is influenced by PTH, calcitriol, estrogen, among other hormones. As bone is mineralized by calcium and phosphorus, osteoblasts become embedded with the mineralized matrix, and, following changes

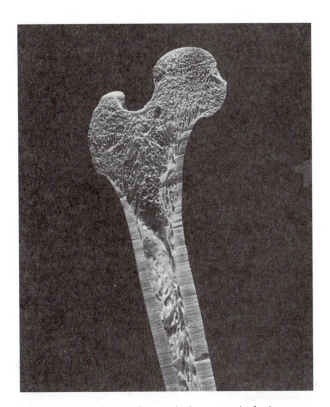

FIGURE 11.1 Trabecular bone is the lacy network of calcium-containing crystals that fills the interior. Cortical bone is the dense, ivorylike bone that forms the exterior shell. *(Whitney EN, Rolfes SR. Understanding Nutrition, 6th ed. St. Paul: West, 1993:396.)*

in morphology and function, become osteocytes. Associated with the osteoblasts is alkaline phosphatase, an enzyme that hydrolyzes phosphate esters to generate free phosphorus. Blood alkaline phosphatase levels increase with increased osteoblast activity. Another type of bone cell is the osteoclast, which resorbs previously made bone. Osteoclasts contain lysosomes that release acid hydrolases capable of dissolving calcium phosphate and attacking bone matrix. Osteoclasts respond to PTH, calcitriol, and calcitonin. Osteoclasts play an important role in helping to maintain normal blood calcium concentrations in times of inadequate calcium intake.

In children and adolescents, skeletal turnover occurs such that formation of bone exceeds resorption of bone. Skeletal turnover continues into adulthood, with peak bone mass occurring between age 30 to 40 years. Bone mass begins to decline during the fifth decade [4]. Although the need for calcium in bone modeling is continuous, its greatest benefits in promoting formation of sturdy skeletal mass occur during linear bone growth and the years immediately following (that is, approximately 10 to 15 years after cessation of linear growth). Roughly from age 18 to 35 years, a person can build

skeletal massiveness, reaching full skeletal maturity at around 35 years [19].

The process of calcification and mineralization of the bone matrix has yet to be clearly delineated. The solubility product of calcium times phosphorus ($Ca^{+2} \times PO_4^{-3}$) is thought to be involved such that, at a certain solubility product, the solution becomes supersaturated and calcium phosphate precipitates. Of the body's phosphorus, 85% is found in bone. Calcium occurs in a mass ratio of 2:1 with phosphorus [4]. Both calcium and phosphorus complex to form calcium phosphate and to form part of the crystal, hydroxyapatite ($Ca_{10} [PO_4]_6 [OH]_2$), which is laid down on collagen in the ossification process of bone formation.

Other Roles The small amount of remaining (not associated with bone, or nonosseous) body calcium, 1%, is found both intracellularly within organelles such as the mitochondria, endoplasmic reticulum (sarcoplasmic reticulum in muscle), nucleus, and vesicles, and extracellularly in the blood, lymph, and body fluids. Of the calcium in the blood plasma, 46 to 50% is ionized (Ca^{+2}), about 40% is bound to proteins, principally albumin [1], and < 10% consists of calcium complexes (for example, calcium citrate, phosphate, and sulfate). Only the ionized calcium is active; therefore, the numerous regulatory functions of calcium are performed by less than one-half of 1% of the total body calcium. Nonosseous calcium is essential for a number of processes, including, for example, the *clotting of blood* (see p. 314 under vitamin K), *nerve conduction, muscle contraction, enzyme regulation,* and *membrane permeability* [4].

Ionized intracellular calcium is maintained at a very low concentration of 100 nmol/L (or approximately 0.0001 of the concentration in the extracellular fluid) [20]. Low intracellular concentrations are maintained by the presence of at least two adenosine triphosphate (ATP)-dependent mechanisms that pump Ca^{+2} out of the cell. In addition, a Ca^{+2} pump can drive Ca^{+2} out of the cytoplasm into the mitochondrial matrix for storage as nonionic calcium phosphate until needed by the cell [20]. Ca^{+2} is also sequestered in the endoplasmic reticulum, or in the case of striated muscle, in the sarcoplasmic reticulum. Figure 11.2 illustrates cellular control of cytosolic-free calcium concentrations.

Raising the concentration of cytosolic Ca^{+2} from intracellular reservoirs or storage sites and through hormone-stimulated transport by a sodium–calcium exchange from extracellular sites allows Ca^{+2} to carry out its cellular functions (Fig. 11.2). Calcium may enter the cell from extracellular sites by transmembrane diffusion, or by one of two channels (voltage dependent or

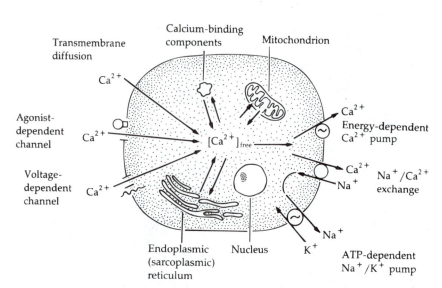

FIGURE 11.2 Cellular control of intracellular free calcium. Free intracellular calcium concentration is influenced by (1) the rate of calcium influx by diffusion across the cell membrane; (2) the passage of calcium through agonist- and voltage-dependent channels; (3) the rate of efflux via the calcium pump and Ca^{2+}/Na^+ exchange; (4) sequestration within the cell by endoplasmic (or sarcoplasmic) reticulum, binding components, and/or mitochondria. (In *Nordin BEC, ed. Calcium in human biology. London: Springer-Verlag, 1988:388. Reprinted with permission.*)

agonist dependent), which are activated by depolarization, neurotransmitters, or hormones). Second messengers may also increase cytoplasmic calcium levels by stimulating release of calcium from intracellular sites such as the endoplasmic reticulum.

Several second messengers act to increase the release of calcium within the cell. Inositol 1,4,5-triphosphate (IP$_3$), which is water soluble, and diacylglycerol (DAG), which is lipid soluble, are two examples of second messengers. IP$_3$ and DAG are derived from phosphatidylinositol 4,5-diphosphate (PIP$_2$), which in turn is derived from phosphatidylinositol, a phospholipid found in cell membranes (Fig. 11.3). Hormone receptor interaction (by first messengers) at the plasma membrane leads to a series of hydrolytic reactions on the phospholipid phosphatidylinositol to generate IP$_3$ and DAG. IP$_3$ functions as a second messenger following diffusion to the endoplasmic reticulum where it triggers the release of calcium into the cytoplasm. DAG also acts as a second messenger where it activates protein kinase C (PKC). PKC is associated with membrane phospholipids [20]. PKC, when associated with phospholipids and DAG, has an increased binding affinity for Ca^{+2} so that the Ca^{+2} requirement of PKC can be met by resting Ca^{+2} concentrations. Without DAG, higher concentrations of Ca^{+2} are needed to activate PKC [21]. The exact role of PKC is unknown, but it is involved in mediating sustained cellular responses [20]. In general, protein kinases catalyze the phosphorylation of amino acids found within proteins, a process that alters the protein's function and thus the cell's function or activity.

Increased free Ca^{+2} concentrations in the cell (through either intracellular release of calcium or by transport of extracellular calcium into the cell) may directly affect the cell; that is, the actions are not mediated through calcium-binding proteins (Fig. 11.3). Increased Ca^{+2} can trigger neutrophils and can activate platelet phospholipase A$_2$. Phospholipase A$_2$ acts on carbon 2 of the glycerol backbone of phospholipids (such as phosphatidylcholine) to liberate fatty acids (such as arachidonic acid from phosphatidylcholine). The arachidonic acid can be metabolized to form thromboxanes, prostaglandins, or leukotrienes (p. 118).

Phosphodiesterase, which hydrolyzes cyclic AMP (cAMP), is dependent on Ca^{+2}. Cyclic AMP formation from ATP is catalyzed by adenylate cyclase, which is found on the plasma membrane. The actions of cAMP and Ca^{+2} are thought to be mutually dependent. Other enzymes that may be affected directly by increased free Ca^{+2} or affected through Ca^{+2} bound to a calcium-binding protein are listed in Table 11.2. Because of calcium's intracellular actions alone or as part of proteins, calcium is sometimes said to function as a second messenger.

In addition to acting alone, increased intracellular Ca^{+2} concentrations promote the binding of calcium to one of several calcium-binding proteins. Calmodulin is one example of a calcium-binding protein and appears to be operative in most cells. Calmodulin consists of two similar globular lobes joined by a long helix. Each lobe contains two Ca^{+2}-binding sites (Fig. 11.4). Binding of Ca^{+2} activates calmodulin by changing its conformation, thereby allowing it to stimulate a variety of macromolecular processes or enzymes. Several enzymes depend on calmodulin for activity. Some examples of the calmodulin-dependent enzymes include (1) myosin

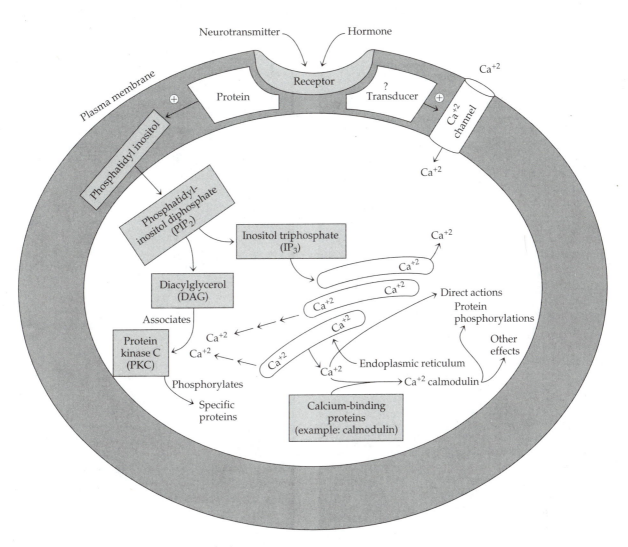

FIGURE 11.3 Some of the intracellular actions of calcium.

light-chain kinase, which phosphorylates the light chain of myosin, and following a sequence of events, causes smooth muscle contraction [22]; (2) phosphorylase kinase which activates phosphorylase; phosphorylase is the enzyme responsible for glycogenolysis, degrading glycogen to glucose 1-PO_4; and (3) calcium calmodulin kinases, of which there are several with several functions. Others are listed in Table 11.2.

A second example of a calcium-binding protein is troponin C, which is found in skeletal muscle. Skeletal muscle stimulated by nerve impulses (acetylcholine as neurotransmitter) triggers increased concentrations of calcium. The calcium can then bind to the troponin C, allowing muscle contraction. The structure of troponin C, with its four binding sites for calcium, closely resembles that of calmodulin. Like calmodulin, the conformational change in troponin C due to Ca^{+2} binding permits

an interaction between actin and myosin, resulting in muscle contraction [20]. Once the plasma membrane repolarizes, calcium is pumped back into the sarcoplasmic reticulum, troponin C releases its bound calcium, and myosin and actin no longer interact [20].

A third calcium-binding protein is calbindin. This protein is synthesized in response to calcitriol and is associated with increased absorption of calcium in the intestine (p. 302).

Figure 11.3 depicts some of the varied actions of increased Ca^{+2} concentrations. Shown in this diagram are some of the roles of IP_3, DAG, calmodulin, and calcium.

Regulation of Calcium Concentrations

Calcium concentrations are tightly controlled both intracellularly and extracellularly. Three main hormones

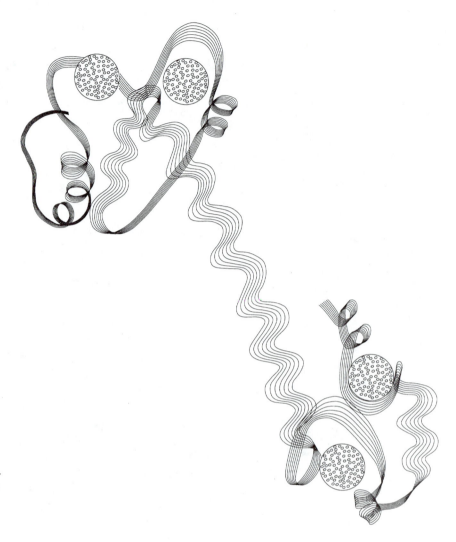

FIGURE 11.4 Schematic representation of the binding of four calcium ions (Ca^{+2}) by the calcium-binding protein calmodulin.

Table 11.2 Selected Enzymes Regulated by Calcium and/or Calmodulin

Adenylate cyclase	Glycogen synthase
Ca^{2+}-dependent protein kinase	Guanylate cyclase
Ca^{2+}/Mg^{2-}-ATPase	Myosin kinase
Ca^{2+}/phospholipid-dependent protein kinase	NAD kinase
Cyclic nucleotide phosphodiesterase	Phospholipase A$_2$
Glycerol 3-phosphate dehydrogenase	Phosphorylase kinase
	Pyruvate carboxylase
	Pyruvate dehydrogenase
	Pyruvate kinase

are involved in calcium homeostasis: PTH, calcitonin, and calcitriol (1,25 [OH]$_2$ D$_3$). PTH acts to increase extracellular fluid–plasma calcium concentration by promoting resorption of calcium from the bone; calcitriol may also be involved in this process. PTH also acts by increasing reabsorption of calcium by kidney tubules, and by increasing the rate of formation of calcitriol in the kidney (see Fig. 10.16, p. 302). 1,25 (OH)$_2$ D$_3$ accelerates absorption of calcium from the gastrointestinal tract as discussed on page 302. PTH is influenced by plasma calcium and phosphorus concentrations. Low plasma calcium concentrations stimulate PTH secretion. Prolonged diets high in phosphorus and low in calcium may result in a mild secondary hyperparathyroidism, and can possibly lead to calcium secretion into the gastrointestinal tract as well as loss from bone. However, studies demonstrating such effects on bone are not available [4,23]. Magnesium inhibits PTH secretion. In contrast to PTH, calcitonin serves to lower serum Ca^{+2} by inhibiting osteoclast activity and preventing mobilization of Ca^{+2} from bone [22].

Alterations in the regulation of systemic and/or cellular Ca^{+2} concentrations have been implicated in the pathogenesis of high blood pressure (hypertension) [22,24], which is discussed further as part of the "Perspective" section at the end of this chapter.

As described on page 329, low calcium (Ca^{+2}) concentrations are maintained within cells through ATP-dependent calcium pumps as well as through storage in the mitochondria, endoplasmic reticulum, nucleus, and vesicles. Following stimulation and release of Ca^{+2} into the cytoplasm, concentrations are returned to their normal low levels by a reversal of the events that raised its concentration. For example, the neurotransmitter may be degraded or the agonist may be released from the cell surface receptor, intracellular second messengers are inactivated, and Ca^{+2} is pumped out of the cell or is once again sequestered by intracellular organelles and binders.

Interactions with Other Nutrients

Calcium interacts with several nutrients not only at the absorptive surface of the intestinal cell, but also within the body. Some interrelationships between calcium and other nutrients (lactose, protein, vitamin D, fat, fiber, phytates, zinc) have been discussed under the section of calcium absorption and transport. Additional interactions are discussed here. *Phosphorus* is particularly interesting in that although it causes loss of calcium by increasing calcium secretion into the gut, it conserves calcium by decreasing the amount of calcium lost in the urine. Because *magnesium* is necessary for the secretion of PTH, it also indirectly influences calcium. Like phosphorus, increased *potassium* consumption also reduces urinary calcium excretion [25–27].

Some nutrients interact with calcium and promote loss of calcium from the body. Dietary protein directly influences calcium [3]; doubling of protein intake without changing intake of other nutrients results in about a 50% increase in urinary calcium [28]. Sulfate generated from metabolism of the sulfur-containing amino acids in the protein may be binding with the calcium and increasing its urinary excretion [26]. Because many protein-containing foods also contain phosphorus, ingestion of foods containing both nutrients tends to minimize negative effects on calcium balance [4]. Relationships between *sodium* and calcium have been documented whereby the sodium load (100 mmol or 2.3 g/day) increases urinary calcium excretion by 1 mmol or 40 mg/day [26,29]. Caffeine (300 to 400 mg) not only increases urinary calcium (0.25 mmol or 10 mg/day) by reducing renal reabsorption, but also causes increased secretion of calcium into the gut, thereby leading to endogenous fecal losses [27,30].

Calcium in the form of dietary supplements (providing 600 mg calcium in various forms such as calcium citrate) or in natural food form appears to decrease

iron—heme and nonheme iron—absorption by 49 to 62% [31]. Calcium is thought to affect iron transfer within the enterocyte and not at the brush border [3]. This relationship has been documented in several studies and occurs primarily when the calcium and iron are ingested together with food [3].

Excretion

Calcium is excreted primarily in the urine and feces, with up to 182 mg (average 60 mg) lost daily from the skin [3,17,32]. Most calcium is filtered and reabsorbed by the kidney such that urinary calcium (50% as ionized calcium and 50% as calcium complexes with sulfate, phosphate, citrate, and oxalate) losses range from 100 to 240 mg day [3]. Urinary calcium excretion, however, is decreased with phosphorus, potassium, and magnesium, but increased with sodium and protein, as discussed under the section of interrelationships with other nutrients. Fecal losses of calcium from endogenous and exogenous sources range from 45 to 100 mg day [3]. Fecal losses may increase with consumption of fiber, phytate, and oxalate, magnesium in excess, and in people with fat-malabsorbing disorders.

Figure 11.5 depicts the average calcium exchange in an adult, as well as showing the role of PTH, calcitriol, and calcitonin. About 1 g of calcium is ingested daily with approximately one-third (0.36 g) of this amount being absorbed. The total amount of calcium in the extracellular fluid pool of the body is about 1 g. Since approximately 0.19 g calcium moves into the intestinal lumen from digestive secretions or as shed epithelial cells, the net absorption from the gastrointestinal tract is about 0.17 g. The same amount (0.17 g) is excreted in the urine of people who are in calcium equilibrium.

Recommended Dietary Allowance (RDA)

During the first year of life, the RDA for calcium is 400 to 600 mg/day, then increasing to 800 mg/day from age 1 year through 10 years. Recommendations further increase to 1,200 mg/day from ages 11 to 24 years, a time for peak bone mineralization [4]; these recommendations represent an increase over the 1980 RDA [33], which were 1,200 mg/day at 11 years but dropped to 800 mg/day once the person reached 18 years. However, the 1989 RDA for calcium for preadolescent and adolescent children has been questioned because it appears to be insufficient to support optimal gains in bone mass during growth and development [34]. Although the exact age at which peak bone mass is achieved is uncertain, it is believed to be no earlier than 25 years [4]. For adults over 25 years, in the opinion of the subcommittee of the tenth

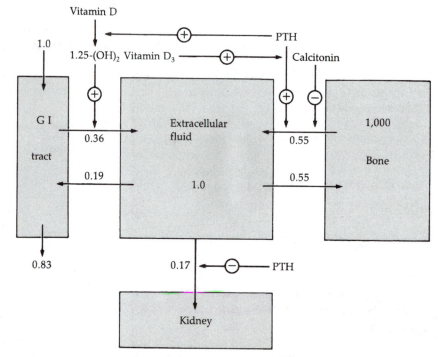

FIGURE 11.5 Calcium exchange and hormonal control of calcium homeostasis. Positive regulation is indicated by ⊕; inhibitory regulation by ⊖. All numerical values are in grams. *(Aurbach JD, Marx SJ, Spiegel AM. Parathyroid hormone, calciforim and the calciferols. In: Wilson JD, Foster DW, eds., Williams textbook of endocrinology, 7th ed. Philadelphia: Saunders, 1985:144, Fig. 29-6.)*

edition of the RDA, a calcium intake of 800 mg/day is sufficient. With pregnancy and lactation, however, an intake of 1,200 mg/day is recommended [4].

The 1989 RDA do not agree with the recommendations emanating from the 1984 National Institutes of Health (NIH) consensus panel on osteoporosis. The NIH panel suggested a calcium intake of 1,000 mg/day by estrogen-replete premenopausal women and postmenopausal women treated with estrogen, and an intake of 1,500 mg/day by untreated postmenopausal women [19]. The distinction between those treated and not treated with estrogen is made because estrogen influences bone mineralization. Postmenopausal women experience a rapid loss of bone minerals without estrogen replacement.

Popularization by the media of the need for calcium, the lack of sufficient calcium in diets of especially women, and the support of the NIH [19] recommendations by many health care providers, have caused the sale of calcium supplements to soar. Although the preferable source of calcium is food, few people are willing to consume as much milk and/or milk products as would be necessary to secure this higher level of calcium intake, thus calcium supplements continue to be marketed heavily.

Numerous calcium supplements are available from which the consumer can choose. Several of these supplements are listed in Table 11.3, along with informa-

Table 11.3 Calcium Absorption from Various Calcium Salts (supplements)

Calcium Salts (listed in decreasing order of solubility)	% Absorption	Amount Supplying 500 mg Elemental Ca (grams)
Calcium acetate	32 ± 4	2.16
Calcium lactate	32 ± 4	3.53
Calcium gluconate	27 ± 3	5.49
Calcium citrate	30 ± 3	2.37
Calcium carbonate	39 ± 3	1.26

Source: Adapted from Sheikh MS, Santa Ana CA, Nicar MJ, et al. Gastrointestinal absorption of calcium from milk and calcium salts. Reprinted by permission of the New England Journal of Medicine. Vol 317; 532–536, 1987.

tion on absorption [2]. Although the differences in absorption are not statistically significant, the variation in the amount of elemental calcium in an equal weight of supplement is clearly significant [2]. Calcium carbonate contains more elemental calcium and consequently requires a smaller dosage; however, absorption appears to vary considerably among people [16].

Although many researchers have demonstrated that current bone calcium loss in adults cannot be correlated with current calcium intake [19], many others are convinced that a present generous intake of the mineral will allow increased absorption via the nonsaturable paracellular route, thereby decelerating the rate of calcium loss from the body [35].

Deficiency

Inadequate intake, poor calcium absorption, and/or excessive calcium losses contribute to inadequate mineralization of bone. Rickets in children occurs when the amount of calcium accretion per unit bone matrix is deficient. Low levels of free ionized Ca^{+2} in the blood (hypocalcemia) may result in tetany. Tetany is manifested by intermittent muscle contractions. Muscle pain, muscle spasms, and paresthesias (numbness or tingling in the hands and feet) are common signs of tetany. In adults deficient in calcium, osteoporosis—the loss of bone mass (protein matrix and bone minerals)—occurs [36]. Two types of osteoporosis have been described: type I, which occurs in postmenopausal women between the ages of 51 and 65 years and affects mainly the vertebrae and distal radius; and type II, which occurs in men and women over the age of 75 years and affects the vertebrae, hip, pelvis, humerus, and tibia [30]. Both types I and II contribute to bone loss in individuals aged 65 to 75 years.

Much of the U.S. population, particularly females over 12 years of age, fails to consume the recommended amounts of calcium. Inadequate calcium intake during the period of bone mineralization is a concern because of (1) the high incidence of osteoporosis among elderly women and the (2) significant correlation shown to exist between present bone density and past calcium intake [4]. Several studies have reported positive effects from calcium supplementation on age-related bone loss [37]. Other populations associated with increased needs for calcium include those with high-protein diets, high-fiber diets, fat malabsorption (which increases fecal calcium excretion), immobilization (promotes calcium loss from bone), decreased gastrointestinal transit time, and long-term use of thiazide diuretics (which increase calcium excretion in the urine).

Deficient (long-term) calcium intakes are also associated with the development of hypertension and colon cancer [37]. An inverse relationship between calcium and blood pressure exists (as intake of calcium decreases, prevalence of hypertension increases), with a steep slope at calcium intakes less than 600 mg/day [24,37]. Calcium supplementation has been shown to lower blood pressure in some hypertensive people previously ingesting a diet inadequate in calcium [37]. Colon cancer also has been linked with calcium-deficient diets [15,37]. Adequate intakes of calcium (> 800 mg/day) are thought to be protective against colon cancer; however, insufficient evidence in humans warrants against the use of calcium to prevent colon cancer [4]. A suggested basis for this effect is the ability of calcium to bind bile acids and free fatty acids, which act as promoters of cancer by inducing colon cell hyperproliferation [4].

Toxicity

Intakes of calcium in amounts up to 2,500 mg appear to be safe for most individuals [4,38]. Constipation has been reported by some [1,4]. Ingestion of calcium in amounts greater than 3,000 mg may result in hypercalcemia [1]; soft tissue calcification is not likely unless the plasma calcium concentration times the plasma phosphorus concentration exceeds 2.2 mmol/L [1]. People with idiopathic hypercalciuria (urinary calcium levels in excess of 4 mg per kg of body weight per day), however, may be at increased risk for development of calcium-containing kidney stones with excessive calcium intakes [39].

Assessment of Nutriture

No routine biochemical method appears to accurately assess calcium status. Serum calcium (composed of protein-bound calcium, diffusible calcium complexes, and ionized calcium) is so exquisitely regulated that it may indicate little about calcium status. Normal serum calcium concentrations range from 8.5 to 10.5 mg/dL for adults, with slightly higher levels in children [9]. Serum ionized calcium, Ca^{+2}, does, however, relate to alterations in calcium metabolism [38], and when albumin concentration is normal the ratio between bound calcium and ionized calcium remains constant. When albumin concentrations are depressed, corrections are needed to adjust for the corresponding decrease that will occur in the protein-bound fraction of calcium. For each 1 g/dL decrease in serum albumin, serum calcium will decrease 0.8 mg/dL. The following equations can be used for estimating protein-bound calcium:

$$\text{Protein-bound calcium (mg/dL)} = 0.44 + 0.76 \times \text{albumin (g/dL) or} = 0.8 \times (\text{normal albumin} - \text{actual albumin}) + \text{measured calcium}$$

Neutron activation, an *in vivo* procedure where gamma rays are counted following administration of ^{48}Ca into the body and exposure of the body to a low neutron flux [38], is one method available to assess total body calcium content. Results of neutron activation correlate with single-photon absorptiometry, which measures total bone mineral content. Single-photon absorptiometry exposes a portion of a limb (usually the radius/forearm or os calcis/heel) to radiation. Dual-photon absorptiometry uses a radioisotope that emits two gamma rays and can be used to measure total bone mineral content of sites such as the vertebrae and proximal femur where variations in soft tissue thickness around the bone needs to be accounted for. In single-photon absorptiometry, the quantity of bone mineral is inversely proportional to the amount of photon energy transmitted from the bone, as measured by a scintillation counter [38]. In addition to photon absorptiometry, bone densitometry can be assessed through computerized tomography (CT) scans [15]. CT, although less accurate and precise than dual-photon absorptiometry, can measure variances in tissue density (such as in vertebral bone). People are placed in a scanner, X rays are taken, and radiation pulses are emitted, collected, and processed to reconstruct the image and calculate density [9].

References Cited for Calcium

1. Arnaud CD, Sanchez SD. Calcium and phosphorus. In: Brown ML, ed. Present knowledge in nutrition, 6th ed. Washington, DC: International Life Sciences Institute Nutrition Foundation, 1990:212–223.
2. Sheikh MS, Santa Ana CA, Nicar MJ, Schiller LR, Fordtran JS. Gastrointestinal absorption of calcium from milk and calcium salts. N Engl J Med 1987;317:532–536.
3. Allen LH, Wood RJ. Calcium and phosphorus. In: Shils ME, Olson JA, Shike M. Modern nutrition in health and disease, 8th ed. Philadelphia: Lea and Febiger, 1994:144–163.
4. National Research Council. Recommended dietary allowances, 10th ed. Washington, DC: National Academy Press, 1989:174–184.
5. Schaafsma G. Calcium in extracellular fluid homeostasis. In: Nordin BEC. Calcium in human biology. London: Springer-Verlag, 1988;241–259.
6. Harland BF, Oberleas D. Phytate in foods. Wld Rev Nutr Diet 1987;52:235–259.
7. Greger JL. Mineral bioavailability/new concepts. Nutr Today 1987;22:4–9.
8. Spencer H. Minerals and mineral interactions in human beings. J Am Diet Assoc 1986;86:864–867.
9. Tilkian SM, Conover MB, Tilkian AG. Clinical implications of laboratory tests, 4th ed. St. Louis: Mosby, 1987.
10. Anderson JJB. Nutritional biochemistry of calcium and phosphorus. J Nutr Biochem 1991;2:300–307.
11. Whiting SJ. Safety of some calcium supplements questioned. Nutr Rev 1994;52:95–97.
12. Bronner F. Intestinal calcium absorption: Mechanisms and applications. J Nutr 1987;117:1347–1352.
13. Bronner F. Transcellular calcium transport. In: Bronner F, ed. Intracellular calcium regulation. New York: Wiley-Liss, 1990; 415–437.
14. Silverberg SJ, Shane E, De La Cruz L, Segre GV, Clemens TL, Bilezikian JP. Abnormalities in parathyroid hormone secretion and 1,25 dihydroxyvitamin D_3 formation in women with osteoporosis. N Engl J Med 1989;320:277–281.
15. Weaver CM. Assessing calcium status and metabolism. J Nutr 1990;120:1470–1473.
16. Recker RR, Bammi A, Barger-Lux MJ, Heaney RP. Calcium absorbability from milk products, an imitation milk and calcium carbonate. Am J Clin Nutr 1988;47:93–95.
17. Peacock M. Calcium absorption efficiency and calcium requirements in children and adolescents. Am J Clin Nutr 1991;54:261S–265S.
18. Raisz LG, Kream BE. Regulation of bone formation. N Eng J Med. 1983;309:29–35.
19. National Institutes of Health. Consensus Development Panel. Osteoporosis. JAMA 1984;252:799–802.
20. Rasmussen H. The calcium messenger system (parts 1 and 2). N Engl J Med 1986;314:1094–1101, 1164–1170.
21. Wasserman RH. Cellular calcium: Action of hormones. In: Bronner F, ed. Intracellular calcium regulation. New York: Wiley–Liss, 1990;385–419.
22. Bukoski RD, Kremer D. Calcium-regulating hormones in hypertension: vascular actions. Am J Clin Nutr 1991;54:220S–226S.
23. Calvo MS. Dietary phosphorus, calcium metabolism and bone. J Nutr 1993;123:1627–1633.
24. McCarron DA, Morris CD, Young E, Roullet C, Drueke T. Dietary calcium and blood pressure: Modifying factors in specific populations. 1991;54:215S–219S.
25. Lemann J, Pleuss JA, Gray RW. Potassium causes calcium retention in healthy adults. J Nutr 1993;123:1623–1626.
26. Massey LK. Dietary factors influencing calcium and bone metabolism: Introduction. J Nutr 1993;123:1609–1610.
27. Massey LK, Whiting SJ. Caffeine, urinary calcium, calcium metabolism and bone. J Nutr 1993;123:1611–1614.
28. Heaney RP. Protein intake and the calcium economy. J Am Diet Assoc 1993;93:1259–1260.
29. Nordin BEC, Need AG, Morris HA, Horowitz M. The nature and significance of the relationship between urinary sodium and urinary calcium in women. J Nutr 1993;123:1615–1622.
30. Harward MP. Nutritive therapies for osteoporosis: The role of calcium. Med Clin N Am 1993;77:889–898.
31. Cook JD, Dassenko SA, Whittaker P. Calcium supplementation: effect on iron absorption. Am J Clin Nutr 1991;53:106–111.
32. Charles P, Eriksen EF, Hasling C, Sondergard K, Mosekilde L. Dermal, intestinal, and renal obligatory losses of calcium: relation to skeletal calcium loss. Am J Clin Nutr 1991;54: 266S–273S.
33. National Research Council. Recommended dietary allowances, 9th ed. Washington, DC: National Academy of Sciences, 1980;125–133.
34. Andon MB, Lloyd T, Matkovic V. Supplementation trials with calcium citrate malate: Evidence in favor of

increasing the calcium RDA during childhood and adolescence. J Nutr 1994;124:1412S–1417S.

35. Heaney RP. In: Peck WA, ed. Bone and mineral research. New York: Elsevier, 1986;255–301.
36. Sowers MF. Epidemiology of calcium and vitamin D in bone loss. J Nutr 1993;123:413–417.
37. Barger-Lux MJ, Heaney RP. The role of calcium intake in preventing bone fragility, hypertension, and certain cancers. J Nutr 1994; 124:1406S–1411S.
38. Gibson RS. Principles of nutritional assessment. New York: Oxford University Press, 1990:487–510.
39. Brown WW, Wolfson M. Diet as culprit or therapy. Stone disease, chronic renal failure, and nephrotic syndrome. Med Clin N Am 1993;77:783–794.

Additional References

Pansu D, Bronner F. Calcium transport and intracellular calcium homeostasis. New York: Springer-Verlag, 1990.
Bronner F. Intracellular calcium regulation. New York: Wiley, 1990.
Nordin BEC. Calcium in human biology. London: Springer-Verlag, 1988.
Cheung WY. Calcium and cell function. Orlando: Academic Press, 1986.
Entire issue J Nutr 1994;124: August supplement.

PHOSPHORUS

Among the inorganic elements, phosphorus is second only to calcium in abundance in the human body. Approximately 85% of the body's phosphorus is in the skeleton, with the remainder associated with organic substances of soft tissue.

Sources

Phosphorus is widely distributed in foods. The best food sources of phosphorus are listed in Table 11.1, and include meat, poultry, fish, eggs, milk, and milk products. Nuts, legumes, cereals, grains, and chocolate also contain phosphorus; however, animal products are superior sources of available phosphorus compared to cereals and soya-based foods. Coffee, tea, and soft drinks also provide small amounts of phosphorus.

Dietary phosphorus occurs in both an inorganic form as well as phosphoproteins, phosphorylated sugars, and phospholipids. The relative amounts of inorganic and organic phosphorus vary with the type of diet. Meats contain phosphorus that is largely organic and thus requires hydrolysis for absorption to occur. Over 80% of the phosphorus in grains such as wheat, rice, and corn is found as phytic acid (hexaphosphoinositol) (Fig. 11.6)

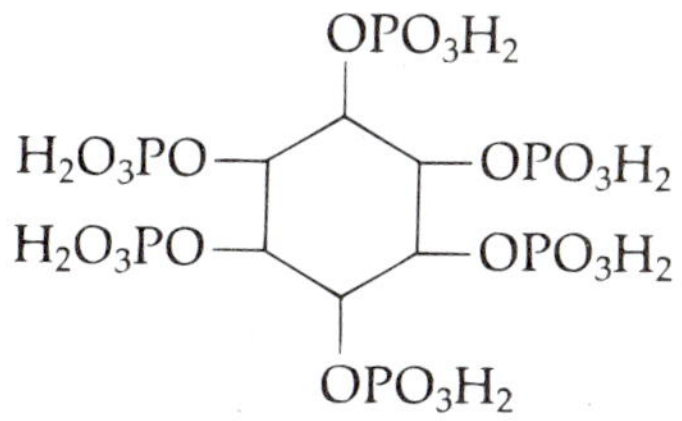

Phytic acid

FIGURE 11.6 Phytic acid.

[1]. About 33% of the phosphorus in milk is in the form of inorganic phosphates [1].

Digestion, Absorption, and Transport

Regardless of its dietary form, most phosphorus is absorbed in its inorganic form. Organically bound phosphorus is hydrolyzed enzymatically in the lumen of the small intestine and released as inorganic phosphate (P_i). Alkaline phosphatase functions at the brush border of the enterocyte to free phosphorus from its bound form. Although alkaline phosphatase can free much of the bound phosphorus, phosphorus as part of phytic acid is not as bioavailable.

Phytic acid is the major form of grain cereal phosphate. The poor bioavailability of phosphorus from phytates is due to the absence of phytase in mammalian digestion. Phytase is a phosphate esterase that liberates phosphate from phytic acid. Yeasts in breads possess phytase and can hydrolyze some of the phytates to yield some phosphorus available for absorption. About 50% of phosphorus from phytates is thought to be absorbed [2].

Magnesium, aluminum, and calcium intakes also impair phosphorus absorption. Phosphorus absorption may be reduced by dietary magnesium and, conversely, a deficiency of luminal magnesium enhances the absorption of phosphate. The two minerals are thought to form a complex within the gastrointestinal tract to render each other unavailable for absorption. Aluminum hydroxide (3 g) given with a meal reduces phosphorus absorption from 70 to 35% [1]. Hypophosphatemia (low blood phosphorus) may result from the prolonged use of nonabsorbable aluminum and magnesium hydroxide gels as found in antacids. In fact, such gels are used as treatment for the hyperphosphatemia associated with chronic kidney failure. Calcium (as calcium acetate or calcium carbonate) also inhibits phosphorus absorption, and is used as a phosphate-binding agent in people on hemodialysis with hyperphosphatemia.

Phosphorus (as inorganic phosphorus, P_i) absorption occurs throughout the small intestine. Between 50 and 70% of phosphorus is absorbed with normal intake, and up to 90% when intake is low [2]. Unlike calcium, the intestinal absorption of phosphorus is not affected by body needs; thus high dietary phosphorus can lead to high serum phosphorus, which leads to increased urinary phosphorus excretion. In other words, maintenance of the phosphate balance is achieved largely through renal excretion.

Radiophosphorus perfusion studies suggest that phosphorus absorption occurs primarily in the duodenum and jejunum. Orally administered radioisotopes of phosphorus appear in the blood within 10 minutes and peak after about an hour.

The mechanisms of phosphorus absorption have not been clearly elucidated. Phosphorus absorption appears to occur by either of two processes: first, a saturable, carrier-mediated active transport system, and the second, a linear, concentration-dependent, diffusion process [1,3]. The active transport system across the intestinal brush border is sodium dependent [1]. Vitamin D as calcitriol stimulates the absorption of phosphorus, especially in the duodenum; however, parathyroid hormone (PTH) is not thought to play a direct role [1].

Absorbed phosphate exists in the plasma in two main forms. About 70% of phosphorus in the plasma is found as part of phospholipids [1]. The remaining phosphorus, about 10%, is bound to protein, about 5% is bound to calcium or magnesium, and the remaining 85% is found as inorganic phosphates, primarily HPO_4^{-2} and to a lesser extent $H_2PO_4^-$ [1]. Inorganic phosphorus is sometimes referred to as *"ultrafilterable phosphate."* In adults, plasma inorganic phosphate ranges between 2.5 and 4.4 mg/dL. Dietary phosphate, age and stage of growth, time of day, hormonal effects, and renal function all contribute to the variability of the serum phosphate concentration. Circulating phosphate is in equilibrium with skeletal and cellular inorganic phosphate and with that of organic phosphates formed in intermediary metabolism. Phosphorus is found in all cells of the body, with bone and muscle containing the majority.

Functions

Phosphate is of prime importance in the development of skeletal tissue, which in itself accounts for 85% of the total phosphate store. In bone, phosphorus is part of calcium phosphate ($Ca_3[PO_4]_2$) and the crystal, hydroxyapatite ($Ca_{10}[PO_4]_6[OH]_2$), which is laid down on collagen in the ossification process of bone formation. See the calcium section of this chapter for a further discussion of bone mineralization and the roles of calcium and phosphorus (p. 328).

Phosphorus that is not part of bone is found in either extracellular fluids or intracellularly. Within cells, phosphorus is involved in a host of processes. Phosphorus is of vital importance in intermediary metabolism of the energy nutrients, contributing to the metabolic potential in the form of high-energy phosphate bonds, such as ATP, and through the phosphorylation of substrates. Many enzymatic activities are controlled by alternating phosphorylation or dephosphorylation. For example, see the discussion of glycogen degradation (p. 82).

Phosphate is also an important component of the nucleic acids DNA and RNA. Phosphorus alternates with pentose sugars to form the linear backbone of these macromolecules.

Cell membranes are made up in part from lipids, including phospholipids, which as their name implies contain phosphorus.

Phosphate also functions in acid–base balance. Filtered phosphate reacts with secreted hydrogen ions, releasing sodium ions in the process. This action increases pH. The sodium ion may be reabsorbed through the kidney tubule under the influence of aldosterone.

$$Na_2HPO_4 + H^+ \longrightarrow NaH_2PO_4 + Na^+$$

Interactions with Other Nutrients

The interactions between phosphorus and *magnesium*, and phytate have been addressed under the section on phosphorus absorption. In addition, the optimal ratio between *calcium* and phosphorus in the diet has been questioned, because animal studies suggest that diets low in calcium–phosphorus ratios lead to progressive bone loss due to phosphorus-induced stimulation of parathyroid hormone (PTH) release. Although such an effect may occur in humans on high-phosphate diets for prolonged periods, studies demonstrating such effects are not available [2,4]. Women ingesting a diet with a calcium-to-phosphorus ratio of 1:4 for a four-week period have been reported to exhibit elevated PTH. And persistent elevations of PTH could lead to loss of minerals from bone [5]; however, studies monitoring bone loss are needed.

Excretion

In contrast to calcium, where approximately two-thirds of its dietary intake is excreted in the feces and one-third in the urine, the reverse is true for phosphorus. About two-thirds of phosphorus is excreted in inorganic form

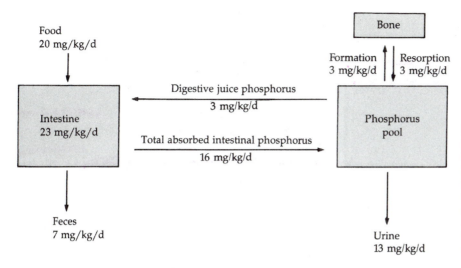

FIGURE 11.7 An overview of phosphorus metabolism for the normal human adult, on an average intake of phosphorus, who is in zero phosphorus balance. *(Wilkinson R. Absorption of calcium, phosphorus, and magnesium. In: Nordin, BEC, ed. Calcium, phosphate and magnesium metabolism. New York: Churchill Livingstone 1976:78. Reprinted with permission.)*

in the urine; about one-third is excreted in the feces. PTH is the primary hormone regulating phosphorus excretion. PTH stimulates urinary phosphorus excretion by inhibiting its tubular reabsorption. Dietary phosphorus intake also influences renal excretion. The amount of dietary phosphorus and absorbed phosphorus is approximately a linear relationship with urinary phosphorus. This relationship is maintained even if intake is increased severalfold. If a person is in zero balance, then urinary excretion of phosphorus is the same as the net absorbed phosphorus, which is defined as the difference between the total amount absorbed in the intestine and that which is secreted in the digestive juice. A scheme of phosphorus metabolism for a normal adult on an average intake and in zero balance is represented in Figure 11.7.

A well-defined diurnal variation in urinary phosphate exists that is not related to feeding patterns but rather to changes in tubular reabsorption. The pattern relates to physical activity, with the nadir of urinary excretion appearing a few hours after the end of sleep. Since this is inversely related to the diurnal fluctuation of the release of adrenal corticotropic hormone and cortisol, both of which peak after a period of sleep, it appears that phosphate excretion may be under the influence of the pituitary and adrenal glands. In fact, tubular reabsorption of phosphate is increased by short-term cortisol therapy. Other hormones that inhibit the tubular reabsorption of phosphorus include the estrogen and thyroid hormones [1].

Recommended Dietary Allowances

Relatively little work has been done to determine phosphorus requirements. Because the body adapts to

changes in dietary phosphorus intake by altering phosphorus excretion and because of the widespread availability of phosphorus in foods, deficiency is rare, as discussed in the next section. It is generally held, probably correctly, that phosphorus intake must be adequate if the intake of other nutrients is adequate. The RDAs for phosphorus are available and they parallel recommendations for calcium in children and adults. Intakes of 300 to 500 mg are suggested for infants. The RDA for phosphorus for children through 10 years is 800 mg, with intakes of 1,200 mg recommended for adolescents and adults through 24 years. For adults aged 25 years and older, the RDA drops to 800 mg.

Deficiency

Phosphorus deficiency is rare, because almost all foods contain phosphorus, and the body adapts to dietary fluctuations by changes in excretion [2]. Premature infants and people who are receiving aluminum hydroxide antacids, which bind phosphorus in the gastrointestinal tract, have exhibited signs of deficiency. People with malabsorptive disorders such as Crohn's disease, those with alcoholism, or uncontrolled diabetes mellitus may exhibit imbalances in phosphorus. Deficiency of phosphorus causes bone loss, or hypophosphatemic rickets, and disturbances in oxygen dissociation from hemoglobin due to a decrease in the formation of 2,3-diphosphoglycerate, which regulates the release of oxygen from hemoglobin. Phosphorus deficiency has also been associated with myopathy, weakness, cardiomyopathy, and neurologic problems, among others [1].

Toxicity

Toxicity from phosphorus is rare, and problems appear to occur only when calcium-to-phosphorus ratios are altered significantly in infants. High-phosphorus human milk substitutes, when given to infants, result in hypocalcemia and tetany [1].

Assessment of Nutriture

The assessment of phosphorus nutriture is not a major consideration due to the rarity of deficiency. Serum phosphorus concentrations may be assessed; however, their specificity and sensitivity are low. Concentrations are affected by several confounding factors that are unrelated to phosphorus status [6].

References Cited for Phosphorus

1. Allen LH, Wood RJ. Calcium and phosphorus. In: Shils ME, Olson JA, Shike M. Modern nutrition in health and disease, 8th ed. Philadelphia: Lea and Febiger, 1994: 144–163.
2. National Research Council. Recommended dietary allowances, 10th ed. Washington, DC: National Academy Press, 1989:184–187.
3. Anderson JJB. Nutritional biochemistry of calcium and phosphorus. J Nutr Biochem 1991;2:300–307.
4. Calvo MS. Dietary phosphorus, calcium metabolism and bone. J Nutr 1993;123:1627–1633.
5. Anderson JJB, Barrett CJH. Dietary phosphorus: The benefits and the problems. Nutr Today 1994;29:29–34.
6. Gibson RS. Principles of nutritional assessment. New York: Oxford University Press, 1990:487–510.

Additional References

Arnaud CD, Sanchez SD. Calcium and phosphorus. In: Brown ML, ed. Present knowledge in nutrition, 6th ed. Washington, DC: International Life Sciences Institute Nutrition Foundation, 1990:212–223.

Shirazi-Beechey S, Gorvel J, Beechey R. Intestinal phosphate transport: Localization, properties, and identification, a progress report. In: Bronner F, Peterlik M, eds. Progress in clinical and biological research. New York: Liss, 1988;252: 59–64.

Danisi G, Caverzasio J, Trechsel U, et al. Phosphate transport adaptation in intestinal brush border membrane vesicles, and plasma levels of 1,25-dihydroxycholecalciferol. In: Bronner F, Peterlik M, eds. Progress in clinical and biological research. New York: Liss, 1988;252:65–66.

MAGNESIUM

Magnesium as a cation in the human body ranks fourth in overall abundance, but intracellularly it is second only to potassium. The normal human body contains 21 to 28 g magnesium, approximately 60% of which is located in bone and the remaining 40% in extracellular fluids and soft tissues [1,2].

Sources

Magnesium is found in a wide variety of foods and beverages. Beverages rich in magnesium are coffee, tea, and cocoa. On the basis of weight, foods and food components particularly high in magnesium are whole-grain cereals, nuts, legumes, spices, and seafoods. On the basis of calories, most fruits and green, leafy vegetables are excellent sources of magnesium. Chlorophyll found in the green, leafy vegetables contains magnesium. Other particularly good food sources of magnesium are listed in Table 11.1.

Food processing and preparation may substantially reduce the magnesium content of foods. For example, the refining of whole wheat with removal of the germ and outer layers can reduce the magnesium content by 80% [1].

Absorption and Transport

Magnesium absorption occurs throughout the small intestine, including both the jejunum and ileum. In contrast to the jejunum, absorption in the ileum appears to be saturable [3]. Absorption in comparison to intake is curvilinear, occurring by simple diffusion with 10 mmol/L or more concentrations as would occur following ingestion of pharmacologic doses of the mineral, or by a saturable, carrier-mediated–facilitative transport system with typical ingestion and thus concentrations of the mineral [3,4]. The colon may also play a role in the absorption of magnesium [3], especially if disease has interfered with magnesium absorption in the small intestine [2].

About 30 to 60% of magnesium is thought to be absorbed in adults with usual intakes [1,5,6]. Magnesium absorption is more efficient when magnesium status is poor or marginal and/or when magnesium intake is low [2].

Magnesium absorption may be influenced by a variety of other factors. For example, dietary phytate and fiber impair magnesium absorption to a small extent [1]. Unabsorbed fatty acids present in high quantities, as occur with steatorrhea, may bind to magnesium, as to calcium, to form soaps. These magnesium–fatty acid soaps are excreted in the feces [5]. Vitamin D increases magnesium absorption, but less than it does calcium absorption [2,5].

In the plasma, most magnesium (55%) is found free, about 32% is bound to protein, and 13% is complexed with citrate, phosphate, or other ions [4]. Concentrations of magnesium in the plasma are maintained between 1.3 to 2.1 mEq/L; however, the homeostatic mechanism of control is unclear. Maintenance of these constant values appears to depend on gastrointestinal absorption, renal excretion, and transmembranous cation flux rather than hormonal regulation [1].

Extracellular magnesium is thought to represent one magnesium pool in the body. At least two other magnesium pools exist in the body [4]. The extracellular magnesium pool exhibits quick turnover. Another intracellular magnesium pool has a turnover rate of about half that of the first pool [2]. The third pool is skeletal magnesium, which has a very slow turnover rate [2].

Functions

Between 60 and 65% of magnesium in the body is found associated with bone. Bone magnesium is divided between that found associated with phosphorus and calcium, as part of the crystal lattice, and that found on the surface. Bone surface magnesium is thought to represent a magnesium pool and to reflect changes in serum levels. In contrast, the magnesium in the crystal lattice is probably deposited at the time of bone formation [3].

Magnesium, which does not function as part of the bone, is found in extracellular fluids (1%) and in soft tissues (34 to 39%), primarily muscle [1,4]. Within cells, magnesium is bound to phospholipids as part of cell membranes (plasma, endoplasmic reticulum, and mitochondria), nucleic acids, protein, and as a complex with ATP.

Overall, magnesium is important for over 300 different enzyme reactions [2,3]. A primary function of magnesium is to bind to phosphate groups in ATP, thereby forming a complex that assists in the transfer of ATP phosphate. Figure 11.8 depicts magnesium as a ligand for the phosphate groups of ATP. Protein kinases transfer the γ-phosphate of magnesium ATP to a substrate [3]. Magnesium also functions within cells as an allosteric activator of enzyme activity and for membrane stabilization [5].

Listed here are some of the many fundamental roles of magnesium in the body [3,6]:

- Glycolysis: hexokinase and phosphofructokinase (p. 84)
- Krebs cycle: oxidative decarboxylation in Krebs cycle
- Hexose monophosphate shunt: transketolase reaction (p. 87 and 241)
- Creatine phosphate formation (p. 180): creatine kinase
- Beta oxidation: initiation by thiokinase (acyl CoA synthetase)

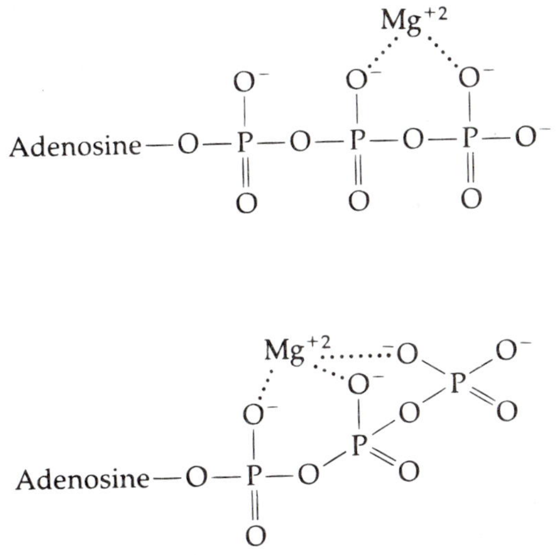

FIGURE 11.8 Modes by which Mg^{+2} provides stability to ATP.

- Activities of alkaline phosphatase and pyrophosphatase
- Nucleic acid synthesis
- DNA synthesis and degradation, as well as the physical integrity of the DNA helix
- DNA and RNA transcription
- Amino acid activation
- Protein synthesis (for example, with ribosomal aggregation and binding messenger RNA to 70S ribosome subunits)
- Cardiac and smooth muscle contractability (both direct action as well as influence on calcium ion transport and use)
- Vascular reactivity and coagulation (possible role)
- Cyclic adenosine monophosphate (cAMP) formation from adenylate cyclase (see Fig. 11.9)—because of its function in formation of cAMP, magnesium is involved in mediating the effects of numerous hormones

Interactions with Other Nutrients

Magnesium has interrelationships with a number of other nutrients. The first relationship that will be discussed is that with *calcium*. Magnesium is needed for PTH secretion, which is important in calcium homeostasis. Moreover, magnesium is needed for PTH effects on the bone, kidney, and gastrointestinal tract. The hydroxylation of *vitamin D* in the liver requires magnesium, and high magnesium levels, like calcium, inhibit PTH secretion [2,6]. Magnesium may mimic calcium by binding to calcium-binding sites and eliciting the appropriate physiologic response [2,6–8]. Magnesium may also cause

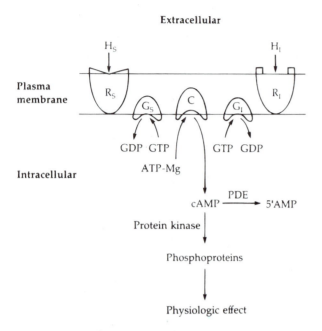

FIGURE 11.9 Schematic outline of the adenylate cyclase–cyclic AMP system that involves magnesium. The membrane-bound adenylate cyclase, stimulated by a wide variety of hormones and metabolic agents, modulates cAMP. Mg^{+2} is very important in this modulation. Abbreviations used: R_S, stimulatory receptors; R_I, inhibitory receptors; G_S, stimulatory guanine nucleotide-binding proteins; G_I, inhibitory guanine nucleotide-binding proteins; PDE, phosphodiesterase; C, catalytic unit of adenylate cyclase. *Reprinted, by permission of the New England Journal of Medicine 312:26–33, 1985.*

an alteration in calcium distribution by changing the flux of calcium across the cell membrane or by displacing calcium on its intracellular binding sites. Magnesium may further inhibit release of calcium from the sarcoplasmic reticulum in response to increased influx from extracellular sites and may activate the Ca^{+2}-ATPase pump to decrease intracellular Ca^{+2} concentrations [8]. The ratio of calcium to magnesium has been shown to affect muscle contraction. Magnesium may compete with calcium for nonspecific binding sites on troponin C and myosin [8]. Additional effects of magnesium are seen in the smooth muscles [6,8]. For example, calcium binding initiates acetylcholine release and smooth muscle contraction; magnesium bound to the calcium sites prevents calcium binding, and inhibits contraction [7]. The magnesium–calcium relationship has implications in people with respiratory disease, because increased intracellular calcium promotes bronchial smooth muscle contraction [7]. Magnesium may also influence the process of blood coagulation. In blood coagulation, calcium and magnesium are antagonistic, with calcium promoting the processes and magnesium inhibiting them [9].

A close interrelationship also exists between magnesium and *potassium*. Magnesium influences the balance between extracellular and intracellular potassium, but its mechanism of action is unclear [2]. One theory is that because magnesium is necessary for the function of Na^+/K^+-ATPase, a deficiency of magnesium would lead to impaired pumping of sodium out of the cell and the movement of potassium into the cell [2]. When magnesium and potassium deficiencies are coexistent, as may occur with some diuretic drug therapies, magnesium infusions, but not potassium infusions, can normalize muscle potassium [2]. Lastly, dietary *protein* intake impacts magnesium retention. Increasing dietary protein to a marginally adequate level in subjects previously ingesting low-magnesium and very low protein diets, improved magnesium retention. When, however, protein intake was further increased, magnesium retention was decreased [2].

Excretion

Absorbed magnesium not retained by the body is lost primarily via the kidneys. Of the serum magnesium, 70 to 80% [4] is ultrafilterable by the kidney; however, 95 to 97% is reabsorbed [3]. Thus only about 3 to 5% of the filtered magnesium is excreted in the urine [2,4]. With a low dietary intake of magnesium, the kidneys are able to conserve magnesium very effectively [2]. Rises in serum magnesium lead to increased filtration and excretion [6].

Fecal magnesium concentrations represent unabsorbed magnesium and a small amount of endogenous magnesium that escaped reabsorption. About 25 to 50 mg of endogenous magnesium may be excreted daily in the feces [1]. Magnesium may also be lost in the sweat, in amounts estimated at about 15 mg/day [2].

Recommended Dietary Allowance

The RDA for magnesium (350 and 280 mg/day for the adult 76-kg male and 62-kg female, respectively) represents a compromise between needs estimated by balance studies and the usual dietary magnesium intake by a population in which magnesium deficiency rarely appears except in pathologic conditions [1]. The RDA for adults of both sexes is 4.5 mg/kg/day [1]. The amount of magnesium furnished by the average U.S. diet is estimated at approximately 120 mg/1,000 kcal [10]. Balance studies indicate that adult needs for magnesium may be as low as 3 mg/kg/day or as high as 4.5 mg/kg/day [1].

Deficiency

Deficiency of magnesium in humans is usually associated with the presence of other illnesses such as alcoholism or renal disease. Pure deficiency of magnesium due to inadequate dietary intake has not been reported, but has been induced in humans under research protocols. Symptoms associated with deficiency include nausea, vomiting, anorexia, muscle weakness, spasms, and tremors, personality changes, and hallucinations, among others. Biochemical changes include low blood concentrations of not only magnesium, but also potassium and calcium [1,4]. Poor magnesium status may also be related to cardiovascular disease, myocardial infarction (heart attack), toxemia of pregnancy, and hypertension [2,3,5,8].

Conditions and populations associated with increased need for magnesium intake include vomiting, diarrhea, alcoholism, protein malnutrition, diuretic use, malabsorption, diabetes mellitus, parathyroid disease, and postsurgical patients.

Toxicity

An excessive intake of magnesium is not likely to cause toxicity except in the case of people with renal insufficiency [11]. Normal kidneys are able to remove magnesium so rapidly that significant increases in serum levels do not occur [3]. Excessive intakes of magnesium salts (3 to 5 g) such as from $MgSO_4$, may, however, have a cathartic effect leading to diarrhea and possible dehydration [10]. Acute magnesium toxicity from excessive intravenous administration of magnesium has resulted in nausea, depression, and paralysis [11].

Assessment of Nutriture

Assessment of magnesium status is difficult, because extracellular magnesium represents only about 1% of the total body magnesium and appears to be homeostatically regulated. Despite low sensitivity and specificity, serum magnesium concentrations are routinely measured to assess magnesium status [5]. Normal serum levels may occur despite severe intracellular deficit [2]. However, when serum magnesium is below normal an inadequate amount of intracellular magnesium is a certainty. Erythrocyte magnesium concentrations may reflect longer-term magnesium status due to the life span of the red blood cell [11]. Peripheral lymphocyte magnesium concentrations correlate with skeletal and cardiac muscle magnesium content and thus represent a possible indicator of magnesium status [5].

More definitive determination of magnesium status may involve measurement of renal magnesium excretion before and after the administration of an intravenous magnesium load. Decreased excretion determined over two 24-hour periods following administration of the magnesium load indicates deficiency [3]. Normal serum and urinary magnesium concentrations are 1.6 to 2.6 mg/dL and 36 to 207 mg/24 hours, respectively.

References Cited for Magnesium

1. National Research Council. Recommended dietary allowances, 10th ed. Washington, DC: National Academy Press, 1989:187–194.
2. Wester PO. Magnesium. Am J Clin Nutr 1987;45(suppl): 1305–1312.
3. Shils ME. Magnesium. In: Shils ME, Olson JA, Shike M. Modern Nutrition in Health and Disease, 8th ed. Philadelphia: Lea and Febiger, 1994:164–184.
4. Shils ME. Magnesium. In: Brown ML, ed. Present knowledge in nutrition, 6th ed. Washington, DC: International Life Sciences Institute Nutrition Foundation, 1990: 224–232.
5. Rude RK. Magnesium metabolism and deficiency. Endocrin Metab Clin N Am 1993;22:377–395.
6. Levine BS, Coburn JW. Magnesium, the mimic/antagonist of calcium. N Engl J Med 1984;310:1253–1255.
7. Landon RA, Yound EA. Role of magnesium in regulation of lung function. J Am Diet Assoc 1993;93:674–677.
8. Iseri LT, French JH. Magnesium: Nature's physiologic calcium blocker. Am Heart J 1984;108:188–193.
9. Weaver K. Magnesium and its role in vascular reactivity and coagulation. Contemp Nutr 1987;12(3).
10. National Research Council. Recommended dietary allowances, 9th ed. Washington, DC: National Academy of Sciences, 1980:134–136.
11. Gibson RS. Principles of nutritional assessment. New York: Oxford University Press, 1990:487–510.

Among the macrominerals, sodium, potassium, and chloride ions represent the major electrolytes, a term that, by definition, indicates that they contribute electrical charges to the fluid compartments of the body. Their concentrations are precisely regulated to assure that a normal electrolyte balance is maintained. In keeping with their role as electrolytes, sodium, potassium, and chloride will be considered again in Chapter 13, which deals specifically with fluid and electrolyte balance. In addition to their electrolyte role, however, these minerals also function as enzyme activators and in the transmission of nerve impulses. Functions, along with food sources and deficiency symptoms of these minerals, are shown in Table 11.1.

SODIUM

Approximately 30% of the 120 mg of sodium in the body is located on the surface of bone crystals. From that site, it can be released into the bloodstream should hyponatremia (low serum sodium) develop. The remainder of the body's sodium is in the extracellular fluid, primarily plasma, and in nerve and muscle tissue. Sodium constitutes about 93% of the cations in the blood, making it by far the most abundant member of this family.

Absorption and Transport

Approximately 95% of ingested sodium is absorbed, with the remaining 5% excreted in the feces. Sodium absorbed in excess of the amount needed is excreted by the kidneys. There are three basic pathways for absorption of sodium across the intestinal mucosa. One of these pathways (the Na^+/glucose cotransport system) functions broadly throughout the small intestine. Another pathway (an electroneutral Na^+ and Cl^- cotransport system) is active in both the small intestine and the proximal portion of the colon), and the third pathway (an electrogenic sodium absorption mechanism) occurs principally in the colon.

The Na^+/glucose cotransport system involves a carrier on the apical membrane of the small intestinal epithelium. Na^+ and glucose bind to the carrier, which shuttles them from the outer surface to the inner surface of the membrane. There, both are released before the carrier returns to the outer surface. Absorbed Na^+ is then pumped out across the basolateral membrane by the Na^+/K^+-ATPase pump (p. 17), while the glucose diffuses across the membrane by a facilitated transport pathway. The Na^+ gradient created by the Na^+/K^+-ATPase pump provides the needed energy to maintain the absorptive direction of the ion. Cotransport of Na^+ by this mechanism can also occur with solutes other than glucose, including amino acids [1], di- and tripeptides, and many B vitamins [2].

The electroneutral Na^+ and Cl^- cotransport mechanism has been proposed because of the observation that a significant portion of sodium uptake requires the presence of chloride, and vice versa [3]. Precisely how this system functions has not yet been established. However, it is believed that the cotransport is composed of Na^+/H^+ exchange working in concert with a Cl^-/HCO_3^- mechanism [4]. The mechanism allows the entrance of both Na^+ and Cl^- into the cell, wherein they are exchanged for H^+ and HCO_3^-. Protons and HCO_3^- are produced within the cell by the action of carbonic anhydrase on CO_2. Absorbed Na^+ is pumped across the basolateral membrane by the Na^+/K^+-ATPase pump, followed by Cl^-, which crosses by diffusion.

The colonic mechanism is called an *electrogenic sodium absorption mechanism* because the absorbed sodium ion is the only ion moving transcellularly, allowing its transport to be monitored by electrical equipment. It enters the luminal membrane of the colonic mucosal cell through Na^+-conducting pathways called Na^+ channels, diffusing inwardly by the downhill concentration gradient of the ion. The absorbed sodium is accompanied by water and anions, resulting in net water and electrolyte movement from the luminal side to the bloodstream side of the colon epithelium. It is pumped out across the basolateral membrane on the bloodstream side of the cell by the Na^+/K^+-ATPase pump.

All three of these mechanisms are depicted schematically in Figure 11.10. It is important to recognize that the common driving force for sodium absorption in all the processes is the inwardly directed gradient maintained by the basolateral Na^+ pump.

Interactions with Other Nutrients

The well-documented interaction of sodium with calcium is worthy of discussion. It has long been recognized (prior to 1940) that dietary sodium intake affects urinary calcium excretion. More currently, research has focused on the association of high dietary sodium intake with increased calcium requirements, increased bone resorption, and possibly osteoporosis. Studies have shown, however, that despite accompanying calciuria, oral sodium loading may not affect calcium balance. This is because the sodium challenge also causes an increase in serum PTH levels and cAMP excretion, along with a significant decrease in fecal calcium excretion. Such calcium-elevating effects may act as compensatory mechanisms to offset the urinary calcium losses. The sodium–calcium interaction and its possible association with osteoporosis have been reviewed [5]. For additional information on this topic, see references 24 and 27 in the "Calcium" section of this chapter.

Regulation and Excretion

As mentioned previously, nearly all (95%) of ingested sodium is absorbed by the mechanisms described. Therefore, much larger amounts are absorbed than are required by the body, the excess being excreted primarily by the kidneys. Sodium losses also take place through the skin via sweating. Under conditions of moderate temperature and level of exercise, sodium losses are small. However, since the sodium content of sweat is

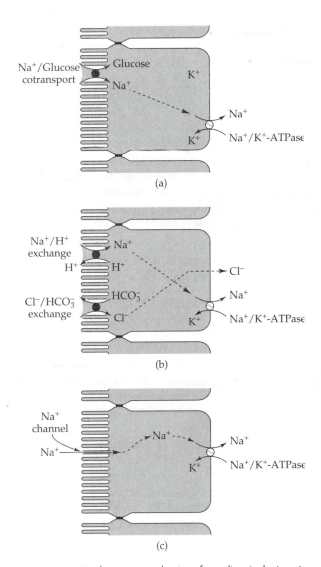

FIGURE 11.10 Absorption mechanisms for sodium in the intestine. (a) Na$^+$/glucose cotransport. A carrier on the luminal membrane of the mucosal cell cotransports sodium together with a solute such as glucose into the cell. Once in the cell, Na$^+$ is pumped across the basolateral membrane by Na$^+$/K$^+$-ATPase, while glucose exits through the membrane by facilitated diffusion. (b) Electroneutral Na$^+$ and Cl$^-$ absorption. The cotransport of Na$^+$ and Cl$^-$ may be linked to a Na$^+$/H$^+$ exchange and a Cl$^-$/HCO$_3^-$ exchange. Sodium is then pumped basolaterally with Cl$^-$ diffusing passively. (c) Electrogenic Na$^+$ absorption. Sodium enters the luminal membrane via a Na$^+$ channel.

about 50 mEq/L, it can be reasoned that conditions of high temperature and/or sustained vigorous exercise can account for significant losses. Renal excretion and retention of sodium are under the control of aldosterone, which promotes the retention (reabsorption) of sodium and the excretion of potassium. The hormone is released from the adrenal cortex in response to low sodium or,

more importantly, high potassium serum concentrations. The renal regulation of sodium, as well as potassium and chloride, is presented in greater detail in Chapter 13.

Recommended Dietary Allowances and Assessment of Nutriture

The major source of sodium in the diet is added salt in the form of sodium chloride. Sodium comprises 39% by weight of sodium chloride. Because salt is so extensively used in food processing and manufacturing, it is estimated that processed foods account for nearly 75% of total sodium consumed. Canned meats and soups, condiments, pickled foods, and traditional snacks are particularly high in added salt. Naturally occurring sources of sodium such as milk, meats, eggs, and most vegetables furnish only about 10% of consumed sodium. Salt added during cooking and at the table provides roughly 15% of total sodium, and water supplies less than 10%.

However unpalatable in a diet, an intake of only 115 mg/day of sodium is probably sufficient to replace obligatory losses and provide for growth. To compensate for wide variations in physical activity and climatic exposure, which account for sodium losses through sweating, the National Research Council recommends an intake of 500 mg/day [6]. Due to the high salt content of a typical diet, however, sodium intake is generally much greater. Depending on the method of assessment used, estimates of ingested sodium range from 1,800 to 5,000 mg/day.

Dietary deficiencies of sodium do not normally occur, due to the abundance of the mineral across a broad spectrum of foods consumed. Serum concentrations of sodium are normally regulated within the range of 135 to 145 mEq/L. It is measured routinely in clinical laboratories to determine electrolyte balance (see Chapter 13) and to identify possible renal disease, which may disturb normal sodium metabolism. Sodium ion in the serum and other biological fluids is usually quantified by the technique of ion-selective electrode potentiometry. The method measures Na$^+$ in the same manner as a pH meter measures protons.

POTASSIUM

In contrast to sodium, 98% of the body's potassium is intracellular. The approximate 270 mg of potassium is located inside the cells, making it the major intracellular fluid cation. Potassium influences the contractility of smooth, skeletal, and cardiac muscle, and profoundly affects the excitability of nerve tissue. It is also important in maintaining electrolyte and pH balance.

Absorption and Transport

The mechanisms by which potassium is absorbed from the gastrointestinal tract are not as clearly understood as those of sodium absorption. Only recently, relative to sodium absorption elucidation, have actual intestinal transport mechanisms for potassium been recognized and investigated. Over 90% of ingested potassium is absorbed, and while the sites along the gastrointestinal tract at which this takes place have not been precisely identified, the colon appears to play a major role in this function [7,8].

It is believed that K^+ may be absorbed through the apical membrane of the colonic mucosal cell by a K^+/H^+ ATPase pump. This would exchange intracellular H^+ for luminal K^+, the mechanism by which H^+ along with Cl^- (secreted via Cl^- channels), is secreted into the stomach as HCl. Alternatively, K^+ may enter the cell via apical membrane channels that serve as secretory pathways as well. The K^+ accumulated in the cell then diffuses across the basolateral membrane via the K^+ channel.

Interactions with Other Nutrients

Like sodium, potassium has an effect on the urinary excretion of calcium. However, its effect is opposite to that of sodium in that it decreases calcium excretion while sodium increases it. There exists a current practice of replacing some of the NaCl in the diet with KCl in order to reduce the amount of NaCl consumed. The finding that potassium is not as calciuric as sodium, and in fact actually reduces the excretory rate of calcium, further supports the practice [9]. For additional information on this subject, see references 23–25 in the "Calcium" section of this chapter.

Regulation and Excretion

Potassium is absorbed from the intestine at an efficiency of greater than 90%. Only small amounts are excreted in the feces. As with sodium, potassium balance is achieved largely through the kidneys, with aldosterone being the major regulatory hormone. Aldosterone acts reciprocally on sodium and potassium. Although it stimulates the reabsorption of sodium in the kidney tubules, it accelerates the excretion of potassium. Renal control of potassium is discussed further in Chapter 13.

Hyperkalemia (abnormally high serum concentration of potassium) is toxic, resulting in severe cardiac arrhythmias and even cardiac arrest. It is nearly impossible to produce hyperkalemia by dietary means in an individual with normal circulation and renal function. This is because of potassium's delicate control within a narrow concentration range. Similarly, hypokalemia (abnormally low serum potassium) does not occur by dietary deficiency, because of the abundance of potassium in common foods. Hypokalemia, associated with muscular weakness, nervous irritability, and mental disorientation can result from profound alimentary fluid loss such as would occur in severe vomiting and diarrhea.

Recommended Dietary Allowances and Assessment of Nutriture

Potassium is widespread in the diet, and is especially abundant in unprocessed foods, fruits, many vegetables, and fresh meats. Also, many salt substitutes contain potassium in place of sodium. The National Research Council recommends a dietary intake of 2,000 mg/day of potassium [6], but states further that 3,500 mg/day may be more desirable in view of the increased intake of fruits and vegetables recommended for prevention and control of hypertension.

The normal serum concentration of potassium, as K^+, is 3.6 to 5.0 mEq/L. It is commonly assayed clinically to identify renal disease and monitor electrolyte balance. Because of its toxicity, reported high values are brought to the attention of the attending physician immediately so that appropriate corrective measures may be taken. Potassium, like sodium, is determined in the serum primarily by the method of ion-selective electrode potentiometry.

CHLORIDE

Chloride is the most abundant anion in the extracellular fluid. Approximately 88% of chloride is found in extracellular fluid, and just 12% is intracellular. Its negative charge neutralizes the positive charge of sodium ions with which it is usually associated. In this respect, it is of great importance in the maintenance of electrolyte balance.

Chloride has important functions in addition to its role as a major electrolyte. It is required for the formation of gastric hydrochloric acid, secreted along with protons from the parietal cells of the stomach. Also, it acts as the exchange anion in the red blood cell for HCO_3^-. Sometimes referred to as the *chloride shift*, this latter process requires a protein transporter that moves

Cl^- and HCO_3^- in opposite directions across the cell membrane. The purpose is to allow the conveying of tissue-derived CO_2 back to the lungs in the form of plasma HCO_3^-. Waste CO_2 from respiring tissues enters the red blood cell, where it is converted to HCO_3^- by carbonic anhydrase. The transporter protein (chloride–bicarbonate exchanger) then transports the HCO_3^- out of the cell into the plasma while it simultaneously transports plasma Cl^- into the cell. In the absence of chloride, bicarbonate transport ceases.

Absorption, Transport, and Secretion

Chloride is almost completely absorbed in the small intestine. Its absorption closely follows that of sodium in the establishment and maintenance of electrical neutrality. The absorptive mechanisms, however, are generally different. For example, in the Na^+–glucose cotransport system (described in the "Sodium" section), chloride follows the actively absorbed Na^+ *passively* through a so-called paracellular, or tight junction, pathway. The absorbed Na^+ creates an electrical gradient that provides the energy for the accompanying, inward diffusion of Cl^-. The electroneutral Na^+ and Cl^- cotransport absorption system also contributes to the movement of chloride into the mucosal cells, although the relative contribution of this system to total chloride absorption is not well established. Sodium absorbed by the electrogenic Na^+ absorption mechanism is also accompanied by chloride, which follows the absorbed sodium passively (paracellularly) to maintain electrical neutrality. It is clear, therefore, that regardless of which absorptive mechanism is functioning, wherever sodium goes chloride cannot be far behind!

Secretory mechanisms for the electrolytes throughout the gastrointestinal tract center on chloride. It is the major secretory product of the stomach and the rest of the gastrointestinal tract. The well-defined mechanism is an electrogenic Cl^- secretion because Cl^- is the only ion actively secreted by the epithelium, and its movement can be monitored by changes in electrical potentials. Cells take up chloride from the blood across the basolateral membrane via a $Na^+/K^+/Cl^-$ cotransport pathway. An appropriate gradient is set up by the Na^+/K^+-ATPase pump, which maintains a low concentration of intracellular sodium. Potassium channels on the basolateral membrane allow potassium recycling out of the cell. Accumulating chloride in the cell exits through the apical membrane into the lumen via the Cl^- channels. Figure 11.11 illustrates the chloride secretory mechanism.

Chloride channels have not been studied extensively because of a lack of chemical blockers specific for the

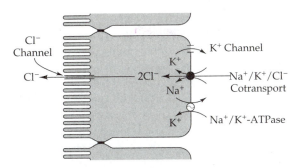

FIGURE 11.11 Intestinal chloride secretory mechanism. Chloride is cotransported along with Na^+ and K^+ from the circulation across the basolateral membrane and into the mucosal cell. Chloride then exits the cell into the lumen through Cl^- channels in the apical membrane. The driving force is provided by active removal of Na^+ by the Na^+/K^+-ATPase pump and the recycling of potassium through K^+ channels on the basolateral membrane..

chloride channel. However, studies on the defective gene of cystic fibrosis (caused by chloride transport dysfunction) have revealed a protein called the "cystic fibrosis transmembrane conductance regulator" (CFTR) [10]. The predicted structure of the protein is that of a channel or channel accessory.

Regulation and Excretion

It is estimated that the average adult consumes between 50 and 200 mEq/day. Chloride output occurs through three primary routes: the gastrointestinal tract, the skin, and the kidneys, with losses through each of these routes reflecting closely that of sodium. Excretion of chloride through the gastrointestinal tract is normally very small (1 to 2 mEq/day for the average adult), in keeping with its extensive absorption in the intestine. Losses through the skin are essentially the same as sodium; that is, normally quite small except in cases of high temperature and vigorous exercise. The major route of excretion is through the kidneys, where it is primarily regulated indirectly through sodium regulation.

Recommended Dietary Allowances and Assessment of Nutriture

Nearly all the chloride consumed in the diet is associated with sodium in the form of NaCl. Therefore, it is abundant in a large number of foods, particularly the snack items and foods that are processed. However, it also is found in eggs, fresh meats, and seafood. Dietary deficiency of chloride therefore does not occur under normal conditions. As in the case of the other electrolytes, the chief cause of deficiency arises through alimentary disturbance such as severe diarrhea and vomiting.

The National Research Council recommends a chloride intake of 750 mg/day [6]. In view of losses through sweating, however, this value may have to be adjusted upward in cases of physically rigorous lifestyles or chronic exposure to high temperatures.

The serum concentration of chloride is 101 to 111 mEq/L. Its measurement is generally used to establish the chloride status of the body. However, like all serum solutes, concentration depends on the body water status. It is possible, for example, that the total body store of chloride may be diminished, yet, if body water accompanies the losses, fluid concentrations of chloride may appear normal and may even be elevated. Two widely used methods for determining chloride in serum are based on ion-selective electrode potentiometry and on a coulometric titration with silver ions.

References Cited for Sodium, Potassium, and Chloride

1. Munck BG. Intestinal absorption of amino acids. In: Johnson LR, et al., eds. Physiology of the gastrointestinal tract. New York: Raven Press, 1981:1097–1122.
2. Rose RC. Intestinal absorption of water-soluble vitamins. In: Johnson LR, et al., eds. Physiology of the gastrointestinal tract. New York: Raven press, 1987:1581–1596.
3. Frizzell RA, et al. Sodium-coupled chloride transport by epithelial tissues. Am J Physiol 1979;236:F1–8.
4. Barrett KE, Dharmsathaphorn K. Transport of water and electrolytes in the gastrointestinal tract: Physiological mechanisms, regulation, and methods of study. In: Maxwell MH, Kleeman CR. Clinical disorders of fluid and electrolyte metabolism. Narins RG, ed. New York: McGraw-Hill, 1994:506–507.
5. Shortt C and Flynn A. Sodium–calcium inter-relationships with specific reference to osteoporosis. Nutr Res Rev 1990;3:101–115.
6. National Research Council. Recommended dietary allowances, 10th ed. Washington DC: National Academy Press, 1989.
7. Hayslett JP, Binder HJ. Mechanism of potassium adaptation. Am J Physiol 1982;243:F103–112.
8. Kliger AS, et al. Demonstration of active potassium transport in the mammalian colon. J Clin Invest 1981; 67:1189–1196.
9. Bell RR, Eldrid MM, Watson FR. The influence of NaCl and KCl on urinary calcium excretion in healthy young women. Nutr Res 1992;12:17–26.
10. Riordan JR, et al. Identification of the cystic fibrosis gene: Cloning and characterization of complementary DNA. Science 1989;245:1066–1075.

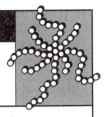

PERSPECTIVE

Macrominerals and Hypertension

The high incidence of osteoporosis among the elderly, particularly women, has implicated a need for generous calcium intakes throughout life. Now another disease, hypertension, which affects as many as 58 million Americans [1] and is particularly prevalent among the elderly, is being linked by some researchers to an inadequate intake of calcium and perhaps other minerals.

Hypertension is an increase in vascular resistance most often due to a decreased luminal diameter of the arteries and/or arterioles. This decrease in luminal diameters is caused by excessive shortening of the vascular smooth muscle actomyosin [2]; the initiator for the contraction (or shortening) is intracellular calcium. At first glance it seems quite incongruous that a deficiency of dietary calcium could be a cause of hypertension.

Attempts to link hypertension to dietary factors and to treat the disorder by dietary manipulations date back to W. Kempner, M.D., [3] and his very low-protein rice–fruit diet, which also proved to be very low in sodium. Dietary factors that have been investigated in relation to hypertension include (in addition to sodium) protein, total calories, fat, alcohol, chloride, potassium, magnesium, and calcium [4]. Intensive research concerning the role of sodium in the development and/or treatment of hypertension has been particularly fruitful because through establishing the fact that a certain population of hypertensives (approximately 30 to 50%) are much more sensitive to an excess of sodium than others, it has strongly suggested that hypertension is a heterogeneous disease, having a variety of precipitating factors.

A possible relationship between calcium and the development of hypertension was first recognized with the discovery in the early 1970s that communities characterized by hard water (high content of calcium) had a lower death rate from cardiovascular disease [5]. Since that time much evidence from epidemiologic studies, laboratory studies, and clinical trials has accumulated to support the relationship between calcium and blood pressure.

Epidemiologic evidence supporting the role of calcium in the control of blood pressure has come from a comparison of the prevalence of gestational hypertension (high blood pressure during pregnancy) in different countries where the intake of calcium varied. The incidence of gestational hypertension was inversely related to calcium intake. Various dietary surveys have also suggested that hypertensives as a group consume

less calcium than normotensives [5]. In the analysis by McCarron et al. [6] of data collected as part of the National Health and Nutrition Examination Survey 1971 to 1974 (NHANES I), calcium emerged as the only nutrient to distinguish hypertensives from normotensives; hypertensives consumed 18% less calcium than people with normal blood pressure. Other investigators [7–9] have challenged the analyses of McCarron et al. [6], and using data gathered from both NHANES I and II, found no association between calcium intake and either the prevalence of hypertension or mean levels of blood pressure [8].

The effect of calcium on blood pressure has been investigated in both animals and humans. Chronic dietary exposure to diets ranging in calcium content from 0.59 to 4.3% have repeatedly been shown to decrease the rate at which blood pressure rises in normal, pregnant, and hypertensive animals [10]. The greatest effect of dietary calcium, however, occurs in animal models of hypertension [10]. The effects of calcium on blood pressure in human studies have been limited in number, but the few conducted on pregnant women generally support the hypothesis that an adequate calcium intake is an important factor in controlling blood pressure. In one study an intake of 2,000 mg calcium per day from the fifteenth week of gestation to time of delivery prevented the rise in blood pressure that is characteristic of the third trimester of pregnancy. Those women receiving a placebo or only 1,000 mg calcium/day experienced the expected rise in blood pressure. Similar results have also been produced in other studies [11].

Not all people with hypertension are affected similarly by calcium supplementation. In a randomized, double-blind crossover trial, 48 hypertensive and 32 matched normotensives received either 1,000 mg of calcium/day (provided as calcium carbonate) or a placebo for eight weeks. After a period of four weeks in which only placebo was given, the treatments were switched and continued for an additional eight weeks. As compared to the placebo, calcium caused an average decrease of 5.6 mm Hg in systolic pressure and 2.3 mm Hg in diastolic pressure. The downward trend in blood pressure became apparent after six weeks of supplementation but was continuing at the end of the eight weeks. Despite the average decrease in blood pressure, not all the hypertensives responded to treatment. Using the criterion of a 10mm Hg decrease in systolic

PERSPECTIVE (continued)

pressure with calcium as compared to placebo, the investigators found that only 44% of the hypertensive subjects responded to calcium therapy. In the remaining hypertensives, blood pressure either remained the same or even increased. Of the normotensive subjects, 19% showed response to treatment [10]. Those subjects responding to calcium supplementation by a reduction in blood pressure exhibited an increase in serum ionized calcium but no exacerbation of urinary calcium. The ineffectiveness of calcium supplements in lowering the blood pressure of most normotensives is not understood, but it is suggested that a high basal intake of calcium may be responsible [12].

The difference in response among hypertensives to oral calcium may be due to the heterogenicity of the disease [13–15]. Only a subset of the people suffering from hypertension are "calcium sensitive." People who appear to benefit from oral calcium therapy are those who have been classified as having low renin activity and being "salt sensitive." For a given dietary salt intake, hypertensive people with low renin levels have a calcium metabolic profile characterized by lower average levels of serum-ionized calcium and higher levels of parathyroid hormone and 1,25-dihydroxy cholecalciferol than those found in normotensive people or other subgroups of hypertensive people. An opposite calcium metabolic pattern is exhibited by hypertensives who are salt insensitive or who have high renin activity. It may be this latter group of hypertensives that respond to calcium supplementation with an increase in blood pressure. Efforts are presently being made to define criteria that can be used to predict those hypertensive people who will be helped by oral calcium supplementation.

How dietary calcium can exhibit an antihypertensive effect in "calcium-sensitive" hypertensives is uncertain beyond the fact that additional calcium in the diet of these people increases serum ionized calcium and does not exacerbate calciuria [10]. On first consideration, calcium would appear to be an unlikely nutrient to lower blood pressure because an increase in the cytoplasmic Ca^{+2} concentration is the immediate stimulus for the contraction of vascular smooth muscle [2]. However, in addition to its initiation of muscle contraction, calcium has a membrane-stabilizing, vaso-relaxing effect on the smooth muscle cells [16].

Calcium may influence blood pressure through a variety of other mechanisms: an effect on the central and peripheral sympathetic nervous system; modification of vascular actions of calcium-regulating hormones (PTH, calcitonin, calcitriol); inductive effect on intracellular calcium pathways such as the cation's interaction with its binding protein calmodulin or the Ca^{+2}-ATPase pump; interaction with other nutrients [17]. Some nutrients with which calcium may interact and thereby effect a blood pressure change include sodium, potassium, and magnesium.

Exchange of sodium and calcium across the cell membrane is interdependent, as is illustrated in Figure 11.2, which shows the cellular control of cytosolic free-calcium concentrations. The relationship between these two cations is quite complex. Although the antihypertensive effect of calcium appears to be enhanced by adequate sodium intake, excessive sodium intake causes an increase in urinary calcium. A high intake of calcium likewise increases the urinary excretion of sodium [1,18]. Research suggests that adequate calcium intakes appear to protect against the hypertensive effects of a high-sodium, low-potassium diet [19].

Potassium is also thought to impact blood pressure. Potassium may induce vascular smooth muscle relaxation and thus peripheral resistance. And potassium is thought to be involved in the kinin system or to affect renin, which affects blood pressure [20]. Higher potassium intakes alone or potassium intake relative to sodium intakes have also been associated with a lower prevalence of hypertension [20].

Magnesium has also been investigated and linked to hypertension because it has direct vasodilatory action [20]. Epidemiologic data suggest a relationship between blood pressure and magnesium intake. The results of studies providing magnesium supplementation to treat hypertension have been contradictory. The link between blood pressure and magnesium may or may not be related to calcium's effect on blood pressure. Some investigators believe that magnesium deficiency leads to increased intracellular calcium concentration, thereby increasing vasoconstriction and blood pressure [21].

The current knowledge about the effect of calcium and other nutrients such as potassium and magnesium on blood pressure is ambiguous, therefore, specific recommendations for dietary intakes that could prove beneficial in the prevention or treatment of hypertension cannot be made. Because inadequate intakes of calcium and potassium appear more positively associated with an increase in blood pressure than do adequate intakes, the most prudent recommendation is that people consume calcium and potassium in an amount suggested by the National Research Council [22]. The Joint National Committee on Detection, Evaluation, and Treatment of High Blood Pressure also suggests maintenance of adequate dietary intakes of calcium, potassium, and magnesium for the treatment of hypertension in their report [23].

PERSPECTIVE (continued)

References Cited

1. Calcium update. Dairy Council Dig 1987;58(3).
2. Van Breemen C, Cauvin C, Johns A, et al. Ca^{+2} regulation of vascular smooth muscle. Fed Proc 1985;45:2746–2751.
3. Dole VP, Dahl LK, Cotzias G, et al. Dietary treatment for hypertension: Clinical and metabolic studies of patients on rice-fruit diet. J Clin Invest 1950; 29:1189–1206.
4. Karanja N, McCarron D. The calcium-blood pressure hypothesis: evidence for its validity. Contemp Nutr 1984;9(11).
5. Henry H, McCarron DA, Morris CD, et al. Increasing calcium intake lowers blood pressure: The literature reviewed. J Am Diet Assoc 1985;85:182–185.
6. McCarron DA. Blood pressure and nutrient intake in the United States. Science 1984;224:1392–1398.
7. Gruchow HW, Sobocinski KA, Barboriak JJ. Alcohol, nutrient intake, and hypertension in US adults. JAMA 1985;253:1567–1570.
8. Sempos C, Cooper R, Kovar MG, et al. Dietary calcium and blood pressure in National Health and Nutrition Surveys I and II. Hypertension. 1986;8: 1067–1075.
9. Kaplan NM, Meese RB. The calcium deficiency hypothesis: A critique. Ann Intern Med 1986;105: 947–955.
10. Karanja N, McCarron DA. Calcium and hypertension. Ann Rev Nutr 1986;6:475–494.
11. Villar J. Calcium supplementation reduces blood pressure during pregnancy: Results of a randomized controlled clinical trial. Obstet Gynecol 1987;70: 317–322.
12. Aalberts JS, Weegels PL, van der Heyden L, et al. Calcium supplementation: Effect on blood pressure and urinary mineral excretion in normotensive male lactoovovegetarians and omnivores. Am J Clin Nutr 1988;48:131–138.
13. Resnick LM. Calcium and hypertension: The emerging connection. Ann Intern Med 1985;103(6, part 1): 944–945.
14. Resnick LM, Nicholson JP, Laragh JH. Calcium metabolism in essential hypertension: Relationship to altered renin system activity. Fed Proc 1985;45: 2739–2745.
15. Barger-Lux MJ, Heaney RP. The role of calcium intake in preventing bone fragility, hypertension, and certain cancers. J Nutr 1994;124:1406S–1411S.
16. Wegener LL, McCarron DA. Calcium and hypertension. Nutr MD 1985;11:1,2.
17. McCarron DA, Morris CD. The calcium deficiency hypothesis of hypertension. Ann Intern Med 1987; 107:919–922.
18. An update on diet and blood pressure. Dairy Council Dig 1986;57(5).
19. Gruchow HW, Sobocinski KA, Barboriak JJ. Calcium intake and the relationship of dietary sodium and potassium to blood pressure. Am J Clin Nutr 1988;48:1463–1470.
20. Stein PP, Black HR. The role of diet in the genesis and treatment of hypertension. Med Clin N Am 1993;77:831–847.
21. Magnesium and blood pressure. Nutr MD 1998; 14(5):1.
22. National Research Council. Recommended dietary allowances, 10th ed. Washington, DC: National Academy Press, 1989.
23. Joint National Committee on Detection, Evaluation, and Treatment of High Blood Pressure. The fifth report. Arch Intern Med 1993;153:154–183.

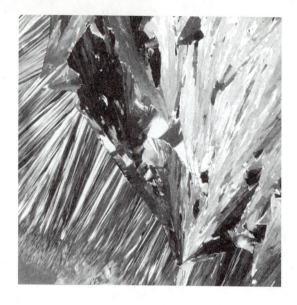

MICROMINERALS

Photo: Photomicrograph of crystallized manganese sulfate

A precise definition for the essential microminerals (or trace minerals) has not been established. Some define an essential microdineral as one that comprises less than one-hundredth of 1 percent of total body weight. Others define it as a nutrient the body needs in concentrations of one part per million or less [1]. These minerals initially gained the nomenclature of "trace" because their concentrations in tissue were not easily quantified by early analytical methods [2]. Iron appears to be the mineral that divides the macrominerals from the microminerals; consequently, some define an essential trace mineral as one that is needed by the body in a concentration equal to or lower than iron [1]. Alternately, trace may be defined as needed by the body in amounts less than 100 mg per day.

The term *essential* as applied to trace elements is also specifed. An element is considered essential if a dietary deficiency of that element consistently results in a suboptimal biological function that is preventable or reversible by physiological amounts of the element [3]. More stringent criteria proposed to establish essentiality of a mineral include [4]:

- It is present in all healthy tissue of living things.
- Its concentration from one animal to the next is fairly constant.
- Its withdrawal from the body induces reproducibly the same physiological and structural abnormalities, regardless of species studied.
- Its addition either reduces or prevents these abnormalities.
- The abnormalities induced by deficiencies are always accompanied by specific biochemical changes.
- These biochemical changes can be prevented or cured when the deficiency is prevented or cured.

For four essential trace minerals (iron, zinc, iodine, and selenium), recommended dietary allowances (RDA) have been set

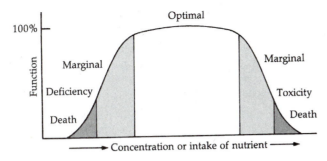

FIGURE 12.1 Dependence of biological function on tissue concentration or intake of a nutrient. (Mertz W. The essential trace minerals. Science, September 18, 1981, 213:1333. Copyright 1981 by the AAAS, reprinted with permission.)

for humans. A range of safe and adequate daily dietary intakes has been estimated for another five essential trace minerals (fluorine, copper, manganese, chromium, and molybdenum). Appendix A provides the RDAs for the microminerals. Very little is known about the need of humans for ultratrace elements, including nickel, silicon, vanadium, arsenic, and boron; therefore, no recommendations for intake exists.

Each essential trace mineral is necessary for one or more functions in the body, and its function(s) is optimal when body concentrations of the nutrient fall within a specific range. Whenever the concentration is too low or too high, function is impaired and death can result. This concept, illustrated in Figure 12.1, is especially important when considering the trace minerals because their optimal range of concentration can be fairly narrow. Moreover, because of the interactions among the essential trace minerals, an excessive intake of one, especially a divalent ion (such as zinc, magnesium, calcium, iron), may inhibit the absorption and cause deficiency of another divalent ion [5]. Conversely, a deficiency of one divalent ion may enhance the absorption of another [6].

This chapter discusses the sources, digestion (when applicable), absorption, transport, functions, interactions with other nutrients, excretion, recommended intakes, deficiency, toxicity, and assessment of nutriture for the microminerals as well as for several ultratrace elements. Table 12.1 provides an overview of selected functions, sources, deficiency symptoms, and recommended intakes for these minerals.

References Cited

1. Tracing the facts about trace minerals. Tufts University Diet and Nutr Letter March 1987;5:3–6.
2. Mertz W. The essential trace elements. Science 1981;213:1332–1338.
3. Nielsen FH. Ultratrace elements in nutrition. Ann Rev Nutr 1984;4:21–41.
4. Underwood EJ, Mertz W. Trace elements in human and animal nutrition. San Diego: Academic Press, 1987;2:1–19.
5. Greger JL. Mineral bioavailability/new concepts. Nutr Today 1987;22:4–9.
6. Finch CA, Huebers H. Perspectives in iron metabolism. N Engl J Med 1982;306:1520–1528.

IRON

The human body contains approximately 2 to 4 grams of iron. Over 65% of body iron is found in hemoglobin, up to about 10% is found as myoglobin, about 1% to 3% is found as part of enzymes, and the remaining body iron is found in the blood or in storage [1]. Table 12.2 (p. 356) gives an approximate distribution of iron per kilogram of body weight in adult males and females. The total amount of iron found in a person is related not only to body weight, but also is influenced by a variety of physiologic conditions including age, gender, pregnancy, and state of growth.

Iron, a metal, exists in several oxidation states varying from Fe^{+6} to Fe^{-2}, depending on its chemical environment. The only states that are stable in the aqueous environment of the human body (and in food) are the ferric (Fe^{+3}) and the ferrous (Fe^{+2}) forms.

Sources

Although iron is widely distributed in food, its content in an average Western diet is estimated to contain no more than 5 to 7 mg iron per 1,000 kcal [2]. Iron is found in one of two forms in foods, heme and nonheme. Heme iron is derived mainly from hemoglobin and myoglobin, and is thus found in meat, fish, and poultry. About 50 to 60% of the iron in meat, fish, and poultry is heme iron; the rest is nonheme iron [2,3]. Nonheme iron is found primarily in plant foods (nuts, fruits, vegetables, and grains) and in dairy products (milk, cheese, eggs). Nonheme iron is usually bound to components of foods and must be hydrolyzed or solubilized prior to absorption.

Foods particularly high in iron, such as liver and organ meats, are not popular items in most Western diets. Some of the more popular foods that are relatively good sources of iron include red meats, dark green, leafy vegetables, and dried fruits. Other good sources of iron are listed in Table 12.1.

TABLE 12.1 The Microminerals: Selected Function, Deficiency Symptoms, Food Sources, and Recommended Intake

Mineral	Selected Physiological Functions	Selected Enzyme Cofactors	Selected Deficiency Symptoms	Selected Food Sources in Rank Order	Adult RDA or ESADDI
Arsenic[a]	In animals: necessary for normal growth and iron use	—	Unknown	Most foods contain less than 0.3 μg/g; seafood is the richest source	—
Boron[a]	Bone composition, structure, and strength		In animals: depressed growth	Fruits, vegetables, legumes, nuts	—
Chromium	Normal use of blood glucose and function of insulin		Glucose intolerance, abnormalities in glucose and lipid metabolism, elevated circulating insulin, glycosuria	Mushrooms, prunes, nuts, asparagus, organ meats, whole-grain bread and cereals, American cheese, beer	50–200 μg
Copper	Required for proper use of iron by the body, amine oxidase, cytochrome oxidase; role in development of connective tissue— lysyl oxidase, ceruloplasmin, tyrosinase, melanin synthesis	In a variety of oxidases; for example, cytochrome oxidase	Fall in serum copper and ceruloplasmin levels, anemia, neutropenia, leukopenia, bone demineralization, failure of erythropoiesis	Liver, shellfish, whole grains, cherries, legumes, chocolate, nuts, eggs, muscle meats, fish, poultry	1.5–3.0 mg
Fluorine	Maintenance of teeth and bone structure	—	Dental caries, osteoporosis, osteosclerosis	Mackerel, sardines, salt pork, salmon, shrimp, meat, sunflower seeds, kale, potatoes, watercress, honey, wheat; drinking water content varies	1.5–4.0 mg
Iodine	Thyroid hormones synthesis	—	Enlargement of thyroid gland, myxedema, cretinism, increase in blood lipids, liver gluconeogenesis, and extracellular retention of NaCl and H_2O	Iodized salt, saltwater seafood, sunflower seeds, mushrooms, eggs, beef liver, peanuts, spinach, pumpkin, broccoli, chocolate	150 μg
Iron	Necessary component of hemoglobin and myoglobin for O_2 transport and cellular use; facilitates transfer of electrons in electron transport chain	Heme enzymes, including catalase, cytochromes, peroxidase, myeloperoxidase Nonheme enzymes	Listlessness, fatigue, palpitations on exertion, sore tongue, angular stomatitis, dysphagia, anemia, decreased serum iron, hematocrit and hemoglobin, decreased resistance to infection	Organ meats (liver), blackstrap molasses, clams and oysters, legumes, nuts and seeds, red meats, dark green, leafy vegetables, dried fruits, enriched and/or whole-grain breads and cereals	10 mg male, 15 mg female
Manganese	Essential for normal brain function; role in enzyme systems, collagen formation, bone growth, urea formation, fatty acid and cholesterol synthesis, and protein digestion	Arginase, pyruvate carboxylase	Known in animals, possibly in humans: impaired growth, skeletal abnormalities, impaired function of central nervous system, defects in lipid and CHO metabolism	Wheat bran, legumes, nuts, lettuce, beet tops, blueberries, pineapple, seafood, poultry, meat	2.5– 5.0 mg

[a]These minerals are essential in animals and very likely are essential for humans.

Table 12.1 (continued)

Mineral	Selected Physiological Functions	Selected Enzyme Cofactors	Selected Deficiency Symptoms	Selected Food Sources in Rank Order	Adult RDA or ESADDI
Molybdenum	Role in metabolism of purines, pyrimidines, pteridines, aldehydes, and oxidation of sulfite	Xanthine dehydro-genase and oxi-dase, aldehyde oxi-dase, sulfite oxidase	Hypermethioninemia, increased urinary xanthine and sulfite excretion, decreased urinary sulfate and urate excretion	Soybeans, lentils, pasta, buckwheat, oats, rice, bread	75–250 μg
Nickel[a]	Possibly involved in hormonal membrane or enzyme activity	—	In animals: changes in liver, anemia	Nuts, legumes, shellfish, cacoa products, hydrogenated solid shortening, spinach, asparagus, grains	—
Selenium	Protect cells against destruction by hydrogen peroxide and free radicals	Glutathione peroxidase, 5'-deiodinase	Myalgia, cardiac myopathy, increased red blood cell fragility, pancreatic degeneration	Grains, meat, poultry, fish, dairy products	70 μg male, 55 μg female
Silicon[a]	Apparent role in formation of connective tissue and bone matrix	Prolyl hydroxylase	In animals: decreased bone collagen, skull deformity, long bone abnormalities	Beer, unrefined grains, plant foods	—
Vanadium	Apparent role in lipid metabolism or reproductive performance	—	In animals: reduced growth, poor reproductive performance, changes in hematological parameters, bone defects, alteration of lipid metabolism	(Food contains very little): shellfish, spinach, parsley, mushrooms, whole grains, dill seeds, black pepper	—
Zinc	Role in energy metabolism, protein synthesis, collagen formation, alcohol detoxification, carbon dioxide elimination, sexual maturation, taste and smell functions	DNA-RNA polymerase, carbonic anhy-drase, carboxy-peptidase, alkaline phos-phatase, deoxy-thymidine kinase	Poor wound healing, subnormal growth, anorexia, abnormal taste and smell, changes in hair, nails, skin inflammation, anemia, retarded development of reproductive system, low plasma zinc levels	Oysters, wheat germ, beef, liver, dark meat of turkey and chicken, whole grains, particularly wheat	15 mg male, 12 mg female

[a]These minerals essential in animals and very likely essential for humans.

In addition to natural amounts of iron found in foods, some foods are fortified with iron. The present standards (1981 FDA Guidelines) for iron enrichment of cereal products are given in Table 12.3 (page 356).

Digestion, Absorption, and Transport

Heme Iron Heme iron must be hydrolyzed from the globin portion of hemoglobin or myoglobin prior to absorption. This digestion is accomplished by proteases in the stomach and small intestine. The heme containing the iron and porphyrin ring is then absorbed intact (as a metalloporphyrin) [3] into the mucosal cell of the small intestine (shown later in Fig. 12.3, page 358).

Absorption of heme iron is influenced by body iron stores. Heme absorption is inversely related to iron stores and may range from 15% with normal iron status to 35% in persons who are iron deficient. Iron absorption can occur throughout the small intestine, but is most efficient in the proximal portion, particularly the duodenum [2]. Within the mucosal cell the absorbed heme is broken down by a heme oxygenase into ferrous iron and protoporphyrin. The released iron moves through the mucosal cells for use by the intestinal cell or for transport and use by other body tissues [2,3].

Nonheme Iron Nonheme iron bound to components of foods must be enzymatically liberated in order for absorption to occur. Gastric secretions and hydrochloric acid aid in the release of nonheme iron from food components and may also stabilize the ionic iron thereby delaying or preventing precipitation (which de-

TABLE 12.2 Approximate Distribution of Iron in Adult Male and Female

		Male (mg/kg body weight)	Female (mg/kg body weight)
Functional compounds	Hemoglobin	31	28
	Myoglobin	4	3
	Heme enzymes	1	1
	Nonheme enzymes	1	1
	Transferrin iron	0.05	0.05
		37.05	33.05
Storage compounds	Ferritin	9	4
	Hemosiderin	4	1
		13	5
Total Iron		50.05	38.05

Sources: Finch CA, Huebers H. Perspectives in iron metabolism. N Engl J Med 1982;306:1520–1528; Leibel RL. Behavioral and biochemical correlates of iron deficiency. J Am Diet Assoc 1977;77:378–404; and Hallberg L. Iron absorption and iron deficiency. Hum Nutr Clin Nutr 1982;36C:259–278.

TABLE 12.3 Current (1981) FDA Standards for Iron Enrichment of Cereal Products

Product	mg Iron/lb Product
Bread, rolls, buns	12.5[a]
Flour	20.0[b]
Corn grits, cornmeal, rice	13–26[c]
Macaroni products	13–16.5[c]

[a] ~28g/slice bread.
[b] 1 tbsp flour ~8g.
[c] 2 oz dry rice and macaroni ~60g.

creases iron absorption) in the small intestine [2]. Absorption of iron is improved if the iron is present in the ferrous (Fe^{+2}) versus the ferric (Fe^{+3}) state. Ferrous iron transverses the glycocalyx and mucous layers of the intestinal brush border better than ferric iron [2]. Reduction to the ferrous form can be accomplished by hydrochloric acid present in gastric juice. However, as the ferrous iron passes into the small intestine, which contains juices with an alkaline pH, ferrous iron may be oxidized (to become ferric iron) and further may form ferric hydroxide. Ferric hydroxide—$Fe(OH)_3$—is relatively insoluble and tends to aggregate and precipitate, making the iron less available for absorption.

Several compounds (chelators, discussed in the next paragraph) may chelate with nonheme iron to either inhibit or enhance its absorption. Chelators are small or-

ganic compounds that form a complex with a metal ion. Whether the chelated iron is absorbed or excreted depends on the nature of the iron–chelate complex. If the iron–chelate complex maintains solubility and the iron is loosely bonded, the iron can be released at the mucosal cell and absorption enhanced. However, if the iron–chelate is strongly bonded and insoluble, the iron will be excreted as part of the chelate [3].

Concomitantly ingested substances such as ascorbic acid, citric acid, lactic acid, tartaric acid, fructose and sorbitol, and meat, fish, or poultry promote absorption of nonheme iron. Meat, poultry, and fish factors that enhance nonheme iron absorption have not been clearly identified. The enhancement is not a general property of animal proteins, but is due to the digestion products from animal tissues that are high in the contractile proteins actin and myosin [4]. Both of these proteins are digested into peptides that contain relatively large amounts of the amino acid cysteine. The cysteine-containing peptides appear to be responsible for the increased absorption of iron [3–5]. It is further suspected that meat is not just a source of solubilizing ligands (ligands are compounds such as the cysteine-containing peptides that bind iron or other minerals), but also may improve iron absorption through stimulation of enhancing intestinal secretions [4]. Other substances known to improve nonheme iron absorption include various acids. Ascorbic acid (vitamin C), for example, acts as a reducing agent and can form a chelate with nonheme ferric iron at an acid pH [4]. This chelate remains soluble in the small intestine and thus can improve nonheme iron absorption [3].

$$\text{Ascorbate} \longrightarrow \text{dehydroascorbate}$$
$$Fe^{+3} \quad Fe^{+2} \longrightarrow \text{ascorbate-}Fe^{+2}\text{ chelate}$$
$$\text{ascorbate}$$

EDTA, while generally shown to inhibit iron absorption, in some cases may improve iron absorption from meals with low iron bioavailability [6].

Knowledge of the amount of the enhancers in a meal has allowed estimation of the iron available for absorption [7,8]; 75 units of ascorbic acid and/or meat, fish, poultry (MFP) factor [one unit = 1.3 g raw or 1 g cooked meat, fish, poultry, or 1 mg ascorbic acid] have been shown to maximize the effect on iron absorption when consumed with the iron source [9]. Units in excess of 75 seem to have no further benefit. Absence of enhancing factors predicts a nonheme iron absorption of only 2 to 3% of the dietary nonheme iron, but 75 units of these factors can increase absorption of nonheme iron to 8% (some suggest up to 20% if the person is also iron deficient) [3]. These estimates of absorption have been based on the assumption of approximately 500 mg iron stores [7,8]. Calculations for the estimation of food iron absorption are found in Appendix B.

Dietary factors such as polyphenols including tannins (in tea), oxalic acid (in spinach, chard, berries, chocolate, tea, among others), phytates (for example, in maize and whole grain), EDTA (a preservative), phosvitin in egg yolks, calcium alone and as calcium phosphate salts, and zinc inhibit the absorption of nonheme iron [4,7,10–12]. Tea (or rather, the phenolic compounds in tea) consumed with a source of iron may reduce iron absorption over 60%. Coffee consumption, with or just after a meal, may reduce iron absorption by 40% [2]. Calcium (600 mg) as calcium phosphate when given with 18 mg iron as ferrous sulfate decreased iron absorption by 62%, possibly through the formation and precipitation of ferric phosphate [13]. Calcium (600 mg) as calcium citrate given with 18 mg iron as ferrous sulfate also decreased iron absorption by 49% [13], thus implicating both phosphorus and calcium as inhibitors of iron absorption. Moreover, these effects are not limited to supplements. Similar reductions in iron absorption have been shown with milk ingestion [14]. Thus, to maximize iron absorption from a supplement, do not take the iron with a source of calcium. Zinc and iron are thought to compete for the same portion of a common absorptive pathway; however, evidence that humans are ingesting sufficient zinc to impair iron absorption has not been generated. Other intraluminal factors that are inhibitory include rapid transit time, achylia (absence of digestive juices), malabsorption syndromes, and excess alkalinization as may occur with excessive use of antacids or with decreased gastric acidity. Overall absorption of iron from the U.S. diet is estimated at 10 to 15% [7,12].

Entry of iron into the body is carefully regulated by its absorption, a complex and poorly understood process. As indicated in Figure 12.2, the regulation of absorption in the healthy individual is closely tied to the level of iron stores. Absorption increases when iron stores are low and decreases as stores become greater; iron absorption can rise to 3 to 6 mg daily when the body is depleted of iron, and can fall to 0.5 mg or less daily when iron stores are high (Fig. 12.2) [2]. Absorption of heme iron is more affected than nonheme iron in iron-deficient states. The rate of erythropoiesis also appears to influence iron absorption [10].

How iron moves through the mucosal cell or is distributed within the cell has not been clearly elucidated. A proposed model is shown in Figure 12.3. Nonheme iron may be taken up in the ionic form, principally ferrous iron, by receptors on the intestinal mucosal cells. The ferrous iron may be converted to ferric iron before

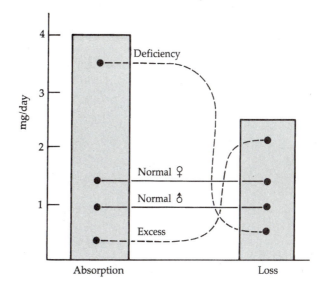

FIGURE 12.2 Absorption and excretion of iron in relation to need.

binding to membrane proteins. Some iron is thought to pass through the mucosal cell by diffusion. In addition, amino acids such as cysteine and histidine may transport ferrous iron across the mucosal cell. Some mucosal iron may be oxidized to ferric iron and bound to mucosal cell apotransferrin to form transferrin [2]. The transferrin then transports the ferric iron across the cytosol of the mucosal cell for release across the basolateral membrane. Iron, not crossing the cell by diffusion, bound to amino acids, or as part of transferrin, may be incorporated into apoferritin. Apoferritin is a protein that acts as a shell in which iron is trapped. This protein further serves as a ferroxidase using oxygen to convert the trapped ferrous iron to the ferric state for deposition and storage. The stored ferric iron can be reduced to the ferrous state and released from the ferritin molecule should iron be needed by the mucosal cell or required for transport to other tissues. If not needed, the iron remains as ferritin and is excreted when the short-lived (two to three days) mucosal cells are sloughed off into the lumen of the gastrointestinal tract. Iron deposition into ferritin may be responsible for the increase or decrease in the amount of iron that passes into the plasma for transport to tissues.

Iron moving through the mucosal cell may be used by the cell for a variety of functions. These functions are discussed in the next section. Transport of iron across the basolateral membrane involves a receptor protein that binds ferrous iron.

Iron in the ferric state is transported in the plasma bound to the glycoprotein transferrin. Ceruloplasmin, a

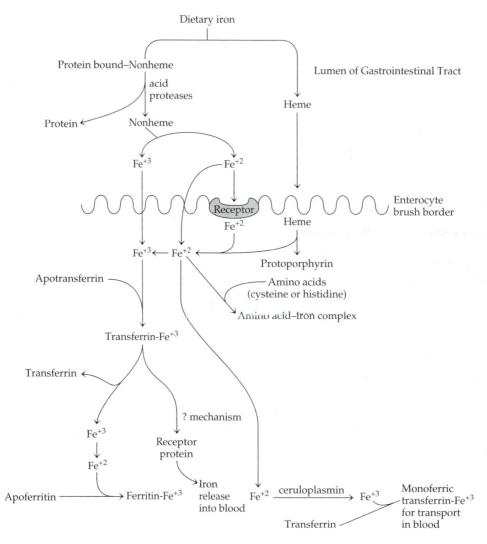

FIGURE 12.3 Proposed transport of iron.

copper-containing protein also with ferroxidase activity, catalyzes the oxidation of ferrous iron to its ferric form so that it can bind tightly to transferrin. Most iron is found in the body bound to protein rather than as free iron. The binding of iron by proteins serves as a defense mechanism, because free iron (Fe^{+2}) readily reacts (Fenton reaction) with hydrogen peroxide (H_2O_2).

$$Fe^{+2} + H_2O_2 \longrightarrow Fe^{+3} + OH^- + OH^{\cdot}$$

This reaction generates a hydroxy anion and a free hydroxy radical ($OH^{\cdot}$), which is extremely reactive and damaging to cells (see Chapter 10, "Perspective" section).

Transferrin, which is made in the liver, has two binding sites for minerals. The binding site near the C-terminal end of transferrin has a high affinity for ferric iron. The binding site near the N-terminal end has a high affinity for ferric iron, but will also bind other minerals such as chromium followed in descending order by copper > manganese > cadmium > zinc and nickel. Tight binding of ferric iron to transferrin also requires the presence of an anion, usually bicarbonate, at each binding site. Transferrin in the plasma is typically one-third saturated with ferric iron. If all binding sites of the transferrin were occupied, then the transferrin would be fully (100%) saturated. Transferrin binds ferric iron following transport across the basolateral membrane of the mucosal cell. Iron is delivered by transferrin to storage sites such as the liver, spleen, and bone marrow, as well as to tissues in need of the iron.

Iron is stored in three principal sites, the liver, bone marrow, and spleen. Transferrin delivers iron to the liver for storage in the parenchyma [2]. Reticuloendothelial (RE) cells also store iron. Reticuloendothelial cells are found in the spleen, liver, bone marrow, and between muscle fibers [15]. Most of the iron stored in reticuloendothelial cells is derived from phagocytosis of red blood cells and degradation of hemoglobin.

Ferritin is the primary storage form of iron in cells. Apoferritin is synthesized in a variety of tissues, including the liver, spleen, bone marrow, and intestine. Cellular iron is thought to influence in part the synthesis of apoferritin. *In vitro* observations suggest that iron deposition in ferritin involves the oxidation of ferrous iron into ferric oxyhydroxide crystals (FeOOH). This oxidation is thought to occur in the pores of the ferritin molecule and requires molecular oxygen as the electron acceptor [2,15]. Ferric oxyhydroxide is deposited in the interior of the protein shell. Apoferritin is shaped as a hollow sphere within which as many as 4,300 iron atoms can be stored [2]. Ferritin is constantly being degraded and resynthesized, thereby providing an available intracellular iron pool. Equilibration between serum ferritin and tissue ferritin occurs, and thus serum ferritin is used as an index of body iron stores; 1 μg ferritin/L serum = 10 mg iron stores [16]. Normal serum ferritin concentrations exceed 12 μg/L for adult females and 15 μg/L for adult males.

Hemosiderin is another iron-storage protein. Hemosiderin is thought to be a degradation product of ferritin, representing, for example, aggregated ferritin or a deposit of degraded apoferritin and coalesced iron atoms. The content of iron in hemosiderin may be as high as 50%. The ratio of ferritin to hemosiderin in the liver varies according to the level of iron stored in the organ, with ferritin predominating at lower iron concentrations and hemosiderin at higher concentrations (iron overload) [2,17]. Although iron in hemosiderin can be labilized to supply free iron, the rate at which iron is released is slower than that from ferritin.

Release of iron from stores (Fig. 12.4) requires reducing substances such as riboflavin (FMNH$_2$), niacin (NADH), and/or vitamin C. Oxidation of iron to enable binding to transferrin for transport to tissues requires ceruloplasmin (Fig. 12.4). The amount of iron taken up by the tissues is dependent on the degree of saturation of the transferrin, with the rate of iron delivery being greater from diferric transferrin than from monoferric transferrin [15].

Uptake of iron by tissues involves the binding of the transferrin to receptors on cells. The complex is thought to be internalized by endocytosis and to form a vesicle in the cytoplasm of the cell. Lysosomal enzymes release the ferric iron and apotransferrin, which is thought to return to the cell surface and plasma [15]. The ferric iron is re-

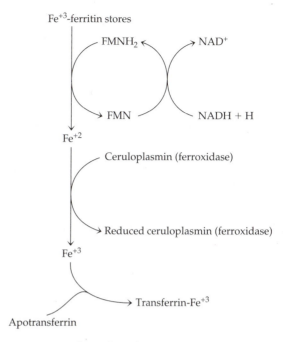

FIGURE 12.4 Release of iron from stores.

duced and transported out of the vesicle and into the cytoplasm of the cell for use. The number of transferrin receptors on cells increases or decreases depending on intracellular iron concentrations. In other words, intracellular iron affects the genetic expression of transferrin receptors on the cell.

Functions

The essentiality of iron is due, in part, to its presence in heme. The atom of iron in the center of the heme molecule allows the transport of oxygen to tissues (hemoglobin); the transitional storage of oxygen in tissues, particularly cardiac muscle (myoglobin); and the transport of electrons through the respiratory chain (cytochromes).

The iron atom in the center of heme is highly reactive and allows the formation of coordinate bonds with six other atoms [18]. In heme, iron forms four bonds with the nitrogen atoms of the four pyrrole rings (Fig. 12.5); these bonds hold the iron atom in the plane of the porphyrin ring. The other coordinate bonds of iron are with atoms of amino acid groups in the protein with which the heme group is associated. However, in heme proteins that bind oxygen—namely, hemoglobin, myoglobin, and cytochrome a−a$_3$ (the last enzyme, which also requires copper, in the electron transport chain)—only one coordinate bond exists between the iron and the protein, so that the sixth coordinate bond is formed

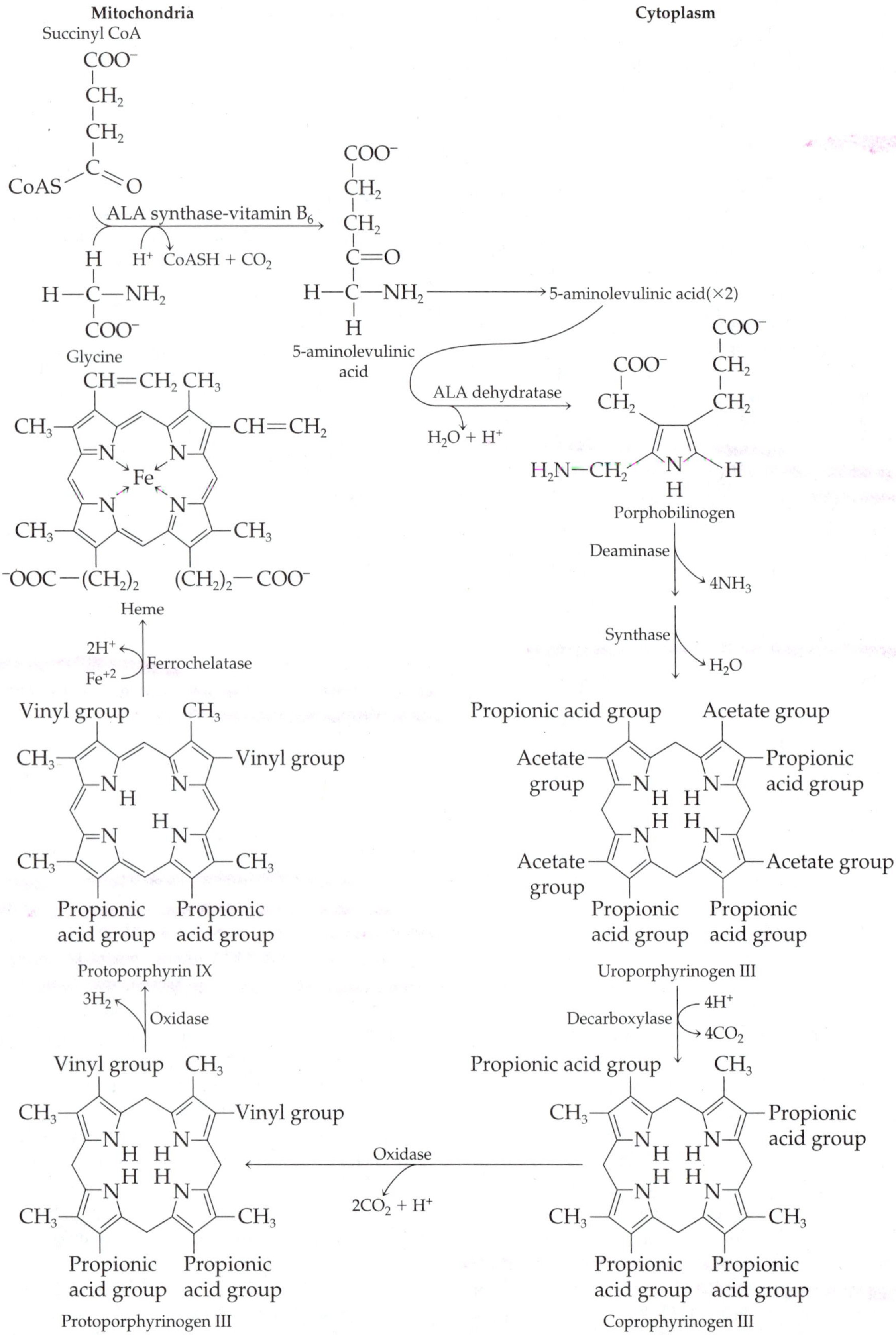

Mitochondria

Succinyl CoA

$$COO^-$$
$$|$$
$$CH_2$$
$$|$$
$$CH_2$$
$$|$$
$$CoAS \overset{\displaystyle C}{\underset{}{\diagdown}} O$$

ALA synthase-vitamin B_6 ⟶

H^+ $CoASH + CO_2$

$$H$$
$$|$$
$$H-C-NH_2$$
$$|$$
$$COO^-$$

Glycine

Cytoplasm

$$COO^-$$
$$|$$
$$CH_2$$
$$|$$
$$CH_2$$
$$|$$
$$C=O$$
$$|$$
$$H-C-NH_2$$
$$|$$
$$H$$

5-aminolevulinic acid ⟶ 5-aminolevulinic acid (×2)

ALA dehydratase

$H_2O + H^+$

Porphobilinogen

Deaminase

$4NH_3$

Synthase

H_2O

Uroporphyrinogen III

Decarboxylase

$4H^+$
$4CO_2$

Coprophyrinogen III

Oxidase

$2CO_2 + H^+$

Heme

$2H^+$
Fe^{+2} Ferrochelatase

Protoporphyrin IX

$3H_2$ Oxidase

Protoporphyrinogen III

FIGURE 12.5 Heme biosynthesis. [Vinyl group: $CH=CH_2$; propionic acid group: $(CH_2)_2COO^-$; acetate group: CH_2COO^-]

with oxygen [18]. The oxygen is held quite loosely so that transfer can be rapid.

The synthesis of heme (Fig. 12.5) and attachment of globin occurs in the bone marrow. Erythropoietic cells possess transferrin receptors on their cell surface. Transferrin delivers the iron for heme synthesis to the erythropoietic cells in the bone marrow. Heme synthesis begins in the mitochondria where glycine and succinyl CoA combine to form δ-aminolevulinic acid (ALA). The reaction is catalyzed by δ-aminolevulinic acid synthase, a vitamin B_6-dependent enzyme that is inhibited by the final end product heme. ALA enters the cytoplasm where a zinc-dependent dehydratase catalyzes the condensation of two ALA molecules to form porphobilinogen. This enzyme is sensitive to lead, which binds to its sulfhydryl groups to inactivate the enzyme. Next, in a series of reactions involving a deaminase, a synthase, and a decarboxylase, four porphobilinogens condense to form a tetrapyrrole that cyclizes. Side chains are modified, and coproporphyrinogen III is formed. This compound then enters the mitochondria and is converted into protoporphyrinogen III. Protoporphyrinogen III is oxidized to form protoporphyrin IX. Lastly, an iron (Fe^{+2}) atom is inserted by ferrochelatase to yield heme.

Other heme-containing cytochromes in the electron transport chain (Fig. 3.12), such as cytochromes b and c, pass along single electrons rather than oxygen. The transfer of electrons along the chain is made possible by the change in the oxidation state of iron. In the reduced cytochromes, the iron atom is in the ferrous state. The iron atom of the reduced cytochrome becomes oxidized to the ferric state when a single electron is transferred to the next cytochrome. The iron atom of the cytochrome receiving the electron becomes reduced. Other iron-containing cytochromes include cytochrome b_5 (involved in lipid metabolism) and cytochrome P_{450} (involved in drug metabolism).

Nonheme iron sulfur enzymes involved in electron transport include NADH dehydrogenase, succinate dehydrogenase, and ubiquinone-cytochrome c reductase. Whether iron is carrying oxygen or transporting electrons, its essentiality in energy transformation is without question.

Other body enzymes involved in a variety of processes, besides the respiratory chain, also require iron. Peroxidase, myeloperoxidase, and catalase contain heme iron. Catalase, with four heme groups, converts hydrogen peroxide to water and molecular oxygen; this enzyme helps prevent cellular damage by hydrogen peroxide (see "Perspective" section in Chapter 10). Myeloperoxidase is found in granules within neutrophils, and aids immune system function. During phagocytosis of bacteria, myeloperoxidase is released into the phagocytic vesicle within the neutrophil. The phagocytic vesicle contains a variety of compounds including hydrogen peroxide (H_2O_2), free hydroxy radicals (OH⁻), and other ions such as chloride (Cl⁻). Myeloperoxidase catalyzes the following reaction:

$$H_2O_2 + Cl^- \longrightarrow H_2O + HOCl$$

The HOCl (hypochlorate) formed in the reaction is a strong toxic oxidant that is important for the destruction of foreign substances such as bacteria. Activity of myeloperoxidase may be impaired with iron deficiency with a resulting increased susceptibility or severity of infection.

Tryptophan dioxygenase (also called a *pyrrolase* and a heme-containing enzyme) converts tryptophan to N-formylkynurenine (Fig. 9.18, p. 249). Iron deficiency has been shown to reduce the efficacy of tryptophan as a precursor of niacin [19]. Phenylalanine hydroxylase (also called *oxygenase*) contains one to two iron atoms, and converts phenylalanine to tyrosine; vitamin C also is involved in this reaction (see Fig. 9.7, p. 231). In tyrosine catabolism, homogentisate oxidase, which converts homogentisate to maleylacetoacetate (p. 231), requires iron (Fig. 9.7). Xanthine dehydrogenase and xanthine oxidase, both nonheme iron- and molybdenum-containing enzymes, convert hypoxanthine to xanthine and then xanthine to uric acid (Fig. 7.11, p. 170). Glycerol phosphate dehydrogenase, a flavoprotein, has a nonheme iron component (p. 87). In the Krebs cycle, aconitase, which converts citrate to isocitrate (p. 90), requires one to two nonheme iron atoms. Phosphoenolpyruvate carboxykinase, important in gluconeogenesis, also requires iron for function. Ribonucleotide reductase (nonheme iron-dependent) converts adenosine diphosphate (ADP) into deoxy ADP (dADP). This reaction is crucial for DNA synthesis and thus cell replication. Iron is also required by two enzymes involved in the synthesis of carnitine (Fig. 9.6, p. 230), which is required for transport of long-chain fatty acids into the mitochondria for oxidation.

Interactions with Other Nutrients

The interactions of iron with *ascorbic acid* in relation to enhancing iron absorption and to maintaining iron in the appropriate valence state for enzyme function have been discussed previously (p. 356 and 359). As shown in Figure 12.4, an interrelationship also exists between iron and *copper* because of the role of the copper-containing ceruloplasmin as a ferroxidase.

Another nutrient with which iron appears to interact is *zinc*. A molar ratio of nonheme iron (ferrous sulfate) to zinc of 25:1 diminished the absorption of zinc from water to 34% in humans; however, when the same ratio of iron to zinc was given with a meal, no inhibitory effects were demonstrated [20]. Ratios of nonheme iron to zinc of 2:1 and 3:1 have also been shown to inhibit zinc absorption, while similar ratios of heme iron to zinc had no effect on zinc absorption [21]. Thus, excessive intake of nonheme iron, as may occur with supplements, may have a detrimental effect on zinc absorption.

Another association is that between *vitamin A* and iron. Iron appears to accumulate in the liver and spleen with a vitamin A deficiency, and iron deficiency anemia appears as evidenced by low hemoglobin and hematocrit indices [22].

Iron and *lead* also interact. Lead inhibits the activity of δ-aminolevulinic acid dehydratase, an enzyme required in heme synthesis (Fig. 12.5). In addition, increased absorption of lead occurs with iron deficiency, especially in children [1].

Interactions between iron and *nickel* are discussed on page 405.

Excretion

Despite the importance of dietary iron in maintaining the long-term adequacy of body iron, the amount of iron absorbed cannot provide the concentration of iron needed were it not for the avid conservation and constant recycling of body iron. The daily enteric absorption of iron amounts to only about 0.06% of the total body iron content or up to about 4 mg per day. Absorption will, however, increase or decrease according to need.

Most of the iron entering the plasma for distribution by transferrin is contributed by sites of hemoglobin destruction (phagocytes such as macrophages of the reticuloendothelial system) and sites of stored iron (ferritin and hemosiderin). The majority of old red blood cells are taken up by macrophages in the spleen and degraded; however, a small amount of red blood cell lysis occurs within the blood. The free hemoglobin and any free heme released in the blood following cell lysis are quickly bound to two proteins, haptoglobin and hemopexin, respectively. These proteins (synthesized by the liver) form complexes with the hemoglobin and heme, and deliver the compounds to the liver. The iron from degraded hemoglobin in red blood cells is reused for erythropoiesis. Red blood cells live for about 120 days and are then trapped and phagocytosed by the reticuloendothelial cells primarily in the spleen. The normal adult releases about 20 to 25 mg iron per day from the catabolism of hemoglobin. The heme portion of the molecule is catabolized by heme oxygenase to biliverdin and subsequently to bilirubin, which is then secreted into the bile for excretion from the body [2].

Unless body stores are exhausted, the supply of iron to the plasma pool can be adjusted within wide limits. The requirement for transferrin iron is determined by the needs of the bone marrow for red blood cell synthesis. Therefore, with chronic hemolysis the quantity of iron passing through the plasma can expand six to eight times normal. In contrast, when erythropoiesis declines dramatically, as occurs on descent from high altitudes, the quantity of iron in the plasma pool may decrease to as little as one-third of normal [15]. Figure 12.6 represents schematically the internal iron exchange in the body.

The external iron exchange (or iron balance) is depicted in Figure 12.2. In the normal adult male, daily iron losses are approximately between 0.9 and 1.0 mg/day (12 to 14 μg/kg/day). Most of these losses are via the gastrointestinal tract (0.6 mg), with about 0.45 mg due to minute (~1 mL) blood loss (which occurs even in healthy people) [2,15] and another 0.15 mg iron due to losses in bile and desquamated mucosal cells. About 0.2 to 0.3 mg iron is lost by desquamation of surface cells from the skin, and a very small amount, about 0.1 mg, is lost in the urine [2,15]. Losses of iron may increase in people with gastrointestinal ulcers or intestinal parasites, or with hemorrhage induced by surgery or due to injury.

Basal iron losses as just described are a bit less in women because of their smaller surface area; total basal losses approach 0.7 to 0.8 mg/day. Total losses of premenopausal women, however, are estimated at about 1.3 to 1.4 mg/day because of iron loss in menses [3]. The average loss of blood during a menstrual cycle is about 35 mL, with an upper limit of about 80 mL. The iron content of blood is about 0.5 mg per 100 mL of blood, which translates into a loss of about 17.5 mg of iron per period. When averaged out over a month, iron loss in menses is about 0.5 mg per day [12]; in some women, however, iron loss due to menses alone may exceed 1.4 mg/day [12]. The increased excretion of iron in healthy people with excessive intakes is due to the above-average concentration of iron in the ferritin of desquamated mucosal cells.

Balancing iron uptake with its loss from the body is very important to health. The high incidence of iron deficiency anemia, the most common nutrition deficiency in humans in the world [23], attests to the fact that iron equilibrium often has not been attained, particularly in many young children, girls, and women of childbearing age.

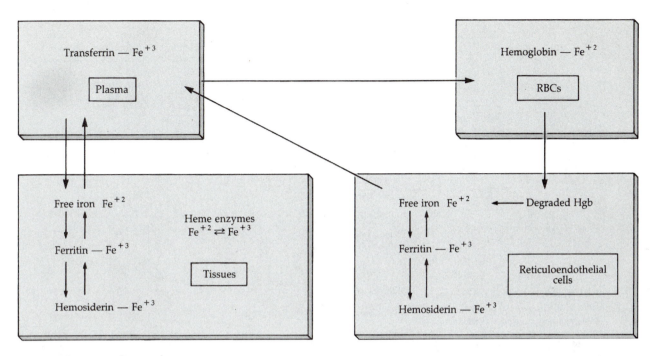

FIGURE 12.6 Internal iron exchange.

Recommended Dietary Allowances

Basal iron losses, which average 0.7 to 1.0 mg/day by the adult male and postmenopausal female plus increased needs for selected populations with increased iron losses, have been considered in formulating the RDA. Assuming an iron absorption of 10%, 10 mg iron (the 1980 and 1989 RDA) for males and postmenopausal females was thought to be adequate [8]. Because of menstrual losses, the 1980 RDA for women during childbearing years was set at 18 mg/day [8].

The subcommittee on the tenth edition of the RDA examined additional survey data that indicated the adequacy of an iron intake of 14 mg/day for approximately 95% of all menstruating women [12]. The RDA for iron for childbearing women was lowered to 15 mg/day, while the RDA for iron for men and postmenopausal women was not changed from the 10 mg recommended in 1980 [12]. Due to the absence of menstruation during pregnancy and the increased or more efficient iron absorption that also occurs with pregnancy, the 1989 RDA suggests 30 mg iron/day for pregnant women [12]. Because 30 mg iron is more than can be normally obtained from the diet, supplements are usually needed.

Because no evidence of iron deficiency exists with iron stores of 300 mg and because absorption increases whenever iron stores are depleted, the 1980–1985 Committee on Recommended Dietary Allowances [7] set the RDI for iron at 15 mg/day, a level that would maintain stores of 300 mg.

Deficiency—Iron Deficiency With and Without Anemia

Iron intake is frequently inadequate in four population groups [7,8,12]: (1) infants and young children (6 months to 4 years) because of the low iron content of milk and other preferred food, rapid growth rate, and body reserves of iron insufficient to meet needs beyond 6 months; (2) adolescents in their early growth spurt because of rapid growth and needs of expanding red cell mass; (3) females during childbearing years because of menstrual iron losses; and (4) pregnant women because of their expanding blood volume, demands of fetus and placenta, plus blood losses to be incurred in childbirth. In addition, many nonpregnant females during childbearing years are falling short of the RDA for iron because their caloric intake is often restricted and because only 5 to 7 mg iron can be expected per 1,000 kcal from an average Western diet [2]. Other conditions and populations associated with increased need for intake due to iron losses or impaired absorption are hemorrhage, protein calorie malnutrition, renal disease, achlorhydria, prolonged use of alkaline-based drugs such as antacids, decreased gastrointestinal transit time, steatorrhea, and parasites.

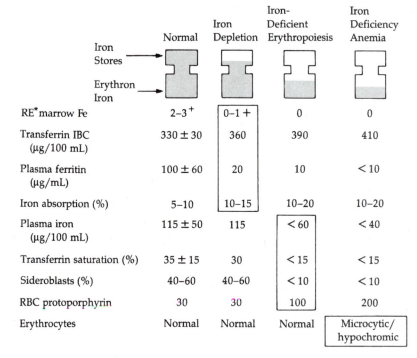

	Normal	Iron Depletion	Iron-Deficient Erythropoiesis	Iron Deficiency Anemia
RE* marrow Fe	2-3+	0-1+	0	0
Transferrin IBC (µg/100 mL)	330 ± 30	360	390	410
Plasma ferritin (µg/mL)	100 ± 60	20	10	< 10
Iron absorption (%)	5-10	10-15	10-20	10-20
Plasma iron (µg/100 mL)	115 ± 50	115	< 60	< 40
Transferrin saturation (%)	35 ± 15	30	< 15	< 15
Sideroblasts (%)	40-60	40-60	< 10	< 10
RBC protoporphyrin	30	30	100	200
Erythrocytes	Normal	Normal	Normal	Microcytic/hypochromic

*RE = reticuloendothelial

FIGURE 12.7 Sequence of changes induced by gradual depletion of iron content of body. *(From Victor Herbert, "Recommended Dietary Intakes (RDI) of Iron in Humans," Am J Clin Nutr 1987, 45:679–686. © Am J Clin Nutr, American Society for Clinical Nutrition.)*

Figure 12.7 depicts the gradual depletion of iron content in the body and demonstrates the fact that anemia does not occur until iron depletion is severe. Iron deficiency without anemia, however, can occur. Symptoms of iron deficiency, mostly demonstrated in children, include pallor, listlessness, behavioral disturbances, impaired performance in some cognitive tasks, some irreversible impairment of learning ability, and short attention span [1,23]. Iron deficiency may impair degradation of γ-amino butyric acid (GABA, an inhibitory neurotransmitter in the brain, p. 183), or may inhibit dopamine producing neurons [23]. Possible impairment of the immune system, decreased resistance to infection and impaired capacity to maintain body temperature have also been shown [1,23,24].

Further discussion of iron deficiency with and without anemia as it relates to changes that occur in indices of iron status are discussed under the section "Assessment of Nutriture."

Toxicity—Hemosiderosis and Hemochromatosis

The term *hemochromatosis* is used to indicate iron overload or toxicity, which is coupled with tissue damage, whereas *hemosiderosis* is the traditional term indicating iron overload without tissue damage [2]. The incidence of iron overload and/or toxicity is not as prevalent in the United States as is iron deficiency, but the consequences can be severe.

Accidental iron overload has been observed in young children following excessive ingestion of iron pills or vitamin and mineral pills. Other people susceptible to iron overload possess the genetically (autosomal recessive) transmitted idiopathic hemochromatotic trait. In the United States it is estimated that about two or three people per 10,000 (or 0.3 to 0.5% of Caucasians) are homozygous for the trait [25,26], while 8 to 15% of Caucasians are heterozygous [26]. Hemochromatosis is most often seen in adult Caucasian males and begins to occur around 20 years of age. The condition is characterized by increased (at least two times normal) iron absorption with deposition of iron as hemosiderin in the parenchymal cells of the liver and other organs, causing damage to the tissues. Heterozygotes for the condition do not develop abnormalities of the liver and heart, but show abnormal iron status [26]. Before the development of a screening test [25], no method existed for identifying people with iron overload until pathologic changes (primarily cirrhosis) occurred at around age 50 years [27]. Treatment of the condition usually involves frequent phlebotomy (removal of blood), and may require administration of deferroxamine, which can chelate iron and increase urinary iron excretion.

Other people who are at particularly high risk for iron overload are those with iron-loading anemias, thalassemia, and sideroblastic anemia. The elevated erythropoiesis in people so affected causes an increased absorption of iron.

Assessment of Nutriture

Numerous measurements are used for the assessment of iron nutriture. The most common indices are hemoglobin and hematocrit. Also used is the characterization of red blood cells as to size and amount of hemoglobin in them. Of the three measurements—mean corpuscular volume (MCV), mean corpuscular hemoglobin (MCH), and mean corpuscular hemoglobin concentration (MCHC)—used to characterize red blood cells, MCV is the most popular and is used often in analysis of large-survey data. Table 12.4a gives the marginal range of hemoglobin and hematocrit levels, and Table 12.4b illustrates the derivation of normal values for MCV, MCH, and MCHC.

The measurements listed in Table 12.4a and b are helpful in identifying severe iron deficiency anemia but may be much less useful in the diagnosis of mild iron deficiency anemia or iron deficiency without anemia. In these conditions, evaluation of iron stores is much more

valuable, because iron deficiency occurs in three stages, beginning with depletion of iron stores.

In the first stages of iron deficiency, iron stores are diminished. Iron stores may be evaluated by the measurement of plasma ferritin; plasma ferritin levels associated with iron deficiency are shown in Figure 12.7. Typically in the second stage of iron deficiency not only will plasma ferritin concentrations be diminished, but also transferrin saturation. The free protoporphyrin concentration in the erythrocyte will rise (protoporphyrin accumulates within red blood cells when iron is not available). Transferrin is normally one-third saturated with ferric iron; however, with iron deficiency, transferrin saturation diminishes to less than 15% as shown in Figure 12.7. Transferrin saturation can be calculated by multiplying the serum iron concentration by 100 and then dividing by the total iron-binding capacity (TIBC). TIBC represents the amount of iron that plasma transferrin can bind; TIBC ranges from about 250 to 450 μg/dL. The amount of iron bound to the transferrin is measured as serum iron with normal values ranging from 60 to 175 μg/dL.

In the final stages of iron deficiency, anemia occurs. Serum ferritin and transferrin saturation remain depressed, free protoporphyrin remains elevated. Serum iron is diminished, TIBC is elevated, and hemoglobin,

TABLE 12.4 Common Measurements of Iron Status

A. Marginal hemoglobin and hematocrit values[a]

Age	Hemoglobin g/dL	Age	Hematocrit (% packed cell volume)
6–23 mo	9.0–9.9	Up to 2 yr	28–30
2–5 yr	10.0–10.9	2–5 yr	30–33
6–12 yr	10.0–11.4	6–12 yr	30–35
13–16 yr (M)	12.0–12.9	13–16 yr (M)	37–39
13–16 (F)	10.0–11.4	13–16 yr (F)	31–35
16+ yr (M)	12.0–13.9	16+ yr (M)	37–43
16+ yr (F)	10.0–11.9	16+ yr (F)	31–37
Pregnant		*Pregnant*	
Second trimester	9.5–10.9	Second trimester	30–35
Third trimester	9.0–10.5	Third trimester	30–33

B. Normal range of calculated values for RBCs (MCV, MCH, and MCHC)

$$MCV = \frac{\text{hematocrit in mL/100 mL}}{\text{RBCs in millions/μL}} \times 10 = 80 \text{ to } 90 \text{ μ}^3$$

$$MCH = \frac{\text{hemoglobin in g/100 mL}}{\text{RBCs in millions/mm}^3} \times 10 = 27 \text{ to } 32 \text{ pg (picograms)}$$

$$MCHC = \frac{\text{hemoglobin in g/100 mL}}{\text{hematocrit in mL/100 mL}} \times 100 = 33\% \text{ to } 38\%$$

[a]Anywhere below lower-range figure indicates deficiency, while value exceeding upper-range figure denotes acceptable level.

hematocrit, MCH, MCHC, and MCV are lower than normal. Red blood cells are pale (hypochromic) and small (microcytosis). Figure 12.7 illustrates the changes that occur in these various measurements.

With the increasing awareness of the inverse relationship between iron status and capacity to do work or exercise as well as scholastic achievement and behavior in children [1,24], perhaps more effort will be directed toward identification of people at risk for iron deficiency and then toward prevention of the deficiency.

References Cited for Iron

1. Dall PR. Iron. In: Brown ML., ed. Present knowledge in nutrition, 6th ed. Washington, DC: International Life Sciences Institute Nutrition Foundation, 1990:241–250.
2. Fairbanks VF. Iron in medicine and nutrition. In: Shils ME, Olson JA, Shike M., eds. Modern nutrition in health and disease, 8th ed. Philadelphia: Lea and Febiger, 1994;185–213.
3. Monsen, ER. Iron nutrition and absorption: Dietary factors which impact iron bioavailability. J Am Diet Assoc 1988;88:786–790.
4. Hurrell RF, Lynch SR, Trinidad TP, Dassenko SA, Cook JD. Iron absorption in humans: Bovine serum albumin compared with beef muscle and egg white. Am J Clin Nutr 1988;47:102–107.
5. Taylor PG, Martinez-Torres C, Romano EL, Layrisse M. The effect of cysteine-containing peptides released during meat digestion on iron absorption in humans. Am J Clin Nutr 1986;43:68–71.
6. MacPhail AP, Ratel RC, Bothwell TH, Lamparelli RD. EDTA and the absorption of iron from food. Am J Clin Nutr 1994;59:644–648.
7. Herbert V. Recommended dietary intakes (RDI) of iron in humans. Am J Clin Nutr 1987;45:679–686.
8. National Research Council. Recommended dietary allowances, 9th ed. Washington, DC: National Academy of Sciences 1980:137–144.
9. Monsen ER, Balintfy JL. Calculating dietary iron bioavailability: Refinement and computerization. J Am Diet Assoc 1982;80:307–311.
10. Finch CA, Cook JD. Iron deficiency. Am J Clin Nutr 1984;39:471–477.
11. Hallberg L, Rossander L, Skanberg A-B. Phytates and the inhibitory effect of bran on iron absorption in man. Am J Clin Nutr 1987;45:988–996.
12. National Research Council. Recommended dietary allowances, 10th ed. Washington, DC: National Academy Press, 1989:195–205.
13. Cook JD, Dassenko SA, Whittaker P. Calcium supplementation: effect on iron absorption. Am J Clin Nutr 1991;53:106–111.
14. Hallberg L, Brune M, Erlandsson M, Sandberg A-S, Rossander-Hulten L. Calcium: Effect of different amounts on nonheme- and heme-iron absorption in humans. Am J Clin Nutr 1991;53:112–119.
15. Bothwell TH, Charlton RW, Motulsky AG. Idiopathic hemochromatosis. In: Stanbury JB, Wyngaarden JB, Fredrickson DS, Goldstein JL, Brown MS, eds. The metabolic basis of inherited disease, 5th ed. New York: McGraw-Hill 1983; 1269–1298.
16. Cook JD, Skikne BS. Serum ferritin: A possible model for the assessment of nutrient stores. Am J Clin Nutr 1982;35:1180–1185.
17. Finch CA, Huebers H. Perspectives in iron metabolism. N Engl J Med 1982;306:1520–1528.
18. Newsholme EA, Leech AR. Biochemistry for the medical sciences. New York: Wiley, 1983.
19. Uduho GW, Han Y, Baker DH. Iron deficiency reduces the efficacy of tryptophan as a niacin precursor. J Nutr 1994;124:444–450.
20. Sandstrom B, Davidsson L, Cederblad A, Lonnerdal B. Oral iron, dietary ligands and zinc absorption. J Nutr 1985;115:411–414.
21. Solomons NW, Jacob RA. Studies on the bioavailability of zinc in humans: Effects of heme and nonheme iron on the absorption of zinc. Am J Clin Nutr 1981;34:475–482.
22. Houwelingen FV, Van Den Berg GJ, Lemmens AG, Sijtsma KW, Beynen AC. Iron and zinc status in rats with diet-induced marginal deficiency of vitamin A and/or copper. Biol Trace Elem Res 1993;38:83–95.
23. Scrimshaw NS. Iron deficiency. Scientific Am 1991;265:46–52.
24. Beard JL. Iron fortification—rationale and effects. Nutr Today 1986;21:17–20.
25. Skikne, BS, Cook JD. Screening test for iron overload. Am J Clin Nutr 1987;46:840–843.
26. Johnson MA. Iron: Nutrition monitoring and nutrition status assessment. J Nutr 1990;120:1486–1491.
27. Finch CA. The detection of iron overload. N Engl J Med 1982; 307:1702–1703.

Additional Reference

Beard JL, Connor JR, Jones BC. Iron in the brain. Nutr Rev 1993;51:157–170.

ZINC

Although the essentiality of zinc in mammalian nutrition was established in 1934, an appreciation for this mineral in human nutrition has developed only during the last 20 to 25 years. Human zinc deficiency was first noted in the early 1960s, but the affected population was adolescents living in the Nile delta of Egypt and in rural Iran, where the diet was composed primarily of cereals and cereal products [1,2]. A 1972 report of marginal zinc deficiency among middle-class children in Denver was a major stimulus for scrutiny of human zinc nutrition in the

TABLE 12.5 Zinc Content of Selected Foods

Food Group (serving)	Food	Zinc (mg)
Seafood (3 oz)	Oysters	8.0
	Crabmeat	3.8
	Shrimp	1.8
	Tuna	0.8
Meat and poultry (3 oz)	Beef liver	4.3
	Chicken, dark meat	2.4
	Ground beef	3.8
	Ham	3.4
	Pork loin	2.6
Eggs and dairy products (2)	Eggs	1.0
(1c)	Milk, low fat	0.9
(1 oz)	Cheddar cheese	0.5
(½ c)	Cottage cheese	0.4
Legumes (½ c)	Black-eyed peas	1.5
(½ c)	Cooked, dried beans	0.9
(2 tbsp)	Peanut butter	1.0
Grains and cereals (1 c)	Oatmeal, cooked	1.2
(1 slice)	Whole-wheat bread	0.5
(1 slice)	White wheat bread	0.2
Fruits and vegetables (1 small = 100g)	Potato, baked	0.6
(½ c)	Broccoli, cooked	0.15
(½ c)	Squash, zucchini, cooked	0.18
(⅔ c)	Strawberries	0.08

Sources: Adapted/Reprinted with permission from Wagner PA. Zinc nutrition in elderly. Geriatrics 1985;40:111–125. Copyright by Advanstar Communications, Inc. Printed in U.S.A.; and Freeland JH, Cousins RJ. Zinc content of selected foods. © The American Dietetic Association. Reprinted by permission from Journal of the American Dietetic Association Vol. 68 (1976), pp. 527–528.

United States [3]. In the 1974 edition of the Recommended Dietary Allowances (RDA), an allowance for zinc appeared for the first time.

Zinc can exist in several different valence states, but it is almost universally found as the divalent ion (Zn^{+2}). The estimated content of zinc in the adult human body ranges from 1.5 to 2.5 g [1]. Zinc is found in all organs and tissues (primarily intracellularly) and in body fluids. Most of the zinc in humans is found in bone, liver, kidney, muscle, and skin [1].

Sources

Zinc is typically associated with the protein fraction and or nucleic acid fraction of food. Zinc forms complexes with amino acids, peptides, proteins, and nucleic acids [1]. The zinc content of foods varies widely (Table 12.5). Very good sources of zinc are red meats (especially organ meats) and seafood (especially oysters and mollusks). Other good sources of zinc include poultry, pork, dairy products, whole grains (especially bran and germ), and vegetables (leafy and root). Poor zinc sources are fruits and refined cereals.

Processing of certain foods may affect the amount of their zinc content that is available for absorption. Heat treatment can cause food zinc to form complexes that are resistant to hydrolysis, and therefore make zinc unavailable for absorption. Maillard reaction products (amino acid–carbohydrate complexes resulting from browning) are particularly notable for their trapping of zinc [1].

Absorption and Transport

Zinc available for absorption and transport comes not only from dietary sources, but also from pancreatic and biliary secretions into the gastrointestinal tract. Most zinc is absorbed in the proximal small intestine. Although the jejunum is thought to contribute most significantly to zinc absorption [1], the relative contribution of the duodenum, jejunum, and ileum toward overall zinc absorption has not been demonstrated [2]. Zinc is thought to be absorbed into the enterocyte by a carrier-mediated process that may [2] or may not require energy (Fig. 12.8) [1,4]. Low intakes of dietary zinc are absorbed more efficiently than higher intakes and thereby suggest carrier involvement [1,4,5]. However, no receptor sites in the enterocytes for zinc have been identified [1]. Uptake of zinc is enhanced with low zinc status, suggesting that the total amount of zinc absorbed is homeostatically regulated. Exactly how zinc status regulates absorption

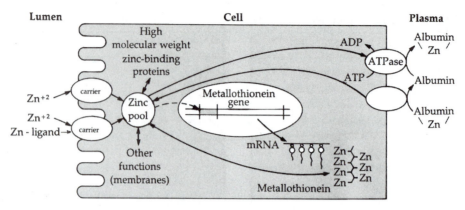

FIGURE 12.8 Schematic representation of zinc absorption by enterocytes. Carrier-mediated transport at the brush border is shown. Interaction of zinc with intracellular macromolecules is indicated as is the effect of zinc pool size on thionein polypeptide synthesis and the formation of metallothionein. Active transport of zinc through the basolateral membrane is shown as is the transfer of cellular zinc to and from its carrier albumin in the plasma. *(Modified from Zinc. In: Solomons NW, Rosenberg, JH, eds. Absorption and malabsorption of mineral nutrients. New York: Liss, 1984:152.)*

of the mineral is unclear [1]. At higher zinc intakes, non-saturable diffusion or paracellular absorption is thought to contribute to zinc absorption [1]; diffusion is not affected by zinc deficiency.

The bioavailability of zinc from foods and food combinations can differ tremendously. Various dietary substances that affect zinc bioavailability appear to form chelates with the mineral. Whether these substances are enhancers or inhibitors depends on the digestibility and absorbability of the zinc chelates formed. Studies have shown that zinc consumed with beverages, certain foods, or meals can vary in absorption from 12 to 59% [2]; a value of 20% was chosen in setting the 1989 RDA [2].

The mechanism of zinc absorption is poorly understood. Zinc is believed to be liberated from food during the digestive process. Whether the freed zinc moves across the brush border as an ion or in a chelated complex is uncertain [4]. The preponderance of evidence supports absorption of zinc as a complex with ligands derived from both exogenous and endogenous sources [1,4]. Possible endogenous ligands are citric acid and picolinic acid [2,4], the latter of which is a metabolite of the tryptophan to niacin pathway (p. 249) as well as prostaglandins [2,4]. Histidine [6], cysteine, and possibly other amino acids (lysine and glycine) or glutathione (a tripeptide composed of cysteine, glutamate, and glycine) may serve as ligands and have been shown to enhance the absorption of zinc especially in the presence of inhibitors such as iron [1,4,7].

Zinc from meat is much more readily absorbed than that from plant sources. Moreover, about 70% of zinc consumed by most people in the United States is provided by animal products such as meat [5]. Enhanced

bioavailability of zinc from animal tissue is believed to be due to the interaction between zinc and products of protein digestion (that is, amino acids such as histidine) [8]. It is postulated that histidine, and the other amino acids listed earlier, form a ligand with zinc that is readily absorbed [4,6,7]. Pancreatic secretions are also thought to contain an unidentified constituent that enhances zinc absorption [2].

Chief among the inhibitors of zinc bioavailability is phytate (inositol hexaphosphate) contributed by plant foods, particularly cereals such as maize and bran, and legumes. Fermentation of bread, however, reduces the phytate content and improves zinc absorption. Phytate alone, however, seems to have little adverse effect on the bioavailability of zinc even at a phytate–zinc ratio of 10:1 [9]. It is in the presence of a high intraluminal calcium that phytate exerts its inhibitory effect on zinc, and this inhibition may occur at phytate–zinc ratios much lower than 10 [9,10]. Orthophosphate, in contrast to polyphosphates, does not appear to inhibit zinc absorption [5]. Because of the high phytate content of legumes, much research has been devoted to the bioavailability of zinc from soy products. Large variation in zinc bioavailability, primarily related to pH, has been demonstrated in soy isolates and concentrates [10]. Decreased zinc absorption from products with a neutral pH is thought to be due to formation of poorly digested protein-phytate-mineral complexes [10].

Other substances shown to inhibit zinc absorption include oxalic acid (in spinach, chard, berries, chocolate, tea, among others), polyphenols such as tannins (in tea), and fiber. Interactions also exist between zinc and the vitamin folic acid and between zinc and a variety of divalent cations (Cd^{+2}, Cu^{+2}, Ca^{+2}, and Fe^{+2}). Cadmium, for example, binds to sites that zinc would normally bind to and disrupts normal zinc functions. Folic acid (350 µg) ingestion for two weeks has been shown to decrease zinc (50 mg) absorption by 21% [11]. The relationship between the divalent cations is very complex, but is probably related to the fact that these cations compete with one another for binding ligands in the intestinal lumen or within the cell, and for receptor sites in the enterocytes.

Ferrous sulfate and zinc sulfate ingested together in a ratio of 2:1 (50 mg:25 mg) and 3:1 (75 mg:25 mg) decreased zinc absorption in humans [12]. Zinc sulfate ingested with heme chloride did not inhibit zinc absorption [12]. Likewise, ingestion of oysters (providing 54 mg zinc) with 100 mg ferrous iron did not inhibit zinc absorption [12]. Iron (100 mg) and folate (350 µg) supplements decreased zinc (25 mg) absorption by 51% in pregnant women [11]. These studies suggest that to maximize zinc absorption from zinc sulfate, the zinc supplement should not be consumed with iron sulfate supplements.

Diminished zinc absorption by calcium has been demonstrated in animals; however, no effects were shown in humans ingesting almost 2 g calcium [13] or 500 mg calcium as calcium carbonate or hydroxyapatite [14]. The effects of calcium on zinc absorption appear to be related more to the combination of calcium and phytate in the diet than to calcium alone.

Evidence for significant interaction between cadmium and dietary zinc is scant [1,15]. Such is not the case, however, for the interaction between zinc and copper. Although copper has the potential for interfering with zinc absorption, this has not been reported. However, zinc supplements can inhibit copper absorption and lead to copper deficiency (see the section on interactions with other nutrients).

Movement of zinc through the enterocyte is not a well-delineated process. As indicated in Figure 12.8, zinc entering the enterocyte contributes to the cellular zinc pool; consequently, its ultimate fate has several possibilities. The zinc may (1) be used within the enterocyte (see the section on functions), (2) pass through the cell and the basolateral membrane into the plasma, a process believed to be energy dependent, or (3) be bound to metallothionein.

Figure 12.8 also demonstrates that a zinc pool expanded by elevated zinc consumption appears to stimulate the synthesis of thionein polypeptides that can complex with zinc to form metallothionein [4]. Metallothionein is viewed as an intracellular binding ligand. The protein has an unusually high content of cysteine (30% cysteine residues). These cysteine residues func-

tion in metal binding. The zinc captured and held as metallothionein in the enterocytes is lost into the lumen with the sloughing of these cells. Reduced zinc absorption is directly correlated with metallothionein formation from orally administered zinc and newly synthesized thionein polypeptides [16]. Gene expression of thionein is induced by diets high in zinc [4].

The zinc actively transported across the basolateral membrane of the enterocyte and into the blood is transported in the blood primarily bound loosely to albumin [1,4]. Other compounds that bind and transport about 15 to 40% of the zinc in the blood include α-2 macroglobulin, transferrin, and immunoglobulin (Ig) G. Two amino acids, histidine and cysteine, also loosely bind 2 to 8% of the zinc to form a ternary (histidine–zinc–cysteine) complex in the blood.

Zinc is complexed and released from its plasma carriers on a continual basis. Some of this released zinc can pass back into the enterocyte and perhaps even through the cell into the intestinal lumen. Zinc passing into portal blood from the intestine is mainly transported by albumin (Fig. 12.8) to the liver where the mineral is initially concentrated. From the liver, zinc is distributed to other tissues. The albumin-bound zinc appears to be that which is most readily taken up by tissues [4], and it is this fraction of plasma zinc that is thought to be important in the regulation of zinc absorption [4].

The mechanism of zinc uptake by tissues is unknown. Multiple passive transport systems have been proposed. Carriers of zinc are not thought to be highly selective. The route of transport may depend in part on the chemical form of zinc presented to the cell [17]. One carrier system is believed to be associated with amino acid use [18]. An increase in amino acid use by tissues leads to an increased uptake of zinc and *vice versa*. Numerous metalloenzymes within the cell require zinc as a component; therefore it is reasonable to assume that enzyme synthesis and zinc uptake are correlated.

No readily available storage form of zinc appears to exist in the body [1]. The zinc content of most soft tissues including muscle, brain, lung, and heart is relatively stable and does not respond (equilibrate with other zinc pools) to changes in dietary zinc intake [2,5]. Bones also release the mineral very slowly and cannot be depended on for a supply of zinc during dietary deprivation. When dietary intake fails to satisfy body needs for zinc, catabolism of the zinc-containing metalloproteins (enzymes) in muscle and other soft tissues is required so that zinc can be redistributed to meet particularly crucial needs for the mineral [1,18]. Liver metallothionein zinc may also be mobilized to provide zinc to other body tissues.

Metallothionein is found in most tissues of the body, including the liver, pancreas, kidney, intestine, and red blood cell. Liver metallothionein-bound zinc diminishes as dietary zinc intake decreases and is thus thought to reflect zinc status or stores. Zinc also appears to affect the gene expression of metallothionein. Lysosomal acid proteases degrade metallothionein to release zinc for use by cells or other tissues. Zinc efflux, however, depends on the glucocorticoid-regulated turnover of the metallothionein [4]. Metallothionein gene expression is also influenced by glucagon and the monokine interleukin 1. Interleukin 1 is synthesized and secreted by monocytes and activated macrophages. This monokine is thought to induce metallothionein gene transcription during infection [19]. During infection, plasma zinc concentrations typically decrease and hepatic zinc concentrations rise; the sequestering of zinc by liver metallothionein in turn prevents bacterial use of zinc for its own replication.

Functions

Zinc as a nutrient has many seemingly divergent functions, probably because of the numerous metalloenzymes of which it is a component. As a component of metalloenzymes, zinc provides structural integrity to the protein and/or participates directly in the reaction at the catalytic site. Zinc is a part of more enzyme systems than the rest of the trace minerals combined, and it affects many fundamental processes of life [1,2]. Enzymes (at least 70 and perhaps over 200) [1,4] from every enzyme class (Table 12.6) have been shown to require zinc. A few of these zinc-dependent enzymes are discussed next.

Carbonic anhydrase, found primarily in the erythrocytes but also the renal tubule, is essential for respiration; it catalyzes the following reaction, thereby allowing rapid disposal of carbon dioxide:

TABLE 12.6 Selected Functions of Zinc

Metalloenzyme roles
  Oxidoreductase
  Hydrolase
  Lyase
  Isomerase
  Transferase
  Ligase
Gene expression
Cell replication
Membrane and cytoskeletal stabilization
Structural role in hormones

$$CO_2 + H_2O \xrightarrow{\text{carbonic anhydrase-Zn}^{+2}}$$

$$H_2CO_3 \xrightarrow{\text{dissociation}} H^+ + HCO_3^-$$

The H^+ dissociated from carbonic acid reduces oxyhemoglobin as oxygen is released to the tissues; the bicarbonate passes into the plasma to participate in buffering reactions. The amount of zinc associated with carbonic anhydrase and carried by the erythrocytes is approximately eight to nine times as much as that distributed to tissues in plasma [4]. Carbonic anhydrase has a very high affinity for the mineral zinc; even with zinc deprivation, catabolism of this enzyme apparently does not occur.

Alkaline phosphatase contains four zinc ions per enzyme molecule. Two of the four are required for enzyme activity. The enzyme lacks substrate specificity, but hydrolyzes monoesters of phosphates from various compounds. Enzyme activity decreases with zinc deficiency [4].

Alcohol dehydrogenase also contains four zinc ions per enzyme molecule, with two of the four being required for catalytic activity and two required for structure and protein conformation. This enzyme is important in the conversion of alcohols to aldehydes such as retinol to retinal, which is needed for the visual cycle and night vision. NADH also participates in the reaction.

Another example of a zinc-dependent enzyme is carboxypeptidase A (Fig. 12.9), an exopeptidase secreted by the pancreas into the duodenum and necessary for the digestion of protein. Zinc is bound tightly to carboxypeptidase A and is essential for enzymatic activity. Carboxypeptidase A activity decreases with zinc deficiency. Also involved in protein catabolism are aminopeptidases that have been shown to contain one zinc atom needed for catalytic activity.

Delta-aminolevulinic acid dehydratase, involved in heme synthesis, is zinc dependent. This thiol (SH)-containing enzyme is made up of eight subunits, each of which binds one zinc atom [20]. Zinc is essential for the maintenance of free thiols in the enzyme. The enzyme catalyzes the condensation of δ-aminolevulinic acid to form porphobilinogen (Fig. 12.5, p. 360).

Superoxide dismutase (SOD) found in the cell cytoplasm requires two atoms each of both zinc and copper for function. This important enzyme catalyzes the removal of superoxide radicals, O_2^-.

$$2O_2^- + 2H^+ \xrightarrow{\text{zinc copper SOD}} H_2O_2 + O_2$$

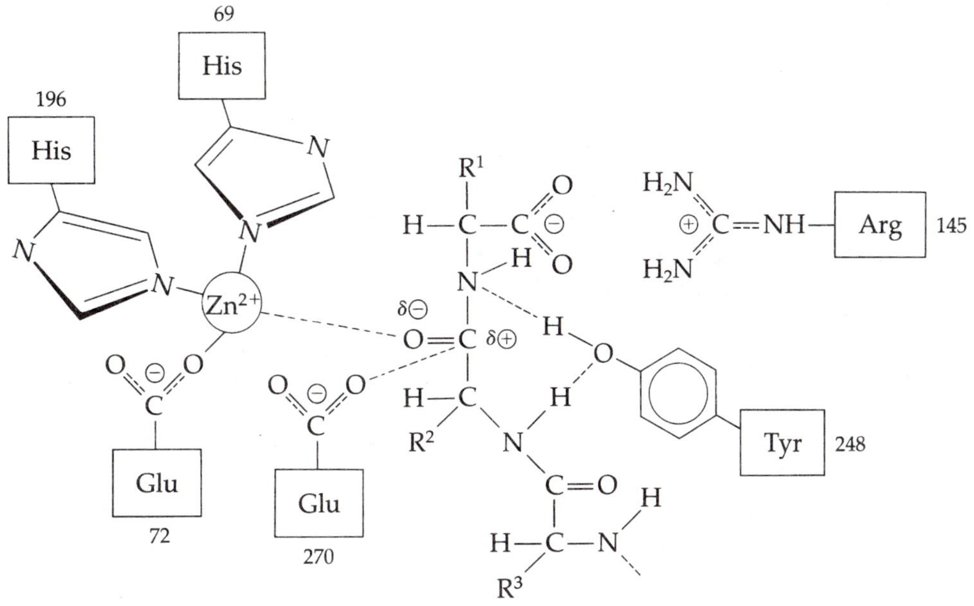

FIGURE 12.9 Partial structure of carboxypeptidase A.

Physiologic functions of zinc include tissue or cell growth, cell replication, bone formation, skin integrity, cell-mediated immunity, and generalized host defense. The role of zinc in tissue growth is related primarily to its function in the regulation of protein synthesis, which includes its influence on polysome conformation as well as the synthesis and catabolism of the nucleic acids. Paramount in nucleic acid synthesis are the zinc metalloenzymes DNA and RNA polymerase and deoxythymidine kinase, the latter being necessary for the conservation or salvaging of thymine, the pyrimidine unique to DNA. Catabolism of RNA appears to be regulated by zinc due to the influence of zinc on ribonuclease activity. Ribonuclease activity increases with a zinc deficiency [21]. Enzymes such as deoxynucleotidyl transferase, nucleoside phosphorylase, and reverse transcriptase also require zinc.

With respect to transcription, zinc appears to interact with nuclear proteins that bind to promoter sequences of specific genes (Fig. 12.10). Thus, zinc helps regulate transcription. Specifically, zinc serves as a necessary structural component of DNA-binding proteins that contain zinc fingers. "Zinc fingers" is a term used to indicate the shape (configuration) of the proteins, which look like fingers, and the presence of the mineral zinc bound to the protein (Fig. 12.10). The fingerlike configuration results from the twisting and coiling of the

cysteine and histidine residues in that segment of the protein. DNA-binding proteins that contain zinc fingers also bind retinoic acid, thyroxine, 1,25-(OH)₂ vitamin D, and other steroid hormones, such as estrogen and androgens. Thus, hormones such as retinoic acid or 1,25-(OH)₂ vitamin D would enter the cell nucleus (see Chapter 10, section on vitamin A) and bind to a specific protein containing zinc fingers. In the presence of zinc, which is required for the binding of the protein to the DNA, the protein (with the hormone attached to it) binds to the DNA to affect gene expression (Fig. 12.10).

The effect of zinc on cell membranes may be through direct effects on membrane protein's conformation and/or on protein to protein interactions [17]. Zinc may affect the activity of several enzymes attached to plasma membranes. Some of these enzymes include alkaline phosphatase, carbonic anhydrase, and superoxide dismutase, among others [17]. These particular enzymes that control the structures and functions of the membranes to which they are attached are in turn controlled by zinc [16]. Zinc itself is believed also to stabilize membrane structure by stabilizing phospholipids and thiol (SH) groups that need to be maintained in a reduced state [20], and to guard the membrane against peroxidative damage by occupying sites on the membrane that might be instead occupied by pro-oxidant metals such as iron or by quenching free radi-

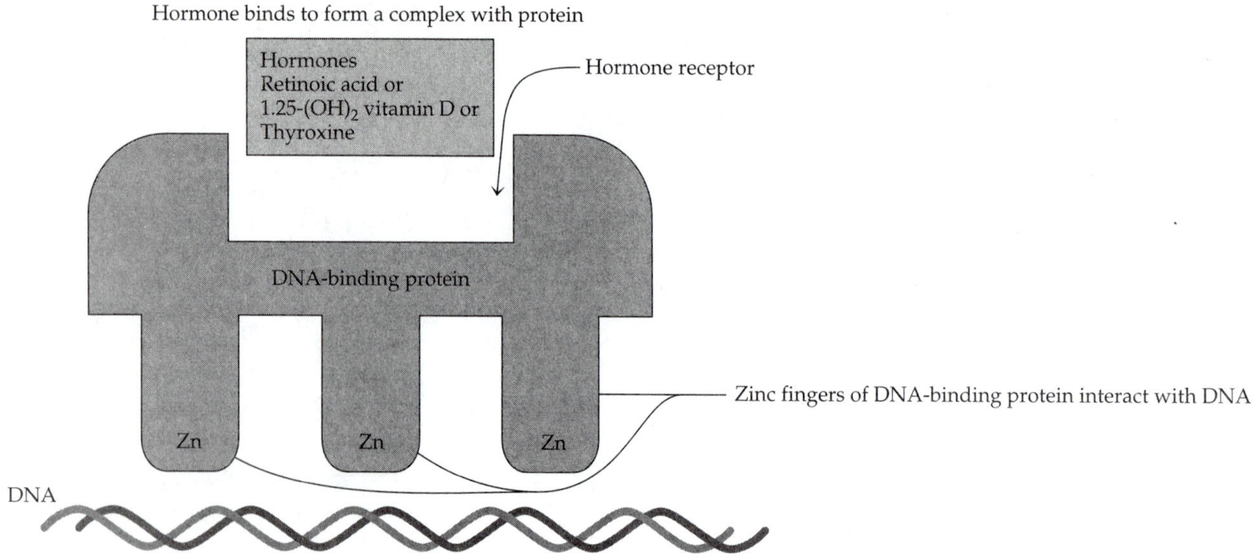

FIGURE 12.10 One role of zinc in gene expression.

cals through association with metallothionein [1]. Zinc may also stabilize membranes by promoting associations between membrane skeletal and cytoskeletal proteins [17].

Zinc influences carbohydrate metabolism. A zinc deficiency causes a decreased insulin response and an impaired glucose tolerance [10]. Zinc also appears to influence the basal metabolic rate (BMR); a decrease in thyroid hormones and BMR has been observed in subjects receiving a zinc-restricted diet [22]. Zinc is important for taste; it is a component of gustin, a protein involved in taste acuity.

Although many of the functions of zinc are known, many roles of zinc are not known. The effects of zinc deficiency on the body fail to explain fully the manifestations of zinc deprivation.

Interactions with Other Nutrients

A discussion of some of the interactions that occur between zinc and several other divalent ions has been previously addressed under the section on absorption. Interrelationships between zinc and *vitamin A* also have been observed. The role of zinc and alcohol dehydrogenase that acts on retinol (vitamin A) has been mentioned earlier under zinc functions. In addition, zinc is necessary for the synthesis of retinol-binding protein, which transports vitamin A in the blood. Zinc deficiency is as-

sociated with decreased mobilization of retinol from the liver as well as decreased concentrations of several transport proteins found in the blood, including albumin, transferrin, and prealbumin [23].

The detrimental effect of excessive zinc intake on *copper* absorption is thought to result from zinc's stimulation of thionein synthesis. Thionein polypeptides have a high affinity for copper and formation of copper metallothionein traps the metal in the enterocyte, preventing its passage into the plasma. Zinc intakes of 18.5 mg daily for two weeks have been shown to impair copper retention in men [24]. Intakes of 25 mg zinc for six weeks decreased superoxide dismutase activity, an indication of impaired copper status [25]. The danger of copper deficiency precipitated by zinc supplementation has led to the recommendation that the maximum therapeutic dose of elemental zinc be limited to 40 mg daily [26].

Diminished *calcium* absorption has occurred with ingestion of zinc supplements when calcium intake is low (230 mg calcium) [13]. However, absorption appears unaffected when calcium intakes are at adequate (recommended) levels [26].

Excretion

The routes of zinc loss from the body are via the body surface, kidney, and gastrointestinal tract. Most of the zinc lost from the body is excreted in the feces. Endogenous zinc entering the gastrointestinal tract is primarily in the form of metalloproteins, which are secreted by the salivary glands, intestinal mucosa, pancreas, and liver [1,2]. Zinc is also contributed to the gastrointestinal lumen by sloughed intestinal cells and possibly by enterocytes that may permit a bidirectional flow of the mineral. A small amount of zinc is excreted via the kidney; urinary zinc averages approximately 400 to 600 μg/day [1]. The zinc appearing in the urine is believed to be derived from the small percentage of plasma zinc that is complexed with histidine and cysteine. Regulation of the renal excretion of these amino acid–zinc complexes is poorly understood, but the majority of zinc filtered is reabsorbed by the kidney tubules [1]. Surface losses of zinc occur with exfoliation of skin and with sweating to total about 1 mg zinc loss/day [1,2,18]. Another minor route of zinc loss is via hair which contains about 0.1 to 0.2 mg zinc/g hair. Total zinc losses approximate about 2.2 to 2.8 mg/day [5]. Obligatory zinc losses decrease with decreased zinc intake [5].

Recommended Dietary Allowance

The subcommittee on the tenth edition of the RDA [5] based zinc recommendations on the intake needed to maintain balance as well as on estimates of zinc absorption and body losses of zinc. Balance studies have indicated that at least 12 mg zinc/day is necessary for achievement of equilibrium in healthy young men. Since zinc losses from healthy young men have been estimated at between 2.2 to 2.8 mg daily, approximately 2.5 mg absorbed zinc is needed for maintenance of equilibrium. In order to allow for less than optimal zinc absorption, an absorption efficiency of only 20% was assumed. The resulting dietary zinc requirement (2.5 mg losses/20% absorption) amounts to 12.5 mg daily. The 1989 RDA for zinc is set at 15 mg/day for young men. An allowance of 12 mg/day is considered adequate for adult women because of their smaller body size [5].

During pregnancy the RDA for zinc is 15 mg/day to cover the calculated need for growth of the fetus and placenta because there is no indication for an increased absorption efficiency in pregnant women [5]. Zinc requirements for lactating women vary according to the zinc content of human milk and the amount of milk produced during the first and second half year. Because of the higher zinc content in the milk as well as the greater milk production during the first 6 months of lactation, the allowance during this period is set at 19 mg/day [5].

For the last half of the year, the zinc allowance drops to 16 mg/day [5].

Deficiency

Because no functional store of zinc appears to exist [1], and because zinc deposited in bones appears to be held quite tenaciously, a deficient intake of zinc results in the catabolism of some of the zinc metalloenzymes [1]. Normally zinc is removed from those metalloenzymes that hold it less securely. Three metalloenzymes shown in experimental animals to be sensitive to zinc deprivation are alkaline phosphatase in bone, carboxypeptidase A in pancreas, and deoxythymidine kinase in subcutaneous connective tissue [21]. The zinc so released is redistributed throughout the body to satisfy the more crucial cellular needs. Certain metalloenzymes, however, such as carbonic anhydrase, which have very high affinity for zinc, may be little influenced by a general zinc deprivation. The extent to which the metalloenzyme will lose zinc during a deficiency depends on the geometry of the nitrogen, oxygen, and/or sulfur atoms that comprise the binding site [4].

Estimates of the average amount of zinc consumed by adults from a mixed U.S. diet range from 6 to 15 mg per day [5]. Several population groups are thought to consume less than adequate amounts of zinc, principally elderly women [27,28]. Other conditions and populations associated with increased need for intake include those with alcoholism, chronic illness, stress, trauma, surgery, malabsorption, lactovegetarians, and children consuming vegetarian diets [27].

Signs and symptoms of zinc deficiency include growth retardation (an early response to zinc deficiency in children) [30], skeletal abnormalities due to impaired development of epiphyseal cartilage [2], defective collagen synthesis and or cross-linking [2], poor wound healing, dermatitis, delayed sexual maturation in children, hypogeusia (blunting of sense of taste), night blindness, alopecia (hair loss), impaired immune function, and impaired protein synthesis [23,31], among others [16]. Also remember, metalloenzymes sensitive to zinc deprivation include alkaline phosphatase in bone, carboxypeptidase A in the pancreas, and deoxythymidine kinase in subcutaneous connective tissue [21].

Toxicity

Excessive intakes of zinc can cause toxicity. An acute toxicity with 1 to 2 g zinc sulfate (225 to 450 mg zinc) can produce metallic taste, nausea, vomiting, epigastric pain, abdominal cramps, and bloody diarrhea [1,5,32]. Chronic ingestion of therapeutic doses or doses as low as 18.5 or 25 mg daily of zinc can result in a copper deficiency due to the competition of these two minerals for intestinal absorption [5,24,25]. Ingestion of 100 to 300 mg zinc daily as prescribed for some patients with sickle cell anemia and other conditions has induced copper deficiency evidenced by hypocupremia, anemia, leukopenia, and neutropenia as well as abnormal cholesterol metabolism [32]. Furthermore, copper deficiency induced by intakes of zinc (110 to 165 mg) for 10 months did not respond to cessation of zinc and 2 months of oral copper supplementation. Cupric chloride given intravenously for five days was needed to correct the deficiency and suggested that elimination of excess zinc by the body is a slow process and will continue to inhibit copper absorption until it is eliminated [32].

Assessment of Nutriture

The strong homeostatic control of body zinc has made the evaluation of zinc nutriture very difficult [33]. A variety of static indices has been used to assess zinc status, including measurements of zinc in red blood cells, leukocytes, neutrophils, and plasma. The most common means for assessment being serum or plasma zinc with fasting concentrations of less than 70 μg/dL suggesting deficiency [30,34]. Zinc (fasting) in the plasma decreases only when the dietary intake is so low that homeostasis cannot be established without use of zinc from the exchangeable pool that includes plasma zinc [1,30]. Low fasting plasma zinc thus indicates that little zinc is present in the exchangeable zinc pool, and reflects a loss of zinc from bone and liver [30]. Interpretation of plasma zinc must be made with caution because concentrations are influenced by many factors, unrelated to zinc depletion, including meals, time of day (diurnal variation), stress, infections, hypoalbuminemia, steroid therapy, and oral contraceptive administration [33,35,36]. Postprandial zinc concentrations have been found to be more sensitive to low dietary zinc intakes than fasting plasma zinc [37].

Although serum metallothionein concentrations are thought to be less sensitive to zinc deficiency than red blood cell concentrations, the latter is thought to detect the initial response to a low dietary zinc intake and may be useful for detecting zinc redistribution among tissues [1,30]. Urinary zinc excretion diminishes with severe zinc deficiency.

Zinc content of hair has been another popular static index used in the assessment of zinc nutriture. Low hair zinc may be associated with chronic intake of dietary zinc in suboptimal amounts [34]. Standardized proce-

dures, however, are needed to eliminate contamination from, for example, shampoo and confounding variables such as variations due to hair color, sampling sites, and so on. The concentration of zinc in hair depends not only on delivery of zinc to the root but also on the rate of hair growth.

The measurement of the activity of zinc-dependent enzymes has also been employed as an index of zinc status. Although carbonic anhydrase activity decreases only after signs of zinc deficiency appear, the activity of alkaline phosphatase decreases much sooner [34]. Measurements of activity before and after zinc supplementation are recommended [34]. An oral zinc tolerance test has also been used to assess zinc absorption from different meals or supplements. The test typically involves ingestion of 25 or 50 mg zinc as zinc acetate with a test meal or supplement. Changes in plasma zinc concentrations are assessed between the different meals [34].

References Cited for Zinc

1. King JC, Keen CL. Zinc. In: Shils ME, Olson JA, Shike M., eds. Modern nutrition in health and disease, 8th ed. Philadelphia: Lea and Febiger, 1994;214–230.
2. Cousins RJ, Hempe JM. Zinc. In: Brown ML., ed. Present knowledge in nutrition, 6th ed. Washington, DC: International Life Sciences Institute Nutrition Foundation, 1990:251–260.
3. Wagner PA. Zinc nutriture in the elderly. Geriatrics 1985;40:111–125.
4. DiSilvestro RA, Cousins RJ. Physiological ligands for copper and zinc. Ann Rev Nutr 1983;3:261–288.
5. National Research Council. Recommended dietary allowances, 10th ed. Washington, DC: National Academy Press, 1989;205–213.
6. Scholmerich J, Freudemann A, Kottgen E, Wietholtz H, Steiert B, Lohle E, Haussinger D, Gerok W. Bioavailability of zinc from zinc-histidine complexes. I. Comparison with zinc sulfate in healthy men. Am J Clin Nutr 1987;45:1480–1486.
7. Sandstrom B, Davidsson L, Cederblad A, Lonnerdal B. Oral iron, dietary ligands and zinc absorption. J Nutr 1985;115:411–414.
8. Greger JL. Mineral bioavailability/new concepts. Nutr Today 1987;22:4–9.
9. Ellis R, Kelsay JL, Reynolds RD, Morris ER, Moser PB, Frazier CW. Phytate:zinc and phytate x calcium:zinc millimolar ratios in self-selected diets of Americans, Asian Indians and Nepalese. J Am Diet Assoc 1987;87:1043–1047.
10. Forbes RM, Erdman JW Jr. Bioavailability of trace mineral elements. Ann Rev Nutr 1983;3:213–231.
11. Simmer K, Iles CA, James C, Thompson RPH. Are iron-folate supplements harmful? Am J Clin Nutr 1987;45:122–125.

12. Solomons NW, Jacob RA. Studies on the bioavailability of zinc in humans: Effects of heme and nonheme iron on the absorption of zinc. Am J Clin Nutr 1981; 34:475–482.

13. Spencer H. Minerals and mineral interactions in human beings. J Am Diet Assoc 1986;86:864–867.

14. Dawson-Hughes B, Seligson FH, Hughes VA. Effects of calcium carbonate and hydroxyapatite on zinc and iron retention in postmenopausal women. Am J Clin Nutr 1986;44:83–88.

15. O'Dell BL. Bioavailability of trace elements. Nutr Rev 1984;42:301–308.

16. Prasad AS. Clinical, biochemical and nutritional spectrum of zinc deficiency in human subjects: An update. Nutr Rev 1983;41:197–208.

17. Bettger WJ, O'Dell BL. Physiological roles of zinc in the plasma membrane of mammalian cells. J Nutr Biochem 1993;4:194–207.

18. Sandstead HH, Evans GW. Zinc. In: Olson RE, Broquist HB, Chichester CO, Darby WJ, Kolbye AC Jr, Stalvey RM, eds. Nutrition Reviews' present knowledge in nutrition, 5th ed. Washington, DC: The Nutrition Foundation 1984;479–505.

19. Bremner I, Beattie JH. Metallothionein and the trace minerals. Ann Rev Nutr 1990;10:63–83.

20. Role of zinc in enzyme regulation and protection of essential thiol groups. Nutr Rev 1986;44:309–311.

21. Prasad AS. Nutritional zinc today. Nutr Today 1981;16: 4–11.

22. Wada L, King JC. Effect of low zinc intakes on basal metabolic rate, thyroid hormones and protein utilization in adult men. J Nutr 1986;116:1045–1053.

23. Bates J, McClain CJ. The effect of severe zinc deficiency on serum levels of albumin, transferrin, and prealbumin in man. Am J Clin Nutr 1981;34:1655–1660.

24. Festa MD, Anderson HL, Dowdy RP, Ellersieck MR. Effect of zinc intake on copper excretion and retention in men. Am J Clin Nutr 1985;41:285–292.

25. Fischer PWF, Giroux A, L'Abbe MR. Effect of zinc supplementation on copper status in adult man. Am J Clin Nutr 1984;40:743–746.

26. Solomons NW. Mineral interactions in the diet. J Dent Child 1982;49:445–448.

27. Pennington JAT, Young BE, Wilson DB, Johnson RD, Vanderveen JE. Mineral content of foods and total diets: The selected minerals in foods survey, 1982 to 1984. J Am Diet Assoc 1986;86:876–891.

28. Pennington JAT, Young BE. Total diet study nutritional elements, 1982–1989. J Am Diet Assoc 1991;91:179–183.

29. Gibson RS. Content and bioavailabilty of trace elements in vegetarian diets. Am J Clin Nutr 1994;59(suppl.): 1223S–1232S.

30. King JC. Assessment of zinc status. J Nutr 1990;120: 1474–1479.

31. Baer MT, King JC, Tamura T, Margen S, Bradfield RB, Weston WL, Daugherty NA. Nitrogen utilization, enzyme activity, glucose intolerance and leukocyte chemo-taxis in human experimental zinc depletion. Am J Clin Nutr 1985;41:1220–1235.

32. Fosmire GJ. Zinc toxicity. Am J Clin Nutr 1990;51: 225–227.

33. Milne DB. Assessment of zinc and copper nutritional status in man. Nutr MD 1987;13(5):1–2.

34. Gibson RS. Principles of nutritional assessment. New York: Oxford University Press, 1990:542–553.

35. Wallock LM, King JC, Hambidge KM, English-Westcott JE, Pritts J. Meal-induced changes in plasma, erythrocyte, and urinary zinc concentrations in adult women. Am J Clin Nutr 1993;58:695–701.

36. King JC, Hambidge KM, Westcott JL, Kern DL, Marshall G. Daily variation in plasma zinc concentrations in women fed meals at six-hour intervals. J Nutr 1994;124: 508–516.

37. Mellman DL, Hambidge KM, Westcott JL. Effect of dietary zinc restriction on postprandial changes in plasma zinc. Am J Clin Nutr 1993;58:702–704.

Additional References

Chesters JK. Trace element-gene interactions with particular reference to zinc. Proc Nutr Soc 1991;50:123–129.

Vallee BL, Auld DS. Zinc coordination, function, and structure of zinc enzymes and other proteins. Biochemistry 1990;29:5647–5659.

COPPER

The copper content of the human adult body is on the order of 50 to 120 mg [1,2]. The amount of tissue copper is age related, with the newborn and very young normally richer in copper per unit of body weight than adults. Copper's pattern of tissue distribution may also vary with age and with copper status, but it is normally found in highest concentration in the liver, with variably lesser amounts in the brain, heart, kidneys, and spleen. In the body, copper shifts between its cuprous state (Cu^{+1}) and cupric state (Cu^{+2}); however, the latter state predominates.

Sources

The copper content of food varies widely reflecting the origin of the food, and the conditions under which the food was produced, handled, and prepared for use. Consequently, analytic values of copper published for a specific food must be used with caution. The broad range of the copper content of selected foods, as listed in Table 12.7, reflects these variations. The richest sources are considered to be organ meats, shellfish,

Table 12.7 Some Food Copper Values

Food	Copper Content (mg/100g)	Food	Copper Content (mg/100g)
Dairy		Vegetables	
Egg, whole	0.07	Potato, without peel	0.07
Milk, whole	0.003	Potato chips	0.35
Yogurt, low-fat, plain	0.004	Potato, sweet	0.18
Cheese, cheddar	0.04	Carrot	0.05
Meat, Fish, Poultry		Broccoli	0.03
Liver, beef	6.09	Spinach	0.08
Chicken	0.07	Peas	0.10
Beef, sirloin	0.14	Lettuce	0.03
Pork	0.09	Tomato	0.06
Tuna, canned	0.05	Corn	0.04
Shrimp, cooked	0.30	Cabbage	0.01
Grains		Fruits	
Macaroni, cooked	0.08	Apple	0.03
Corn grits, cooked	0.01	Banana	0.14
Rice, white, cooked	0.08	Grapes	0.09
Roll, white	0.14	Peach	0.06
Bread, whole-wheat	0.25	Pear	0.09
Nuts		Pineapple	0.05
Peanut	0.68	Orange	0.04
Pecan	1.24	Raisins	0.32
		Prunes	0.29

Source: Pennington JAT, Young BE, Johnson RD, and Vanderveen JE. Mineral content of foods and total diets: The selected minerals in foods survey, 1982 to 1984. Reprint from JOURNAL OF THE AMERICAN DIETETIC ASSOCIATION. Vol. 86:876–891, 1986.

nuts, seeds, legumes, dried fruits, as well as a few select vegetables.

Absorption and Transport

Although copper is absorbed throughout the small intestine especially the duodenum [2], the stomach also appears to possess a substantial absorptive capacity. This may be attributable to the solubilizing effect of the acidic environment on copper, thereby facilitating its transport across the gastric mucosa.

The biochemical mechanisms for the absorption of copper across the brush border of the small intestine are not completely understood. It is possible that luminal copper must be bound to more absorbable ligands for effective transport, and even if copper is transported in the free ionic form, such ligands may present the metal to brush border receptors in a way that increases uptake.

Copper absorption ranges from about 12% with intakes of about 7.5 mg to 56% with intakes of 0.8 mg [1,3]. Copper absorption may be as high as 71% as observed in women consuming 0.9 to 1.2 mg copper per day [4]. Copper appears to be absorbed by two mechanisms, one saturable, involving an active transport system, and the other a nonsaturable, passive diffusion process. As is true for other transport systems, low concentrations of dietary copper are primarily transported via the active pathway, while the diffusion process accommodates higher concentrations.

Copper transport across the brush border membrane may be influenced by a variety of dietary components, some exerting a positive effect and some influencing its absorption negatively. Examples of substances that facilitate copper absorption include amino acids, especially histidine, which may bind to copper and allow absorption through an amino acid transport system, as well as citrate and gluconate, which are thought to act as binding ligands [5]. Several substances impede copper absorption. Zinc in amounts as low as 18.5 mg has been shown to impair copper absorption in men [6]; at slightly higher intakes (25 mg zinc for six weeks), superoxide dismutase activity decreased, suggesting impaired copper status [7]. The detrimental effect of excessive zinc intake on copper absorption is thought to result from zinc's stimulation of thionein synthesis. Thionein, a protein that possesses an unusually high proportion (25 to 30%) of thiol groups in the form of cysteine, avidly binds copper as well as other metals to form metallothionein. Intestinal metallothionein may function as a negative modulator of copper absorption and in this respect acts as a detoxifying agent, binding copper and reducing its transmucosal flux (passage into the plasma) when the dietary intake and therefore luminal concentration of the metal is excessive [12]. At normal intake levels of copper, however, the regulatory role of the protein remains unclear.

Antacid ingestion (up to 15 antacid tablets per day containing oxides of bismuth, aluminum, silica, magnesium, and sodium) may result in precipitation of copper at the alkaline pH, and thus inhibit copper absorption to induce copper deficiency [8]. Also suggesting the inhibitory role of an alkaline environment on copper absorption is the improved copper absorption experienced by people with pancreatic insufficiency, and thus a lower intestinal pH than normal.

Calcium (2,382 mg as calcium gluconate) and phosphorus (2,442 mg as glycerol phosphate) have been shown to increase fecal copper excretion, compared to diets containing only moderate amounts of calcium (780 mg as calcium gluconate) with either high phosphorus (2,442 mg as glycerol phosphate) or moderate phosphorus (843 mg as glycerol phosphate) [9]. Urinary copper losses were also significantly greater on the high-calcium, high-phosphorus diet than on the moderate-calcium, moderate-phosphorus diet [9].

Dietary carbohydrates and amino acids also affect copper absorption. Copper balance was greater in men consuming 20% fructose as compared to starch [10]. In chicks, cysteine administration inhibited the absorption of copper–amino acid complexes [11].

Luminal copper concentrations also influence absorption, with high luminal copper concentrations inhibiting absorption, and low luminal copper concentrations as well as poor copper status improving absorption. Intestinal cell thionein concentrations affect the delivery of copper from the intestinal cell into the plasma.

Once within the intestinal cell, copper may be used by the cell (see section on functions) or may be transported through the cell for subsequent transport across the basolateral membrane.

From the intestinal cell, copper is transported to the liver bound loosely to albumin, and possibly to transcuprein (Tc) [13,14] and/or amino acids such as histidine [5]. The observations that the uptake of copper by the hepatocytes is a saturable, temperature-dependent process and that no competition with other metal ions occurs suggest that a specific, facilitated diffusion mechanism is in effect. Transport across the cell membrane may involve the formation of certain amino acid–copper complexes, and may also involve albumin [14].

Once within cells, more than half of the accumulated copper is found in the supernatant fraction and one-fourth within the nuclei. It first appears to bind to metallothionein, then is slowly transferred to the copper enzymes such as superoxide dismutase (SOD), which appears to be given high priority with respect to the use of cellular copper. Experimentally, a tenfold reduction in hepatic copper resulted in only a twofold decrease in SOD activity [15]. In the liver, copper also binds to apoceruloplasmin. Four to six copper ions (Cu^{+2}) are attached tightly to apoceruloplasmin to form ceruloplasmin. Copper is found at the protein's active site and gives the protein a blue color. Ceruloplasmin is released into the blood from the liver, and constitutes 70 to 80% of circulating copper in the blood after meals [5,13,14]. The remaining copper in the blood circulates loosely bound to albumin, transcuprein, and histidine. The basic aspects of mammalian copper metabolism are summarized in Figure 12.11.

Uptake of ceruloplasmin copper by extrahepatic cells involves binding of ceruloplasmin to specific receptors. The copper is reduced to Cu^{+1} and dissociates from the ceruloplasmin, then enters the cells. Ascorbic acid enhances copper transfer, and is probably involved in the reduction of the copper.

Copper is found within a variety of cells and tissues in the body, including the liver and kidney, which rapidly extract copper from the blood. Other tissues that take up copper include bone, muscle, skin, brain, intestine, heart, spleen, among others. Within cells and tissues, copper is bound to amino acids or proteins. The liver appears to be the main storage site for copper, which is thought to be bound to metallothionein [1]. The amount of copper available to extrahepatic tissues is thought to be regulated by the liver through the synthesis of ceruloplasmin, through copper incorporation into metallothionein, and through excretion of copper into the bile [5].

Functions

The essentiality of copper is due, in part, to its participation as an enzyme activator in crucial reactions. Several copper-requiring metalloenzymes and the reactions they catalyze are described next.

Ceruloplasmin is not simply a transporter of plasma copper; it is also a multifaceted oxidative enzyme. Ceruloplasmin, also known as *ferroxidase I*, is responsible for the oxidation of minerals, most notably ferrous (Fe^{+2}) iron, but also manganese (Mn^{+2}). The oxidation of Fe^{+2} to Fe^{+3} is needed in order for iron to bind to transferrin. Transferrin then transports the mobilized iron from its

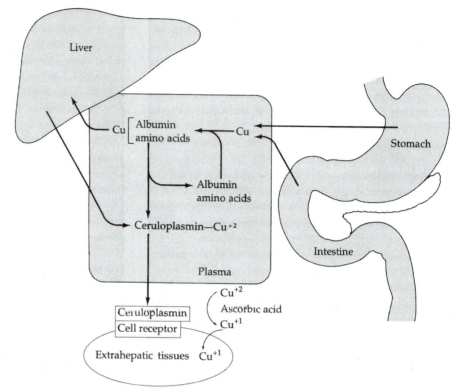

FIGURE 12.11 Basic aspects of copper metabolism. Absorbed copper is transported in portal plasma bound principally to albumin and amino acids. In the systemic circulation, copper is part of ceruloplasmin, in which form it is delivered to extrahepatic tissues.

hepatic stores to tissues that need the mineral. Ceruloplasmin also modulates the inflammatory process as an acute-phase protein. Ceruloplasmin concentrations rise in the blood with, for example, infection. During infections, phagocytosis of invading organisms by white blood cells generates superoxide radicals, which must be eliminated to prevent further damage to body cells. Superoxide radicals also are generated in normal metabolism. *Superoxide dismutase* (SOD) found in the cytosol of cells is copper and zinc dependent and catalyzes the removal of the superoxide radicals (O_2^-).

$$2O_2^- + 2H^+ \xrightarrow{\text{zinc copper SOD}} H_2O_2 + O_2$$

Superoxide radicals can cause peroxidative damage of phospholipid components of cell membranes (see "Perspective" section in Chapter 10). SOD therefore assumes a very important protective function. SOD is found in most cells of the body. Increased peroxidation of cell membranes is found with copper deficiency.

Several *amine oxidases* are also copper dependent. The amine oxidases are found both in the blood and in body tissues. The amine oxidases function to catabolize amines such as tyramine, histamine, and dopamine to form aldehydes.

$$RCH_2NH_2 \xrightarrow{\text{amine oxidase-Cu}} RCH\!\!=\!\!O + NH_3$$

Tyramine and dopamine can be oxidized by monoamine oxidase. Diamine oxidase inactivates histamine.

Cytochrome oxidase contains two to three copper atoms per molecule. This enzyme is the terminal oxidative step in mitochondrial electron transport (p. 62), where it transfers an electron. O_2 is reduced to form water and ATP is produced.

In *tyrosine metabolism* (Fig. 9.7, p. 231), three reactions depend on copper. First, the enzymatic conversion by tyrosine hydroxylase of tyrosine to 3,4-dihydroxyphenylalanine (L-dopa), which may be further metabolized to dopamine or may be used for the synthesis of the pigment melanin found in eyes, skin, and hair, requires copper. Although the conversion of L-dopa to dopamine does not require copper, the conversion of dopamine to norepinephrine by dopamine hydroxylase requires vitamin C and up to eight copper atoms per molecule (p. 231). Also in tyrosine catabolism, the conversion of hydroxyphenylpyruvate to homogentisate requires a copper-dependent hydroxylase and vitamin C.

In connective tissues (collagen, elastin), *lysyl oxidase* catalyzes the removal of the epsilon amino group of lysyl residues of a polypeptide and the oxidation of the terminal carbon atom of an aldehyde. This reaction is necessary for the biosynthesis of connective tissue. The lesions of copper deficiency that affect bone and connective tissue are likely due to a deficiency of this enzyme.

Copper plays a variety of other roles in the body that may or may not involve enzymes. Neurologic disorders such as ataxia and neuropathy appear to be affected by copper. For example, copper status strongly affects the levels of neuropeptides, enkephalins, and endorphins [16], but it is not clear if or how this effect is related to any of the metalloenzymatic functions of copper. Decreased concentrations of norepinephrine are found in the brain with copper deficiency. Myelination is also decreased with copper deficiency.

Interactions with Other Nutrients

Copper is known to interact with a number of inorganic and organic dietary constituents. Among organic dietary substances, *ascorbic acid* (1.5 g for 64 days) resulted in decreased serum ceruloplasmin activity, however, concentrations still remained within the normal range [17]. Intakes of 605 mg vitamin C for three weeks also resulted in a 21% decrease in serum ceruloplasmin oxidase activity [18]. The effects of vitamin C may be mediated through the reduction of the cupric ion to its cuprous form by the ascorbate or through the formation of a poorly absorbable complex, or both.

It is well established that a strong, mutual antagonism exists between copper and *zinc*, most likely caused by the induction of intestinal metallothionein by zinc. This results in excessive intracellular binding of the copper, reducing its luminal-to-serosal flux, and entry into the blood. Zinc intakes ranging from 18.5 mg to 300 mg daily have resulted in a copper deficiency [6,7,19]. Furthermore, copper deficiency induced by intakes of zinc (110 to 165 mg) for 10 months did not respond to cessation of zinc and 2 months of oral copper supplementation. Cupric chloride given intravenously for five days (total dose 10 mg) was needed to correct the deficiency and suggested that elimination of excess zinc by the body is a slow process and will continue to inhibit copper absorption until it is eliminated [20].

In addition to the interference of copper absorption by zinc, another interaction of copper having practical importance involves *iron*. The importance of copper in normal iron metabolism is evidenced by the anemia that results from prolonged copper deficiency. It is known that the anemia is caused by an impaired mobilization and use of iron due to the reduced ferroxidase activity of ceruloplasmin, which is responsible for oxidation of iron

to its trivalent (Fe^{+3}) state. Only as Fe^{+3} can iron be coordinated to its transport protein transferrin.

Dietary copper also forms complexes with molybdenum and sulfur. More specifically, in animals (rats and ruminants) tetrathiomolybdate $(MoS_4)^{-2}$ has been shown to form an insoluble complex with copper to inhibit its absorption in the gastrointestinal tract. Such findings have not been reported in humans; however, urinary copper excretion in humans has been shown to rise from 24 µg/day to 77 µg/day as molybdenum intake increased from 160 µg to 1,540 µg/day [3]. No changes in fecal copper excretion were noted, suggesting perhaps that molybdenum increased copper mobilization from tissues and promoted excretion [3].

Copper and selenium also appear to interact. Copper deficiency has been shown to decrease the activity of the selenium-dependent enzymes glutathione peroxidase and 5′-deiodinase [21].

Antagonistic interactions between copper and excessive amounts of cadmium, silver, and mercury have been described but have more theoretical than practical importance [22].

Excretion

Most ingested copper is excreted from the body in the feces. Most of this copper is unabsorbed copper, but active excretion via the bile also occurs. The relative amounts of unabsorbed and excreted copper depend on factors such as its dietary form and its interaction with other food components. A small amount of copper is also excreted in the urine. Adults normally excrete from 10 to 30 µg of copper daily through the kidneys [1]. Small amounts (50 µg) of copper are also lost in sweat and with desquamation of the skin [1]. Only trace amounts of copper are lost in normal menstrual flow so that a woman's copper status, unlike her iron status, is not compromised by menstruation.

Estimated Safe and Adequate Daily Dietary Intake

In the 1980 edition of the RDA, a recommendation for an Estimated Safe and Adequate Daily Dietary Intake (ESADDI) for copper was first made by the Food and Nutrition Board. The 1989 Committee on the RDA recommends a daily copper intake for infants of 75 µg/kg of body weight [23]. This figure allows for the feeding of formulas in which copper is less bioavailable than in breast milk and is therefore higher than the amount recommended for strictly breastfed infants. For children and adults, for whom recommended intake is based on balance studies, the Food and Nutrition Board established a safe and adequate range for copper intake of 1.5 to 3 mg/day [23].

Deficiency

Various conditions associated with copper deficiency are now recognized, including hypochromic, microcytic anemia, neutropenia, leukopenia, depigmentation of skin and hair, impaired immune function, and skeletal demineralization, all of which are reversible by copper administration. The normal concentration of serum copper ranges from 64 to 156 μg/dL [1]. Serum copper and ceruloplasmin (normal concentration about 18 to 40 mg/dL) as well as red blood cell SOD (normal 0.47 to 0.067 mg/g) activity typically decrease with copper deficiency [1]. Decreased activity of glutathione peroxidase has also been reported although the mechanism of action is unclear [24]. In copper-deficient animals, hypercholesterolemia is found [25,26]. Elevated plasma cholesterol has also been shown with low copper intakes in some humans [23]. Conditions and populations associated with increased need for intake include excessive antacid ingestion, nephrosis, and malabsorptive disorders such as celiac disease, tropical sprue, and protein-losing enteropathies. Low copper intakes have been reported for several age groups from infants through older adults [3,27].

Toxicity

Copper intakes of 64 mg (250 mg copper sulfate) have resulted in nausea, vomiting, and diarrhea. The exact amount of copper known to cause more serious complications is not known; however, copper toxicity has been observed in patients on hemodialysis and in infants following consumption of water high in copper [1]. Wilson's disease, a genetic disorder, is characterized by copper accumulation in organs. Disturbed organ function occurs especially in the liver, kidney, and brain. While the exact biochemical defect is unknown, treatment of Wilson's disease involves avoidance of high copper foods and D-penicillamine therapy to bind body copper and increase its excretion [28].

Assessment of Nutriture

Serum or red blood cell copper is frequently used to assess copper status. Response of serum ceruloplasmin to copper supplements is also thought to be useful as an index of copper status. Ceruloplasmin will increase following supplementation only in copper-deficient subjects [29]. SOD activity is sensitive to copper deficiency; SOD activity decreases prior to changes in serum copper and ceruloplasmin. Hair copper concentrations have not been shown to correlate with either serum or organ copper, and thus do not appear to be useful indicators of copper status [29].

References Cited for Copper

1. Turnlund JR. Copper. In: Shils ME, Olson JA, Shike M., eds. Modern nutrition in health and disease, 8th ed. Philadelphia: Lea and Febiger 1994;231–241.
2. O'Dell B. Copper. In: Brown ML., ed. Present knowledge in nutrition, 6th ed. Washington, DC: International Life Sciences Institute Nutrition Foundation 1990:261–267.
3. Turnlund JR. Copper nutriture, bioavailability, and the influence of dietary factors. J Am Diet Assoc 1988;88: 303–308.
4. Johnson PE, Milne DB, Lykken GI. Effects of age and sex on copper absorption, biological half-life, and status in humans. Am J Clin Nutr 1992;56:917–925.
5. DiSilvestro RA, Cousins RJ. Physiological ligands for copper and zinc. Ann Rev Nutr 1983;3:261–288.
6. Festa MD, Anderson HL, Dowdy RP, Ellersieck MR. Effect of zinc intake on copper excretion and retention in men. Am J Clin Nutr 1985;41:285–292.
7. Fischer PWF, Giroux A, L'Abbe MR. Effect of zinc supplementation on copper status in adult man. Am J Clin Nutr 1984;40:743–746.
8. Conditioned copper deficiency due to antacids. Nutr Rev 1984;42:319–321.
9. Snedeker SM, Smith SA, Greger JL. Effect of dietary calcium and phosphorus levels on the utilization of iron, copper, and zinc by adult males. J Nutr 1982;112: 136–143.
10. Reiser S, Smith JC, Mertz W, Holbrook JT, Scholfield DJ, Powell AS, Canfield WK, Canary JJ. Indices of copper status in humans consuming a typical American diet containing either fructose or starch. Am J Clin Nutr 1985;42:242–251.
11. Aoyagi S, Baker DH. Copper-amino acid complexes are partially protected against inhibitory effects of L-cysteine and L-ascorbic acid on copper absorption in chicks. J Nutr 1994;124:388–395.
12. Cousins, RJ. Absorption, transport and hepatic metabolism of copper and zinc: Special reference to metallothionein and ceruloplasmin. Physiol Rev 1985;65:238–244.
13. Frieden E. Perspectives on copper biochemistry. Clin Physiol Biochem 1986;4:11–19.
14. Harris ED. The transport of copper. In: Prasad AS, ed. Essential and toxic trace elements in human health and disease: An update. New York: Wiley-Liss, 1993;163–179.
15. Chung K, Romero N, Tinker D, Keen CL, Amemiya K, Rucker R. Role of copper in the regulation and accumulation of superoxide dismutase and metallothionein in rat liver. J Nutr 1988;118:859–864.
16. Bhathena SJ, Recant L, Voyles NR, Timmers KI, Reiser S, Smith JC, Powell AS. Decreased plasma enkephalins in copper deficiency in man. Am J Clin Nutr 1986;43:42–46.

17. Finley EB, Cerklewski FL. Influence of ascorbic acid supplementation on copper status in young adult men. Am J Clin Nutr 1983;37:553–556.

18. Jacob RA, Skala JH, Omaye ST, Turnlund JR. Effect of varying ascorbic acid intakes on copper absorption and ceruloplasmin levels of young men. J Nutr 1987;117: 2109–2115.

19. Fosmire GJ. Zinc toxicity. Am J Clin Nutr 1990; 51:225–227.

20. Hoffman HN, Phyliky RL, Fleming CR. Zinc-induced copper deficiency. Gastroenterology 1988;94:508–512.

21. Olin KL, Walter RM, Keen CL. Copper deficiency affects selenoglutathione peroxidase and selenodeiodinase activities and antioxidant defense in weanling rats. Am J Clin Nutr 1994;59:654–658.

22. O'Dell BL. Bioavailability of trace elements. Nutr Rev 1984;42:301–308

23. National Research Council. Recommended dietary allowances, 10th ed. Washington, DC: National Academy Press 1989;224–230.

24. Jenkinson SG, Lawrence RA, Burk RF, Williams DM. Effects of copper deficiency on the activity of the selenoenzyme glutathione peroxidase and on excretion and tissue retention of $^{75}SeO_3{}^{2-}$. J Nutr 1982;112:197–204.

25. Lei KY. Dietary copper: Cholesterol and lipoprotein metabolism. Ann Rev Nutr 1991;11:265–283.

26. Copper deficiency and hypercholesterolemia. Nutr Rev 1987;45:116–117.

27. Pennington JAT, Young BE. Total diet study nutritional elements, 1982–1989. J Am Diet Assoc 1991;91:179–183.

28. Smithgall JM. The copper-controlled diet: Current aspects of dietary copper restriction in management of copper metabolism disorders. J Am Diet Assoc 1985;85: 609–611.

29. Gibson RS. Principles of nutritional assessment. New York: Oxford University Press, 1990:542–553.

SELENIUM

Selenium, a nonmetal, exists in several oxidation states, for example, as selenide or selenoamino acids Se^{-2}, as selenite Se^{+4}, and as selenate Se^{+6} [1]. Total body selenium content is approximately 15 mg.

Sources

Perhaps more than any other essential trace element, selenium varies greatly in its soil concentration throughout the regions of the world. This, in turn, relates directly to its concentration in food plants. Actually, this heterogeneous distribution has had scientific benefit in that it has provided a clear correlation between those selenium-poor regions of the world (such as China) and the incidence of disease associated with selenium deficiency.

Defining those geographic regions specifically throughout the world that are selenium poor or selenium rich will not be a part of this discussion. However, Figure 12.12 is offered to illustrate, in part, the large difference in regional soil concentrations and how that difference is reflected in the blood selenium concentration of the local population. For further information, the interested reader is referred to the review by Levander [2] on global selenium nutrition.

Due to the wide disparity in soil selenium concentrations, tables listing the mineral's content in assorted

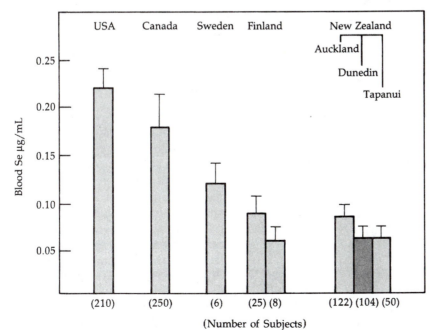

FIGURE 12.12 Blood selenium concentrations of healthy adults in the United States, Canada, Sweden, Finland, and New Zealand. *(Thomson CD, Robinson MF. Am J Clin Nutr 1980;33: 307–323. © Am J Clin Nutr, American Society for Clinical Nutrition.)*

foods are generally inappropriate and therefore not readily available. Those that are available are regionally specific. However, generally, animal products (especially organ meats) are thought to contain more selenium than plant sources. Seafood is also thought to represent one of the better sources of selenium, although the bioavailability of selenium from fish containing mercury is thought to be low due to the formation of unabsorbable mercury–selenium complexes [3,4]. Bioavailability of selenium from fish low in mercury, however, may also be low [3,4].

Digestion, Absorption, and Transport

The enteric absorption of selenium depends, to a great extent, on its dietary form. It occurs naturally in foods almost exclusively in the form of organic compounds, primarily selenomethionine, selenocystine, selenocysteine, and Se-methyl selenomethionine. These forms are thought to represent selenium analogs of sulfur-containing amino acids, the element substitution made possible by the chemical similarity between selenium and sulfur. These selenium analogs become incorporated into plant proteins.

In those parts of the world where selenium levels in natural foodstuffs are low, animal feeds are generally supplemented with sodium selenite (Na_2SeO_3). Therefore, this may also be an important dietary form of selenium in addition to the seleno-organic structures. Adding to the importance of selenite in selenium nutrition is the fact that selenium consumed in organic form is released as selenite during postabsorptive metabolism.

The organic forms of selenium as well as selenite are all efficiently absorbed, although to different extents, from the gastrointestinal tract, primarily at sites in the duodenum. Less absorption occurs in the jejunum and ileum, and virtually none in the stomach. Balance and stable isotopic tracer studies have generally shown that selenium, as selenomethionine, is more effectively absorbed than selenite [5]. Selenoamino acid absorption is estimated at 50 to 80%, while absorption from selenites is thought to be between 44 to 70%. Selenomethionine is thought to be better absorbed than selenocysteine, and selenates are thought to be better absorbed than selenites [6].

Factors enhancing selenium absorption include vitamins C, A, and E, as well as the presence of reduced glutathione in the intestinal lumen [1]. Heavy metals, such as mercury [4,7], and phytates are thought to inhibit selenium absorption through chelation and precipitation.

In the blood, selenium binds to alpha and beta globulins. Specifically, lipoproteins such as VLDL (an α-2

globulin) and LDL (a β globulin) have been shown to contain and transport selenium. Additional selenium transport proteins have been identified in some animals. The selenocystine-containing plasma protein called *selenoprotein P* has been isolated in the rat and appears to function as a selenium transport and possibly a storage protein [8].

Absorbed selenium becomes incorporated into a wide variety of proteins that may assume both transport and storage roles. The synthesis of these proteins appears to be induced by selenium. The rise and fall in concentration of various selenoproteins with time suggests that the proteins may be important in selenium flux among tissues [9].

The mechanism by which selenium is freed from plasma transport proteins is not known. Tissues containing relatively high selenium concentrations include the kidney, liver, heart, pancreas, and muscle [1]. The lungs, brain, bone, and red blood cells also contain selenium. Uptake of selenium into the red blood cell is thought to occur by diffusion with selenite uptake exceeding selenate, which in turn exceeds selenomethionine uptake [1].

Higher tissue concentrations of selenium have resulted when selenium was administered as selenomethionine as opposed to selenite. But the reverse is true with respect to the uptake of selenium by its major metalloenzyme glutathione peroxidase. That is to say, dietary selenium in the inorganic form such as selenite leads to greater incorporation of the mineral into glutathione peroxidase than when selenomethionine, the organic form, is the dietary form [10].

Organic selenoamino acids, not incorporated into proteins, are catabolized by a lyase to free the selenium for use by enzymes. Selenocysteine lyase, for example, hydrolyzes selenocysteine into alanine and H_2Se.

Functions

Various incompletely understood roles for selenium in mammalian metabolism have been postulated. Some of the less defined roles include its involvement in the maintenance or induction of the *cytochrome P450 system*, in *pancreatic function*, in *DNA repair and enzyme activation*, in *immune system function*, and in *detoxification of heavy metals*.

A clearly established function of selenium, however, is as an essential, tightly bound, cofactor for *glutathione peroxidase* (GSH-Px). Glutathione peroxidase uses reduced glutathione (GSH) and catalyzes the reduction of both organic peroxides ROOH (such as lipid peroxide LOOH) and hydrogen peroxide (H_2O_2) [11]. Glutathione is a tripeptide of glycine, cysteine, and glutamate. It is found in most cells of the body and furnishes reducing equivalents in reactions. Glutathione peroxidase is found mainly (about 70%) in the cytosol of cells, and to a lesser extent (approximately 30%) in the mitochondrial matrix. The enzyme is also found in the plasma where it is thought to originate from the renal proximal tubule cells [12]. Selenium availability has been shown to affect mRNA concentrations of glutathione peroxidase in the liver. With selenium deficiency, less mRNA for hepatic glutathione peroxidase is made and enzyme activity is diminished [7]. With selenium supplementation, there is a rapid increase in mRNA to control levels, but a gradual increase in enzyme activity.

Glutathione peroxidase catalyzes the following reaction:

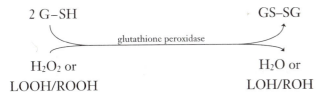

GS—SG represents oxidized glutathione, LOH represents an hydroxylipid, and ROH represents the hydroxy form of an organic compound. The reaction, catalyzed by glutathione peroxidase, neutralizes or eliminates hydrogen peroxide and organic (including lipid) peroxides. These peroxides, if not removed, could damage cellular membranes. The generation of hydrogen peroxides, lipid and organic peroxides, as well as the interdependent roles of selenium (as part of glutathione peroxidase), vitamin E, iron (as catalase), and zinc and copper (as superoxide dismutase (SOD)) are shown in the "Perspective" section at the end of Chapter 10.

The regeneration of reduced glutathione from its oxidized state is imperative. Glutathione reductase catalyzes the reduction in a reaction dependent on $NADPH + H^+$ and shown here:

GS-SG   2 G-SH
            glutathione reductase

$NADPH + H^+$ $NADP^+$

NADPH is derived from the hexose monophosphate shunt.

Selenium also appears to be necessary for iodine metabolism. 5'-*iodothyronine deiodinase* (type I) has been shown to be a selenoprotein with a single selenium atom at its active site [7]. The enzyme is found in the endoplasmic reticulum of the liver and kidney [7]. 5'-iodothyronine deiodinase catalyzes the deiodination of thyroxine

(T_4) to form tri-iodothyronine (T_3) as well as the conversion of reverse (r) T_3 to 3,3'-di-iodothyronine.

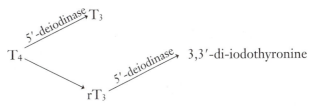

For further information regarding thyroid hormone metabolism, see the section of this chapter on iodine.

Interactions with Other Nutrients

The interrelationship between selenium and the other antioxidant nutrients is discussed in the "Perspective" section at the end of Chapter 10. *Lead* and selenium appear to react such that subclinical amounts of lead intake are found to lower significantly the tissue concentration of selenium. Although this mechanism is unclear, the fact that both elements bind to sulfhydryl groups provides reason for speculation [13]. *Iron* deficiency in rats has been shown to decrease the synthesis of hepatic glutathione peroxidase and to decrease selenium concentrations in the liver [14]. The mechanism(s) of action are unclear but are thought to reflect, in part, decreased transcription of the gene for glutathione peroxidase. Copper and selenium also appear to interact. Copper deficiency has been shown to decrease the activity of the selenium-dependent enzymes glutathione peroxidase and 5'-deiodinase [15]; whether the interaction is related to iron is unclear.

An interaction also occurs between selenium and the amino acid *methionine*. Because dietary selenium can be found as selenomethionine, and, as such, is readily bioavailable in most organisms, the potency of selenium in this form may be reduced if a situation of methionine deficiency exists [4]. The explanation for this observation is that if methionine is deficient, seleno-methionine substitutes for it in the synthesis of body proteins [4,16]. Selenium then becomes available only as these proteins subsequently become degraded in the course of normal turnover.

Excretion

The major routes of selenium excretion are urinary (50 to 67% of total amount excreted) and fecal (40 to 50% of total excretory output). Renal clearance comparison studies on people having a low body store of selenium and on those with much higher levels indicate that the kidneys play an important role in selenium homeostasis in humans [17]. Only a few (for example, trimethyl se-lenonium ion) of the several metabolites of selenium have been identified in the urine.

With excessive selenium intake, selenium loss from the body may occur by the skin and lungs. Pulmonary elimination of selenium occurs with exhalation of a volatile (garlicky smell) selenium compound, dimethylselenide [$(CH_3)_2Se$].

Recommended Dietary Allowance

Balance studies as well as repletion studies of men with selenium deficiency in regions of China have aided researchers in the formulation of a RDA for selenium. The balance study technique alone is of little help in determining the selenium requirements of humans, because humans can seemingly adjust their selenium homeostatic mechanisms to remain in balance despite a wide range of dietary intakes. Results of balance studies by Levander [18] at the U.S. Department of Agriculture found fecal and urinary selenium losses were about 82 μg and 62 μg in men and women, respectively; selenium intake of the men and women was 90 μg and 74 μg, respectively. In the repletion studies, the selenium requirement was estimated to be 10 μg selenium to prevent Keshan disease (described in the Deficiency section that follows), while intake of 40 μg/day improved and plateaued glutathione peroxidase activity [18]. A so-called physiological requirement, based on the amount of dietary selenium required to maximize plasma glutathione peroxidase activity, is thus considered to be 40 μg/day. Following corrections for body weight and individual variation, this method resulted in a recommended dietary selenium intake of 70 and 55 μg/day for adult male and females, respectively, in the United States [18,19].

Deficiency

Selenium deficiency has been linked to a number of livestock animal diseases, and also to regional human diseases such as Keshan disease and Kashin-Beck's disease in China [20]. Keshan disease is characterized by cardiomyopathy involving cardiogenic shock and/or congestive heart failure, along with multifocal necrosis of heart tissue, which becomes replaced with fibrous tissue [20]. Kashin-Beck's disease is characterized by osteoarthropathy involving degeneration and necrosis of the joints and epiphyseal-plate cartilages of the legs and arms [20]. Several factors, including selenium deficiency, are thought to contribute to the development of Kashin-Beck's disease.

Selenium deficiency has also been observed in people receiving total parenteral nutrition [21–23]. Predominant symptoms of deficiency included muscle pain and weakness, along with loss of pigmentation of hair and skin, and whitening of nail beds.

A possible connection between selenium deficiency and cardiovascular disease and cancer has been postulated. In short, such studies are inconclusive, but are summarized thoroughly in the review by Levander [24–25].

Toxicity

The suggested maximum for selenium intake as inorganic salts is about 550 μg per day, and slightly higher intakes of 775 μg from seleniferous foods and/or organic selenium compounds [1]. Intakes of 750 μg per day may result in biochemical abnormalities and intakes of 27.3 mg or more per day have produced physical manifestations [19]. Selected signs and symptoms of toxicity include nausea, vomiting, fatigue, hair and nail loss, changes in nail beds, and interference in sulfur metabolism (primarily oxidation of sulfhydryl groups), and inhibition of protein synthesis [19,26].

Assessment of Nutriture

Serum or plasma selenium concentrations are thought to be indicative of short-term changes in dietary selenium intake and will respond more quickly to changes in selenium intake or supplementation than whole-blood selenium. Whole-blood selenium or red blood cell selenium represents an index of longer-term selenium status than plasma [19], and is useful for populations with habitually low selenium intakes.

The activity of glutathione peroxidase in platelets is also used as an indicator of selenium status [27]. The enzyme in platelets has a relatively rapid turnover, a high selenium content, and enzyme activity responds rapidly to changes in selenium intake [3]. Enzyme activity plateaus, however, as intake increases therefore serving as an index of selenium status in populations with low intake [19]. Good correlations between blood or plasma selenium concentration (up to a concentration of about 1.0 μmol/L) and glutathione peroxidase activity in red blood cells has been shown and suggests that plasma selenium can be used to assess selenium status as long as plasma selenium is less than 1 μmol/L [28]. Toenail clippings have also been suggested as being reflective of selenium status six to nine months prior to sampling; however, further studies are needed for validation [29]. Urinary selenium concentrations most appropriately identify selenium toxicity.

References Cited for Selenium

1. Combs GF, Combs SB. The role of selenium in nutrition. Orlando: Academic Press, 1986.
2. Levander OA. A global view of human selenium nutrition. Ann Rev Nutr 1987;7:227–250.
3. Levander OA. Considerations in the design of selenium bioavailability studies. Fed Proc 1983;42:1721–1725.
4. Forbes RM, Erdman JW. Bioavailability of trace mineral elements. Ann Rev Nutr 1983;3:213–231.
5. McAdam PA, Lewis SA, et al. Absorption of selenite and L-selenomethionine in healthy young men, using a ^{74}Se tracer. Fed Proc 1985;44:1671.
6. Thomson CD, Robinson MF. Urinary and fecal excretions and absorption of a large supplement of selenium: Superiority of selenate over selenite. Am J Clin Nutr 1986;44:659–663.
7. Burk RF, Hill KE. Regulation of selenoproteins. Ann Rev Nutr 1993;13:65–81.
8. Motsenbocker MA, Tappel AL. A selenocystine containing selenium transport protein in rat plasma. Biochim Biophys Acta 1982;719:147–153.
9. Evenson JK, Sunde RA. Selenium incorporation into seleno proteins in the selenium-adequate and selenium-deficient rat. Proc Soc Exp Biol Med 1988;187:169–180.
10. Whanger PD, Butler JA. Effects of various dietary levels of selenium as selenite or selenomethionine on tissue selenium levels and glutathione peroxidase activity in rats. J Nutr 1988;118:846–852.
11. Stadtman TC. Selenium biochemistry. Ann Rev Biochem 1990;59:111–127.
12. Avissar N, Ornt DB, Yagil Y, Horowitz S, Watkins RH, Kerl EA, Takahashi K, Palmer IS, Cohen HJ. Glutathione peroxidase activity in human plasma originates mainly from kidney proximal tubular cells. FASEB J 1993;7:A277.
13. Neatherly MW, Miller WJ, Gentry RP, et al. Influence of high dietary lead on selenium metabolism in dairy calves. J Dairy Sci 1987;70:645–652.
14. Moriarty PM, Picciano MF, Beard J, Reddy CC. Iron deficiency decreases Se-GPX mRNA level in the liver and impairs selenium utilization in other tissues. FASEB J 1993;7:A277.
15. Olin KL, Walter RM, Keen CL. Copper deficiency affects selenoglutathione peroxidase and selenodeiodinase activities and antioxidant defense in weanling rats. Am J Clin Nutr 1994;59:654–658.
16. Waschulewski IH, Sunde RA. Effect of dietary methionine on utilization of tissue selenium from dietary selenomethionine for glutathione peroxidase in the rat. J Nutr 1988;119:367–374.
17. Robinson JR, Robinson MF, Levander OA, Thomson CD. Urinary excretion of selenium by New Zealand and North American human subjects on different intakes. Am J Clin Nutr 1985;41:1023–1031.
18. Levander OA. Scientific rationale for the 1989 recommended dietary allowance for selenium. J Am Diet Assoc 1991;91:1572–1576.
19. National Research Council. Recommended dietary allowances, 10th ed. Washington, DC: National Academy Press, 1989;217–224.
20. Ge K, Yang G. The epidemiology of selenium deficiency in the etiological study of endemic diseases in China. Am J Clin Nutr 1993;57:259S–263S.
21. Abrams CK, Siram SM, Galsim C, Johnson-Hamilton H, Munford FL, Mezghebe H. Selenium deficiency in long-term total parenteral nutrition. Nutr Clin Prac 1992;7:175–178.
22. van Rij AM, Thomson CD, McKenzie JM, Robinson MF. Selenium deficiency in total parenteral nutrition. Am J Clin Nutr 1979;32:2076–2085.
23. Vinton NE, Dahlstrom KA, Strobel CT, Ament ME. Macrocytosis and pseudoalbinism: Manifestations of selenium deficiency. J Pediatr 1987;111:711–717.
24. Levander OA. Selenium. In: Mertz W, ed. Trace elements in human and animal nutrition. Orlando, FL: Academic Press, 1986;2:209–279.
25. Virtamo J, Huttunen JK. Minerals, trace elements, and cardiovascular disease. Ann Clin Res 1988;20:102–113.
26. Lane HW, Lotspeich CA, Moore CE, Ballard J, Dudrick SJ, Warren DC. The effect of selenium supplementation on selenium status of patients receiving chronic total parenteral nutrition. JPEN 1987;11:177–182.
27. Neve J, Vertongen F, Capel P. Selenium supplementation in healthy Belgian adults: Response in platelet glutathione peroxidase activity and other blood indices. Am J Clin Nutr 1988;48:139–143.
28. Diplock AT. Indexes of selenium status in human populations. Am J Clin Nutr 1993;57:256S–258S.
29. Ovaskainen ML, Virtamo J, Alfthan G, Haukka J, Pietinen P, Taylor PR, Huttunen JK. Toenail selenium as an indicator of selenium intake among middle-aged men in an area with low soil selenium. Am J Clin Nutr 1993;57:662–665.

Additional Reference

Arthur JR, ed. Interrelationships between selenium deficiency, iodine deficiency, and thyroid hormones. Am J Clin Nutr 1993;57:235S–318S.

CHROMIUM

Chromium, a metal, exists in several oxidation states, from Cr^{-2} to Cr^{+6}. Cr^{+3} is the most stable of the oxidation states and is thought to be of the most importance in humans [1].

Sources

In foods, most chromium exists in the trivalent form (Cr^{+3}). The better sources of chromium are thought to include meats (especially organ meats) and whole grains [2]. Other foods providing relatively high amounts of chromium include cheese, mushrooms, prunes, nuts, asparagus, beer, and wine [2]. Brewer's yeast is notable because of its high suspected content of the biologically active organic form of chromium known as *glucose tolerance factor (GTF)* [3].

Numerous analytic difficulties and biological uncertainties have been associated with the determination of chromium in food. Therefore, existing values for total chromium in foods should be considered qualitative rather than quantitative. Thus, these values allow only relative comparisons of chromium intake.

Food processing and refining can cause certain foods such as grains, cereals, and sugar cane to lose most of their chromium [2]. In contrast, the preparation of foods in stainless steel cookware may increase the amount of the mineral available for ingestion [2]. Chromium is leached from stainless steel, particularly by the action of acid foods [2].

Absorption and Transport

Chromium is thought to be absorbed throughout the small intestine, especially in the jejunum [4]. The mode of absorption is thought to be carrier mediated, with diffusion contributing to absorption with high intakes of the mineral.

Absorption appears to differ between the two forms of the mineral found in food. The absorption of inorganic Cr^{+3} seems to be poor, with reported values ranging from 0.4 to 2% [1,2]. About 1.8% of chromium was absorbed in two humans from a mixed diet containing about 37 μg chromium [5]. The biologically active organic complex of chromium (known as *glucose tolerance factor*) apparently is absorbed by animals at a much higher rate (10 to 25%) [6], but it is uncertain whether humans possess that same efficiency of absorption [1,2]. Although high rates of absorption of the organic complex by humans have been proposed, much of the evidence presented for the increased absorbability has been circumstantial [3].

In the blood, inorganic Cr^{+3} binds competitively with transferrin, and is transported in the blood along with iron bound to transferrin. If transferrin sites are unavailable for chromium, albumin along with globulins and possibly lipoproteins are thought to transport the mineral [1]. Chromium may be stored with ferric iron due to its transport by iron-rich transferrin [1].

Exactly how the organically complexed chromium is transported in the blood is uncertain, but it is rapidly available to cells after absorption. Moreover, only the organically complexed chromium (GTF) is active; therefore, absorbed inorganic chromium must be transported to a site where its incorporation into the organic complex can occur. The liver is proposed as a possible site for the synthesis of the metabolically active molecule [7], and use of the inorganic chromium for potentiation of insulin action is delayed until organic complexing has occurred [1,2,7].

Metabolically active chromium is believed to be held in a body pool from which the active molecule can be released for use as needed. The adult body pool size is estimated to be approximately 4 to 6 mg [8]. Organically complexed chromium in food can enter this body pool immediately on absorption. Tissues high in chromium include the kidney, liver, muscle, spleen, heart, pancreas, and bone.

Functions

The biological action of chromium is believed due to its complexing with nicotinic acid and amino acids to form the organic compound glucose tolerance factor (GTF). GTF is thought to initiate the disulfide bridging between insulin and the insulin receptor (Fig. 12.13). The

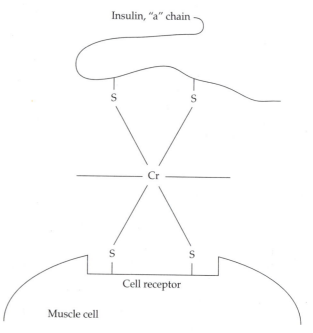

FIGURE 12.13 Proposed interaction of Cr as part of GTF to insulin and cell's insulin receptor. *(Modified from Mertz W, Toepfer EW, Roginski EE, Polansky MM. Present knowledge of the role of chromium. Fed Proc 1974;33:2276.)*

effectiveness of insulin is greater in the presence of chromium than in its absence [9]. Thus the primary function of GTF is to potentiate insulin action, thereby affecting cellular glucose uptake, and intracellular carbohydrate and lipid metabolism.

GTF was first identified in brewer's yeast. Although this factor has never been purified or its exact structure characterized, complexes with good biological activity have been synthesized from niacin, chromium, and glutathione. None of the synthetic complexes, however, exactly duplicate the naturally occurring organically complexed chromium. Moreover, absorption and transport of the synthetic products are less efficient than that of the naturally occurring complex [1,2]. Nevertheless, the belief remains that the biologically active molecule is a dinicotinato chromium complex coordinated with amino acids that stabilize the complex. Mertz [7] proposed that the initial product of *in vivo* synthesis is a tetra-aquo dinicotinato chromium complex, as shown in Figure 12.14. Because this complex is unstable in the alkaline pH of the organism, Mertz proposed that the coordinated

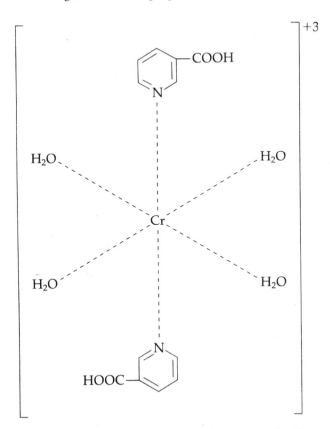

FIGURE 12.14 Tetra-aquo-di-nicotinato chromium complex. Water molecules are believed to be replaced by amino acids (glutamic acid, cysteine, and glycine) to stabilize the complex. *(From Nutrition Reviews 33(1975):129–135. © International Life Sciences Institute-Nutrition Foundation. Used with permission.)*

water molecules are replaced by ligands (amino acids), thereby stabilizing the complex and preventing its precipitation. The amino acids acting as ligands are believed to be those making up glutathione (glutamic acid, cysteine, and glycine). The exact coordination of the amino acids with the chromium is uncertain.

GTF, contained in a body pool, is believed by Mertz [7] to resemble a hormone being released into the blood in response to a physiologic stimulus. In the case of chromium, the stimulus is insulin. After release from the body pool, the active Cr^{+3} as GTF is transported to the periphery, where it exerts a marked biological action by potentiating the action of insulin. The failure to identify the precise action of GTF in potentiation of insulin activity has, however, raised a question about the essentiality of chromium. Although the insulin receptor has been purified and characterized, no evidence has been uncovered for chromium as a component of the receptor's subunits, as part of an accessory protein for insulin binding, or as a second messenger in mediating the effect of insulin [8].

Chromium may have additional roles, or may exhibit its influence through the actions of insulin. Roles particularly in *lipid metabolism* have been suggested for chromium. For example, chromium may affect lipoprotein lipase activity and in some unknown way affect cholesterol metabolism [1,2]. Several studies have reported improvements in blood lipid profiles of people following chromium supplementation. Significant increases in blood HDL cholesterol along with decreases in total and LDL cholesterol concentrations have been demonstrated with chromium supplementation [9]. The mechanism by which chromium exerts its effects requires further research.

Another proposed role for chromium is in relation to *nucleic acid metabolism*. It is postulated that Cr^{+3} is involved in maintaining the structural integrity of nuclear strands and in the regulation of gene expression [2]. RNA synthesis *in vitro* as directed by DNA is enhanced by chromium binding to the template [1].

Excretion

Chromium released into the plasma in response to a glucose challenge is excreted from the body via the kidneys. Although urinary chromium normally appears to average less than 1 µg daily, this amount represents about 95% of the daily chromium excretion [1]. Consumption of diets high in simple sugars (35% simple sugars, 15% complex carbohydrates) has been shown to raise urinary chromium in some subjects to 300%, in contrast to consumption of diets high in complex (starch) carbohydrates (35% complex carbohydrates, 15% simple sugars) [2,10].

Estimated Safe and Adequate Daily Dietary Intake

The estimated safe and adequate intake for chromium was first reported in the 1980 edition of the RDA [2,11]. Ingestion of 200 μg chromium per day has been proposed based on the following. First, the daily losses of chromium approximate 1 μg/day. Second, an absorbability of only 0.5% is assumed to occur with ingestion of inorganic chromium. Thus, ingestion of 200 μg chromium per day with 0.5% absorbability would provide the 1 μg needed to replenish losses. However, because food chromium is believed to be a mixture of inorganic and organic forms of the mineral, absorption of chromium is likely to exceed 0.5%.

In the 1989 edition of the RDA, a recommended estimated safe and adequate daily dietary intake range for chromium of 50 to 200 μg/day is given for adults and adolescents. This recommendation is based on the fact that the average intake of 50 μg/day appears sufficient to prevent signs of chromium deficiency in most of the U.S. population [11].

Deficiency

According to Anderson [12], signs and symptoms of chromium deficiency in the general population appear widespread. Concern has existed about chromium nutriture in the United States because (1) some segments of the population (especially the elderly) are consuming less than the recommended chromium intake [13,14]; (2) tissue chromium levels appear to decline with age; and (3) the evidence of impaired glucose tolerance increases among the aged [13]. Metabolic balance studies, carried out to learn more about the daily intake and requirement of chromium by healthy elderly people, revealed that intakes well under 50 μg/day were sufficient for chromium equilibrium among most subjects [13]. The conclusion of the authors is that the healthy elderly must have chromium absorption rates exceeding 2%; therefore, chromium intake less than the safe and adequate range suggested in the 1980 RDA issue may be acceptable.

Chromium needs may very well be increased in certain diseases, such as diabetes and coronary heart disease, although a link between chromium and these diseases is not conclusive [2,15]. Chromium deficiency results in insulin resistance characterized by hyperinsulinemia. Hyperinsulinemia has been implicated as a risk factor for coronary heart disease [16]. Mild chromium deficiency also has been shown to be a risk factor for a group of symptoms (except hypertension) similar to Syndrome X [17]. Syndrome X represents a constellation of abnormalities that increase the risk of coronary heart disease and include hyperinsulinemia, resistance to insulin-stimulated glucose uptake, glucose intolerance, hypertriglyceridemia, decreased blood HDL concentrations, and hypertension [18].

Severe trauma and stress appear to increase the need for chromium. Stress, for example, elevates the secretion of hormones, which alters glucose metabolism, and apparently affects chromium metabolism [15].

In people receiving total parenteral nutrition without chromium, symptoms of deficiency included impaired glucose tolerance with high blood glucose and glucose excretion in the urine, neuropathy, high-plasma free fatty acid concentrations, among others.

Toxicity

Oral supplementation with chromium up to 800 μg appears to be safe [1,2,11]. The danger of toxicity seems to be associated with exposure to industrial hexavalent forms (Cr^{+6}) of chromium that may be absorbed through the skin or that may enter the body through inhalation [2]. Inhalation or direct contact with hexavalent chromium may result in respiratory disease, and in dermatitis and skin ulcerations, respectively. Liver damage may also occur.

Assessment of Nutriture

No specific tests are currently available to determine chromium status prior to supplementation [9]. Although a chromium plasma level of approximately 0.5 ng/mL is considered normal, the chromium content of physiologic fluids is not indicative of status [19]. Fasting plasma chromium is not in equilibrium with tissue chromium. Responses of plasma chromium to an oral glucose load are inconsistent. Urinary chromium also appears to reflect recent intake, but does not reflect status [19]. Hair chromium concentrations may indicate the status of a large population, but not of individuals [9].

Relative chromium status can be evaluated retrospectively through following the effects of chromium supplementation on adults. Adult subjects, showing improvement in glucose (lower plasma glucose) and/or lipid parameters (such as increased HDL, decreased total and LDL cholesterol concentrations) after supplementation with approximately 200 μg chromium/day for one to three months, can be considered as having been in a marginally low chromium status [20].

References Cited for Chromium

1. Nielsen FH. Chromium. In: Shils ME, Olson JA, Shike M., eds. Modern nutrition in health and disease. Philadelphia: Lea and Febiger, 1994;264–268.

2. Stoecker BJ. Chromium. In: Brown ML, ed. Present knowledge in nutrition. Washington, DC: International Life Sciences Institute Nutrition Foundation, 1990;287–293.

3. Forbes RM, Erdman JW Jr. Bioavailability of trace mineral elements. Ann Rev Nutr 1983;3:213–231.

4. Anderson RA. Chromium. In: Mertz W, ed. Trace elements in human and animal nutrition, 5th ed. San Diego: Academic Press, 1987;1:225–244.

5. Offenbacher EG, Spencer H, Dowling HJ, Pi-Sunyer FX. Metabolic chromium balances in men. Am J Clin Nutr 1986;44:77–82.

6. Ware GW. Reviews of environmental contamination and toxicology. New York: Springer-Verlag, 1989;107:34–52.

7. Mertz W. Effects and metabolism of glucose tolerance factor. Nutr Rev 1975;33:129–135.

8. Is chromium essential for humans? Nutr Rev 1988;46: 17–20.

9. Mertz W. Chromium in human nutrition: A review. J Nutr 1993; 123:626–633.

10. Kozlovsky AS, Moser PB, Reiser S, et al. Effects of diets high in simple sugars on urinary chromium losses. Metabolism 1986;35:515–518.

11. National Research Council. Recommended dietary allowances, 10th ed. Washington, DC: National Academy Press, 1989;241–243.

12. Anderson RA. Recent advances in the clinical and biochemical effects of chromium deficiency. In: Prasad AS, ed. Essential and toxic trace elements in human health and disease: An update. New York: Wiley-Liss, 1993;221–234.

13. Bunker VW, Lawson MS, Delves HT et al. The uptake and excretion of chromium by the elderly. Am J Clin Nutr 1984;39:797–802.

14. Anderson RA, Kozlovsky A. Chromium intake, absorption, and excretion of subjects consuming self-selected diets. Am J Clin Nutr 1985;41:1177–1183.

15. Nielsen FH. Nutritional significance of the ultratrace minerals. Nutr Rev 1988;46:337–341.

16. Zavaroni I, Bonora E, Pagliara M, Dall'aglio E, Luchetti L, Buonanno G, Bonati PA, Bergonzani M, Gnudi L, Passeri M, Reaven G. Risk factors for coronary artery disease in healthy persons with hyperinsulinemia and normal glucose tolerance. N Eng J Med 1989;320:702–706.

17. Reaven GM. The role of insulin resistance and hyperinsulinemia in coronary heart disease. Metabolism 1992:41: 16–19.

18. Reaven GM. The role of insulin resistance in human disease. Diabetes 1988;37:1595–1607.

19. Anderson RA, Polansky MM, Bryden NA, Patterson KY, Veillon C, Glinsmann WH. Effects of chromium supplementation on urinary chromium excretion of human subjects and correlation of chromium excretion with selected clinical parameters. J Nutr 1983;113:276–281.

20. Anderson RA, Polasky MM, Bryden NA, Canary JJ. Supplemental chromium effects on glucose, insulin, glucagon, and urinary chromium losses in subjects consuming controlled low chromium diets. Am J Clin Nutr 1991;54:909–916.

IODINE

Iodine is typically found and functions in its ionic form iodide. Hence the term *iodide* is used throughout this discussion of the trace element. Iodide, which is not a metal, is one of the heaviest elements in living organisms. About 15 to 20 mg iodide is found in the human body [1].

Sources

The iodide concentration in human foods is extremely variable because, as is so often the case, it reflects the regionally variable soil concentrations of the element and the amount and nature of fertilizer used in plant cultivation. The amount of iodide in the drinking water is an indication of the iodide content of the rocks and soils of a region, and it parallels closely the incidence of iodine deficiency among the inhabitants of that region. Numerous investigations, spanning decades, have demonstrated unequivocally the relationship of low levels of iodide in drinking water to the incidence of goiter (see section on iodine deficiency). One such study, by Karmarkar et al. [2], found that the iodide content of water from goitrous areas in India, Nepal, and Ceylon ranged from 0.1 to 1.2 μg/L compared to 9.0 μg/L found in nongoitrous Delhi [1,2].

Seafood is particularly rich in iodide; however, large differences in content exist between seawater and freshwater fish. Edible sea fish may contain from 300 to 3,000 μg I/kg, in contrast to only 20 to 40 μg I/kg freshwater fish.

An additional source of iodide is from breads and grain products made from bread dough. Dough oxidizers or conditioners contain iodates (IO_3^-) as food additives to improve cross-linking of the gluten. Such iodates provide about 500 μg I^- per 100 g bread [3].

Digestion, Absorption, and Transport

Dietary iodine (I) is primarily in the form of iodide (I^-) or is converted to iodide in the gastrointestinal tract. For example, iodate is reduced to iodide by glutathione [4]. Iodates are found in bread.

Iodide is absorbed rapidly and completely throughout the gastrointestinal tract, including the stomach. Very little iodide appears in the feces. The small quantities of iodinated amino acids and other organic forms of iodide are absorbed, but not as efficiently as the iodide ion. The thyroid hormones thyroxine (T_4) and triiodothyronine (T_3) also are absorbed unchanged, therefore allowing T_4 medication to be administered orally.

Following absorption, free iodide appears in the blood (Fig. 12.15). Iodide is distributed throughout the

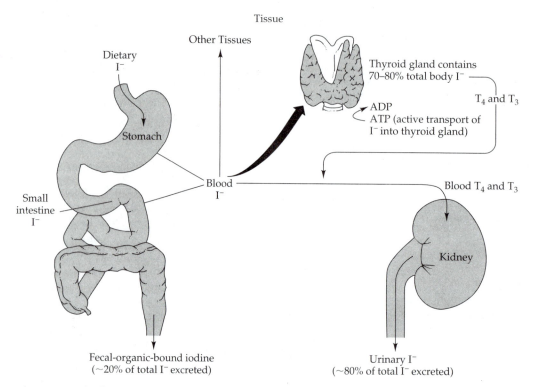

FIGURE 12.15 Overview of iodine metabolism.

extracellular fluid from which it is capable of permeating all tissues. The element selectively concentrates, however, in the thyroid, salivary, and gastric glands. Lesser amounts of iodide are found in mammary glands, ovaries, placenta, and skin. It is the thyroid gland that traps iodide most aggressively, doing so by way of a sodium-dependent, active transport system against an iodide gradient that is often 40 to 50 times the plasma concentration. The thyroid gland contains 70 to 80% of the total body iodide and takes up about 120 μg iodide per day.

Since the thyroid gland and its synthesis of the thyroid hormones are the focal points of iodide metabolism, information on the transport of iodide into nonthyroidal tissue is sparse. It is likely, however, that salivary gland uptake proceeds by an active transport mechanism similar to that of the thyroid [5].

Functions

The main function of iodide is for the synthesis of the thyroid hormones by the thyroid gland. The thyroid gland is made of multiple acini, also called *follicles*. The follicles are spherical in shape and are surrounded by a single layer of thyroid cells. The follicles are filled with colloid, a proteinaceous material. The thyroid cells collect the iodide actively. The thyroid gland must trap approximately 60 μg of iodide daily against a steep gradient of the element to ensure an adequate supply of hormones [1]. Figure 12.16 illustrates the synthesis of thyroid hormones. The trapping mechanism operates through a Na^+ (in)–K^+ (out) ATPase pump, confirmed in studies on transport in plasma membrane vesicles [6]. Also occurring within the thyroid cells is the synthesis of thyroglobulin (a glycoprotein), the oxidation of iodide (I^-) to iodine (I), and the binding of iodine to the number 3 position of tyrosyl residues of thyroglobulin (a process called "organification" of the iodine). The binding of iodine to the tyrosyl residue of thyroglobulin is catalyzed by thyroid peroxidase and generates 3-monoiodotyrosine (MIT) (Fig. 12.16b). Hydrogen peroxide acts as the electron acceptor. MIT is iodinated in the number 5 position to form 3,5-di-iodotyrosine (DIT). In the colloid, two DIT condense or couple to form 3,5,3′,5′-tetraiodothyronine (T_4) (Fig. 12.16b) with the elimination of an alanine side chain. Small amounts of DIT condense with MIT to form 3,5,3′-tri-iodothyronine (T_3) (Fig. 12.16b) and reverse (r) T_3.

To release the thyroid hormones into the blood, iodothyroglobulin must be resorbed in the form of col-

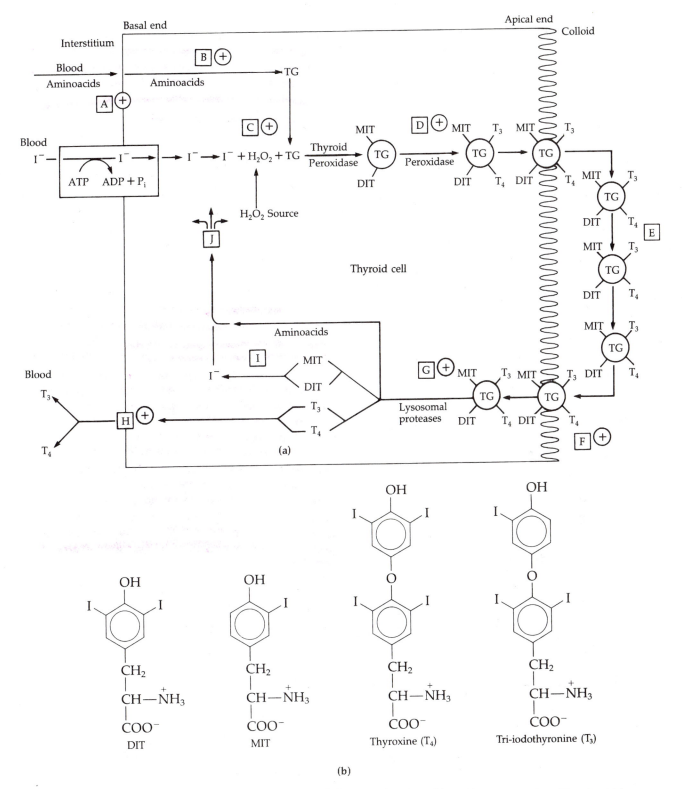

FIGURE 12.16 (a) Schematic representation of a thyroid cell illustrating the stages of thyroid hormonogenesis and intrathyroidal iodine metabolism. Symbols: A, iodine transport; B, thyroglobulin (TG) synthesis; C, iodine organification; D, intrathyroglobulin coupling; E, storage; F, endocytosis; G, hydrolysis; H, hormone secretion; I, intrathyroidal deiodination; J, recycling; the steps influenced by the thyroid-stimulating hormone (TSH) are represented by the symbol ⊕ Structures of MIT, DIT, T₃, and T₄ are shown in (b).

loid droplets by endocytosis back into the thyroid cell. Within the thyroid cell, the iodothyroglobulin is hydrolyzed by lysosomal proteases, and T_4 and T_3 are released into the blood. In the blood, T_4 and T_3 associate with transport proteins, and are distributed to target cells in peripheral tissues. Thyroid-binding globulin, found in the plasma, has the smallest capacity, but the greatest affinity for T_4 and T_3. Albumin and transthyretin (formerly called *prealbumin*) also transport the thyroid hormones. A very small fraction ($< 0.1\%$) of the blood T_4 and T_3 is not bound to transport proteins, and it is this free form that is available to the cell receptors, and therefore is hormonally active. The plasma concentration of T_4 is nearly 50 times that of T_3, and therefore is considered to be the major thyroid hormone, despite the fact that T_3 is many times more potent on an equal molar basis. For a more in-depth review of thyroid hormone synthesis, the reader is referred to the review by Taurog [7].

DIT and MIT not used for thyroid hormone synthesis in the thyroid cells are deiodinated, and the iodine is made available for recycling in the formation of new iodothyroglobulin. Several tissues, the liver, kidney, brain, pituitary, and brown adipose tissue to name a few, can deiodinate T_4 to generate T_3 and rT_3. Most T_3 in the blood has been synthesized in the liver from T_4. A 5'-selenium-dependent deiodinase generates T_3, and a 5-deiodinase generates rT_3. Conversion of T_4 to T_3 is impaired with selenium deficiency.

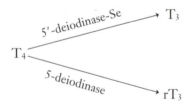

The multiple effects of the thyroid hormones result from the hormones' occupancy of nuclear receptors, with subsequent effects on gene expression. The receptors appear to be the same in all tissues, binding T_3 more avidly than T_4 and requiring fivefold to sevenfold higher concentrations of T_4 to achieve comparable physiologic effects. Zinc may play a role in the binding of the zinc fingers of the receptor protein (which in turn is influenced by thyroid hormones) to the DNA.

Although mechanisms of action of the thyroid hormones are unclear, biological effects are in response to increased messenger RNA (mRNA) and protein synthesis triggered by the hormone receptor attachment. Numerous hypotheses for mechanisms have been proposed, including modulation of (Na^+/K^+-ATPase) transport systems, of adrenergic receptor sensitivity, and of neu-

rotransmitters. The review by Sterling [8] provides more comprehensive reading on this topic.

Effects of thyroid hormones on metabolism are many and varied. They stimulate the basal rate of metabolism, oxygen (O_2) consumption, and heat production, and they are necessary for normal nervous system development and linear growth. Directly or indirectly, most organ systems are under the influence of these substances.

Interactions with Other Nutrients

The discovery that *selenium* was required for 5'-deiodinase has prompted a flurry of research, as reviewed in the February 1993 supplement of the *American Journal of Clinical Nutrition* [9]. Interactions between iodine and *arsenic* are discussed on page 412–413.

A more established interaction is that between iodide and goitrogens. Substances that interfere with iodide metabolism in any way that inhibits thyroid hormonogenesis are termed *goitrogens* because their effect is to secondarily augment TSH release and consequently thyroid gland enlargement. Goitrogens may affect iodide uptake by the gland, organification of the iodide, or hormone release from the thyroid cells.

Most goitrogenic compounds act by competing with iodide in its active transport process into the thyroid cells. Halide ions such as bromide (Br^-) and astatide (At^-) function in this way, as do thiocyanate (SCN^-), perrhenate (ReO_4^-), and pertechnetate (TcO_4). Perchlorate (ClO_4^-), along with perrhenate, and pertechnetate interfere with organification as well as uptake; and lithium (Li^-), used to treat some psychiatric disorders, inhibits hormone release from the gland.

That some natural foods are goitrogenic was evidenced many years ago when it was discovered that rabbits fed a fresh cabbage diet developed goiters that could be reversed by iodine supplementation. It was later shown that vegetables of the cabbage family contained, along with small quantities of thiocyanates, a potent goitrogen that later became known as *goitrin* (Fig. 12.17).

FIGURE 12.17 Goitrin.

A long list of edible plants contain goitrin, including cabbage, kale, cauliflower, broccoli, rutabaga, turnips, brussels sprouts, and mustard greens. It is doubtful, however, if these foods are consumed in sufficient quantity to implicate them in the etiology of endemic goiter. Perhaps the only food to be identified directly with goiter etiology is cassava, which is consumed in large quantities in Third World countries [10]. It contains cyanogen glucosides, of which thiocyanates are a major metabolite.

Excretion

The kidneys have no mechanism to conserve iodide, and therefore provide the major route (about 80 to 90%) for iodide excretion. The urinary output of iodide correlates closely with the plasma iodide concentration and in fact has been used to monitor iodide status in populations. For example, it has been suggested that iodide excretion of 50 μg I/g creatinine in a representative sample of a population is indicative of endemic goiter within that population [11].

Fecal excretion of iodide (up to 20% of the total excreted) in humans is relatively low, ranging from 6.7 to 42.1 μg/day [12]. Some iodide is also lost in sweat, and this can be of consequence in hot, tropical regions where iodide intake is marginally adequate.

Recommended Dietary Allowance

Because of its important link to thyroid function, iodide nutriture has been investigated thoroughly for over half a century. Dating as far back as the 1930s, results of intake requirements have been published based on balance studies and on calculations of average daily urinary losses. Adult daily requirements established by those early studies were in the range of 100 to 200 μg. The estimates have not changed significantly over the years. The 1989 RDA is 150 μg/day for adults of both sexes and provides a margin of safety to allow for unquantified levels of goitrogens in the diet [3]. Although the recommendations apply equally to both sexes, iodide needs are higher during pregnancy and lactation. The minimum amount (requirement) of iodide to prevent goiter is estimated between 50 to 75 μg/day or about 1 μg I/kg body weight.

Deficiency

Thyroid Hormone Release as Related to Iodide Deficiency The release of thyroid hormones by the thyroid gland is controlled. Thyrotropin-releasing hormone released from the hypothalamus acts on the pituitary gland to stimulate thyroid-stimulating hormone (TSH). TSH, in response to thyrotropin-releasing hormone, is secreted from the anterior pituitary and increases the activity of the thyroid gland. Simple goiter is associated most often with dietary insufficiency of iodine and is characterized by enlargement of the thyroid gland. Enlargement of the thyroid gland is caused by its overstimulation by TSH, the output of which is regulated by T_4 through negative feedback to the pituitary. Iodine deficiency causes depletion of thyroid iodine stores, and therefore reduced output of T_4 and T_3. The decline in the blood level of T_4 triggers release of pituitary TSH, resulting in hyperplasia of the thyroid. The growth of the gland is self-restricting, however, because in its enlarged state it traps and processes available iodide more efficiently. The gland returns to normal size as dietary iodine is increased to adequate amounts.

Iodine Deficiency and Iodine Deficiency Disorders Iodine deficiency prevails in many areas of the world, and is associated most often with dietary insufficiency of iodine. Iodine deficiency is the main cause of goiter (although other factors such as ingestion of goitrogens may cause the disorder). Goiter is characterized by enlargement of the thyroid gland, caused by its overstimulation by TSH as already discussed. Iodide deficiency causes depletion of thyroid iodine stores and therefore reduced output of T_4 and T_3. The decline in the blood level of T_4 triggers release of pituitary TSH, resulting in hyperplasia of the thyroid gland. When the prevalence of goiter in any population exceeds 10%, it is called *endemic goiter* [13].

Because of the effects of iodide deficiency on growth, development, and other health problems, the term *iodide deficiency disorders* (IDD) has been implemented. Iodine deficiency in a fetus results from iodide deficiency of the mother; cretinism, of which there are two types, results. Neurologic cretinism is characterized in the infant by mental deficiency, hearing loss or deaf mutism, and motor disorders such as spasticity and muscular rigidity [1,13]. Hypothyroid cretinism results in thyroid failure.

The addition of iodide to table salt and the administration of iodized oil has done much to alleviate the problem of endemic goiter in some goitrous regions of the world. Yet iodide deficiency continues to be a major health problem in many underdeveloped countries, and in China may be coupled with selenium deficiency [14].

Toxicity

No adverse effects from iodide intakes of up to about 2 mg/day have been reported [1,3].

Assessment of Nutriture

Iodide nutritional status assessment is generally directed at populations living in areas suspected to be iodide deficient. The assessment is based on both the physical examination and chemical testing of individuals. The data collected for assessment studies are extensive and include at least the following:

- Total population count including the number of children <15 years of age
- The incidence of goiter as established by physical examination and cretinism in the population
- The quantification of urinary iodide excretion
- The quantification of iodide in the drinking water
- Determination of serum T_4 levels in various age groups

The chemistry of tests measuring urinary iodide excretion is based on the ability of iodide ion to reduce cerric ion, which is yellow, to its colorless, cerrous state as shown here:

$$2 \text{ iodide (I}^-) \longrightarrow I_2$$

$$2 \text{ cerric (Ce}^{+4}) \text{ (yellow)} \qquad 2 \text{ cerrous (Ce}^{+3}) \text{ (colorless)}$$

The extent of the color change, which is directly proportional to the iodide concentration in the specimen, is monitored spectrophotometrically. All iodine in the specimen, therefore, must first be reduced to iodide. Urinary iodine concentrations less than 50 μg/g creatinine are considered at risk [15]. However, the use of iodine–creatinine ratio in casual urine samples has been shown to be unsuitable as an indicator for evaluating iodine status in some populations [16].

Radioactive iodide (^{131}I) uptake may also be measured to assess thyroid function. The greater the overall uptake and the quicker the uptake of the radioactive iodide by the thyroid gland, the greater the likelihood of iodide deficiency [15].

References Cited for Iodine

1. Clugston GA, Hetzel BS. Iodine. In: Shils ME, Olson JA, Shike M., eds. Modern nutrition in health and disease. Philadelphia: Lea and Febiger, 1994;252–263.
2. Karmarkar MG, Deo MG, Kochupillai N, Ramalingaswami V. Pathophysiology of Himalayan endemic goiter. Am J Clin Nutr 1974;27:96–103.
3. National Research Council. Recommended dietary allowances, 10th ed. Washington, DC: National Academy Press, 1989;213–217.
4. Taurog A, Howells EM, Nachimson HI. Conversion of iodate to iodide in vitro and in vivo. J Biol Chem 1966;241:4686–4693.
5. Harden RMcG, Alexander WD, Shimmins J, Kostalas H, Mason DK. Quantitative aspects of the inhibitory effect of the iodide ion on parotid salivary iodide and pertechnetate secretion in man. J Lab Clin Med 1968;71:92–100.
6. O'Neill B, Magnolato D, Semenza G. The electrogenic, Na$^+$-dependent I$^-$ transport system in plasma membrane vesicles from thyroid glands. Biochim Biophys Acta 1987;896:263–274.
7. Taurog A. Hormone synthesis: Thyroid iodine metabolism. In: Ingbar SH, Braverman LE, eds. Werner's the thyroid. Philadelphia: Lippincott 1986;53–97.
8. Sterling K. Thyroid hormone action at the cellular level. In: Ingbar SH, Braverman LE, eds. Werner's the thyroid. Philadelphia: Lippincott 1986;219–233.
9. Arthur JR, ed. Interrelationships between selenium deficiency, iodine deficiency, and thyroid hormones. Am J Clin Nutr 1993; 57:235S–318S.
10. Maberly GF, Waite KV, Eastman CJ, et al. In: Ui N, Torizuka K, Nagataki A, et al., eds. Current problems in thyroid research. Amsterdam: Excerpta Medica 1983:341.
11. Stanbury JB, Ermans AM, Hetzel BS, et al. Endemic goitre and cretinism: Public health significance and prevention. WHO Chron 1974;28:220–228.
12. Vought RL, London WT, Lutwak L, Dublin TD. Reliability of estimates of serum inorganic iodine and daily fecal and urinary iodine excretion from single casual specimens. J Clin Endocr Metab 1963;23:1218–1228.
13. Lamberg BA. Iodine deficiency disorders and endemic goitre. Eur J Clin Nutr 1993;47:1–8.
14. Ma T, Guo J, Wang F. The epidemiology of iodine-deficiency diseases in China. Am J Clin Nutr 1993;57:264S–266S.
15. Gibson RS. Principles of nutritional assessment. New York: Oxford University Press, 1990;527–532.
16. Furnee CA, Haar FVD, West CE, Hautvast JGAJ. A critical appraisal of goiter assessment and the ratio of urinary iodine to creatinine for evaluating iodine status. Am J Clin Nutr 1994;59:1415–1417.

MANGANESE

Although widely distributed in nature, manganese occurs in only trace amounts in animal tissues. The body of a healthy 70-kg man is estimated to contain a total of 10 to 20 mg of the metal.

Sources

Whole-grain cereals, dried fruits, nuts, and leafy vegetables are among the manganese-rich common foods. Tea also contains large amounts of manganese; however, manganese in tea is not well absorbed [1,2]. A wide con-

Table 12.8 Manganese Content of Selected Food and Beverages

Food Group	Manganese Content (mg/100g)	
	Mean	Range
Cereals	0.677	0.24–1.4
Meat	0.059	0.035–0.11
Fish	0.085	0.045–0.13
Milk	<0.010	—
Fats	<0.020	—
Root vegetables	0.134	0.05–0.22
Other vegetables	0.151	0.10–0.22
Fruit and sugars	0.167	0.04–0.36
Beverages		
Beer	0.01	0.01–0.05
Wine		
White	0.88	0.03–2.34
Red	1.44	0.53–1.95
Coffee (instant)	2.0	1.3–3.9
Tea	61.0	35–90

Modified from: Wenlock RW, Buss DH, Dixon EJ. Trace nutrients. 2. Manganese in British food. Br J Nutr. 1979;41:253–261.

tent range of the mineral in cereal grains is due partly to plant species differences and partly to the efficiency with which the milling process separates the manganese-rich and manganese-poor parts of the grain. Patent flour, for example, has a much lower manganese concentration than the wheat grain from which it was produced. Table 12.8 lists the manganese contents of selected foods.

Absorption and Transport

Little information is available on the mechanism of manganese absorption, although it has been established that the process occurs equally well throughout the length of the small intestine [3]. Dietary manganese absorption varies considerably with values of 3% up to 50% reported. The absorption process itself appears to be quickly saturable and probably involves a low-capacity, high-affinity, active transport mechanism as demonstrated in rats [4–6]. Within the duodenum, ingested manganese as Mn^{+2} is thought to be converted to Mn^{+3} [4].

There is evidence for the enhancement of absorption by low molecular weight ligands such as histidine and citrate [6]. In addition, in a manner reminiscent of iron absorption in iron deficiency (p. 357), increased manganese absorption takes place when intake is low, and reduced absorption accompanies a high intake [4].

Animal studies suggest that fiber, phytate, oxalic acid, calcium, and phosphorus may precipitate the manganese, making it unavailable for absorption [2,6]. Iron competes

with manganese for absorption, and may thus inhibit its absorption if present in sufficient concentrations [3].

Manganese entering into the portal circulation from the gastrointestinal tract may either remain free or become bound as Mn^{+2} to α-2 macroglobulin before traversing the liver, where it is almost totally removed. From the liver, some Mn^{+2} may be oxidized by ceruloplasmin to Mn^{+3} and may complex with transferrin. Mn^{+3} bound to transferrin is taken up by extrahepatic tissues.

Manganese is cleared rapidly from the blood and accumulates preferentially in the mitochondria of tissues, a process that may be mediated by a Ca^{+2} carrier [7]. Within the mitochondria, manganese is present as hydrate Mn^{+2}, Mn^{+3}, and as $Mn_3(PO_4)_2$, a matrix precipitate [8]. Manganese is found in most organs and tissues, and does not tend to concentrate significantly in any particular one, although its concentration is highest in bone, liver, pancreas, and kidney. Hair can also accumulate manganese.

Functions

At the molecular level, manganese, like other trace elements, can function both as an enzyme activator and as a constituent of metalloenzymes, but the relationship of these functions to the gross physiologic changes observed in manganese deficiency is not well correlated. Reviews pertaining to this topic have been published [9].

In the activation of enzyme-catalyzed reactions, the metal can act by binding to the substrate (such as ATP) or to the enzyme directly, with induction of conformational changes. Enzymes that can be activated by manganese in this manner are numerous and diverse in function. They include hydrolases, kinases, decarboxylases, and transferases. The activity of most of these enzymes is not, however, affected by a manganese deficiency, largely because the activation is not manganese specific. The metal can be replaced by other divalent cations, primarily magnesium. One exception to this apparent lack of specificity is the manganese-specific activation of the glycosyl transferases that catalyze the transfer of a sugar moiety from uridine diphosphate (UDP) to an acceptor, as shown by the general reaction:

$$\text{UDP-sugar + acceptor} \xrightarrow{\text{glycosyl transferase}} \text{UDP + acceptor-sugar}$$

Manganese also activates prolidase, a dipeptidase with specificity for dipeptides, and phosphoenolpyruvate carboxykinase (PEPCK); in manganese-deficient animals, the activity of PEPCK was low [5].

Compared to the manganese-activated enzymes, there are few manganese metalloenzymes. They include arginase (containing four manganese atoms per molecule), the cytosolic enzyme responsible for urea formation (p. 172); pyruvate carboxylase, which also contains 4 manganese atoms and converts pyruvate to oxaloacetate (p. 92); and manganese-dependent superoxide dismutase (Mn-SOD), which like copper- and zinc-dependent SOD (p. 370), can prevent lipid peroxidation by superoxide radicals. Manganese SOD, however, is found in the mitochrondria, whereas copper zinc SOD is found in the cytoplasm. It is likely that the cell ultrastructural abnormalities associated with manganese deficiency may be due to unchecked lipid peroxidation in the cellular membranes due to reduced Mn-SOD activity [2]. Low-manganese diets in animals have been shown to decrease arginase and Mn-SOD activities; however, because magnesium can replace manganese in pyruvate carboxylase, minimal changes in pyruvate carboxylase (which converts pyruvate to oxaloacetate for gluconeogenesis) activity occur [5,10]. Glutamine synthetase (Fig. 7.14) may be a manganese metalloenzyme or simply activiated by manganese or magnesium [4,5].

Manganese may also act as a modulator of second messenger pathways in tissues. For example, manganese increases cAMP accumulation through binding to ATP and ADP. Manganese can activate guanylate cyclase, and manganese may affect cytoplasmic calcium levels and thus regulate calcium-dependent processes (see Fig. 11.3) [8].

Interactions with Other Nutrients

There are only a few interactions of manganese with other trace elements that may be of significance nutritionally. Among them, the manganese–*iron* interaction has received the most attention. Unequivocal symptoms of iron deficiency anemia have been found in the case of excessive manganese supply. When iron intake is inadequate, even a small excess of manganese may be sufficient to elicit symptoms of iron deficiency. However, in a person with normal iron status, the dietary manganese content would have to be extremely high, in the range of 500 to 2,000 mg/kg dry diet, to affect the iron status to the point of causing iron deficiency anemia [11].

The interaction of manganese and iron is at the level of absorption, at which competition for common binding sites occurs among manganese, iron, and cobalt ions. This explains why the absorption of manganese as well as iron is enhanced in situations in which iron deficiency is manifested. Likewise, the absorption and retention of manganese from foods low in iron, such as milk, is rela-

tively high; and if the milk is supplemented with iron, the absorption of manganese is then reduced [12].

Some degree of interaction between manganese and *calcium* and between manganese and *zinc* may also occur in such a way as to affect the bioavailability of manganese [13]. However, because of the paucity of information and the divergent results of some of the relevant studies, the nature of such interactions remains inconclusive.

Excretion

The homeostatic regulation of tissue manganese is chiefly by way of both biliary excretion and absorption (the latter was discussed previously). The mechanisms are interdependent, and their relative contribution in the overall excretion of manganese depends on the extent of dietary intake. Biliary excretion constitutes the major route of elimination under ordinary conditions, but if dietary overloading of manganese occurs, auxiliary gastrointestinal routes participate. In an overload situation, the excess manganese is apparently excreted into the duodenum and jejunum and, to a lesser extent, the terminal ileum [14]. There is an overall bile-to-plasma concentration ratio of greater than 150, suggesting that manganese transport into the bile must be active. To some extent the excretion of manganese also occurs by way of the pancreatic juice. This route assumes greater importance if the biliary tree is obstructed or if overloading with manganese occurs. Very little manganese is excreted in the urine, even when dietary intake of the mineral is excessive. However, excretion of manganese through the sweat and skin desquamation has been shown to contribute to manganese losses [15].

Estimated Safe and Adequate Daily Dietary Intake

Estimations of the human requirement for manganese are based on balance studies; however, multiple problems with this approach as well as with the factorial method have been reported [1,13]. A provisional dietary recommendation has been set at 2 to 5 mg per day and is thought to represent a dietary intake level achieved by most individuals who exhibit no signs of deficiency or toxicity [1,4].

Deficiency

Studies on a wide variety of species have demonstrated that manganese deficiency is associated with striking and diverse physiologic malfunctions. Manganese deficiency generally does not develop in humans unless the mineral is deliberately eliminated from the diet. Human studies in which men received either 0.11 mg manganese per day for 39 days (however, the diet was also devoid of vitamin K, making it difficult to separate the effects of the manganese and vitamin K deficiencies) or 0.35 mg manganese per day, resulted in negative manganese balance [1,4,5,15,16]. Symptoms and signs of deficiency included nausea, vomiting, dermatitis, decreased serum manganese, decreased fecal manganese excretion, increased serum calcium, phosphorus, and alkaline phosphatase (thought to be associated with skeletal bone changes), decreased growth of hair and nails, changes in hair and beard color, and low blood cholesterol concentrations [1,4,15]. Other effects reported include the occurrence of neonatal ataxia and loss of equilibrium, cell ultrastructure abnormalities, compromised reproductive function, abnormal glucose tolerance, and impaired lipid metabolism [1,2,5]. In rats, dietary manganese deficiency also altered plasma ammonia and urea concentrations in association with decreased arginase activity [10].

Toxicity

No evidence of manganese toxicity has occurred in people receiving as much as 9 mg manganese via food per day [1]. Miners who have inhaled dust fumes high in manganese experience Parkinsonism-like symptoms [4].

Assessment of Nutriture

The normal range of serum manganese concentration is approximately 0.04 to 1.4 µg/dL, but laboratory tests that reliably assess body manganese status have not yet been established. For this reason it becomes difficult to correlate serum concentrations with specific diseases or disorders. Body fluid (plasma, blood, urine) manganese is commonly assayed, as is hair, with blood manganese possibly being indicative of body manganese status [1,17]. In animals, mitochondrial Mn-SOD activity has been shown to be diminished with a low manganese intake; however, application of this finding to humans requires further study.

References Cited for Manganese

1. National Research Council. Recommended dietary allowances, 10th ed. Washington, DC: National Academy Press, 1989;230–235.
2. Kies C. Copper, manganese and zinc: Micronutrients of macroconcern. Food Nutr News 1989;61:50–52.
3. Thomson ABR, Olatunbosun D, Valberg LS. Interrelation of intestinal transport system for manganese and iron. J Lab Clin Med 1971;78:642–655.
4. Nielsen FH. Ultratrace minerals. In: Shils ME, Olson JA, Shike M, eds. Modern nutrition in health and disease. Philadelphia: Lea and Febiger, 1994;269–286.
5. Keen CL, Zidenberg-Cherr S. Manganese. In: Brown ML, ed. Present knowledge in nutrition. Washington, DC: International Life Sciences Institute Nutrition Foundation, 1990;279–286.
6. Garcia-Aranda JA, Wapnir RA, Lifshitz F. In vivo intestinal absorption of manganese in the rat. J Nutr 1983;113:2601–2607.
7. Jeng AY, Shamoo AE. Isolation of a Ca^{+2} carrier from calf heart inner mitochondrial membrane. J Biol Chem 1980;255:6897–6903.
8. Korc M. Manganese as a modulator of signal transduction pathways. In: Prasad AS, ed. Essential and toxic trace elements in human health and disease: An update. New York: Wiley-Liss, 1993;235–255.
9. Keen CL, Lonnerdal B, Hurley LS. Manganese. In: Frieden E, ed. Biochemistry of the essential trace elements. Norfolk, VA: Plenum 1984;89–132.
10. Brock AA, Chapman SA, Ulman EA, Wu G. Dietary manganese deficiency decreases rate hepatic arginase activity. J Nutr 1994;124:340–344.
11. Kirchgessner M, Schwarz FJ, Schnegg A. Interactions of essential metals in human physiology. In: Prasad AS, ed. Current topics in nutrition and disease: Clinical, biochemical and nutritional aspects of trace elements. New York: Liss, 1982:495–499.
12. Keen CL, Frannson GB, Lonnerdal BL. Supplementation of milk with iron bound to lactoferrin using weanling mice: Effects on tissue manganese, zinc, and copper. J Pediatr Gastroenterol Nutr 1984;3:256–261.
13. Forbes RM, Erdman JW. Bioavailability of trace mineral elements. Ann Rev Nutr 1983;3:213–231.
14. Bertinchamps AJ, Miller ST, Cotzias GC. Interdependence of routes excreting manganese. Am J Physiol 1966;211:217–224.
15. Friedman BJ, Freeland-Graves JH, Bales CW, Behmardi F, Shorey-Kutschke RL, Willis RA, Crosby JB, Trickett PC, Houston SD. Manganese balance and clinical observations in young men fed a manganese-deficiency diet. J Nutr 1987;117:133–143.
16. Freeland-Graves JH, Behmardi F, Bales CW, Dougherty V, Lin P-H, Crosby JB, Trickett PC. Metabolic balance of manganese in young men consuming diets containing five levels of dietary manganese. J Nutr 1988;118:764–773.
17. Keen CL, Clegg MS, Lonnerdal B, Hurley LS. Whole blood manganese as an indicator of body manganese. N Engl J Med 1983;308:1230.

MOLYBDENUM

Essentiality of a given trace element generally is established when faulty growth or development or other symptoms of nutritional disorders in an organism correlate with dietary deprivation of that element. In the case of molybdenum, establishing such a correlate has been problematic because of the difficulty in producing molybdenum deficiency in laboratory animals. This is because it is nearly impossible to eliminate traces of the element from synthetic diets and also because of its apparently low daily requirement.

The need for molybdenum was established through the observation that a genetic deficiency of such enzymes as sulfite oxidase and xanthine oxidase (dehydrogenase), which require molybdenum as a cofactor, resulted in severe pathology in human patients [1]. These enzymes are discussed further in the section dealing with the physiologic function of the metal.

Sources

Molybdenum is widespread among the natural foods consumed in typical Western diets. Like other minerals, the molybdenum content of a given plant food may vary greatly, depending on the concentration of molybdenum in the soil. Therefore, it would follow that the metal's content in meats would in turn reflect its concentration in the regional forage. The molybdenum content ranges for selected foods are listed in Table 12.9. Better sources of the mineral include meats (especially organ meats) legumes, cereals, and grains [2,3].

Absorption and Transport

Little is known about the absorption and transport of molybdenum. Sites of molybdenum absorption are thought to include both the stomach and small intestine, with the proximal small intestine responsible for more absorption than the distal section. Active carrier-mediated transport is thought to occur with low molybdenum intakes and diffusion at higher concentrations.

Table 12.9 The Molybdenum Content of Selected Foods

	Molybdenum Content (µg/100g food)
Meat, fish, and poultry	< 1–129
Legumes	16–184
Nuts	11–34
Grains and grain products	2–117
Milk, yogurt, and cheese	2–10
Vegetables	< 1–33
Fruits and fruit juices	0–12

Source: Pennington JAT, Jones JW. Molybdenum, nickel, cobalt, vanadium, and strontium in total diets. Reprinted from JOURNAL OF THE AMERICAN DIETETIC ASSOCIATION Vol.87:1646, 1987.

The range of estimated absorption is wide at 25 to 80% [4,5].

From animal model studies, however, it is understood that the metal is rapidly absorbed from most diets in many of its inorganic forms, including sodium and ammonium molybdate, and even the insoluble compounds molybdenum trioxide and calcium molybdate. In contrast, it is not absorbed effectively as its sulfate salt, presumably because of a competition between molybdenum and inorganic sulfate for common absorption sites [6].

Transport of molybdenum in the blood is thought to occur as molybdate (MoO_4^{-2}). The mineral may be bound to albumin and/or α-2 macroglobulin.

The molybdenum content of human tissues is quite low under normal dietary conditions, averaging 0.1 to 1.0 µg/g wet weight. The liver, kidney, adrenal glands, and bone contain the most molybdenum in terms of absolute amount as well as concentration [7]. Other tissues, such as the small intestine, lungs, spleen, brain, thyroid glands, and muscle, also contain molybdenum.

Functions

The biochemical role of molybdenum centers around the redox function of the element and its necessity as a cofactor for three metalloenzymes: xanthine dehydrogenase, xanthine oxidase, aldehyde oxidase, and sulfite oxidase, all of which catalyze oxidation reduction reactions. The molybdenum cofactor, molybdopterin (Fig. 12.18), consists of a molybdenum atom attached to an organic moiety [8].

The identification and characterization of molybdopterin has been one of the more exciting revelations in molybdenum biochemistry. It is an alkylphosphate-substituted pterin to which molybdenum is coordinated through two sulfur atoms [8,9]. It is through molybdopterin that the molybdenum is anchored to the apoenzyme at its catalytic site. The biosynthetic pathway of molybdopterin has not yet been elucidated.

Xanthine dehydrogenase and xanthine oxidase are nonheme-containing enzymes that also require FAD and molybdopterin. Xanthine dehydrogenase is found in a variety of tissues, including the liver, lungs, kidneys, intestine, among others. Xanthine oxidase is found in the intestine, thyroid cells, and possibly other tissues. Healthy tissues may contain about 10% of their total xanthine enzymes in the oxidase form [10]. Conversion of xanthine dehydrogenase into xanthine oxidase may occur following oxidation of essential sulfhydryl groups or by proteolysis of the dehydrogenase form.

The xanthine dehydrogenase and oxidase enzymes are capable of hydroxylating various purines, pteridines,

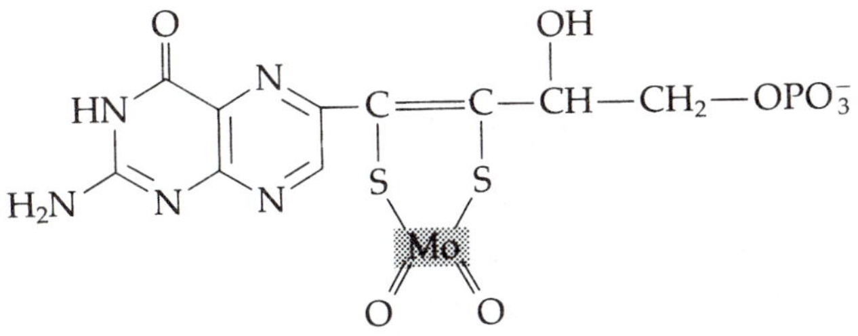

Molybopterin

FIGURE 12.18 Molybdopterin.

pyrimidines, and other heterocyclic nitrogen-containing compounds. Hypoxanthine is derived from purine catabolism, and in most tissues is oxidized by xanthine dehydrogenase to generate xanthine and then uric acid. Xanthine dehydrogenase transfers electrons from the substrate onto NAD^+ to form $NADH + H^+$.

$$Hypoxanthine \xrightarrow{\text{xanthine dehydrogenase}} xanthine$$
$$O_2 \quad H_2O \quad NAD^+ \quad NADH + H^+$$

$$Xanthine \xrightarrow{\text{xanthine dehydrogenase}} uric\ acid$$
$$O_2 \quad H_2O \quad NAD^+ \quad NADH + H^+$$

Modification of xanthine dehydrogenase by proteases can result in the formation of xanthine oxidase. Oxidation of hypoxanthine and xanthine by xanthine oxidase also results in uric acid; however, in these reactions O_2 accepts the electrons and hydrogen peroxide (H_2O_2) is formed.

$$Hypoxanthine \xrightarrow{\text{xanthine oxidase}} xanthine$$
$$O_2 \quad H_2O \quad H_2O_2$$

$$Xanthine \xrightarrow{\text{xanthine oxidase}} uric\ acid$$
$$O_2 \quad H_2O \quad H_2O_2$$

Although low-molybdenum diets or inclusion in the diet of tungstate, a molybdenum antagonist, predictably reduces the level of xanthine oxidase activity in rat intestine and liver, it is interesting to note that no apparent clinical effects result from the perturbation. Furthermore, the human inheritable disorder xanthinuria provides additional evidence for the body's ability to tolerate low xanthine dehydrogenase or oxidase activity. The condition is essentially free of clinical manifestations, except for the possible development of kidney calculi (stones) caused by the high urinary xanthine concentration. Therefore, it is not firmly established if any of the reactions catalyzed by xanthine dehydrogenase or oxidase are necessary for human health [11].

The effects of xanthine oxidase activity, however, have been shown to be quite damaging in people being treated for ischemia (local or temporary deficiency of blood supply and thus relative oxygen deprivation), for example. Degradation of ATP in hypoxic tissue yields hypoxanthine. Reperfusion of the intestine with oxygen (as occurs with medical treatment of for example intestinal ischemia) helps to prevent total destruction of the tissue due to lack of oxygen and nutrients, but also provides xanthine oxidase with the oxygen needed to oxidize the relatively large concentrations of hypoxanthine. Oxidation of hypoxanthine generates large amounts of hydrogen peroxide which further induces tissue damage (see "Perspective" section in Chapter 10).

Sulfite oxidase, a mitochondrial enzyme found in many body tissues, has two molybdopterin and two cytochrome b_5-type residues. The enzyme catalyzes the terminal step in the metabolism of sulfur-containing amino acids (methionine and cysteine), at the same time exhibiting a narrow substrate specificity in its oxidation of sulfite (SO_3^{-2}) to sulfate (SO_4^{-2}). Cytochrome c is the physiologic electron acceptor for this reaction.

Aldehyde oxidase is distinct from the group of aldehyde dehydrogenases. It is a molybdoenzyme that is very similar to xanthine oxidase in size, cofactor composition, and substrate specificity. It presumably functions as a true oxidase, using molecular oxygen as its physiological electron acceptor. The enzyme's primary substrates *in vivo* are not known, although the enzyme may be important for drug metabolism [12]. Also unclear is the effect of variation in molybdenum intake on its activity.

In addition to its biochemical role, molybdenum appears to modulate (likely inhibit through direct interaction) the glucocorticoid receptor complex [13].

Interactions with Other Nutrients

Tungsten has long been recognized as a potent antagonist of molybdenum [14], and in fact its administration into test animals has become the major means for artificially creating a state of molybdenum deficiency. Another interaction involves molybdenum, sulfur, and *copper*. It has been shown, particularly in ruminants, that a high dietary intake of sulfate or molybdenum depressed the tissue uptake of copper and conversely that sulfate and copper decrease molybdenum retention [15]. The proposed explanation for this is that sulfide and hydrosulfide ions are generated in the rumen by reduction of ingested sulfate. The reactive sulfide then displaces oxygen from molybdate ions, yielding oxythiomolybdates and tetrathiomolybdates. Molybdenum is not readily absorbed in the form of thiomolybdates, and furthermore, thiomolybdates bind copper avidly, rendering that metal less physiologically available [16]. It is important to recognize, however, that in humans and other nonruminants, such an interaction is not as important because of the low yield of sulfides and hydrosulfides resulting from sulfate reduction during digestion. However, the feeding of tetrathiomolybdates to nonruminant test animals does result in a compromised uptake of copper. Therefore, it appears that the antagonistic effect of molybdenum or sulfate on copper availability is due to the tendency of molybdenum to sequester reactive sulfide groups. These groups subsequently bind copper ions, which then become less available.

A relationship between molybdenum intake and copper excretion has been documented in humans [17]. Urinary copper excretion in humans has been shown to rise from 24 μg/day to 77 μg/day as molybdenum intake increased from 160 μg to 1,540 μg/day [17]. No changes in fecal copper excretion were noted, suggesting perhaps that molybdenum increased copper mobilization from tissues and promoted excretion [17].

Other nutrients and substances that appear to affect molybdenum availability by mechanisms not yet understood include *manganese, zinc, iron, lead, ascorbic acid, methionine, cysteine, and protein*. A possible relationship with *silicon* is discussed on page 407.

Excretion

Retention of molybdenum in the body is low when dietary intake is high, with urinary excretion as a molybdate ion being the major route of elimination and the regulator of retention [18]. Less than 30% of an ingested dose of molybdenum is retained in the body within three hours following ingestion. Molybdenum is also excreted from the body in the feces by way of the bile and small amounts of molybdenum can be lost in sweat and in hair.

Estimated Safe and Adequate Daily Dietary Intake

Molybdenum is among those ultratrace elements for which no RDA has been established on the basis of present knowledge. Instead, estimated ranges of adequate but safe intake have been proposed, primarily according to balance studies. The ESADDI for molybdenum for adults is 75 to 250 μg [19]. Infants and children probably require proportionately more of the element if intake per unit of body weight is the basis of assessment.

Deficiency

Molydenum deficiency is rarely encountered unless the diet is particularly rich in antagonistic substances such as sulfate, copper, or tungstate. Deficiency in humans has been documented in a patient maintained on total parenteral nutrition for 18 months [20]. The patient exhibited high blood methionine, hypoxanthine, and xanthine concentrations, as well as low blood levels of uric acid. Urinary concentrations of sulfate were low and of sulfite were high. Treatment with 300 μg of ammonium molybdate (163 μg molybdenum) resulted in clinical improvement and normalization of sulfur amino acid metabolism and uric acid production.

The importance of sulfite oxidase, and therefore molybdenum, in human nutrition is evidenced by the neurologic disorders associated with a genetic deficiency of sulfite oxidase in children [1,21]. Elevated urinary sulfite and thiosulfate, along with biochemical manifestations reflecting aberrant sulfur amino acid metabolism and sulfite oxidation were observed.

Toxicity

Molybdenum is relatively nontoxic to humans, although symptoms such as gout (inflammation of the joints due to accumulation of uric acid) have appeared in some people due to high blood uric acid concentrations, which have likely arisen from increased xanthine dehydrogenase activity, and accumulation of the uric acid in and around joints [4,5,19]. Because moderate intakes of molybdenum appear to increase urinary copper excretion [17], further research is needed before intakes can be recommended.

Assessment of Nutriture

Molybdenum appears to distribute itself fairly equally between the plasma and red blood cells. Although a few studies have reported the molybdenum concentrations of human plasma and blood, the use of these as indicators of molybdenum status has not been validated.

References Cited for Molybdenum

1. Johnson JL, Waud WR, Rajagopalan KV, Duran M, Beemer FA, Wadman SK. Inborn errors of molybdenum metabolism: Combined deficiencies of xanthine oxidase in a patient lacking the molybdenum cofactor. Proc Natl Acad Sci USA 1980;77:3715–3719.
2. Tsongas TA, Meglen RR, Walravens PA, Chappell WR. Molybenum in the diet: An estimate of average daily intake in the United States. Am J Clin Nutr 1980;33:1103–1107.
3. Schroeder HA, Balassa JJ, Tipton IH. Essential trace metals in man: Molybdenum. J Chron Dis 1970;23:481–499.
4. Nielsen FH. Ultratrace minerals. In: Shils ME, Olson JA, Shike M., eds. Modern nutrition in health and disease. Philadelphia: Lea and Febiger, 1994;269–286.
5. Nielsen FH. Other trace elements. In: Brown ML, ed. Present knowledge in nutrition. Washington, DC: International Life Sciences Institute Nutrition Foundation, 1990;294–307.
6. Cardin CJ, Mason J. Molybdate and tungstate transfer by rat ileum: Competitive inhibition by sulfate. Biochim Biophys Acta 1976;455:937–944.
7. Scott KC, Turnlund JR. Compartmental model of molybdenum metabolism in adult men fed five levels of molybdenum. FASEB J 1993;7:A288.
8. Kramer SP, Johnson JL, Ribeiro AA, Millington DS, Rajagopalan KV. The structure of the molybdenum cofactor. J Biol Chem 1987;262:16357–16363.
9. Rajagopalan KV. Molybdenum: An essential trace element in human nutrition. Ann Rev Nutr 1988;8:401–427.
10. McCord JM. Free radicals and myocardial ischemia: Overview and outlook. Free Radicals & Medicine 1988;4:9–14
11. Coughlan MP. The role of molybdenum in human biology. J Inher Metab Dis 1983;6(suppl. 1):70–77.
12. Beedham C. Molybdenum hydroxylases as drug-metabolizing enzymes. Drug Metab Rev 1985;16:119–156.
13. Bodine PV, Litwack G. Evidence that the modulator of the glucocorticoid-receptor complex is the endogenous molybdate factor. Proc Natl Acad Sci USA 1988;85:1462–1466.
14. Johnson JL, Rajogopalan KV. Molecular basis of the biological function of molybdenum. J Biol Chem 1974;249:859–866.
15. Suttle NF. The interactions between copper, molybdenum, and sulphur in ruminant nutrition. Ann Rev Nutr 1991;11:121–140.
16. Mills CF, Davis GK. Molybdenum. In: Mertz W, et al. Trace elements in human and animal nutrition. San Diego: Academic Press, 1987;1:449–454.
17. Turnlund JR. Copper nutriture, bioavailability, and the influence of dietary factors. J Am Diet Assoc 1988;88:303–308.
18. Turnlund JR, Keyes WR, Peiffer GL. Absorption, retention, and excretion of a stable isotope of molybdenum in young men during molybdenum depletion and repletion. FASEB J 1993;7:A279.
19. National Research Council. Recommended dietary allowances, 10th ed. Washington, DC: National Academy Press, 1989;243–246.
20. Abumrad N, Schneider AJ, Steel D, Rogers LS. Amino acid intolerance during prolonged total parental nutrition reversed by molybdate therapy. Am J Clin Nutr 1981;34:2551–2559.
21. Johnson JL, Wuebbens MM, Mandell R, Shih VE. Molybdenum cofactor deficiency in a patient previously characterized as deficient in sulfite oxidase. Biochem Med Metab Biol 1988; 40:86–93.

FLUORINE

Whereas fluorine (F) is a gaseous chemical element, fluoride is composed of fluorine bound to either a metal, nonmetal, or organic compound. Fluoride predominates in nature and exerts physiologic effects in the body. The term *fluoride* will be used throughout this section. Analogous to this terminology is the use of the terms *iodide* and *chloride*.

Sources

Community drinking water fluoridation has been practiced for nearly fifty years in the United States following the discovery in 1942 of the inverse relationship of fluoride intake and the incidence of dental caries [1,2]. This has in turn affected the distribution of fluoride in human foods and beverages. The content of fluoride in most food groups (Table 12.10) is low compared to most nutrients. However, not shown are tea and marine fish, which if consumed with the bones are relatively high in fluoride [1]. Ready-to-use infant formulas are made with fluoridated water, thereby providing infants with a source of fluoride. Other beverages vary greatly in their fluoride content, contingent on the use or nonuse of fluoridated water in their processing. It is important that fluoride supplementation of water and foods achieves an *in vivo* level sufficiently high to effect dental and skeletal benefit but not so high as to cause toxicity.

Absorption and Transport

Even at high intakes, soluble fluorides are almost completely absorbed from the gastrointestinal tract at a rate

Table 12.10 Fluoride Content of Various Food Groups

Food Group	Fluoride Content Range (ppm)
Dairy products	0.05–0.07
Meat, fish, poultry	0.22–0.92
Grain, cereal products	0.29–0.41
Potatoes	0.08–0.14
Green, leafy vegetables	0.10–0.15
Legumes	0.15–0.39
Root vegetables	0.09–0.10
Other vegetables, vegetable products	0.06–0.17
Fruits	0.06–0.13
Fats, oils	0.13–0.24
Sugar adjuncts	0.21–0.35

Source: Rao GS. Dietary intake and bioavailability of fluoride. Ann Rev Nutr 1984;4:120. Reproduced with permission, © 1984.

that varies with the chemical form of the element and the presence of other dietary factors. Aqueous solutions of fluorides, such as sodium fluoride and sodium fluorosilicate, which are used in water fluoridation, are almost completely absorbed.

The availability of fluoride in solid foods is, however, generally reduced with only about 50 to 80% of fluoride absorbed from foods. Fluoride bound to proteins in foods is less available for absorption. Fluoride is also relatively poorly absorbed (37 to 54%) from insoluble sources such as bone meal [3].

Humans, given small amounts of soluble fluoride, achieve maximum blood fluoride levels within about 30 minutes to one hour. This rapidity of absorption is accounted for by the fact that it occurs to a great extent in the stomach, a rather unique characteristic among the elements. It is also absorbed throughout the small intestine but at a reduced rate. Fluoride absorption is believed to occur by passive diffusion, and its rapid gastric absorption can be explained by the fact that it exists primarily as hydrogen fluoride (HF) at the low pH of the gastric contents rather than as ionic fluoride. Rate of diffusion across membranes, in general, correlates directly with the lipid solubility of the diffusing substance, and the diffusion of undissociated HF across the gastric mucosa would therefore be predictably rapid [4]. Hydrogen fluoride is a weak acid with a pKa (the negative logarithm of an acid dissociation constant, Ka) of 3.45, dissociating according to the equation

$$HF \longrightarrow H^+ + F^-$$
$$(200) \qquad\qquad (1)$$

Assuming a gastric pH of approximately 1.5, the ratio of HF to F^-, readily calculable from the Henderson-Hasselbalch equation (p. 434), would be nearly 200 to 1, as indicated. The gastric luminal form of fluoride is therefore largely diffusible. In support of the theory that low pH facilitates the gastric absorption of fluoride is the finding [5] that its absorption is enhanced by a high-protein diet, which increases gastric acidity.

Fluoride absorption does not appear to be influenced by its plasma levels except at a very high, perhaps toxic, concentration [6,7]. Furthermore, as a result of studies on possible fluoride–chloride interactions, it was found that fluoride absorption was not inhibited by high chloride intake [8].

Fluoride is transported in the blood in a nonionic, organic form and as ionic fluoride. Organically bound fluoride occurs in variable concentrations that are independent of total fluoride intake and plasma ionic fluoride levels. What is not known is the extent to which environmental contamination by industrially generated fluorocarbons may contribute to the variability. Ionic fluoride concentration, in contrast, correlates directly with the dietary intake even up to very large oral doses, indicating that plasma ionic fluoride is not precisely controlled by homeostatic mechanisms.

Absorbed fluoride leaves the blood very quickly and is distributed rapidly throughout the body, particularly to the hard tissues, where it is sequestered in bones and teeth by apatite. Apatite is a basic calcium phosphate having the theoretic formula $Ca_{10}(PO_4)_6(OH)_2$. Mineralized tissues account for nearly 99% of total body fluoride, with bone being by far the major depot. As the amount of absorbed fluoride increases, so does the quantity taken up by hard tissue. But the percentage retained at high absorption rates becomes less because of accelerated urinary excretion [5]. Skeletal growth rate influences fluoride balance, exemplified by the fact that young, growing people incorporate more fluoride into the skeleton than adults and excrete less in the urine.

Functions

The major functions of fluoride are related to its effects on the mineralization of teeth and bones. Specifically, it promotes mineral precipitation from metastable solutions of calcium and phosphate, leading to the formation of apatite. The apatite is deposited as crystallites within an organic (protein) matrix.

Fluoride can be incorporated into the apatite structure by replacement of hydroxide ions. This can occur during initial crystal formation or by displacement from previously deposited mineral, according to the equation

$$Ca_{10}(PO_4)_6(OH)_2 + xF^- \longrightarrow Ca_{10}(PO_4)_6(OH)_{2-x}F_x^-$$

The extent of fluoride incorporation varies with animal species, age, fluoride exposure, and rate of tissue turnover. In bone and dental enamel of humans and other higher mammals, the substitution of F^- for OH^- is approximately 1:20 to 1:40.

Evidence has been presented for the high affinity of an enamel matrix protein for fluoride, leading to the speculation that fluoride's major role in mineralization may be its participation in the nucleation of crystal formation rather than its association with the mineral phase [9].

Attempts to relate other biochemical defects, such as anemia and impaired growth and reproduction in experimental animals, to fluoride deficiency are ambiguous and not well documented. However, beneficial effects, such as its ability to decrease bone resorption, of fluoride supplementation (typically 50 mg/day), have justified its use in the treatment of osteoporosis [1].

Interactions with Other Nutrients

It has been reported that *aluminum, calcium, magnesium, and chloride* all interact with fluoride in such a way as to reduce its uptake and use, while *phosphate* and *sulfate* increase its uptake [10]. The mechanisms of the interactions are not established, but a given interaction may affect fluoride use at either the level of absorption or skeletal uptake. For example, although it has been found [8] that plasma chloride levels do not affect the absorption of dietary fluoride, ingested sodium chloride does decrease the skeletal uptake of fluoride [11]. This is of interest, since kitchen or table salt has been used as a vehicle for fluoride supplementation in some countries.

The effect of aluminum-containing antacids in sharply reducing the absorption of fluoride, as well as calcium and phosphorus, has received attention in view of the deleterious effect this would have on osteoporosis [12]. It is speculated that aluminum forms insoluble complexes with fluoride in the intestine [12], but the contribution of the pH effect of the antacid on fluoride availability may require further investigation.

Excretion

Excretion of fluoride takes place rapidly via the urine, which accounts for approximately 90% of total excretion. Fecal elimination accounts for the bulk of the remainder, with minor losses occurring in sweat. Some renal tubular reabsorption occurs by passive diffusion of undissociated HF. Since the amount of HF is increased relative to that of F^- as acidity is increased, tubular reabsorption and urinary pH are therefore inversely related.

Estimated Safe and Adequate Daily Dietary Intake

The U.S. National Research Council has recommended 1.5 to 4.0 mg fluoride/day as an estimated "safe and adequate" intake for adults [1]. In the interest of optimizing dental health, the Council on Dental Therapeutics of the American Dental Association has advised fluoride supplementation based on existing drinking water concentrations and the age of the subjects [13,14]. The optimum fluoride concentration in fluoridated drinking water is 1 to 2 ppm.

Deficiency

Fluoride deficiency in test animals has been reported to result in curtailed growth, infertility, and anemia. But these findings are not well documented and clearly cannot be extrapolated in predicting similar effects on humans. In humans, what is unequivocal is that an optimal level of fluoride is necessary to reduce the incidence of dental caries and perhaps also to maintain the integrity of skeletal tissue. It is on this basis that the element is considered essential.

Toxicity

Chronic toxicity of fluoride is referred to as *fluorosis* and is characterized by changes in bone, kidney, and possibly nerve and muscle function [3,14]. Mottling of teeth (dental fluorosis) has been observed in children receiving 2 to 8 mg fluoride/kg [2]. Acute toxicity manifested as nausea, vomiting, acidosis, cardiac arrhythmias, and death has been reported following ingestion of between 5 to 10 g of sodium fluoride [14].

Assessment of Nutriture

Normal ranges for ionic fluoride have been established at 0.01 to 0.2 μg F^-/mL plasma and 0.2 to 1.1 μg F^-/mL urine. The element is most commonly determined in its ionic form by fluoride ion-specific electrode potentiometry, a technique analogous to the hydrogen ion-specific electrode potentiometry of the common pH meter.

References Cited for Fluorine

1. National Research Council. Recommended dietary allowances, 10th ed. Washington, DC: National Academy Press, 1989;235–240.

2. Ophaug RH. Fluoride. In: Brown ML, ed. Present knowledge in nutrition. Washington, DC: International Life Sciences Institute Nutrition Foundation, 1990;274–278.

3. Krishnamachari KAVR. Fluoride. In: Mertz W, ed.: Trace elements in human and animal nutrition. San Diego: Academic Press, 1987;1:365–415.

4. Whitford GM, Pashley DH. Fluoride absorption: The influence of gastric acidity. Calcif Tissue Int 1984;36:302–330.

5. Boyde CD, Cerklewski FL. Influence of type and level of dietary protein on fluoride bioavailability in the rat. J Nutr 1987;117:2086–2090.

6. Whitford GM, Williams JL. Fluoride absorption: Independence from plasma fluoride levels. Proc Soc Exp Biol Med 1986;181:550–554.

7. Ekstrand J. Relationship between fluoride in the drinking water and the plasma fluoride concentration in man. Caries Res 1978;12:123–127.

8. Cerklewski FL, Ridlington JW, Bills ND. Influence of dietary chloride on fluoride bioavailability in the rat. J Nutr 1986;116:618–624.

9. Crenshaw MA, Bawden JW. Fluoride binding by organic matrix from early and late developing bovine fetal enamel determined by flow rate dialysis. Arch Oral Biol 1981;26:473–476.

10. Rao GS. Dietary intake and bioavailability of fluoride. Ann Rev Nutr 1984;4:115–136.

11. Ericsson Y. Influence of sodium chloride and certain other food components on fluoride absorption in the rat. J Nutr 1968;96:60–68.

12. Spencer H, Kramer L. Osteoporosis: Calcium, fluoride, and aluminum interactions. J Am Coll Nutr 1985;4:121–128.

13. American Dental Association. Accepted dental therapeutics, 39th ed. Chicago: American Dental Association, 1982.

14. Heifetz SB, Horowitz HS. The amounts of fluoride in current fluoride therapies: Safety considerations for children. J Dent Child 1984;51:257–269.

NICKEL

Possible signs of nickel deprivation in experimental animals were first reported in the 1970s, but the early findings were subject to question because they were obtained under conditions that did not permit optimal growth among the animals. Also, early studies were fraught with inconsistencies believed to be due, in part, to variables such as the iron status of the animals, which is now known to influence nickel metabolism [1].

Since the year 1975, experimental diets have been greatly improved so as to allow optimal growth and survival, affording greater credibility to research results.

Table 12.11 Nickel Content of Selected Food Groups

Food Group	Nickel Content μg range/100 g
Milk, Yogurt, Cheese	0–8.2
Eggs	0–1.4
Meat, Fish, Poultry	0–14.3
Grains and Grain Products	0.3–228.5
Fruits and Fruit Juices	0–47.7
Vegetables	0.2–40.5

Source: Pennington JAT and Jones JW. Molybdenum, nickel, cobalt, vanadium, and strontium in total diets. Reprinted from JOURNAL OF THE AMERICAN DIETETIC ASSOCIATION 87:1644–1650, 1987.

Signs of nickel deprivation continue to be described for at least six animal species. Included among the more consistent signs are depressed growth, rough hair coat, and impaired hematopoiesis, which probably is due to altered iron metabolism.

Sources

Foods of plant origin have a significantly higher nickel content than foods of animal origin. Nuts are particularly rich in the metal, as indicated in Table 12.11, which lists selected food groups of high nickel content. Grains, cured meats, and vegetables are generally of intermediate nickel content, and foods of animal origin, such as fish, milk, and eggs, are generally low [2].

The chemical form of nickel in foods is unknown, but in plants it is probably largely inorganic and is dependent on the nickel content of the soil. Dietary nickel derived from contamination of processed foods would likely be inorganic as well.

Absorption and Transport

Most of the information on the influence of dietary factors on nickel absorption has come from human studies. Nickel added to beverages such as coffee, tea, cow's milk, and orange juice is absorbed to a lesser extent than if added to water alone [2]. In the same investigation, it was shown that phytate did not reduce absorption despite the fact that nickel ions form stable complexes with phytate *in vitro*. About 50% of nickel is absorbed from water. In contrast, less than 10% of nickel is absorbed from a typical diet [3,4].

The transport of ingested nickel across the intestinal brush border is believed to occur via an energy-dependent mechanism rather than by passive diffusion. Nickel ions appear to compete with iron for a common transport system in the proximal small intestine [5].

Transport across the basolateral membrane is thought to occur by diffusion or as part of a complex with an amino acid or binding ligand.

On entering the blood, nickel becomes bound to albumin [6] and to several different amino acid ligands. These amino acid ligands are believed to include histidine, cysteine, and aspartic acid. Other serum proteins that bind nickel, and that therefore may be involved in its transport and metabolism, are histidine-rich glycoprotein (HRG) and nickeloplasmin. Although it has been found [7] that 43% of total serum nickel in humans is complexed strongly to nickeloplasmin, the physiologic significance of the protein is unclear.

Although nickel is widely distributed among human tissues, its concentration throughout the body is extremely low, occurring at ng/g levels. The highest concentrations of nickel are found in hair, bone, soft tissues such as the lungs, heart, kidneys, and liver, and two glands, the thyroid and adrenal glands.

Functions

A specific role of nickel in human and animal nutrition has not yet been defined, although roles for nickel in plants (such as a cofactor for urease, which catalyzes the hydrolysis of urea into carbon dioxide and ammonia) and micro-organisms have been documented [9,10]. The element, however, can substitute for other metal ion activators *in vitro*. This is not surprising, because, like other ions of the first transition series, Ni^{+2} has the ability to complex with many substances of biological importance.

In the several enzyme systems in which nickel substitution has been demonstrated experimentally, magnesium is most commonly the metal replaced. An example of such a replacement is the formation of the C3 convertase enzyme (C3b,Bb and C4b,2b) of the human complement system, which classically requires Mg^{+2} for activity. The substitution of nickel in place of magnesium in this complex enhanced both the stability and activity of the enzyme [11], therefore raising the question as to nickel's possible physiologic role in the complement system.

It has also been demonstrated that nickel can substitute for zinc in the carboxypeptidases and in horse liver alcohol dehydrogenase. Nickel may be involved with vitamin B_{12} and act as a cofactor for an enzyme in the propionate pathway of branched-chain amino acid and odd-chain fatty acid metabolism [12]. Nielson has suggested that the need for nickel in animals and humans will most likely become evident under situations in which a propionate pathway enzyme, such as the vita-

min B_{12}-dependent methylmalonyl mutase, demands are elevated [13].

Interactions with Other Nutrients

It has already been pointed out in the preceding section that nickel shares with other metals the property of being readily chelated by, and complexed with, a wide variety of ligands. It follows that nickel can compete with those ions for ligand sites. The list of ions with which nickel interacts in this manner is long, including as many as 13 essential minerals. But the only interactions that are of particular nutritional interest are those involving *iron, copper, and zinc*.

The most biologically significant interaction of nickel and iron probably occurs at the level of intestinal absorption, although the mechanism is not well understood. It appears to be either a synergistic or an antagonistic interaction depending on the valence state of the dietary iron. When ferric sulfate alone was used in iron supplementation experiments on nickel-deprived, marginally iron-deficient rats, liver iron content was depressed. But if supplementation was with a ferrous–ferric sulfate mixture, the liver content of iron increased. Furthermore, nickel was shown to interact synergistically with iron as ferric sulfate only, but not as a mixture of ferric and ferrous sulfates in affecting hematopoiesis. The interpretation of these findings is that nickel facilitates the use of ferric ion, but somehow antagonizes ferrous ion absorption, particularly in severe iron deficiency. The enhancement of Fe^{+3} absorption by nickel is not understood. Due to the insolubility of the ferric ion in the duodenum, it either needs to be converted by reduction to Fe^{+2}, which is readily absorbed, or complexed to a soluble, absorbable ligand. There is speculation that nickel may function as a cofactor in enhancing the complexing of the Fe^{+3} with a bioligand, or it may act in an enzyme system that converts Fe^{+3} to Fe^{+2}.

That nickel interacts antagonistically with copper *in vivo* is based on the finding that in copper-deficient rats, physiologic signs of the deficiency are exacerbated by nickel supplementation. The antagonism appears not to occur during absorption of copper but more likely is due to nickel's replacement of copper at certain functional sites.

Deficient or toxic levels of nickel also affect zinc metabolism, possibly by causing redistribution of zinc in the body, rather than by competing with zinc at sites of zinc function. In some instances signs of zinc deficiency in animals were partially alleviated by supplemental nickel, while other symptoms were unaffected by the resulting tissue redistribution. Nielsen [14] has reviewed the interactions of nickel with iron, copper, and zinc.

Excretion

Most of the absorbed nickel is excreted in the urine. Since urinary excretion is the major route for elimination of absorbed nickel, retention of the element in the kidney probably reflects the organ's excretory role. However, within the renal cells, nickel is complexed nonspecifically with uronic acid and neutral sugar oligosaccharides and specifically with an acidic peptide [8]. Since these peptides are not present in plasma, a ligand exchange must take place after glomerular filtration.

Small amounts of absorbed nickel may also be excreted through the bile and also via the sweat glands. Dermal loss of nickel may be significant during episodes of profuse sweating.

Recommended Intake and Assessment of Nutriture

The fact that humans require nickel is postulated from extrapolated data from animal studies, and although a RDA for humans has not been established, it can be approximated from the apparent requirement of animals. For rats and chicks, the requirement for nickel is estimated to be about 50 µg/kg of diet, or 16 µg/1,000 kcal [15], corresponding to a hypothetical human need of approximately 35 µg/day. A requirement of less than 10 µg/day has also been proposed [12].

The reference range for nickel in the serum or plasma of healthy adults is 1 to 21 ng/mL, and the urinary excretion has been reported to be 0.1 to 20 µg/day. Like most of the ultratrace metals, the preferred technique for nickel determination is flameless atomic absorption spectrophotometry. It offers the degree of sensitivity necessary for determination in the nanogram range.

References Cited for Nickel

1. Nielsen FH. The importance of diet composition in ultratrace element research. J Nutr 1985;115:1239–1247.
2. Solomons NW, Viteri F, Shuler TR, Nielsen FH. Bioavailability of nickel in man: Effects of foods and chemically-defined dietary constituents on the absorption of dietary nickel. J Nutr 1982;112:39–50.
3. Nielsen FH. Other trace elements. In: Brown ML, ed. Present knowledge in nutrition. Washington, DC: International Life Sciences Institute Nutrition Foundation, 1990;294–307.
4. Nielsen FH. Ultratrace minerals. In: Shils ME, Olson JA, Shike M., eds. Modern nutrition in health and disease. Philadelphia: Lea and Febiger, 1994;269–286.
5. Nielsen FH. Studies on the interaction between nickel and iron during intestinal absorption. In: Anke M, Bauman W, Braunlich H, et al., eds. Spurenelement—Symposium Leipzig, East Germany: Karl-Marx-Universität, 1983;11–98.
6. Sunderman SW, Jr. In: Bronner CF, Coburn, JW, eds. Disorders of mineral metabolism. New York: Academic Press, 1981: 201–232.
7. Nomoto S. In: Brown SS, Sunderman FW Jr, eds. Nickel toxicology. New York: Academic Press, 1980:89–90.
8. Templeton DM, Bibudhendra S. Peptide and carbohydrate complexes of nickel in human kidney. Biochem J 1985;230:35–42.
9. Walsh CT, Orme-Johnson WH. Nickel enzymes. Biochemistry 1987; 26:4901–4906.
10. Nielsen FH. Nickel. In: Mertz W, ed. Trace elements in human and animal nutrition. San Diego: Academic Press, 1987;1: 245–273.
11. Fishelson Z, Muller-Eberhard HJ. C3 convertase of human complement: Enhanced formation and stability of the enzyme generated with nickel instead of magnesium. J Immunol 1982;129:2603–2607.
12. Nielsen FH. Nutritional requirements for boron, silicon, vanadium, nickel, and arsenic: Current knowledge and speculation. FASEB J 1991;5:2661–2667.
13. Nielsen FH. Ultratrace elements of possible importance for human health: An update. In: Prasad AS, ed. Essential and toxic trace elements in human health. New York: Wiley-Liss, 1993;355–376.
14. Nielsen FH. Nickel. In: Frieden E, ed. Biochemistry of the essential ultratrace elements. New York: Plenum Press, 1984:301–304.
15. Nielsen FH. Possible future implications of nickel, arsenic, silicon, vanadium, and other ultratrace elements in human nutrition. Curr Top Nutr Dis 1982;6:379–404.

SILICON

Silicon occupies a unique position among the essential trace elements in that it is second only to oxygen in earthwide abundance. Quartz, which is crystallized silica, is the most abundant mineral in the earth's crust. The element occurs naturally as its dioxide, silica (SiO_2), and as water-soluble silicic acid, $Si(OH)_4$, formed by hydration of the oxide. In plants, silicon is deposited as the solid, hydrated oxide, $SiO_2 \cdot nH_2O$, known as *silica gel*, following polymerization of silicic acid.

Early investigations concentrated on silicon's toxicity, such as silicon-related urolithiasis and particularly silicosis, caused by the inhalation of dust. But research in the early to mid 1970s established the mineral's essentiality, its specific requirement for the normal growth and development of connective tissue, mucopolysaccharides, cartilage, elastin, and bone. The investigations that led to these findings are thoroughly reviewed by Carlisle [1].

Sources

Data on the distribution of silicon in human foods and diets are sparse. It is known, however, that foods of plant origin are normally much richer in silicon than those of animal origin. High-fiber cereal grains [2] and root vegetables appear to be especially rich sources of the element [3].

Absorption and Transport

The mechanism of the absorption of silicon is not well understood, and future studies will likely be complicated by the fact that its dietary forms are so diverse. Silica, monosilicic acid, and silicon found in organic combination, such as pectin and mucopolysaccharides, are a few of its ingestible forms. The most soluble form of silicon is metasilicate; this form has been commonly used in supplementation studies.

Absorption ranges from 10 to 70% depending on the form of silicon used [3]. Moreover, the extent of absorption of the element appears to correlate with the production of its soluble forms in gastric fluids [4], a finding that is supported by the observation that silicic acid in foods and beverages is readily absorbed in humans and rapidly excreted in the urine.

The fiber content of the diet has also been reported to influence the absorbability of silicon in humans. Nearly 97% of dietary silicon contained in a high-fiber diet remained unabsorbed and was lost in the feces, compared with a fecal excretion of only 60% when a low-fiber diet was consumed [2]. In studies on rats, changes in absorption were shown to relate also to age, sex, and the activity of various endocrine glands [5].

Silicon, as silicic acid, is freely diffusible throughout tissue fluids. Once silicic acid is absorbed into the blood, it is almost entirely nonprotein bound, therefore accounting for its rapid decrease in plasma concentration, its diffusion into tissue fluids, and its rapid urinary excretion. When ^{31}Si silicic acid was administered intravenously (IV) to normal rats, 77% of the compound was recovered in the urine within four hours [6]. In that same study the initial uptake of the label was most rapid in liver, lung, skin, and bone, with slower entry occurring in heart, muscle, spleen, and testes. Negligible uptake into the brain was reported, indicating active exclusion by the blood–brain barrier.

Functions

The physiologic role of silicon is focused on the normal growth and development of bone, connective tissue, and cartilage, functioning both in a metabolic and a struc-

tural capacity. The effect of silicon on bone is to hasten mineralization as well as to promote growth. In test animals, high-silicon diets were associated with increased calcium content of the bone and an accelerated bone maturity. Silicon deficiency also resulted in smaller, less flexible long bones and in deformation of the skull. In studies on chicks, the skull deformation was subsequently found to be due to a significantly reduced collagen content in the connective tissue matrix [7].

The detrimental effect of silicon deficiency on collagen formation is linked to the mineral's requirement in the synthesis of proline and hydroxyproline, the residues of which are of particular importance in collagen's primary structure. Proline is incorporated as such into the procollagen peptide but becomes hydroxylated posttranslationally by prolyl hydroxylase. The reaction (Fig. 12.19) also requires iron and vitamin C. Silicon is required for maximal prolyl hydroxylase activity [8], mechanistically not yet understood, and is probably also required for the synthesis of proline itself [9].

In addition to its positive influence on collagen synthesis, silicon is also needed for the formation of glycosaminoglycans, such as hyaluronic acid, chondroitin sulfate, and keratin sulfate. Glycosaminoglycans are linked covalently to proteins as components of the extracellular ground substance that surrounds the collagen, elastic fibers, and cells. A structural role for silicon in glycosaminoglycan formation may also be proposed, since it has been found to be chemically linked within the glycosaminoglycan framework.

Interactions with Other Nutrients

The only mineral element in a normal diet that may be of any consequence in affecting the availability of silicon is *molybdenum*. The interaction was first discovered when silicon supplementation of a diet high in liver failed to elevate significantly the plasma silicon concentration, and both plasma and tissue silicon levels were subsequently shown to be markedly and inversely affected by molybdenum intake [10]. The reverse is also true—that silicon supplementation reduces the plasma concentration and cellular uptake of dietary molybdenum. Until the mechanism of intestinal absorption of the two elements is better understood, the manner in which they interact remains unknown.

Excretion

The kidney is the major excretory organ of absorbed silicon in experiments in which the element was consumed as silicic acid. Urinary output of silicon generally increases as intake increases up to fairly well-defined lim-

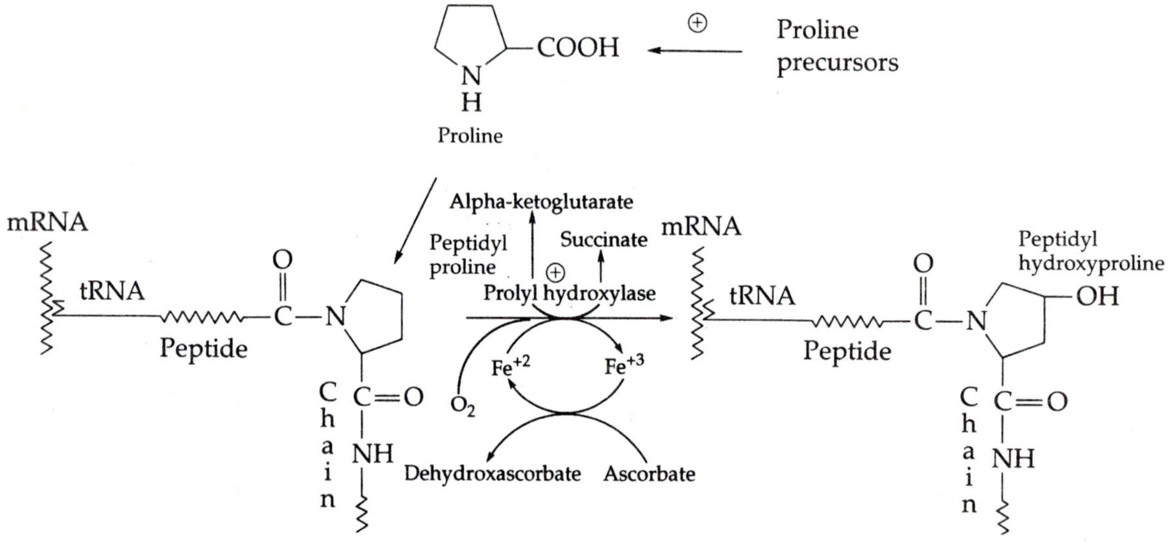

FIGURE 12.19 The posttranslational hydroxylation of peptidyl proline in a growing procollagen chain. In addition to prolyl hydroxylase, the reaction also requires ascorbate, α-ketoglutarate, ferrous iron, and oxygen. The symbol $\oplus$ designates the sites at which silicon positively affects collagen synthesis.

its that do not appear to be imposed by the kidney's inability to excrete more.

Recommended Intake and Assessment of Nutriture

The minimum silicon requirement compatible with human health is largely unknown, as are the dietary forms that render the mineral most available. Requirement assessment has been largely confined to the relationship of dietary intake of silicon, expressed as $\mu g/g$ of dry diet, to observed growth and skeletal development in test animals. Such studies indicate that the dietary silicon requirement may be relatively high compared to that of other trace elements. Estimates of the requirement for silicon for humans ranges from 5 to 20 mg silicon per day [10].

As in the case of most of the trace elements, levels of silicon in biological fluids of healthy adults have been reported, but may not accurately represent nutriture. Chemical assessment is generally performed on serum or plasma, which contains 0.4 to 10.0 $\mu g/mL$. Mass spectrometry, emission spectroscopy, and atomic absorption spectrophotometry are a few of the techniques for determining silicon concentration in biological specimens. Of these, atomic absorption spectrophotometry has been the method of choice for most laboratories.

References Cited for Silicon

1. Carlisle EM. Silicon. In: Frieden E, ed. Biochemistry of the essential trace elements. New York: Plenum Press, 1984;257–291.
2. Kelsay JL, Behall KM, Prather ES. Effect of fiber from fruits and vegetables on metabolic responses of human subjects II. Calcium, magnesium, iron, and silicon balances. Am J Clin Nutr 1979;32:1876–1880.
3. Nielsen FH. Ultratrace minerals. In: Shils ME, Olson JA, Shike M, eds. Modern nutrition in health and disease. Philadelphia: Lea and Febiger, 1994;269–286.
4. Benke GM, Osborn TW. Urinary silicon excretion by rats following oral administration of silicon compounds. Food Cosmet Toxicol 1978;17:123–127.
5. Charnot Y, Peres G. Silicon, endocrine balance and mineral metabolism. In: Bendz G, Lindquist I, eds. Biochemistry of silicon and related problems. New York: Plenum Press, 1978:269–280.
6. Adler AJ, Etzion Z, Berlyne GM. Uptake, distribution, and excretion of [31]silicon in normal rats. Am J Physiol 1986;251:E670–673.
7. Carlisle EM. A silicon requirement for normal skull formation in chicks. J Nutr 1980;110:352–359.
8. Carlisle EM. Silicon: A requirement in bone formation independent of vitamin D. Calc Tissue Intern 1981;33:27–34.
9. Carlisle EM, Alpenfels WF. The role of silicon in proline synthesis. Fed Proc 1984;43:680.
10. Carlisle EM. A silicon-molybdenum interrelationship in vivo. Fed Proc 1979;38:553.

Additional Reference

Evered D, O'Connor M. Silicon biochemistry. New York: John Wiley, 1986.

VANADIUM

The deliberate or adventitious administration of vanadium is known to produce a number of discernible physiologic effects, including toxicity. But in spite of this, its essentiality is not firmly established because of nebulous results of deprivation studies on animals. It may be appropriate to again review (first given in the overview at the beginning of the chapter) the proposed criteria for essentiality that have evolved from trace element research. The following are true about the element: (1) it is present in all healthy tissue of all living things; (2) its concentration from one animal to the next is fairly constant; (3) its withdrawal from the body induces reproducibly the same physiologic and structural abnormalities, regardless of the species studied; (4) its addition either reduces or prevents these abnormalities; (5) the abnormalities induced by deficiencies are always accompanied by specific biochemical changes; and (6) these biological changes can be prevented or cured when the deficiency is prevented or cured.

Elements established as essential may not necessarily comply with all those criteria listed, due in part to limitations imposed by the degree of sophistication of the analytical methodology available. Proof of essentiality is therefore technically easier for elements that occur in relatively high concentration than for those ultratrace elements occurring at very low concentrations and having a low requirement.

Controlled depletion of vanadium has been reported to adversely affect growth rate, perinatal survival, physical appearance, hematocrit, and other manifestations in various animal species [1]. However, none of these were consistently induced by deprivation in repeated experiments, thereby failing to comply with that criterion for essentiality. Nevertheless, its widespread distribution throughout the organs and tissues of animals and humans and the fact that deprivation is accompanied by the effects mentioned has led investigators to declare vanadium's essentiality, at least in the chicken and the rat. On this basis, and in anticipation that its essentiality will eventually be established for the human, vanadium will be reviewed here.

Vanadium exists in several oxidation states, V^{+2} to V^{+5}. In solutions, vanadium produces a range of colors. In its pentavalent state, it is yellowish orange whereas in its divalent state it is blue [2]. In biological systems, vanadium is found in primarily the pentavalent state known as *vanadate* (VO_3^- or $H_2VO_4^-$) or in the tetravalent state vanadyl ion (VO^{+2}).

Sources

The content of vanadium in foods is very low, and consequently so is its average dietary intake. Using neutron activation analysis, Byrne and Kosta [3] found that most fats and oils, fruits, and vegetables contained particularly low levels of the mineral, less than 1 ng/g. Cereals, liver, and fish tended to have intermediate levels of about 5 to 40 ng/g. A few items such as spinach, black pepper, parsley, mushrooms, and oysters contained relatively high concentrations, and shellfish was particularly rich in the element, having greater than 400 ng/g dry basis. Pennington and Jones [4] reported that foods containing relatively high amounts of vanadium included breakfast cereals, canned fruit juices, fish sticks, vegetables, sweets, wine, and beer.

Absorption and Transport

There is limited information on the absorption of vanadium. This is due in part to the fact that its multiform state of oxidation complicates such studies. Dietary composition and the form of vanadium administered predictably affect the percentage absorbed.

According to most animal studies and even relatively older investigations using human subjects, vanadium appears to be poorly absorbed, generally less than 5% [5,6]. Moreover, vanadium is thought to be reduced to vanadyl in the stomach before absorption, yet in contrast to vanadyl, vanadate is 3 to 5 times more efficiently absorbed [5,6].

Studies on vanadium absorption in rats [7] have documented absorption ranging from 10% to as high as 40%. These rat studies suggest caution in assuming that vanadium will always be poorly absorbed.

In plasma and other body fluids, vanadium or vanadate is converted into vanadyl. Glutathione, NADH, and ascorbic acid can act as reducing agents for vanadate. Once formed, vanadyl binds to iron-containing proteins to form vanadyl–transferrin and vanadyl–ferritin complexes. Such complexes also exist in hepatocyte cytosol; it is interesting that while binding occurs with nonheme iron metalloproteins, vanadyl is not significantly attached to hemoproteins.

Vanadium is presumably thought to enter cells as vanadate through transport systems for phosphate, which it mimics chemically, and possibly other anions. Similar to reactions in the plasma, intracellular vanadate is reduced by glutathione to the cation vanadyl, which is then almost exclusively bound to a variety of ligands, many of which are phosphates [8].

Little vanadium is found in the body. Most tissues contain less than 10 ng V/g tissue. Distribution studies indicate that while kidney cells retain most of the absorbed mineral soon after its administration, accumulation later shifts principally to bone, with somewhat lesser amounts in spleen and liver. This is understandable in view of the high content in bone of inorganic phosphate, to which vanadyl binds tenaciously [8].

Functions

Vanadium is very active pharmacologically, exerting a broad assortment of effects that are well documented. However, the reader is cautioned not to confuse essentiality with pharmacologic activity, since the latter is generally manifested only above a concentration threshold that is considerably greater than that required to fulfill the need for essentiality.

No specific biochemical function has been identified for vanadium. Many of vanadium's effects *in vivo* are predictable from a consideration of its aqueous chemistry. As vanadate, it will compete with phosphate at the active sites of phosphate transport proteins, phosphohydrolases, and phosphotransferases. As vanadyl, it will compete with other transition metal ions for binding sites on metalloproteins and for small ligands such as adenosine triphosphate (ATP). Third, it will participate in redox reactions within the cell, particularly with substances that can reduce vanadate nonenzymatically, such as glutathione.

A few of the more thoroughly investigated pharmacologic effects of vanadium are discussed briefly next. Vanadium inhibits Na^+/K^+-ATPase, an enzyme involved in the phosphorylation by ATP of the carrier protein for sodium ions, permitting the transport of the ions against a concentration gradient. Vanadate is known to inhibit the enzyme by binding to its ATP hydrolysis site. Subsequently it was suggested that vanadate might function as a regulator of sodium pump activity [9].

Vanadium, as vanadate, is believed to stimulate adenylate cyclase by promoting an association of an otherwise inactive guanine nucleotide regulatory protein (G protein) with the catalytic unit of the enzyme [10]. Adenylate cyclase catalyzes the formation of cyclic 3′,5′-adenosine monophosphate (cAMP) from ATP. Cyclic AMP then stimulates protein kinases, which catalyze the phosphorylation of various enzymes and other cellular proteins in cytoplasm, membranes, mitochondria, ribosomes, and the nucleus. The phosphorylation is nearly always stimulatory, and it results secondarily from the hormone-induced stimulation of adenylate cyclase. This is the basis for cAMP's putative role as a second messenger of hormone action.

The effect of vanadate on the transport of amino acids across the intestinal mucosa exemplifies both its inhibitory effect on Na^+/K^+-ATPase and its stimulation of adenylate cyclase. At higher concentrations, vanadate inhibits the mucosal-to-serosal flux of alanine, commensurate with a decrease in Na^+/K^+-ATPase function. However, at a lower concentration (too low to affect Na^+/K^+-ATPase), it is stimulatory to alanine transport, attributable to an increase in adenylate cyclase activity and cAMP formation [11].

Vanadium appears to affect glucose metabolism by mimicking the action of insulin. Vanadium thereby stimulates glucose uptake into cells and enhances glucose metabolism for glycogen synthesis. Studies on animals, for example, have shown that vanadate can control high blood glucose and prevent the decline in cardiac performance associated with diabetes [12]. The insulin-mimicking effect of vanadate is linked in part to its stimulation of protein kinase activity. As an example, like insulin, it promotes the phosphorylation of tyrosyl residues in the insulin receptor, preparatory to the expression of insulin activity [13]. The revelation that vanadate can inhibit phosphotyrosine phosphatase, thereby prolonging the activity of phosphorylated enzymes, forms the basis for other proposed mechanisms [14]. There is evidence, too, that sodium vanadate exerts an insulinotropic effect by stimulating the release of insulin from rat islet cells [15].

Although vanadate's chemical similarity to phosphate accounts in large part for its biochemical action, vanadium, as the vanadyl cation, has also been shown to be physiologically active, particularly in its substitution for other metals such as Zn^{+2}, Cu^{+2}, and Fe^{+3} in metalloenzyme activity.

Recent studies examining vanadium deficiency have suggested that the element is associated with iodine metabolism and/or thyroid gland function [16].

Excretion

Most ingested vanadium is excreted in the feces, and most of this represents unabsorbed vanadium. Renal excretion is the major route for the elimination of absorbed vanadium.

Recommended Intake and Assessment of Nutriture

The human requirement for vanadium is not established, although estimates range from 10 to 25 µg/day [6]. Vanadium intake in the U.S. diet is thought to range from 10 to 60 µg/day [2]. Daily intakes up to 100 µg are thought to be safe [2]. Toxicity has been shown in humans with intakes of 10 mg or more. Toxic manifestations include green tongue (due to deposition of green-colored vanadium in the tongue), diarrhea, gastrointestinal cramps, and disturbances in mental function [2,6].

Reported levels of vanadium in healthy adults are 0.02 to 10 ng/mL in plasma or serum, 0.01 to 2.2 µg/g in hair, and 0 to 10 µg/day excreted in the urine. Current analytic techniques for the determination of vanadium in biological specimens are inadequate. The techniques most commonly used are neutron activation analysis and flameless atomic absorption spectrophotometry, the latter being the practical choice for most analytic laboratories.

References Cited for Vanadium

1. Nielsen FH. Vanadium. In: Mertz, W, ed. Trace elements in human and animal nutrition. San Diego: Academic Press, 1987;1:275–300.
2. Harland BF, Harden-Williams BA. Is vanadium of human nutritional importance yet? J Am Diet Assoc 1994;94: 891–894.
3. Byrne AR, Kosta L. Vanadium in foods and in human body fluids and tissues. Sci Total Environ 1978;10:17–30.
4. Pennington JAT, Jones JW. Molybdenum, nickel, cobalt, vanadium, and strontium in total diets. J Am Diet Assoc 1987;87:1644–1650.
5. Nielsen FH. Other trace elements. In: Brown ML, ed. Present knowledge in nutrition. Washington, DC: International Life Sciences Institute Nutrition Foundation, 1990;294–307.
6. Nielsen FH. Ultratrace minerals. In: Shils ME, Olson JA, Shike M, eds. Modern nutrition in health and disease. Philadelphia: Lea and Febiger, 1994;269–286.
7. Bogden JD, Higashino H, Lavenhar MA, Bauman JW, Kemp FW, Aviv A. Balance and tissue distribution of vanadium after short-term ingestion of vanadate. J Nutr 1982;112:2279–2285.
8. Nechay BR, Nanninga LB, Nechay PSE, Post RL, Grantham JJ, Macara IG, Kubena LF, Phillips TD, Nielsen FH. Role of vanadium in biology. Fed Proc 1986;45:123–132.
9. Macara IG, Kustin K, Cantley LC. Glutathione reduces cytoplasmic vanadate: Mechanism and physiological implications. Biochim Biophys Acta 1980;629:95–106.
10. Krawietz W, Downs RW, Spiegel AM, Aurbach GD. Vanadate stimulates adenylate cyclase via the guanine nucleotide regulatory protein by a mechanism differing from that of fluoride. Biochem Pharmacol 1982;31: 843–848.
11. Hajjar JJ, Fucci JC, Rowe WA, Tomicic TK. Effect of vanadate on amino acid transport in rat jejunum. Proc Soc Exp Biol Med 1987;184:403–409.
12. Heyliger CE, Tahiliani AG, McNeill JH. Effect of vanadate on elevated blood glucose and depressed cardiac performance of diabetic rats. Science 1985;227:1474–1477.
13. Tamura S, Brown TA, Whipple JH, Fujita-Yamaguchi Y, Dubler RE, Cheng K, Larner J. A novel mechanism for the insulin-like effects of vanadate on glycogen synthase in rat adipocytes. J Biol Chem 1984;259:6650–6658.
14. Stankiewicz PJ, Gresser MJ. Inhibition of phosphatase and sulfatase by transition-state analogues. Biochemistry 1988;27:206–212.
15. Fagin JA, Ikejiri K, Levin SR. Insulinotropic effects of vanadate. Diabetes 1987;36:1448–1452.
16. Nielsen FH. Ultratrace elements of possible importance for human health: An update. In: Prasad AS, ed. Essential and toxic trace elements in human health. New York: Wiley-Liss, 1993;355–376.

ARSENIC

More than any other essential trace mineral, arsenic conjures an image of toxicity rather than nutritional essentiality. The malevolent aspect of arsenic continues to attract the most attention, since a great deal more of the arsenic literature addresses its toxicologic rather than its nutritional properties. Nevertheless, there is accumulating evidence that arsenic is an essential element in vertebrates [1].

Arsenic is present throughout the earth's continental crust at an estimated concentration of 1.5 to 2.0 µg/g. It is present in all soils, although its concentration varies considerably from region to region, affected by the geologic history of a particular soil and, more importantly, by pollution from unnatural sources. Fallout sources such as pesticides, smelters, and coal-fired power plants can, through aerosols and floating dust, enrich a particular area with arsenic. It then affects humans and animals through its incorporation into foods and feedstuffs, which, however, usually contain less than 0.3 µg/g on a dry basis and rarely exceed 1.0 µg/g. Ranges of arsenic content in various foods and feeds are listed in Table 12.12, from which it is clear that foods of marine origin are much richer in arsenic than other foods.

Arsenic exists in nature in both the trivalent and pentavalent ionic states but in much greater quantity as organoarsenicals, specifically, methylated forms. Some commonly occurring, natural forms of arsenic are illus-

Table 12.12 Arsenic Content of Selected Foods

Food Category	Range (μg/g)
Forage crops	0.1–1.0
Cereals	0.05–0.4
Vegetables	0.05–0.8
Fruits	0.03–1.0 (dry weight)
Meat	0.005–0.1 (fresh weight)
Milk	0.01–0.05
Eggs	0.01–0.1 (fresh weight)
Fish	2.0–80
Oysters	3.0–10
Mussels	Up to 10,120

Source: Anke M. Arsenic. In: Mertz W, ed. Trace elements in human and animal nutrition. Orlando, FL: Academic Press, 1986;2:360.

trated in Figure 12.20. Of these, inorganic arsenite and trivalent organoarsenicals are the most toxic to animals. The pentavalent, methylated arsenic compounds are far less toxic, and are readily absorbed and used.

Absorption and Transport

Absorption, as well as retention and excretion, of arsenicals vary with their chemical form, the quantity administered, and the animal species involved in the study. The major arsenicals found in foods, including those represented in Figure 12.20, are readily absorbed. For example, of the organic arsenicals, over 90% of arsenobetaine and between 70 and 80% of arsenocholine are absorbed. Absorption of organic arsenicals is thought to occur by simple diffusion across the intestinal mucosa. The greater the lipid solubility of the arsenical, the greater the likelihood of its transmucosal passage by simple diffusion.

Inorganic arsenate and arsenite fed in water solutions are also readily absorbed. Although the mechanism of absorption is not well understood, it has been reported [2] that arsenic, as arsenate, is absorbed in a manner similar to phosphorus, as phosphate. Solubility of the inorganic arsenic compound also influences its absorption.

From the intestine, inorganic arsenic is taken up by the liver. Humans and other mammalian species metabolize absorbed inorganic arsenic, shown in Figure 12.20. Arsenate is reduced to arsenite [3–5], which is then methylated. Less toxic methylated forms include methylarsonic acid and dimethylarsinic acid.

Organic arsenic that is absorbed apparently undergoes little or no chemical change, as indicated by the fact that the urinary arsenic excreted following the ingestion of arsenic-rich seafoods remained in the original, organically bound form [6].

Arsenic in the blood is found in two forms, methylated and protein bound. Tissues that contain the most arsenic include skin, hair, and nails. Arsenic is found bound primarily to sulfhydryl (SH) groups of proteins within these tissues.

Functions

Arsenic appears to play a role in methionine as well as in arginine metabolism; however, arsenic has not been shown to be an activator or inhibitor of a specific enzyme. Metabolism of methionine is impaired with arsenic deficiency and the activity of S-adenosylmethionine (SAM) decarboxylase (p. 176, Fig. 7.19) is diminished suggesting a role in certain decarboxylation reactions [7].

The effect of arsenic on arginine metabolism is ambiguous because it is dependent on the arginine and zinc status of the animal. This suggests that the effect of arsenic on the enzyme may somehow be mediated through the nutrients. In studies on kidney arginase activity in chicks, using supplemental arginine, arsenic, and zinc as variables, the following interesting observation resulted. When dietary arginine was increased by supplement, plasma urea and kidney arginase were substantially elevated. However, the elevation of those two parameters was influenced significantly by dietary arsenic and zinc. Zinc deficiency prevented the rise in plasma urea and kidney arginase activity in arsenic-deprived animals, but, in contrast, zinc deficiency increased the elevation of those parameters in arsenic-supplemented animals. In another study, when dietary zinc was marginally adequate, arsenic deprivation caused depressed growth and elevated hematocrits in chicks. However, during zinc deficiency, growth was more markedly depressed and hematocrit values higher in arsenic-supplemented than in arsenic-deprived chicks. The review by Uthus et al. [8] is recommended as additional reading about this interaction among arsenic, zinc, and arginine. There is a need to ascertain how, and at which metabolic sites, this interaction occurs.

Arsenic may also have a role similar to that of phosphorus in lipids, as suggested by the occurrence in marine organisms of organic arsenicals such as arsenocholine, arsenobetaine, and the novel membrane phospholipid, O-phosphatidyltrimethylarsonium lactic acid. Also, in higher animals arsenocholine can replace choline in some of its functions.

Interactions with Other Nutrients

Arsenic seems to interact antagonistically with *selenium* and *iodine*. Because selenate and arsenate are both oxyanions with similar chemical properties, they may com-

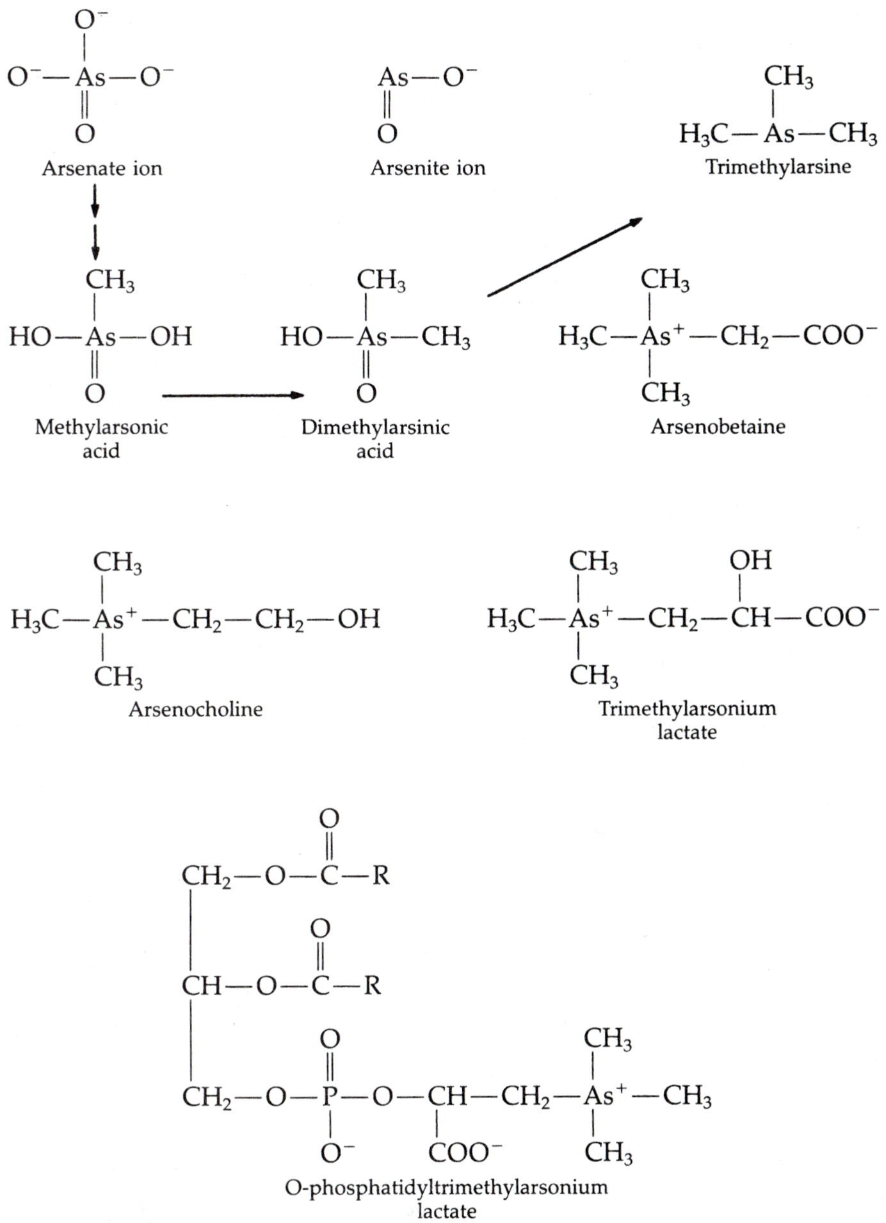

FIGURE 12.20 Some biologically important forms of arsenic.

petitively inhibit the uptake and tissue retention of each other. The interaction of arsenic with iodine is exemplified by the observation that it is goitrogenic in mice. Arsenic is believed to antagonize the mechanism of iodine uptake by the thyroid, causing compensatory goiter.

Excretion

Ingested arsenic is excreted rapidly via the kidneys, with increased intake resulting in an increased excretory rate. The latter therefore can provide a useful index of exposure. The rate of urinary excretion in humans depends on the dietary form of the arsenical. For example, methylarsonic acid and dimethylarsinic acid are excreted at about the same rate—approximately 76% of the ingested amount within a four-day period. Excretion of inorganic arsenite, in contrast, is markedly slower, approximating 46% of the intake over the same period of time. This corroborates the observation [9] that arsenite, compared to other forms, is bound very strongly to tissues.

The results of studies on dogs [4] have shown that intravenously (IV) administered arsenate, at what the authors considered medium dosage, was excreted as arsenite at first, but that later, dimethylarsinic acid became the major urinary metabolite.

Deficiency and Toxicity

Reported effects of arsenic deprivation in test animals have included curtailed growth, reduced conception rate, and increased neonatal mortality.

Organic forms of arsenic are less toxic than inorganic forms of the element. The fatal acute dose of arsenic trioxide appears to be 0.76 to 1.95 mg [10].

Recommended Intake and Assessment of Nutriture

There are insufficient data to estimate a human dietary requirement for arsenic, although 12–15 μg have been suggested [10]. Most diets, however, would be expected to provide an adequate intake of the mineral, due to its ubiquitous occurrence. Recent food surveys indicate intakes of 20 to 140 μg/day in the United States, but this range would be significantly elevated if relatively large amounts of seafood are consumed.

Reported levels of arsenic in body fluids include 2–62 ng/mL whole blood, 1–20 ng/mL plasma or serum, and 5–50 μg excreted daily in urine from healthy adults. Hair arsenic levels are 0.1–1.1 μg/g. Chronic or acute exposure to the metal would elevate these values, and hair analysis has been particularly useful in this respect. This is because hair arsenic content, unlike that of the fluids, represents an average content over an extended period and would not fluctuate in parallel with intermittent exposure to the element.

The current method of choice for the determination of arsenic in biological fluids is atomic absorption spectrometry, although mass spectrometry, neutron activation analysis, and emission spectroscopy have been used successfully.

References Cited for Arsenic

1. Nielsen FH. Evidence of the essentiality of arsenic, nickel, and vanadium, and their possible nutritional significance. In: Draper HH, ed. Advances in nutritional research. New York: Plenum Press 1980;3:157.
2. Klevay LM. Pharmacology and toxicology of heavy metals: Arsenic. Pharmacol Ther 1976;1:189–209.
3. Lerman SA, Clarkson TW, Gerson RJ. Arsenic uptake and metabolism by liver cells is dependent on arsenic's oxidation state. Chem Biol Interact 1983;45:401–406.
4. Tsukamoto H, Parker HR, Peoples SA. Metabolism and renal handling of sodium arsenate in dogs. Am J Vet Res 1983;44:2331–2335.
5. Anke M. Arsenic. In: Mertz W, ed. Trace elements in human and animal nutrition. Orlando, FL: Academic Press, 1986;2:347–372.
6. Tam GKH, Charbonneau SM, Bryce F, Sandi E. Excretion of a single oral dose of fish-arsenic in man. Bull Environ Contam Toxicol 1982;28:669–673.
7. Nielsen FH. Ultratrace elements of possible importance for human health: An update. In: Prasad AS, ed. Essential and toxic trace elements in human health. New York: Wiley-Liss, 1993;355–376.
8. Uthus ED, Cornatzer WE, Nielsen FH. Consequences of arsenic deprivation in laboratory animals. In: Lederer WH, ed. Arsenic symposium, production and use, biomedical and environmental perspectives. New York: Van Nostrand Reinhold, 1983;173–189.
9. Vahter M, Marafante E. Intracellular interaction and metabolic fate of arsenite and arsenate in mice and rabbits. Chem Biol Interact 1983;47:29–44.
10. Nielsen FH. Ultratrace Minerals. In: Shils ME, Olson JA, Shike M, eds. Modern nutrition in health and disease. Philadelphia: Lea and Febiger, 1994;269–286.

BORON

Evidence for the essentiality of boron in animals has been mounting since the 1980s. The element was first considered essential for plants back in the early 1920s.

Sources

Foods of plant origin such as fruits, leafy vegetables, nuts, and legumes are rich in boron, which appears in foods as sodium borate or boric acid. In addition, wine, cider, and beer contribute to dietary intake. Meat and fish are poor sources of the element.

Absorption, Transport, and Excretion

Greater than 90% of ingested boron is thought to be rapidly absorbed [1]; however, most of the absorbed boron is excreted in the urine. Little is known with respect to boron transport and metabolism. Boron is found in body tissues, especially bone and spleen among others [2].

Functions

Boron acts directly or indirectly to influence the composition, structure, and strength of bones [3]. Although the mechanism of action is not known, boron affects variables associated with calcium metabolism including vitamin D and magnesium. For example, a vitamin D deficiency enhances the need for boron, and boron normalizes abnormalities associated with a magnesium deficiency [2].

Boron inhibits two groups of enzymes. One group inhibited by boron is the pyridine or flavin nucleotide requiring oxidoreductases (such as aldehyde dehydrogenase, xanthine dehydrogenase, and cytochrome b_5 reductase) [1]. A second group of enzymes, included in which are chymotrypsin and glyceraldehyde 3-phosphate dehydrogenase, is also affected by borate or boronic acid, which binds to the active site of these enzymes [1].

Boron complexes with organic compounds containing hydroxy groups (OH); therefore, many nutrients, including sugars, pyridoxine, riboflavin, and dehydroascorbic acid, can be bound by boron [1]. In fact, boron toxicity is associated with increased urinary riboflavin excretion in humans [2,4].

Deficiency and Toxicity

Although the most consistent sign of boron deficiency in animals is depressed growth, in humans, a low-boron diet is associated with increased urinary calcium and magnesium excretion and with alterations in steroid hormone metabolism.

Acute toxicity of boron in humans results in nausea, vomiting, diarrhea, dermatitis, and lethargy. Increased urinary excretion of riboflavin has also been reported [2,4].

Recommended Intake and Assessment of Nutriture

Intakes of 1 to 3 mg, and perhaps up to 10 mg boron, have been suggested as safe [1]. A requirement has been estimated at 1 mg daily [4].

Measurement of boron in biological fluids is still being investigated. Inductively coupled plasma emission spectrometry has been used to determine plasma and other body fluid concentrations of the element; however, whether these tissue concentrations are indicative of nutritional status is unknown.

References Cited for Boron

1. Nielsen FH. Ultratrace minerals. In: Shils ME, Olson JA, Shike M, eds. Modern nutrition in health and disease. Philadelphia: Lea and Febiger, 1994;269–286.
2. Nielsen FH. Other elements. In: Mertz, W, ed. Trace elements in human and animal nutrition. San Diego: Academic Press, 1987;2: 415–463.
3. Nielsen FH. Ultratrace elements of possible importance for human health: An update. In: Prasad AS, ed. Essential and toxic trace elements in human health. New York: Wiley-Liss, 1993;355–376.
4. Nielsen FH. Other trace elements. In: Brown ML, ed. Present knowledge in nutrition. Washington, DC: International Life Sciences Institute Nutrition Foundation, 1990;294–307.

COBALT

There is little evidence that there is a role for cobalt in human nutrition other than its being a part of vitamin B_{12} (cobalamin). Although it is true that ionic cobalt can substitute for other metals in metalloenzyme activity *in vitro*, a fact that will be reviewed briefly, there is no evidence for its acting in that capacity *in vivo*. In this respect the metal is unique among the essential trace elements in that the requirement in the human is not for an ionic form of the metal but for a preformed metallovitamin, which cannot be synthesized from dietary metal. Therefore it is the vitamin B_{12} content of foods and diet that is of importance in human nutrition rather than the ionic cobalt status.

There have been reports regarding the dependency of certain enzymes on cobalt as an activator or on the metal's ability to substitute for other metal ion activators. Cobalt, in the form of $CoCl_2$, for example, appears to regulate the activity of certain phosphoprotein phosphatases, such as casein and phosvitin phosphatases [1,2]. In another study on phosphoprotein phosphatases, only Co^{+2} and Mn^{+2} could reactivate enzymes inactivated by ATP, ADP, and PP_i, with cobalt being significantly the more potent as a reactivator [3]. Cobalt, along with Mn^{+2} and Ni^{+2} can also substitute for Zn^{+2} in the metalloenzymes, angiotensin-converting enzyme [4], carboxypeptidase [5], and carbonic anhydrase [6].

The reader is cautioned against interpreting such findings as an implication of the possible essentiality of ionic cobalt. There is no evidence from deprivation studies on animals that the metal is a requirement for these enzymes *in vivo*.

References Cited for Cobalt

1. Japundzic I, Levi E, Japundzic M. Cobalt-dependent protein phosphatases from human cord blood erythrocytes. I. Submolecular structure and regulation of activity of E_3 casein phosphatase. Enzyme 1988;39:134–143.
2. Japundzic I, Levi E, Japundzic M. Cobalt-dependent protein phosphatases from human cord blood erythrocytes. II. Further characterization of E_2 casein phosphatase. Enzyme 1988; 39:144–150.

3. Khandelwal RL, Kamani SAS. Studies on inactivation and reactivation of homogeneous rabbit liver phosphoprotein phosphatases by inorganic pyrophosphate and divalent cations. Biochim Biophys Acta 1980;613:95–105.

4. Bicknell R, Holmquist B, Lee FS, Martin MT, Riordan JF. Electronic spectroscopy of cobalt angiotensin converting enzyme and its inhibitor complexes. Biochemistry 1987;26:7291–7297.

5. Auld DS, Holmquist B. Carboxypeptidase A. Differences in the mechanisms of ester and peptide hydrolysis. Biochemistry 1974;13:4355–4361.

6. Lindskog S. Carbonic anhydrase. In: Spiro TG, ed. Zinc enzymes. New York: Wiley 1983;86–97.

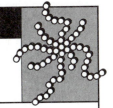

PERSPECTIVE

Hypoferremia and Infection: When Are Iron Supplements Advisable?

As indicated in Figure 1 (at base of triangle), nutritional deficiency is believed to be deleterious and to impair defense mechanisms against infections. This view has been challenged especially with respect to iron, because a normal physiologic response to infection is a decrease in serum iron [1,2]. The reason for this shift of iron from circulation into storage is not understood, but some researchers believe the function of the shift is to protect the host by decreasing the availability of iron to invading micro-organisms [3]. Micro-organisms (with the exception of lactobacilli [2]) cannot multiply without a source of iron. Whether or not the likelihood of human infection can be reduced by iron withholding is highly controversial; nevertheless, effective sequestering of the host's readily available iron from pathogens for their own use is an established fact.

To solubilize and assimilate ferric iron (Fe^{+3}) for their use, bacteria produce siderophores, which chelate the iron and bring it into the cell. Within the cell, iron is released from the chelate by enzymatic reduction to ferrous iron (Fe^{+2}), the usable form of the mineral [3]. The siderophores produced by bacteria invading the host are inhibited in their sequestering of the host's iron by two (or perhaps more) glycoproteins synthesized by the host. The two known glycoproteins are lactoferrin, a major component in human milk and also found in many other mammalian exocrine secretions, and transferrin, the iron-binding protein in the serum that transports iron from the intestine to other tissues of the body [3,4]. Lactoferrin and transferrin each can bind two atoms of iron per molecule of protein and provide the host with what Weinberg [4] terms "nutritional immunity."

As mentioned, infection of the host is characterized by a decrease in serum levels of iron. Unsaturated lactoferrin, which is a major protein component of circulating neutrophils (leucocytes) [4], mediates the iron uptake from the serum. Lactoferrin is released into the plasma from activated neutrophils, binds iron, and the resulting complex is cleared from circulation, thereby causing hypoferremia. The iron complexed by lactoferrin is removed from circulation by mononuclear phagocytes, and the sequestered iron ultimately becomes part of iron storage compounds such as hemosiderin [1]. Much of the iron removed from circulation is stored in the liver [1,5]. Fever also appears to be a deterrent to the securing of iron by bacteria; ele-

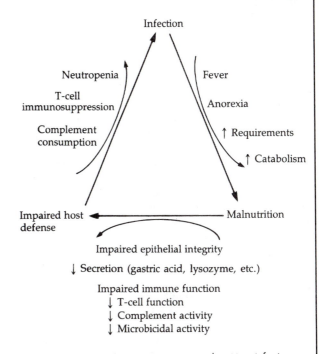

FIGURE 1 Triangle of interaction among malnutrition, infection, and host defense. *(Reproduced with permission from the Annual Review of Nutrition, Vol. 6, © 1986, by Annual Reviews Inc.)*

vated temperatures decrease the production of siderophores [3].

The positive relationship between the availability of iron to bacteria and the likelihood of infections is particularly evident in people suffering from various diseases characterized by iron overload (hyperferremia). People subject to hyperferremic episodes are those suffering from (1) destruction of liver cells containing ferritin, as might occur in viral hepatitis; (2) hemolytic anemia, as can occur in malaria, sickle cell disease, and leukemia; and (3) overload of iron from exogenous sources, which is particularly possible in neonates [5]. These people are more susceptible to infection than their nonhyperferremic counterparts; furthermore, during acute hyperferremic episodes they have greater susceptibility to bacterial and fungal pathogens than they do when their plasma iron is within normal range [5]. Transferrin concentration does not usually rise; therefore, hyperferremia is usually characterized by an elevated iron saturation of circulating transferrin.

PERSPECTIVE (continued)

Weinberg [4,5] postulates that a transferrin saturation of greater than 50% allows an easier removal of the host's iron by the siderophores of pathogens.

Of particular concern is the possible oversupplementation of healthy, full-term neonates who are born with an abundance of iron, as indicated by the degree of transferrin saturation. At birth, mean transferrin saturation is 69%; but by two months healthy infants have decreased the degree of saturation to 34% and by 6 months to 25% [4]. The decrease in saturation is due primarily to increased transferrin being synthesized by the healthy, maturing infant. The normal iron saturation level averages approximately 20 to 30% [4].

The inadvisability of a routine, vigorous treatment of neonates with supplemental iron to prevent iron deficiency has been emphasized by some tragic experiences with prophylactic parenteral iron. About 20 years ago it was a common practice in some New Zealand clinics to administer parenterally an iron–dextran complex to infants during their first week of life to protect them against iron deficiency anemia [1,3,6]. The practice was stopped when it was found that the incidence of bacterial septicemias and meningitis was eight times higher in the treated infants than in those who received no iron supplementation [3,6]. The great majority of affected infants were healthy at birth and did not suffer any recognized perinatal event likely to lead to infection; the increase in the incidence of infections appeared due to iron supplementation [6].

Another group of children at particular risk from exogenous iron are those suffering with kwashiorkor. These children, although actually hypoferremic, have transferrin saturation values of over 100% due to hypotransferrinemia. Because of their inability to synthesize transferrin, these children, when supplemented with iron before correction of their protein deficiency, are very susceptible to iron overload. Circulating free iron in these malnourished children appears to allow a greatly increased incidence of bacterial infections, infections often severe enough to cause death [5,6].

Despite the advantages that possibly could be accrued through iron withdrawal from the host so that bacteria cannot multiply, the dangers associated with iron deficiency anemia cannot be overlooked. Iron deficiency anemia is considered one of humanity's most crucial nutritional problems [7], and many studies suggest that iron deficiency in infants and children predisposes to infection, particularly involving the respiratory and gastrointestinal tracts [1]. Furthermore, these studies suggest that administration of iron in some circumstances can reduce infection rates [1]. Many of these studies, however, have been uncontrolled or poorly controlled and therefore permit no reliable

conclusions about the influence of iron alone in the development or resolution of the infection [1]. Nevertheless, the effect of iron on the host's immune system cannot be overlooked; cell-mediated responses in particular are susceptible to iron deficiency. Not only have defective macrophage functions been observed [8], but also a reduction in the proliferation of T-cells. The proliferation of T-cells requires acquisition of transferrin-bound iron, and, as demonstrated by experimental iron deficiency, transferrin saturation can fall below the value needed for optimal proliferation [2]. Too low a level of transferrin saturation can result in atrophy of lymphoid tissues, with depletion of lymphocytes in general. Therefore a decrease in humoral immunity (production of antibodies) as well as cell-mediated immunity can occur [9].

Developing a unifying hypothesis to explain the two different views regarding iron status and susceptibility to infection is very difficult [1]. Although iron deficiency may increase the host's ability to withhold iron from invading pathogens ("nutritional immunity"), this advantage may be overshadowed by impairment of the host's cell-mediated and humoral immune responses [2]. Keusch and Farthing [1] propose that iron deficiency in an otherwise well-nourished individual with normal serum transferrin should probably require iron supplements orally to remove the risk of an impaired immune system with a consequent risk of increased infections. In contrast, great care should be exercised in supplementing children with severe protein–energy malnutrition. Iron supplementation in these children with very low transferrin values could result in rapid increases in circulating free iron, thereby promoting the growth of invading pathogens. In their opinion, the "physiologic," mild iron deficiency often observed in early infancy can be considered an intermediate state. This physiologic anemia is not harmful to the immune system and at the same time allows less iron to be available to pathogens. The common practice of vigorously treating mild hypoferremia in infants prone to low-grade infections may be ill advised.

The desirable iron balance is one in which iron is not readily accessible to invading microorganisms yet is sufficient for optimal operation of the host's immune system [2]. Although transferrin plays a key role in both mechanisms involved in a desirable balance, the role that the percent iron saturation of transferrin has in making iron available to the siderophores of pathogens remains controversial [2,4].

References Cited

1. Keusch GI, Farthing MJG. Nutrition and infection. Ann Rev Nutr 1986;6:131–154.

PERSPECTIVE (continued)

2. Brock JH. Iron and the outcome of infection. Br Med J 1986;293:518–520.
3. Emery T. Iron metabolism in humans and plants. Am Sci 1982;70:626–632.
4. Weinberg ED. Iron withholding: A defense against infection and neoplasia. Physiol Rev 1984;64:65–102.
5. Weinberg ED. Iron and susceptibility to infectious disease. Science 1974;184:952–956.
6. Weinberg ED. Iron and susceptibility to infectious disease. Science 1975;188:1039.
7. Regenauer J, Saltman P. Iron and susceptibility to infectious disease. Science 1975;188:1038–1039.
8. Beisel WR, Edelman R, Nauss K, et al. Single nutrient effects on immunologic functions. JAMA 1981; 245:53–58.
9. Myrvic QN. Nutrition and immunology. In: Shils M, Young V, eds. Modern nutrition in health and disease, 7th ed. Philadelphia: Lea and Febiger, 1988: 585–616.

HOMEOSTATIC MAINTENANCE

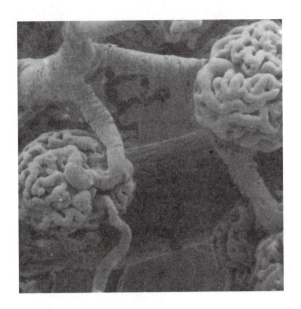

BODY FLUID AND ELECTROLYTE BALANCE

Photo: Glomeruli and associated arterioles

Chapter 1, in particular, and the subsequent chapters dealing with nutrient metabolism have emphasized the specialized nature of cells comprising the organ systems of the body. Despite the great diversity of specialized cellular functions, the composition of the body fluids (the internal environment) enveloping the cells remains relatively constant under normal conditions. This constant composition, or homeostasis, of the internal environment is necessary for optimal activity of the cells. It is maintained by homeostatic mechanisms involving most of the body's organ systems, the most important of which are those of circulation, respiration, and renal excretion, as well as central nervous system (CNS) and endocrine regulation. Many minor disturbances inevitably occur in water distribution, electrolyte balance, and pH of the body fluids during metabolism. As they arise, compensatory mechanisms of the regulatory organs make appropriate corrections in order to maintain the homeostatic state.

WATER DISTRIBUTION IN THE BODY

Water accounts for approximately 60% of the total body weight in a normal adult, making it the most abundant constituent of the human body. In terms of volume, the total body water in a man of average weight (70 kg) is roughly 40 L. Water provides the medium for the solubilization and passage of a multitude of nutrients, both organic and inorganic, from the blood to the cells and the return of metabolic products to the blood. It also serves as the medium in which the vast number of intracellular metabolic reactions take place.

Total body water can theoretically be compartmentalized into two major reservoirs, the intracellular compartment, which includes all water enclosed within cell membranes, and the extracellular compartment, which includes all water external to cell membranes. Of the 40 L of total body water, the intra-

TABLE 13.1 Fluid Compartment Volumes

	Percentage of Body Weight	Percentage of Total Body Water	Volume (L) in 70-kg Man
Total body water	60%	—	42
Extracellular water	20	33%	14
Plasma	5	8	3.5
Interstitial fluid	15	25	10.5
Intracellular water	40	67	28

cellular and extracellular compartments account for about 25 L and 15 L, respectively. The anatomic extracellular water is functionally subdivided into the plasma, which is the cell-free, intravascular water compartment, and the interstitial fluid (ISF). The ISF directly bathes the extravascular cells and provides the medium for the passage of nutrients and metabolic products reciprocally from the blood to those cells. In addition, there are potential spaces in the body (that is, pericardial, pleural, peritoneal, and synovial) that are normally empty except for a small volume of viscous lubricating fluid that needs to be considered as part of the interstitial fluid compartment. The body water compartment volumes are summarized in Table 13.1 for a 70-kg man.

The fraction of total body weight that is water and the percentage of total body water that is extracellular or intracellular do not remain constant during growth. Expressed as a percentage of body weight, total body water decreases during gestation and early childhood, reaching adult values by about 3 years of age. During this time the extracellular water (expressed as a percentage of body weight) decreases while the intracellular water (percentage of body weight) increases (p. 456).

MAINTENANCE OF FLUID BALANCE

Most of the daily intake of water enters by the oral route as beverages and as liquids contained in foods. A relatively small amount of water is also formed within the body as a product of metabolic reactions. These two sources together account for the daily intake of approximately 2,500 mL of fluid, of which the oral route contributes about 2,300 mL, more than 90%.

The routes by which water is lost from the body can vary according to environmental and physiological conditions such as ambient temperature and extent of physical exercise. At an ambient temperature of 68°F, about 1,400 mL of the 2,300 mL taken in is normally lost in the urine, 100 mL is lost in the sweat, and 200 mL in the feces. The remaining 600 mL leaves the body as *insensi-*

ble water loss, so called because the subject is not aware of the water loss as it is occurring. Evaporation from the respiratory tract and diffusion through the skin are examples of insensible water loss.

One of the more important factors determining the distribution of water among the water compartments of the body is osmotic pressure. When a membrane permeable to water but impermeable to solute particles separates two fluid compartments of unequal solute concentrations, there is a net movement of water through the membrane from the solution with higher water (lower solute) concentration toward the solution with lower water (higher solute) concentration. The movement of water is called *osmosis*, and it can be opposed by applying an external pressure across the membrane in the opposite direction. The amount of pressure required to exactly oppose osmosis into a solution across a semipermeable membrane separating it from pure water is the osmotic pressure of the solution.

The *theoretic osmotic pressure* of a solution is proportional to the number of solute particles per unit volume of solution. This concentration is expressed in terms of the osmolarity, or osmoles per liter, of solute particles. One mole of a nonionic solute, such as glucose or urea, is the same as 1 osm, but 1 mol of a solute that dissociates into two or more ions is equivalent to two or more osm. For example, 1.0 mol of sodium chloride equals 2.0 osm because of its dissociation into sodium and chloride ions. The theoretic osmotic pressure presupposes that the solute particles are unable to pass freely through the membrane. When the membrane is permeable to a solute, it does not contribute to the actual, or *effective*, osmotic pressure. The higher the permeability of a membrane to a solute, the lower the effective osmotic pressure of a solution of that solute at a given osmolarity. As an example, cell membranes are much more permeable to a nonionic substance such as urea than to sodium and chloride. Therefore, the effective osmotic pressure of a solution of urea across the cell membrane would be much less than a solution of sodium chloride of the same osmolarity.

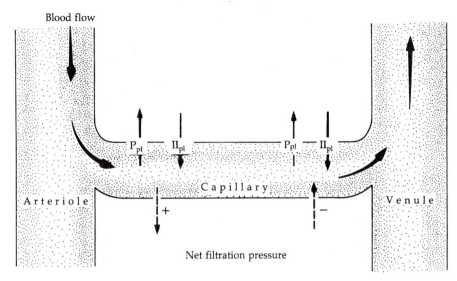

Blood flow

Arteriole

P_{pl} — Π_{pl} P_{pl} — Π_{pl}

Capillary

Venule

+   −

Net filtration pressure

FIGURE 13.1 Starling's hypothesis of water distribution between plasma and interstitial fluid compartments. The relative magnitudes of the pressures, P_{pl} (plasma hydrostatic pressure) and Π_{pl} (plasma osmotic pressure), are represented by the thickness of their respective arrows. There is a positive net filtration pressure at the arteriolar end of the capillary and a negative net filtration pressure at the venule end. *(Kleinman LI, Lorenz JM. Physiology and pathophysiology of body water and electrolytes. In: Kaplan LA, Pesce AJ. Clinical chemistry: theory, analysis, and correlation, 2nd ed. St. Louis: Mosby, 1989:373.)*

The term *osmolality* is sometimes encountered in the expression of osmotic pressure. Like *osmolarity*, it denotes the concentration of solute particles. However, rather than a weight-per-volume expression of concentration, *osmolality* refers to solute concentration on a weight-per-weight basis. Specifically, it is the moles of solute particles per kilogram of solvent. Although it is less convenient than molarity as a unit of concentration, osmolality has the advantage of being unaffected by temperature, which can cause expansion or contraction of solvent volume.

The effective osmotic pressure of plasma and interstitial fluid across the capillary endothelium that separates them is mainly due to large molecules such as proteins that cannot permeate the endothelium. Protein concentration is much higher in the plasma than in the interstitial fluid, therefore conferring on the plasma a relatively high osmotic pressure, or water-attracting property. Proteins and other macromolecules too large to traverse the capillary endothelium are sometimes called *colloids*, and the osmotic pressure attributed to them is appropriately termed the *colloid osmotic pressure*.

Water distribution across the capillary endothelial surface is controlled by the balance of forces that tend to move water from the plasma to the interstitial fluid (filtration forces) and by forces that move water from the interstitial fluid into the plasma (reabsorption forces). The major filtration force in the capillaries is hydrostatic pressure (P_{pl}) caused by the pumping of the heart, while a much weaker filtration force is the ISF colloid osmotic pressure (Π_{isf}). This force is weak because of the negligible concentration of protein in the ISF. Another weak filtration force is a small, *negative*, ISF hydrostatic pres-

sure (P_{isf}). The major reabsorption force, countering the filtration forces, is the plasma osmotic pressure (Π_{pl}), which is approximately 28 mm Hg.

At the arteriolar end of the capillaries, the average values of these forces are P_{pl}, 25 mm Hg; Π_{isf}, 5 mm Hg; P_{isf}, −6 mm Hg; Π_{pl}, 28 mm Hg. The net result of these four forces can be described by Starling's equation:

$$\text{Filtration pressure} = (P_{pl} + \Pi_{isf}) - (\Pi_{pl} + P_{isf})$$

Substituting the values,

$$\begin{aligned}
\text{Filtration pressure} &= (25 + 5) - (28 + (-6)) \\
&= (25 + 5) - (28 - 6) \\
&= 30 - 28 + 6 \\
&= +8 \text{ mm Hg}
\end{aligned}$$

This positive filtration pressure indicates that a net filtration of water from the plasma to the ISF occurs at the arteriolar end of the capillaries. When filtration pressure is negative, this indicates that a net reabsorption of water from the ISF to the plasma will take place. This would be the situation at the venule end of the capillaries, where the P_{pl} is significantly reduced while the concentration of plasma protein, and therefore the Π_{pl}, correspondingly increases. The net effect of these forces on the water distribution between plasma and ISF along the course of the capillary is shown in Figure 13.1.

From what has been discussed to this point, it is important to understand that osmotic pressure, together with proper intake of fluids and their output by body mechanisms, is a most important factor in the maintenance of fluid balance and compartmentalization. The body's extracellular water volume, for example, is determined mainly by its osmolarity. The osmolarity, in turn,

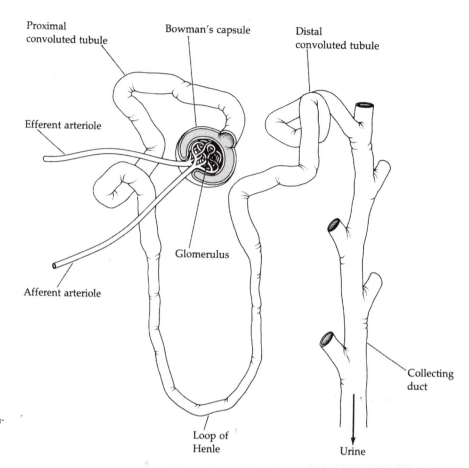

Proximal
convoluted tubule

Bowman's capsule

Distal
convoluted tubule

Efferent arteriole

Glomerulus

Afferent arteriole

Collecting
duct

Loop of
Henle

Urine

FIGURE 13.2 A schematic representation of the major components of the nephron.

acts as the signal to the regulatory factors that are responsible for maintaining fluid homeostasis. The regulation of extracellular water osmolarity and volume is largely the responsibility of the hypothalamus, the renin–angiotensin–aldosterone system, and the kidney. The kidney is central to the regulatory mechanisms, and its function will now be briefly reviewed. For a more detailed account of renal anatomy and physiology, consult a text dealing more specifically with that subject.

The functional unit of the kidney is the nephron, approximately 1 to 1.5 million of which are found in each of the two kidneys. The five components of the nephron are the Bowman's capsule, proximal convoluted tubule, loop of Henle, distal convoluted tubule, and collecting duct. Bowman's capsule is the blind, dilated end of the renal tubule, encapsulating a tuft of approximately 50 capillaries linking the afferent and efferent arterioles. This capillary network is called the *glomerulus*, and it accounts for the particularly rich blood supply that the kidney enjoys. It is estimated that 25% of the volume of blood pumped by the heart into the systemic circulation is circulated through the kidneys. This is particularly significant in view of the fact that the kid-

neys constitute only about 0.5% of total body weight. The assembly of the components of the nephron is schematically shown in Figure 13.2.

The glomerular capillary network acts as a filter in removing water and other substances, including electrolytes, glucose, amino acids, and metabolic waste products from plasma. The filtered substances make up what is known as the *glomerular filtrate*. In the absence of disease, no blood cells, or proteins that exceed a molecular weight of approximately 50,000 daltons, normally enter the glomerular filtrate because their larger size prevents their passage through the pores of the capillary endothelium. Each of the segments of the tubules is functionally distinct in its permeability to water and the solutes of the glomerular filtrate. The tubular segments are surrounded by a network of capillaries into which glomerular filtrate materials can be selectively reabsorbed into the bloodstream as a salvage mechanism. These peritubular capillaries may also secrete certain substances from the blood into the renal tubule. The removal of potentially toxic waste products is a major function of the kidneys and is accomplished through the formation of urine. The basic processes involved in urine formation are *filtration,* through which the glomerular filtrate is formed, *reabsorption* of selected filtrate substances into the bloodstream, and *secretion* of materials into the tubules from the surrounding capillaries. It is through these processes also that the kidneys are able to regulate fluid and electrolyte homeostasis for the proper functioning of cells throughout the body.

In healthy individuals the kidneys are highly sensitive to fluctuations in diet and in fluid and electrolyte intake, and they compensate by varying the volume and consistency of the urine. The glomerular capillaries differ from other capillaries in the body in that the hydrostatic pressure within them is approximately three times greater than in other capillaries. As a result of this high pressure, substances are filtered through the semipermeable membrane into Bowman's capsule at a rate of approximately 130 mL/min. This amounts to over 187,000 mL of filtrate formed per day, yet only about 1,400 mL of urine are produced during this time. This means that less than 1% of the filtrate is excreted as urine, with the remaining 99% being reabsorbed into the blood.

It has already been mentioned that it is the hypothalamus, the renin–angiotensin–aldosterone system, and the kidney that are responsible for maintaining extracellular fluid volume and osmolarity. Actually, the three work in concert because the hypothalamic hormone, antidiuretic hormone (ADH), also called *vasopressin,* and aldosterone, produced in the adrenal cortex, exert their effects through the kidney.

Antidiuretic hormone is produced in the supraoptic nucleus of the hypothalamus but is stored in and secreted by the posterior pituitary gland. It is a potent water-conserving hormone, its action being to increase the water permeability of the distal convoluted tubule and the collecting duct, thereby facilitating the reabsorption of water into the peritubular capillaries. The mechanism by which the hormone exerts this effect is not completely understood. However, ADH increases the activity of adenylate cyclase in the tubular epithelial cells, and the resulting elevation in cyclic AMP (cAMP) concentration is believed to result in the recruitment of water transport units that become inserted into the luminal membrane of the cells [1]. Evidence for the involvement of cAMP in the process is that exogenously administered cAMP or inhibitors of phosphodiesterase, which prolong cAMP activity, mimic the action of ADH. The release of ADH from the posterior pituitary is triggered by increases in extracellular water osmolarity or by decreased intravascular volume. The hypothalamic response to high extracellular fluid osmolarity is attributed to a shrinkage of neurons within the gland caused by the

movement of water out of the neurons into the higher osmotic interstitial fluid. This shrinkage then acts as the signal to the posterior pituitary to release the hormone.

A decrease in blood volume affects the activity of distention receptors and baroreceptors at various sites throughout the vascular network, and this information is relayed to the hypothalamus. Another hormone, angiotensin II, released indirectly by distention receptor relaxation (reduced blood volume) in renal arterioles, stimulates the hypothalamus directly with the release of more ADH.

Increased extracellular fluid osmolarity or decreased blood volume therefore influence what is known as the *water output areas* of the hypothalamus. The term *water output function* refers to the fact that because of the resulting increase in ADH, renal tubular reabsorption of water increases and the output of urine decreases. However, these factors also stimulate the *water intake area* of the hypothalamus as well, resulting in the conscious sensation of thirst. A greater intake of water therefore follows, resulting in a dilution of extracellular fluid and increased blood volume. This, in turn, reduces the release of ADH as fluid homeostasis is restored. The release of ADH and the induction of the thirst sensation in response to plasma osmolarity are illustrated graphically in Figure 13.3. More comprehensive information on the subject of the osmoregulation of ADH is available [2].

Another hormone that plays an important role in the maintenance of fluid balance is aldosterone, which is produced and secreted by the adrenal cortex and, like ADH, exerts its effect through the kidney. It stimulates the active reabsorption of sodium ions in the distal and collecting tubules via a mechanism that involves the transcription and translation of new proteins, which may be Na^+ channels in the luminal membrane, certain mitochondrial enzymes, or Na^+/K^+-ATPase [3]. That protein induction is indeed a part of the mechanism of aldosterone action is evidenced by the inhibition of electrolyte balance regulation by actinomycin D and puromycin, which are inhibitors of protein synthesis. By stimulating sodium reabsorption, aldosterone increases extracellular fluid osmolarity, thereby promoting fluid retention by the body via the hypothalamus–ADH mechanism already discussed. This is why diets high in sodium are contraindicated for those individuals whose fluid "balance" is already upset by excessive retention of water, as in cases of hypertension and edema.

There are several different substances that, according to their plasma concentration, influence the release of aldosterone. They are listed here, and discussed again in the following section on maintenance of electrolyte

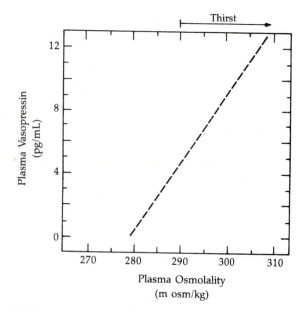

FIGURE 13.3 Relationship of plasma vasopressin to plasma osmolality. The arrow indicates the plasma osmolality at which the sensation of thirst is stimulated. *(Vokes T. Water homeostasis. Ann Rev Nutr 1987;7:386.)*

balance. Listed in decreasing order of their potency in stimulating aldosterone release, they are

1. Increased angiotensin II—this potent polypeptide hormone is a participant in the renin–angiotensin pathway of aldosterone stimulation. It reacts with receptors on adrenal cell membranes, stimulating the synthesis and release of aldosterone.

2. Decreased atrial natriuretic peptide—ANP is a peptide hormone synthesized in atrial cells and released in response to increased arteriolar stretch, indicative of elevated blood pressure. It functions in opposition to aldosterone in that it inhibits sodium reabsorption in the kidney, and thereby promotes sodium excretion [4].

3. Increased potassium concentration.

4. Increased ACTH.

5. Decreased sodium.

Angiotensin II is particularly important in stimulating aldosterone release, and therefore the renin–angiotensin–aldosterone system will now be discussed in greater detail.

Renin is a proteolytic enzyme synthesized, stored, and secreted by cells in the juxtaglomerular bodies of the kidney. Its secretion is stimulated by decreased renal perfusion pressure that is sensed by the distention re-

ceptors and baroreceptors within those bodies. Renin hydrolyzes angiotensinogen (a freely circulating protein synthesized by the liver) to angiotensin I, an inactive decapeptide. Angiotensin I is then acted on by a second proteolytic enzyme, angiotensin-converting enzyme, synthesized in vascular endothelial cells, particularly those in the blood vessels of the lung, producing the potent octapeptide angiotensin II. Angiotensin II then interacts with specific receptors on adrenal cortical cells, leading to the release of aldosterone. Along with its sodium-retaining activity, aldosterone promotes the urinary excretion of potassium.

It may be appropriate to review very briefly the mechanism of action of angiotensin II in increasing the synthesis and release of aldosterone from the adrenal cortex. Stimulatory signals resulting from polypeptide hormone-receptor interactions generally follow one of two major routes. One operates through an accelerated synthesis of cAMP with a consequent increase in protein kinase activity (p. 15). The second mechanism involves signals mediated by hydrolytic products of phospholipids along with increased intracellular calcium concentrations. The second of these, described as follows, applies in the case of angiotensin II action.

As a result of the interaction of angiotensin II with its receptor, a sequential cascade of reactions follows, involving G proteins, phospholipase C, and inositol triphosphate. Phospholipase C raises intracellular Ca^{+2} concentration by increasing Ca^{+2} conductance through Ca^{+2} channels, and inositol triphosphate releases Ca^{+2} from its storage in the endoplasmic reticulum. The elevated concentration of intracellular Ca^{+2} is stimulatory to appropriate synthetic enzymes, mediated through the Ca^{+2}-binding protein calmodulin [5]. Calmodulin is present in all eukaryotic cells. Figure 11.3 illustrates this type of hormonal mechanism.

The sequence of the events that comprise the renin–angiotensin–aldosterone system is illustrated in Figure 13.4. Although not shown in the figure, angiotensin II can be hydrolyzed further to angiotensin III by the hydrolytic removal of an aspartic acid residue by a plasma aminopeptidase. Angiotensin III is also physiologically active. In fact, it has been observed to be more potent than angiotensin II in its aldosterone-stimulating ability [6]. However, its plasma concentration is significantly less than that of angiotensin II, and therefore its contribution to the maintenance of fluid balance is less dramatic. In addition to its role in the conservation of body water through aldosterone action, angiotensin II is also a potent vasoconstrictor, reducing

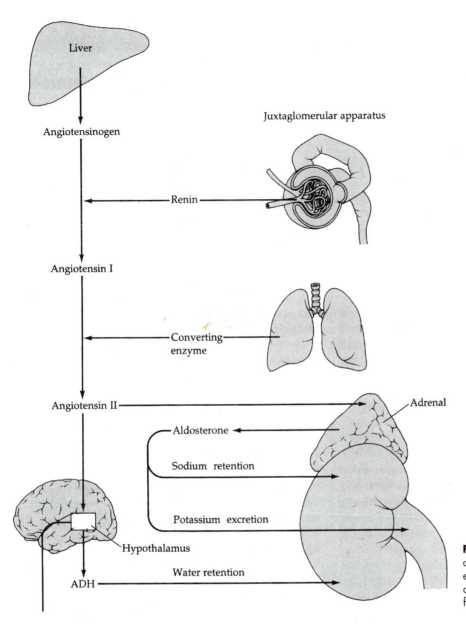

FIGURE 13.4 The renin–angiotensin–aldosterone system illustrating the cooperation of kidneys, liver, lungs, adrenals, and hypothalamus in this mechanism of fluid homeostasis.

the glomerular filtration rate and therefore the filtered load of sodium. Also, it will be recalled that it stimulates the hypothalamic thirst center and the release of ADH, both of which increase body water volume. Figure 13.5 illustrates the central role of the hypothalamus and the action of angiotensin II in the hormonal regulation of fluid homeostasis.

Alterations in food intake can profoundly affect water and electrolyte balance. During the initial days of a period of fasting, for example, there is a marked increase in the renal excretion of sodium, whereas pro-

longed fasting tends to conserve the ion. Refeeding causes a marked retention of sodium, probably due to the ingestion of carbohydrate. Consequently, a rapid regain in body weight follows, caused by an increase in total body water secondary to the stimulation of vasopressin and thirst by the rise in plasma osmolarity. These alterations in sodium and water balance in subjects as a result of early-phase fasting and refeeding account for the weight loss and weight regain to a far greater extent than would be predicted from the changes in caloric balance [7].

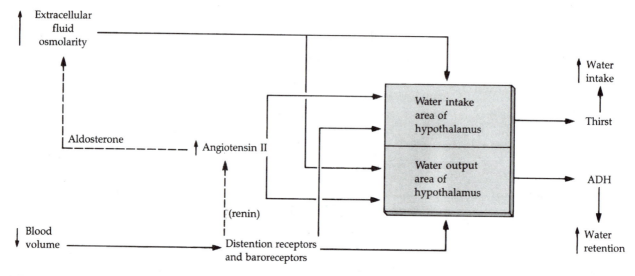

FIGURE 13.5 A summary of the mechanisms by which fluid homeostasis is maintained. Water depletion stimuli such as increased extracellular fluid osmolarity or decreased blood volume can stimulate the hypothalamus either directly or through the production of angiotensin II, formed by the action of the renal protease renin. The renin–angiotensin–aldosterone system (shown by dashed arrows) increases extracellular fluid osmolarity by promoting renal tubular reabsorption of sodium.

MAINTENANCE OF ELECTROLYTE BALANCE

The term *electrolytes* refers to the anions and cations that are distributed throughout the fluid compartments of the body. They are distributed in such a way that within a given compartment, the blood plasma for example, electrical neutrality is always maintained, with the anion concentration exactly balanced by the cation concentration.

The cationic electrolytes of the extracellular fluid include sodium, potassium, calcium, and magnesium, and these are electrically balanced by the anions, chloride, bicarbonate, and proteins, along with relatively low concentrations of organic acids, phosphate, and sulfate. The major electrolytes are listed in Table 13.2. Most of them are categorized nutritionally as macrominerals, and as such, have already been discussed in Chapter 11 from the standpoint of their absorption, function, dietary requirements, and food sources. The maintenance of pH and electrolyte balance, which is the focus of this chapter, is a responsibility that belongs almost exclusively to the kidney.

All filterable substances in plasma—that is, all the plasma solutes except the larger proteins—freely enter the glomerular filtrate from the blood. Some of these substances are metabolic waste products and are excreted in the urine with little or no reabsorption in the tubules. However, most of the materials in the glomerular filtrate must be salvaged by the body, and this is accomplished through their tubular reabsorption by either active or passive mechanisms, or both. Active transport, it will be recalled (p. 17), allows substances to pass across membranes against concentration gradients by the action of ATP-dependent membrane transport systems. Glucose is a prime example of a solute that can be actively transported across the tubular cells from the urine into the blood even though the blood concentration of glucose is normally 20 times that of urine. Another group of solutes, including ammonium, potassium, and phosphate ions, occurs in relatively high concentration in urine compared with blood. These substances are transported from blood into the tubular cells also against a concentration gradient. Passive transport is not energy demanding and is simply the diffusion of a material across a membrane from a compartment of higher concentration of the material to a compartment of lower concentration. This process, too, functions within the renal tubular cells. A brief account of the renal regulation of several major electrolytes will now be considered.

Sodium

Sodium is freely filtered by the glomerulus. About 70% of the filtered sodium is reabsorbed by the proximal tubule, 15% by the loop of Henle, 5% by the distal convoluted tubule, and about 10% by the collecting ducts. It is the major cation found in extracellular fluid.

Active reabsorption of sodium ions in the proximal tubule results in the passive reabsorption of chloride ions, bicarbonate ions, and water. The accompanying

TABLE 13.2 Electrolyte Composition of Body Fluids

	Plasma (mEq/L)	Interstitial Fluid (mEq/L H_2O)	Intracellular Water (mEq/L H_2O)
Cations	153	153	195
Na^+	142	145	10
K^+	4	4	156
Ca^{+2}	5	(2–3)	3.2
Mg^{+2}	2	(1–2)	26
Anions	153	153	195
Cl^-	103	116	2
HCO_3^-	28	31	8
Protein	17	—	55
Others	5	(6)	130
Osmolarity (m osm/L)		294.6	294.6
Theoretic osmotic pressure (mm Hg)		5685.8	5685.8

transfer of the anions chloride and bicarbonate with the cation sodium is required to maintain the necessary electrical neutrality of the extracellular fluid, while the water transfer ensures a normal osmotic pressure. Virtually all cells contain a relatively high concentration of potassium and a low concentration of sodium, whereas the blood plasma and most other extracellular fluids have high sodium and low potassium concentrations, as can be seen in Table 13.2. Clearly, energy must be expended to maintain this gradient across the cell membrane; otherwise, each ion would simply diffuse through the membrane until their intracellular and extracellular concentrations were the same. The gradient is maintained by the Na^+/K^+-ATPase pump, which has already been discussed in Chapter 1. It is the mechanism by which the renal tubular cells "pump" sodium into the blood in exchange for potassium in such a way as to conserve sodium while allowing a constant loss of potassium in the urine.

Active reabsorption of sodium occurs in the distal convoluted tubule under the influence of aldosterone. The mechanism is highly selective for sodium ion, and there is little accompanying water diffusion. This makes it an important system for the regulation of extracellular fluid osmotic pressure. The increased retention of sodium by this mechanism is, however, accompanied by water retention also. This is because the greater extracellular fluid osmotic pressure stimulates tubular water reabsorption through ADH release (Fig. 13.5).

Chloride

The concentration of chloride in the extracellular fluid parallels that of sodium, and chloride generally accompanies sodium in transmembrane passage. However, it will be recalled that chloride reabsorption is passive in the proximal tubule, and it is probably reabsorbed actively in the ascending limb of the loop of Henle and the distal tubule.

Potassium

Potassium is the chief cation of intracellular fluid, and maintenance of a normal level is essential to the life of the cells. The normal person maintains potassium balance by excreting daily an amount of the cation equal to the amount ingested minus the small amount excreted in the feces and sweat.

Potassium is freely filtered at the glomerulus, and its active tubular reabsorption occurs throughout the nephron, except for the descending loop of Henle. Only about 10% of the filtered potassium enters the distal tubules, which, along with the collecting ducts, are able to both secrete and reabsorb potassium. The distal tubule is the site at which changes in the amount of potassium excreted are achieved, and several mechanisms are involved in this control.

The first of these mechanisms is dependent on the cellular potassium content. When a high-potassium diet is consumed, the concentration of potassium rises in cells, including the distal renal tubular cells, providing a concentration gradient that favors the secretion of the cation into the lumen of the tubule. This results in an increase in potassium excretion.

Another important factor in the regulation of potassium balance is the hormone aldosterone, which, besides stimulating distal tubular reabsorption of sodium, simultaneously enhances potassium secretion at that site. In fact, the elevated plasma level of potassium directly stimulates the production and release of aldosterone from the adrenal cortex. Recall that another mechanism for effecting aldosterone release is through decreased renal perfusion pressure and the associated renin–angiotensin–aldosterone pathway.

A third mechanism of renal conservation of potassium occurs in the collecting duct, and involves its active reabsorption coupled to the secretion of protons at that site [8]. The movement of K^+ into the cells of the collecting duct from the urine, and the movement of H^+ in the opposite direction is catalyzed by an H^+/K^+-activated adenosine triphosphatase (H^+/K^+-ATPase), functioning similarly to the Na^+/K^+-ATPase pump discussed previously.

Calcium and Magnesium

Tubular reabsorption of calcium is associated with the reabsorption of sodium and phosphate in the proximal tubule, and the rate of reabsorption of all three ions, as well as fluid, occurs in parallel. Renal tubular reabsorption of calcium is closely linked to the action of parathyroid hormone (PTH) (p. 302). This hormone exerts parallel inhibition of the reabsorption of calcium, sodium, and phosphate in the proximal tubules. However, PTH markedly stimulates reabsorption of calcium in the distal tubules disproportionate to that of sodium and phosphate.

The major pathway of calcium excretion is the intestinal tract. Urinary excretion, approximating 150 mg/d for the average adult, amounts to only about 1% of that filtered by the glomerulus, the remaining 99% being effectively reabsorbed at proximal and distal tubular sites.

Calcium balance is achieved largely by the control of the intestinal absorption of the ion rather than by the regulation of its urinary excretion. The percentage of ingested calcium absorbed decreases as the dietary calcium content increases, and so the amount absorbed remains relatively constant. The slight increase in absorption that occurs with a high-calcium diet is reflected in an increased renal excretion of the cation.

The filtration of magnesium at the glomerulus and its subsequent active reabsorption through the tubular cells parallel that of calcium.

Homeostatic regulation of the ions discussed is crucial to many body functions. For example, greatly decreased extracellular potassium (hypokalemia) produces paralysis, while elevated potassium levels (hyperkalemia) can result in cardiac arrhythmias. Excessive extracellular sodium (hypernatremia) causes fluid retention, and decreased plasma calcium (hypocalcemia) produces tetany (intermittent spasms of the muscles of the extremities) by increasing the permeability of nerve cell membranes to sodium. Magnesium deficiency is also associated with tetany.

Table 13.2 lists the fluid electrolytes and their approximate, normal, compartment concentrations. In terms of electrolyte balance only, it is clear that the contribution of sodium to the total cation milliequivalents is quite large compared to that of potassium, calcium, and magnesium and that a correspondingly high percentage of anion milliequivalents is contributed by chloride and bicarbonate together. The concentration of these three major ions is used to calculate the so-called anion gap, a clinically useful parameter for establishing metabolic disorders that can alter the electrolyte balance. The value is calculated by subtracting the measured anion (chloride + bicarbonate) concentration from the measured cation (sodium) concentration:

$$\text{Measured cations } (Na^+) - \text{measured anions}$$
$$(Cl^- + HCO_3^-) = 12 \text{ mEq/L}$$

Under normal conditions, the value is approximately 12 mEq/L, but may range from 8 to 18 mEq/L. Deviation from a normal anion gap is most commonly associated with increases or decreases in the concentration of certain unmeasured anions such as proteins, organic acids, phosphate, or sulfate. For example, the production of excessive amounts of organic acids, such as would occur in lactic acidosis or ketoacidosis, increases the unmeasured anion concentration at the expense of the measured anion bicarbonate which is neutralized by the acids. Such a condition would therefore cause a greater anion gap.

Considering the effect of plasma osmolarity on water intake and retention, it is logical that if for any reason sodium ion should accumulate in the body water, a concomitant rise in blood pressure (essential hypertension) would result. Clinical evidence for this correlation is the hypertension experienced by patients with adrenal adenomas, whose high levels of aldosterone cause excessive retention of sodium. There is also an apparent causal relationship between dietary intake of sodium (as sodium chloride) and the etiology of hypertension, as suggested by studies conducted through one or more of the following designs:

- Relating salt consumption to the prevalence of hypertension
- Development of hypertension in animals fed high-salt diets
- Response of hypertensive patients fed low-salt diets

There is an abundance of reported observations that deal with the positive correlation of salt intake and hypertension among societies that ingest salt to variable extents. Such observations have led to the generally accepted conclusion that the incidence of hypertension is predictable from the average daily sodium intake among the societies [9]. Also, convincing animal studies dating back to the 1950s have demonstrated a direct correlation between sodium chloride and hypertension [10]. But in spite of these findings, there is a lack of evidence that a cause-and-effect relationship exists among the individuals of a normotensive population. In fact, investigations on the effect of sodium chloride loading on blood pressure among normotensives have revealed no correlation between high-salt intake and hypertension. Furthermore, among subjects with borderline essential hypertension, a low-sodium diet is minimally effective in lowering the blood pressure. This suggests that plasma sodium concentrations are unalterable if the homeostatic mechanisms controlling it are intact. It has become generally accepted that the differences between those who respond to sodium diet therapy and those who do not, have a genetic foundation.

People who are salt sensitive are called *responders*, and those showing salt insensitivity are labeled *nonresponders*. The condition of nonresponders who have essential hypertension does not improve on low-salt diets. Likewise, normotensive nonresponders can consume as much as 4,600 mg of sodium daily (somewhat higher than that of the typical Western diet) without risk. Among the genetically disposed individuals, a comparable intake would likely favor the development of hypertension. For people in this population, a restriction to approximately 1,400 mg or less is recommended [11].

Although a genetic link to salt sensitivity is generally accepted, biochemical mechanisms of the condition are not clearly understood. This is not for a lack of relevant research. A literature review of the many investigations designed to explain the biochemical basis of salt sensitivity and nonsensitivity is available [12].

In summary, the implication of sodium in hypertension remains controversial. It is unlikely that it functions alone in the etiology of the disease, and it may be a contributing factor only in the wake of other biochemical disturbances. The involvement of other cations such as calcium, magnesium, potassium, and cadmium cannot be overlooked [12].

ACID–BASE BALANCE: THE CONTROL OF HYDROGEN ION CONCENTRATION

The hydrogen ion concentration in body fluids must be controlled within a narrow range, its regulation being one of the most important aspects of homeostasis. This is because merely slight deviations from normal acidity can cause marked alteration in enzyme-catalyzed reac-

tion rates in the cells. Hydrogen ion concentration can also affect both the cellular uptake and regulation of metabolites and minerals and the uptake and release of oxygen from hemoglobin.

The degree of acidity of any fluid is determined by its concentration of protons (H^+). The hydrogen ion concentration in body fluids is generally quite low, as it is regulated at approximately 4×10^{-8} mol/L. Concentrations can vary from as low as 1.0×10^{-8} mol/L to as high as 1.0×10^{-7} mol/L, but values outside of this range are not compatible with life. From these values it is apparent that expressing H^+ in terms of its actual concentration is awkward. The concept of pH, which is the negative logarithm of the H^+ concentration, was devised to simplify the expression. It allows concentrations to be expressed as whole numbers rather than as negative exponential values:

$$pH = -\log [H^+]$$

Bracketed values symbolize concentrations. This designation will be used to signify concentrations of other substances as well as protons throughout this discussion. The pH of extracellular fluid, wherein the H^+ concentration may be assumed to be approximately 4×10^{-8} mol/L, can therefore be calculated as follows:

$$pH = -\log (4 \times 10^{-8})$$
$$\text{or } pH = \log \frac{1}{4 \times 10^{-8}}$$
$$(\text{dividing}) = \log (.25 \times 10^8)$$
$$= \log .25 + \log 10^8$$
$$(\text{taking logs}) = -.602 + 8$$
$$pH = 7.4$$

It can be seen that as the value of the negative exponent of 10 becomes larger—that is, the molar concentration of H^+ being smaller—the pH correspondingly increases. Low acidity therefore denotes low H^+ concentration and high pH, while high acidity is associated with a high H^+ concentration and low pH.

An acid, as it relates to fluid acid–base regulation, may be defined as a substance capable of releasing protons. The metabolism of the major nutrients continuously generates acids, which must be neutralized. It has already been explained in Chapter 4 how lactic acid and pyruvic acid can accumulate in periods of oxygen deprivation, and in Chapter 6, how fatty acids are released from triacylglycerols during lipolysis. Also, the acidic ketone bodies, acetoacetic acid and β-hydroxybutyric acid, can increase significantly during periods of prolonged starvation or low carbohydrate intake. Carbon dioxide, the product of complete oxidation of energy nutrients, is itself indirectly acidic, since it forms carbonic acid, H_2CO_3, on combination with H_2O. Acidic salts of sulfuric and phosphoric acids are also generated metabolically from sulfur- or phosphorus-containing substances.

The term *acidosis* refers to a rise in extracellular (principally plasma) H^+ concentration beyond the normal range. Abnormally low H^+ concentration, in contrast (that is, high plasma pH) results in the condition of alkalosis. To guard against such fluctuations in pH, three principal regulatory systems are available: (1) *buffer systems* within the fluids that immediately neutralize acidic or basic compounds, (2) the *respiratory center*, which regulates breathing and the rate of exhalation of CO_2; and (3) *renal regulation*, by which either an acidic or alkaline urine can be formed in order to adjust body fluid acidity.

ACID–BASE BUFFERS

A buffer is a chemical solution designed to resist changes in pH despite the addition of acids or bases. Usually a buffer consists of a weak acid, which can be represented as (HA), and its conjugate base (A^-). The conjugate base is therefore the residual portion of the acid following the release of the proton. The conjugate base of a weak acid is basic, because it tends to attract a proton and to regenerate the acid. Therefore, the dissociation of a weak acid and the reunion of its conjugate base and proton is an equilibrium system:

$$HA \rightleftharpoons H^+ + A^-$$

The equilibrium expression for this reaction is called the *acid dissociation constant* (K_a) and is represented as

$$K_a = \frac{[H^+][A^-]}{[HA]}$$

The equation can be rearranged to

$$[H^+] = K_a \frac{[HA]}{[A^-]}$$

Taking the negative logarithm of both sides of the equation,

$$-\log [H^+] = -\log K_a -\log \frac{[HA]}{[A^-]}$$

These values become

$$pH = pK_a + \log \frac{[A^-]}{[HA]}$$

This is referred to as the *Henderson-Hasselbalch equation*. It can be seen from the equation how a buffer system

composed of a weak acid and its conjugate base resists changes in pH if either strong acid or base is added to the system. To illustrate this very briefly, if the molar concentrations of the conjugate base and the acid are equal, then the ratio $[A^-]/[HA]$ is 1.0, and the log of this ratio is 0, making the pH of the system equal to the pK_a of the acid. The pK_a, which is the negative logarithm of the acid dissociation constant (K_a), of any weak acid is a constant for that particular acid, and simply reflects its strength (its tendency to release a proton). If a strong acid or base is added to this system, the ratio of $[A^-]$ to $[HA]$ changes and therefore changes the pH, but only slightly. Suppose, for example, that both the conjugate base and free acid are present at 0.1 mol/L concentrations, and suppose also that the pK_a of the acid is 7.0. It follows that the pH is also 7.0 under these conditions. Addition of a strong acid such as hydrochloric acid to a final concentration of 0.05 mol/L will convert an equivalent amount of $[A^-]$ to $[HA]$ because, as a completely dissociated acid, it is contributing 0.05 mol/L H^+ as well. The new $[A^-]$ concentration therefore becomes 0.05 mol/L, and the $[HA]$ will be 0.15 mol/L. The logarithm of this new ratio (0.05/0.15, or 0.33) is -0.48, and inserting this value into the Henderson-Hasselbalch equation, it can be seen that the pH decreases by only this amount. In other words, the pH decreased from 7.0 to 6.52 by making the system 0.05 mol/L hydrochloric acid. In contrast, this same concentration of HCl in an unbuffered, aqueous solution would produce an acid pH between 1.0 and 2.0.

The physiologically important buffers that maintain the narrow pH range of extracellular fluid at approximately 7.4 are proteins and the bicarbonate (HCO_3^-)-carbonic acid (H_2CO_3) system. Proteins have the most potent buffering capacity among the physiologic buffers, and because of its high concentration in whole blood, hemoglobin is most important in this respect. It is crucial for the pH regulation necessary for the normal uptake and release of oxygen in the erythrocyte. As amphoteric substances, meaning that they possess both acidic and basic groups on their amino acid side chains, proteins are capable of neutralizing either acids or bases. For instance, the two major buffering groups on a protein are carboxylic acid (R—COOH) and amino (R—NH$_3^+$) functions, which dissociate as shown:

1. $R—COOH \rightleftharpoons R—COO^- + H^+$
2. $R—NH_3^+ \rightleftharpoons R—NH_2 + H^+$

At physiologic pH, the carboxylic acid is largely dissociated into its conjugate base and a proton so that the equilibrium as shown is shifted strongly to the right. At that same pH, however, the amino group, being much weaker as an acid (a stronger base), is only weakly dissociated, and its equilibrium greatly favors the right-to-left direction. If protons, in the form of a strong acid, are added to a protein solution, they are neutralized by reaction 1, because their presence will cause a shift in the equilibrium toward the undissociated acid (right to left). Strong bases, as contributors of hydroxide (OH^-) ions, will likewise be neutralized because as they react with the protons to form water, the equilibrium of reaction 2, as illustrated, shifts to the right to restore the protons that were neutralized.

The bicarbonate–carbonic acid buffer system is of particular importance because it is through this system that respiratory and renal pH regulation is exerted. It is composed of the weak acid carbonic acid (H_2CO_3), and its salt, or conjugate base, bicarbonate ion (HCO_3^-). The acid dissociates reversibly into H^+ and HCO_3^-,

$$H_2CO_3 \rightleftharpoons H^+ + HCO_3^-$$

its buffering capacity being due to the fact that either protons or hydroxide ions added will be neutralized by corresponding shifts in the equilibrium, similar to the carboxy–amino group buffering by proteins described earlier. The H_2CO_3 can be formed not only from the acidification of HCO_3^-, as shown in the right-to-left reaction just shown, but also from the reaction of dissolved CO_2 with water. It will be recalled that CO_2 is formed as a result of total oxidation of the energy nutrients as well as various decarboxylation reactions. The gas diffuses from tissue cells into the extracellular fluids and then into erythrocytes, where its reaction with water to form H_2CO_3 is accelerated by the zinc metalloenzyme, carbonic anhydrase (p. 370). The overall reaction involving carbon dioxide, carbonic acid, and bicarbonate ion occurs as follows:

3. CO_2 (gas) $\rightleftharpoons$ CO_2 (dissolved) $\rightleftharpoons$
   $H_2CO_3 \rightleftharpoons H^+ + HCO_3^-$

In the lungs, these equilibrium reactions are shifted strongly to the left in the circulating erythrocytes due to the release of protons from hemoglobin as hemoglobin acquires oxygen to become oxyhemoglobin. This shift allows the exhalation of carbon dioxide.

Normally the ratio of the concentration of HCO_3^- to H_2CO_3 in plasma is 20 to 1, and the apparent pK_a value for H_2CO_3 is 6.1. It can be shown by the Henderson-Hasselbalch equation how a normal plasma pH of 7.4 results from these values:

$$pH = pK_a + \log \frac{[HCO_3^-]}{[H_2CO_3]}$$
$$= 6.1 + \log \frac{20}{1}$$
$$= 6.1 + 1.3$$
$$pH = 7.4$$

Alterations in the 20-to-1 ratio of $[HCO_3^-]/[H_2CO_3]$ clearly change the pH. Next we show how respiratory and renal regulatory systems function to keep this ratio, and therefore pH, relatively constant.

RESPIRATORY REGULATION OF pH

Should plasma levels of CO_2 rise, perhaps because of accelerated metabolism, more H_2CO_3 will be formed, which, in turn, will cause a fall in pH as it dissociates to release protons (reaction 3). The elevated CO_2 itself, as well as the resulting increase in hydrogen ion concentration, is detected by the respiratory center of the brain, resulting in an increase in the respiratory rate. This hyperventilation significantly increases the amount of CO_2 loss and therefore decreases the amount of H_2CO_3. By reducing H_2CO_3, this mechanism therefore increases the HCO_3^-/H_2CO_3 ratio, elevating the pH to a normal value. Conversely, if plasma pH rises for any reason, due either to an increase in HCO_3^- or a decrease in H_2CO_3, the respiratory center is signaled accordingly and causes a restraint in ventilation. As CO_2 then accumulates, the H_2CO_3 concentration rises, and the pH decreases.

RENAL REGULATION OF pH

Although the intact respiratory system acts as an immediate regulator of the HCO_3^-/H_2CO_3 system, long-term control is exerted by renal mechanisms. The kidneys regulate pH by controlling the secretion of hydrogen ions, by conserving bicarbonate, and through ammonia synthesis. The secretion of hydrogen ions occurs in conjunction with the tubular reabsorption of sodium ions through the mechanism of countertransport. This is an active process involving a common Na^+/H^+ carrier protein and energy sufficient to move the protons from the tubular cells into the tubule lumen against a concentration gradient of protons. In subjects on a normal diet, about 50 to 100 mEq of hydrogen ions are generated daily. Renal secretion of the protons is necessary to prevent a progressive metabolic acidosis.

The renal tubules are not very permeable to bicarbonate ions because of the charge and relatively large size of the ions. They are therefore reabsorbed by a special process. The hydrogen ions in the glomerular filtrate convert filtered bicarbonate ions into H_2CO_3, which dissociates into CO_2 and H_2O. The CO_2 diffuses into the tubular cell, where it combines with water, a reaction catalyzed by carbonic anhydrase, to form H_2CO_3. The rel-

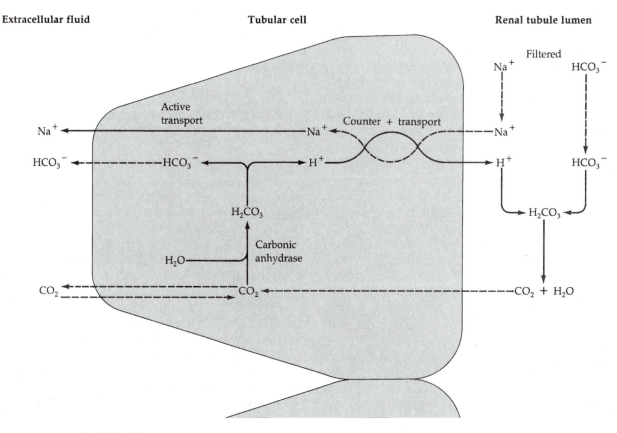

Extracellular fluid   **Tubular cell**   **Renal tubule lumen**

FIGURE 13.6 Renal tubular cell reactions illustrating the origin of and the active secretion of hydrogen ions in exchange for sodium ions, as well as the mechanism for tubular reabsorption of bicarbonate. Solid arrows indicate reactions or active transport, while dashed arrows signify diffusion.

atively high tubular-cell pH allows the dissociation of the H_2CO_3 into HCO_3^- and H^+, after which the bicarbonate re-enters the extracellular fluid, and the proton is actively returned to the lumen by the Na^+/H^+ carrier. These events, by which hydrogen ions are secreted against a concentration gradient in exchange for sodium ions, and bicarbonate is returned to the plasma from the glomerular filtrate, are summarized in Figure 13.6.

The pH of the urine normally falls within the range 5.5 to 6.5, despite the active secretion of hydrogen ions throughout the tubules. This is largely due to the partial neutralization of the hydrogen ions by ammonia, which is secreted into the lumen by the tubular cells. Ammonia is produced in large amounts from the metabolic breakdown of amino acids, and although most of it is excreted in the form of urea, some is delivered to the kidney cells in the form of glutamine. In the renal tubule cells, ammonia is hydrolytically released from the glutamine by the enzyme glutaminase and is secreted into the urine (p. 171). Since it is a basic substance, ammonia immediately combines with protons in the collecting ducts

to form ammonium ions (NH_4^+), which are excreted in the urine primarily as their chloride salts.

Should metabolic acidosis occur, such as in starvation or diabetes, an increase in the urinary excretion of ammonia occurs concomitantly in compensation. This is because the diminished intake and use of carbohydrate stimulates gluconeogenesis and therefore an enhanced excretion of ammonia formed from the higher rate of amino acid catabolism.

Like respiratory regulation, renal regulation of pH is also directed at the maintenance of a normal $[HCO_3^-]/[H_2CO_3]$ ratio. In a situation of alkalosis, for example, in which the plasma *ratio* of HCO_3^- to H_2CO_3 increases as the pH rises above 7.4, the ratio of HCO_3 ions filtered into the tubules to the hydrogen ions secreted into the tubules increases also. This increase occurs because the high extracellular HCO_3^- concentration increases its filtration, while the relatively low concentration of H_2CO_3 decreases the secretion of H^+. Therefore, the fine balance between the HCO_3^- and H^+, that normally exists in the tubules, no longer is in effect. Also, since no HCO_3^- ions can be reabsorbed without first reacting with H^+ (Fig. 13.6), all the excess HCO_3^- will pass into the urine, neutralized by sodium ions or other cations. In effect, therefore, HCO_3^- is removed from the extracellular fluid, restoring the normal HCO_3^-/H_2CO_3 ratio and pH. In acidosis, the ratio of plasma HCO_3^- to H_2CO_3 decreases, meaning that the rate of H^+ secretion rises to a level far greater than the rate of HCO_3^- filtration into the tubules. As a result, most of the filtered HCO_3^- will be converted to H_2CO_3 and reabsorbed as CO_2 (Fig. 13.6), while the excess H^+ is excreted in the urine. As a consequence, the extracellular fluid $[HCO_3^-]/[H_2CO_3]$ ratio increases, and so does the pH.

The importance of the kidney in the homeostatic control of body water, as well as electrolyte and acid–base balance, has been emphasized in this chapter. The material has been presented as a review of the principles involved in such control and the effect of diet on fluid and electrolyte homeostasis. Although a detailed account of renal physiology is not within the scope of this text, excellent sources that deal specifically with this subject are, of course, available. The text, *Handbook of Physiology*, renal physiology section, is quite comprehensive in its coverage of the subject [13].

SUMMARY

The maintenance of body fluid and electrolytes is of vital importance for sound health and nutrition. Intracellular fluid provides the environment for the myriad of metabolic reactions that take place in cells. The interstitial fluid compartment of the extracellular fluid mass allows the migration of nutrients into cells from the blood stream and the return to the bloodstream of metabolic waste products from the cells. These fluids contain the electrolytes, dissolved minerals that have important physiologic functions. Their concentrations and their intracellular and extracellular distribution must be precisely regulated, and the mechanism for achieving this are exerted largely through the kidney. The homeostatic maintenance of fluid volume is also the responsibility of this organ.

Fluid volume control by the kidney is mostly hormone mediated. ADH, produced in the hypothalamus, stimulates the tubular reabsorption of water from the glomerular filtrate. Aldosterone, a product of the adrenal cortex, increases the reabsorption of sodium ions, which indirectly stimulate ADH release through the resulting rise in extracellular fluid osmotic pressure. Thirst centers in the brain, which respond to fluctua-

tions in blood volume or extracellular fluid osmolarity, are also important regulators of fluid balance by their influence on the amount of fluid intake.

The macrominerals sodium and potassium, and other ions of nutritional importance such as calcium, magnesium, and chloride are freely filtered by the renal glomerulus, but are selectively conserved by tubular reabsorption via active transport systems. Potassium is an example of a mineral that is regulated in part by tubular secretion into the filtrate. Secretion of the ion from the distal tubular cells increases as its concentration in those cells rises, due, perhaps, to a heightened dietary intake. Potassium, like sodium, is regulated by aldosterone. Elevated plasma potassium stimulates the release of aldosterone, which exerts opposing renal effects on the two minerals—the enhanced reabsorption of sodium and an increase in potassium excretion. Normal physiologic function depends on proper control of the body fluid acid–base balance. Many metabolic enzymes have a narrow range of pH at which they function adequately, and these catalysts are intolerant of pH swings more than several tenths of a unit from the average normal value of 7.4 for extracellular fluids. The plasma is well buffered, primarily by proteins and by the bicarbonate–carbonic acid system. However, conditions of acidosis or alkalosis can result in certain situations such as an overproduction of organic acids, as would occur in diabetes or starvation, or respiratory aberrations that may cause abnormal carbon dioxide ventilation. Therefore, restoration of normal pH may be necessary, and is accomplished through compensatory mechanisms of the kidneys and lungs. These organs function to maintain a normal ratio of bicarbonate to carbonic acid. The bicarbonate concentration is under the control of the kidneys, which can either conserve the ion, by reabsorbing it to a greater extent, or increase its excretion, depending on whether the ratio needs to be decreased or increased to compensate for a pH disturbance. The carbonic acid value is controlled by the respiratory center. It can be increased or decreased in concentration by changes in the respiratory rate. Hyperventilation, for example, lowers the value by "blowing off" carbon dioxide, while a slowing of respiration retains carbon dioxide and therefore raises the carbonic acid level. From their effects on the bicarbonate–carbonic acid ratio, it can be reasoned that hyperventilation can raise the pH, and respiratory suppression can lower the pH in a compensatory manner.

References Cited

1. de Sousa RC. Cellular modes of action of vasopressin. In: Robinson RR, ed. Nephrology, Vol I. New York: Springer-Verlag 1984:407–416.

2. Robertson GL, Berl T. Water metabolism. In: Brenner BM, Rector FC, eds. The kidney, 3rd ed. Philadelphia: Saunders 1985:385–432.

3. Goodman HM. Basic medical endocrinology. New York: Raven Press 1994:84–87.

4. Van de Stolpe A, Jamison RL. Micropuncture study of the effect of ANP on the papillary collecting duct in the rat. Am J Physiol 1988;254:F477–483.

5. Hadley ME. Endocrinology, 3rd ed. Englewood Cliffs, NJ; Prentice Hall 1992:77–91.

6. David JO, Freeman RH. The other angiotensins. Biochem Pharmacol 1977;26:93–97.

7. Vokes T. Water homeostasis. Ann Rev Nutr 1987;7: 383–406.

8. Wingo CS, Cain BD. The renal H-K-ATPase: Physiological significance and role in potassium homeostasis. Annu Rev Physiol 1993;55:323–347.

9. Altschul AM, Grommet JK. Sodium intake and sodium sensitivity. Nutr Rev 1980;38:393–402.

10. Meneely GR, Ball COT. Experimental epidemiology of chronic sodium chloride toxicity and the protective effect of potassium chloride. Am J Med 1958;25:713.

11. Tobian L. The relationship of salt to hypertension. Am J Clin Nutr 1979;32:2739–2748.

12. Luft FC. Salt and hypertension: Recent advances and perspectives. J Lab Clin Med 1989;114:215–221.

13. Windhager EE, ed. Handbook of physiology. Section 8, Renal physiology, Vols I, II. New York: Oxford University Press, 1992.

Suggested Reading

Vokes T. Water homeostasis. Annu Rev Nutr 1987;7:383–406.
This is a discussion of the mechanisms of water balance regulation and the pathology associated with deficiencies in the regulatory system.

Kaplan NM. Dietary aspects in the treatment of hypertension. Ann Rev Public Health 1986;7:503–519.
This is a discussion of hypertension from the standpoint of dietary mineral intake regulation.

Kleinman LI, Lorenz JM. Physiology and pathophysiology of body water and electrolytes. In: Kaplan LA, Pesce AJ, eds. Clinical chemistry: Theory, analysis, and correlation. St. Louis: Mosby, 1984:363–386.
This is a clearly written clinical approach to fluid and electrolyte homeostasis, with diagrammatic illustrations of the regulatory mechanisms of fluid and electrolyte control.

Sherwin JE, Bruegger BB. Acid–base control and acid–base disorders. In: Kaplan LA, Pesce AJ, eds. Clinical chemistry: Theory, analysis, and correlation. St. Louis: Mosby, 1984:387–402.
This is a brief introduction to the physiologic buffer systems and a clinical approach to the regulation of acid–base balance.

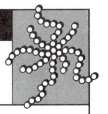

Fluid and Electrolyte Balance in the Athlete

The optimization of physical performance in endurance athletics has received considerable attention during the past couple of decades and has been the focus of extensive research. This fact is evidenced by the number of new journals that have recently emerged dealing with the subject of sports medicine and exercise physiology. The subject has attracted the attention of nutritionists and physiologists alike because of the relevance of these disciplines to the needs of, and the effects on, the human body during prolonged periods of strenuous exertion. The Chapter 4 "Perspective" section dealt with the energy needs of the endurance athlete and how glycogen stores, as available energy sources, can be maximized prior to an athletic event. This "Perspective" section relates to the need for proper fluid and electrolyte balance during prolonged periods of exercise. Even with adequate energy nutrient loading, the performance of the athlete would be seriously compromised by an uncorrected disturbance of this balance.

About 80% of the energy released during exercise is in the form of heat. If this is not removed from the body, the heat load due to metabolic activity, combined with environmental heat during strenuous exercise, could lead to a dramatic increase in body temperature, a condition called *hyperthermia*. Hyperthermia can result in lethal heat injury.

The major mechanism for heat loss is the evaporation of sweat, and it is estimated that nearly 600 kcal are eliminated by the cooling effect of the evaporation of 1 L of sweat. A second, less important means of heat loss is radiation. Heat generated in the working muscles is transported by blood flow to the skin, from which it can be subsequently exchanged with the environment. For either of these thermoregulatory mechanisms, body water is clearly the major participant, and there has been considerable interest in assessing various strategies for its replacement during strenuous exercise.

There is firm evidence that depletion of body water from sweating beyond 2% of body weight can cause significant impairment of endurance through deficiencies in thermoregulatory and circulatory functions. The most likely explanations for this impairment are (1) a reduced plasma volume and therefore reduced hemodynamic capacity to achieve maximal cardiac output and peripheral circulation, and (2) altered sweat gland function, whereby sweating ceases in an autonomic control attempt to conserve body water. As a result, body temperature rises quickly, drastically increasing the chance of cramps, exhaustion, and even heat stroke, the latter having a mortality rate of 80%. Sweat losses of 1.5 L/hour are commonly encountered in endurance sports, and under particularly hot conditions, sweat rates exceeding 2.5 L/hour have been measured in fit individuals. Marathon runners can lose 6 to 8% of body weight in water during the 26.2-mile event, and plasma volume may fall 13 to 18%. It would not be uncommon, therefore, for a 150-lb runner to lose ½ lb of water per mile in a hot environment (equivalent to an 8-oz glass of water).

Dehydration results when fluid loss exceeds intake, the degree of dehydration being directly proportional to this disparity. It is difficult for the endurance athlete to avoid a negative water balance because it is both impractical and distasteful to attempt to replenish the copious amount lost in the course of a marathon. It is distasteful because the necessary intake far exceeds the thirst desire, a stimulus that is delayed behind rapid dehydration. However, the force-feeding of fluids to exactly balance that which was lost is ideal from the standpoint of athletic performance, although the dramatic effects of lesser amounts of fluid replenishment during exercise are also well documented. The experimental design on which these conclusions are based generally is a comparison of the extent of fluid intake with performance and certain physiologic parameters such as heart rate and body temperature. Study groups are generally comprised of subjects who, in the course of prolonged exercise, are (1) force-fed fluids beyond the thirst desire, (2) allowed to drink fluid *ad libitum* (as desired), and (3) deprived of fluid intake. Force-fed subjects display superior performance, lower heart rate, and lower body core temperature than the other groups, and the *ad libitum* group outperforms the deprived group in these parameters.

An imposing question in sports nutrition, and one that has been surrounded by some controversy, is whether electrolyte replacement is necessary during prolonged exercise. Based on the knowledge that sweat contains electrolytes (sodium, potassium, chloride, and magnesium), it was reasoned that significant losses of these occurred during endurance athletics and that their replacement was necessary to optimize performance. In the 1970s, sports drinks supplemented with electrolytes and sometimes glucose (GE drinks) began

PERSPECTIVE (continued)

to appear on the market and were sold under such names as Gatorade, Sportade, and Body Punch. The answer as to whether such supplementation is necessary depends on the extent of depletion of the electrolytes, which, in turn, is a function of the electrolyte composition of sweat and of the total sweat loss [1].

The electrolyte content of sweat in the average individual is very low compared to the body fluids. This is shown in Table 13.3, which compares the electrolyte concentrations of sweat and blood serum. In the case of sodium and chloride, dehydration through sweating has the effect of concentrating these electrolytes in extracellular and intracellular water because of the relatively low concentration of these ions in sweat. Therefore in marathon-level exertion, in which a total sweat loss of 5 to 6 L or less is incurred, rehydration with water alone is adequate, since only about 200 mEq of sodium and chloride would be lost from a relatively large body store. Furthermore, pure water, because of its negligible osmolarity, would leave the stomach and be absorbed more quickly than a hypotonic salt solution, thereby restoring rapidly the normal osmolarity of the body fluids. Although some researchers regard potassium losses during exercise in the heat as constituting a potential health problem, this too is controversial in view of the relatively small amount of the ion lost. On the basis of the potassium content of sweat, shown in Table 1, it can be estimated that a 5-L sweat loss would induce a potassium deficit of less than 20 mEq, or well under 1% of the estimated total body store of 3,000 mEq for a 70-kg man.

Although such arguments are valid for the acclimatized athlete exercising at or less than the equivalent exertional demands of a marathon, conditions do exist where electrolyte loss, particularly sodium, can be significant. Foundry workers and miners working 8-hour shifts in very hot environments may suffer from "miner's cramps," intense skeletal muscle contractions thought to be caused by sodium depletion. In extreme situations such as this, in which sodium loss may exceed 8 g/d, the consumption of GE solutions or salt tablets would be indicated. The environmental conditions, fitness and acclimatization of the workers, and magnitude of sweat loss are factors to be considered in the evaluation of electrolyte supplementation.

TABLE 1 Average Electrolyte Concentrations in Sweat and Blood Serum (mEq/L)

	Na^+	K^+	Cl^-	Mg^{++}
Sweat	40–45	3.9	39	3.3
Blood serum	140	4.0	110	1.5–2.1

Another type of electrolyte disturbance can occur when only water is consumed during particularly long periods of physical activity such as triathalons and ultramarathons. In some instances, weight gains have been reported in these athletes, due simply to voluntary overhydration with water or hypotonic salt solutions during the exercise period (>7 hours). When water intake exceeds water loss to this extent, water intoxication can occur [2]. This is a lay term describing the condition of hyponatremia, or abnormally low plasma concentration of sodium. Afflicted subjects may suffer diarrhea, exhaustion, mental confusion, syncope, and even convulsions. It is not clearly understood why the *hypervolemia* would not be corrected by increased urinary loss mediated through osmoreceptor and ADH mechanisms, but it may be due to a water and sodium conservation mechanism activated by prolonged exercise during the period of exercise and up to 48 hours later.

Enhancement of athletic performance through proper nutrition continues to be the target of a great deal of research, and fluid and electrolyte balance is a most important factor in this pursuit. Pertinent review articles are available to the reader who is interested in exploring this subject in greater depth [3–5].

References Cited

1. Costill DL. Sweating: Its composition and effects on body fluids. Ann NY Acad Sci 1977;301:160–174,183.
2. Noakes TD. Water intoxication: A possible complication during endurance exercise. Med Sci Sports Exerc 1985;17:370.
3. Senay LC, Pivarnik JM. Fluid shifts during exercise. Exerc Sports Sci Rev 1985;13:335–387.
4. Herbert WG. Water and electrolytes. In: Williams MH, ed. Ergogenic aids in sport. Champaign, IL: Human Kinetics Publishers, 1983:56–98.
5. Nieman DC. The sports medicine fitness course. Palo Alto, CA: Bull Publishing, 1986:156–159.

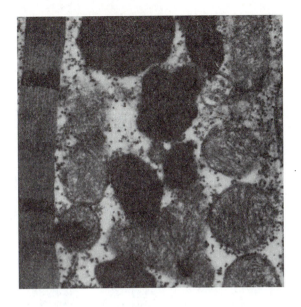

BODY COMPOSITION

Photo: A heart muscle fiber and dark lipofuscin granules

An innate characteristic of maturation and aging is a change in body composition. These compositional changes occur throughout the life cycle, beginning with the embryo and extending through old age. Rapid growth entails not only an increase in body mass but also a change in the proportions of components making up this mass. Young adulthood is a period of relative homeostasis, but in some people modifications of body composition can occur. Following the more or less homeostatic period of young adulthood is the period of progressive aging, when some undesirable changes in body composition inevitably occur. Throughout the life cycle, environment can modify body composition, and one of the most important environmental factors is food. Some knowledge of body composition is needed by nutrition professionals so that they may be better prepared to determine nutrient needs and to identify health risks of people throughout the life cycle.

At any point in time an individual's body composition is a major determinant of his or her nutrient and energy needs. Furthermore, a body composition profile can suggest disease such as malnutrition, osteoporosis, the eating disorder anorexia nervosa, or a person's relative risk for diseases associated with obesity. Excess body fat that is disproportionately placed in a particular area of the body may pose an increased risk for hyperlipidemia, diabetes mellitus, and hypertension (risk factors of cardiovascular disease). Therefore, body composition information has relevance both for disease prevention and therapeutic regimens.

BODY WEIGHT: WHAT SHOULD WE WEIGH?

Recognition of body weight as an indicator of health status is probably universal and as old as humanity itself. Only recently, however, have scientists and health professionals been concerned about determining the optimal weight to minimize susceptibility to disease. The first step to determine acceptable weight for height was taken in 1846 by an English surgeon, John Hutchinson, who published a height–weight table on a sample of 30-year-old Englishmen [1]. Hutchinson urged that future census taking include information on each person's height and weight because he believed such information would be valuable in promoting health and detecting disease [1].

Insurance companies looking to insure those individuals likely to live a long life became interested in heights and weights of people at various ages. Standard weight for height at a particular age was the average weight of those people who applied and were accepted for insurance over a period of several years [1]. However, subsequent studies of the relationship between mortality and weight revealed that average weights were not necessarily the standards that should be used by insurance companies in estimating longevity in applicants. Although the norm appeared to be an increase in weight with aging, mortality statistics suggested that lower weights after about the age of 30 years were beneficial.

In 1942 and 1943, the Metropolitan Life Insurance Company introduced the concept of "ideal" weights for women and men, respectively. No longer was aging a consideration in estimating an acceptable weight for an adult. A weight within the normal range for a person 25 to 30 years of age became the ideal weight for an adult of any age. Body frame size was introduced as a factor in body weight. Unfortunately, no guidelines were provided for determining frame size.

The possible health benefit of an adult's maintaining a lower-than-average weight for height was introduced in the 1959 revision (Table 14.1) of the 1942, 1943 Metropolitan Insurance Company tables. Revision of the tables came as a result of a study by the Society of Actuaries (build and blood pressure study), indicating that lower-than-average weight for height, even for young adults, could be associated with longevity. In the revised tables, weights considered appropriate for the various heights and frame sizes were termed "desirable" rather than ideal. Again the method for determining frame size was omitted. Nevertheless, dividing a person's actual weight by the midpoint of the weight range for his or her roughly estimated frame size became a popular method for identifying people who might be at risk because of overweight or obesity (or, in rare cases, because of underweight). This index, referred to as the Metropolitan Relative Weight (MRW) or relative body weight (RBW), is still in use [2].

The latest height–weight table is the one based on the Actuary Body Build Study [3] and published by the

TABLE 14.1 Desirable Weights for Men and Women, Metropolitan Life Insurance Company, 1959

Height (with shoes)	Weight (in indoor clothing)		
	Small Frame	Medium Frame	Large Frame
Men			
5' 2"	112–120 lb	118–129 lb	126–141 lb
5' 3"	115–123	121–133	129–144
5' 4"	118–126	124–136	132–148
5' 5"	121–129	127–139	135–152
5' 6"	124–133	130–143	138–156
5' 7"	128–137	134–147	142–161
5' 8"	132–141	138–152	147–166
5' 9"	136–145	142–156	151–170
5'10"	140–150	146–160	155–174
5'11"	144–154	150–165	159–179
6' 0"	148–158	154–170	164–184
6' 1"	152–162	158–175	168–189
6' 2"	156–167	162–180	173–194
6' 3"	160–171	167–185	178–199
6' 4"	164–175	172–190	182–204
Women			
4'10"	92– 98 lb	96–107 lb	104–119 lb
4'11"	94–101	98–110	106–122
5' 0"	96–104	101–113	109–125
5' 1"	99–107	104–116	112–128
5' 2"	102–110	107–119	115–131
5' 3"	105–113	110–122	118–134
5' 4"	108–116	113–126	121–138
5' 5"	111–119	116–130	125–142
5' 6"	114–123	120–135	129–146
5' 7"	118–127	124–139	133–150
5' 8"	122–131	128–143	137–154
5' 9"	126–135	132–147	141–158
5'10"	130–140	136–151	145–163
5'11"	134–144	140–155	149–168
6' 0"	138–148	144–159	153–173

Source: Courtesy of Metropolitan Life Insurance Company. Reprinted with permission.

Metropolitan Life Insurance Company in 1983 (Table 14.2). Unlike its predecessors, this table is accompanied by instructions for estimating frame size. People with small, medium, or large frames may be identified by measurement of elbow breadth (Table 14.3 and Fig. 14.1). Approximately 50% of the population falls within the medium-frame category, with the other 50% rather evenly divided between the small-frame and large-frame designations.

In this 1983 table, the weight-for-height figures are designated as "acceptable" rather than ideal or desirable and are somewhat higher than those found in the earlier height–weight tables. The increase of approximately 10% in shorter people and about 5% in people of medium height [4] is a reflection of the mortality data

TABLE 14.2 1983 Metropolitan Life Insurance Company Height and Weight Tables

Height	Small Frame	Medium Frame	Large Frame
Men[a]			
5' 2"	128–134 lb	131–141 lb	138–150 lb
5' 3"	130–136	133–143	140–153
5' 4"	132–138	135–145	142–156
5' 5"	134–140	137–148	144–160
5' 6"	136–142	139–151	146–164
5' 7"	138–145	142–154	149–168
5' 8"	140–148	145–157	152–172
5' 9"	142–151	148–160	155–176
5'10"	144–154	151–163	158–180
5'11"	146–157	154–166	161–184
6' 0"	149–160	157–170	164–188
6' 1"	152–164	160–174	168–192
6' 2"	155–168	164–178	172–197
6' 3"	158–172	167–182	176–202
6' 4"	162–176	171–187	181–207
Women[b]			
4'10"	102–111 lb	109–121 lb	118–131 lb
4'11"	103–113	111–123	120–134
5' 0"	104–115	113–126	122–137
5' 1"	106–118	115–129	125–140
5' 2"	108–121	118–132	128–143
5' 3"	111–124	121–135	131–147
5' 4"	114–127	124–138	134–151
5' 5"	117–130	127–141	137–155
5' 6"	120–133	130–144	140–159
5' 7"	123–136	133–147	143–163
5' 8"	126–139	136–150	146–167
5' 9"	129–142	139–153	149–170
5'10"	132–145	142–156	152–173
5'11"	135–148	145–159	155–176
6' 0"	138–151	148–162	158–179

[a]Weights at ages 25 to 59 years based on lowest mortality. Weight in pounds according to frame (in indoor clothing weighing 5 lb, shoes with 1-in heels).
[b]Weights at ages 25 to 59 years based on lowest clothing weighing 3 lb, shoes with 1-in heels).
Source: Courtesy of Metropolitan Life Insurance Company. Reprinted with permission.

TABLE 14.3 How to Determine Your Body Frame by Elbow Breadth

Height (in 1-in heels)	Elbow Breadth	Height (in 2.5-cm heels)	Elbow Breadth
Men			
5' 2"–5' 3"	$2\frac{1}{2}$–$2\frac{7}{8}$ in	158–161 cm	6.4–7.2 cm
5' 4"–5' 7"	$2\frac{5}{8}$–$2\frac{7}{8}$	162–171	6.7–7.4
5' 8"–5' 11"	$2\frac{3}{4}$–3	172–181	6.9–7.6
6' 0"–6' 3"	$2\frac{3}{4}$–$3\frac{1}{8}$	182–191	7.1–7.8
6' 4"	$2\frac{7}{8}$–$3\frac{1}{4}$	192–193	7.4–8.1
Women			
4' 10"–4' 11"	$2\frac{1}{4}$–$2\frac{1}{2}$ in	148–151 cm	5.6–6.4 cm
5' 0"–5' 3"	$2\frac{1}{4}$–$2\frac{1}{2}$	152–161	5.8–6.5
5' 4"–5' 7"	$2\frac{3}{8}$–$2\frac{5}{8}$	162–171	5.9–6.6
5' 8"–5' 11"	$2\frac{3}{8}$–$2\frac{5}{8}$	172–181	6.1–6.8
6' 0"	$2\frac{1}{2}$–$2\frac{3}{4}$	182–183	6.2–6.9

Note: This table lists the elbow measurements for men and women of medium frame at various heights. Measurements lower than those listed indicate that you have a small frame, while higher measurements indicate a large frame.
Source: Courtesy of Metropolitan Life Insurance Company. Reprinted with permission.

Guidelines for Americans (3rd edition, 1990) provides suggested weights for adults. These weights for heights are given in ranges whereby the higher weights in the ranges apply to men and the lower weights in the range apply to women.

Determination of appropriate weight for an individual is influenced by a variety of factors, including genetic makeup and health status. For instance, a person who has a genetic predisposition toward diabetes mellitus might very well benefit from weight reduction, even though his or her present weight falls within the acceptable range. Yet another person identified as obese but with a stationary weight and no other identifiable risk factors may derive no benefit from loss of weight [4].

Using data from the 1979 Actuary Build Study, Andres [5] determined that the body mass index or Quetelet's index, weight measured in kilograms divided by height measured in meters and raised to a power of 2 or squared (wt/h^2), was associated with the lowest mortality for men and women between the ages of 20 and 70 years. The body mass index is considered a good index of total body fat in both men and women. Andres's analysis demonstrated that the 1983 Metropolitan Life Insurance Company table is appropriate primarily for people in their thirties and forties. According to his figures, weights listed as acceptable in the 1983 table are higher than insurance data would justify for young adults but lower than justifiable in older adults. Age,

collected in the 1979 actuary build study [3]. This study showed that insured men and women under 30 years of age tended to be heavier than their counterparts of the 1959 build and blood pressure study. Of particular interest, however, was the reduced mortality found to be associated with mild-to-moderate overweight in shorter-than-average people. Increased weights for height that appear commensurate with good health according to the 1979 Actuary Build Study support the opinion of researchers who question the use of height–weight tables in determining the optimal weight for an individual. Table 14.4 from the USDA's *Dietary*

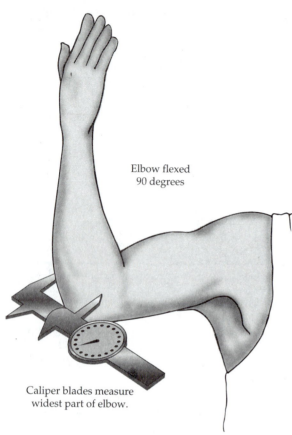

Elbow flexed
90 degrees

Caliper blades measure
widest part of elbow.

Upper arm parallel to floor

FIGURE 14.1 Measurement of elbow breadth. Extend your arm and bend the forearm upward at a 90-degree angle. Keep the fingers straight, and turn the inside of your wrist toward the body. Place the calipers on the two prominent bones on either side of the elbow. Measure the space between the bones with the caliper. Compare this measurement with the measurements shown in Table 14.3.

TABLE 14.4 Suggested Weights For Adults

Height[a]	Weight in pounds[b]	
	19 to 34 years	35 years and over
5'0"	97–128	108–138
5'1"	101–132	111–143
5'2"	104–137	115–148
5'3"	107–141	119–152
5'4"	111–146	122–157
5'5"	114–150	126–162
5'6"	118–155	130–167
5'7"	121–160	134–172
5'8"	125–164	138–178
5'9"	129–169	142–183
5'10"	132–174	146–188
5'11"	136–179	151–194
6'0"	140–184	155–199
6'1"	144–189	159–205
6'2"	148–195	164–210
6'3"	152–200	168–216
6'4"	156–205	173–222
6'5"	160–211	177–228
6'6"	164–216	182–234

[a]Without shoes.
[b]Without clothes.
Source: U.S. Department of Agriculture, U.S. Department of Health and Human Services. Dietary guidelines for Americans, 3rd ed. Washington, DC: USDA, 1990; 9.

however, is also thought to be a determinant in acceptable weight and should be factored into the height–weight tables once again [6].

Although determination of an appropriate weight for an individual must be based on the person's unique characteristics including present health status, activity level, and medical and/or family history, standard weights for height can be quite useful in identifying people who are possibly at risk because of their weight. People at risk include those individuals with weight for height well below the lowest end of the acceptable range or well above the highest end of the acceptable range. Extremes in either direction more than likely pose some health risks. Figures 14.2 and 14.3 illustrate acceptable weight for height based on the body mass index.

Although measuring both height and weight is relatively easy to do and can provide information on growth and nutritional status, neither weight for height nor body mass index is always a valid indicator of the degree of body fatness. The failure of weight as a valid measure of fatness became clear in World War II. Behnke, a Navy physician, was able to demonstrate by hydrostatic weighing that several football players who had been found unfit for military service because of excessive weight actually had less body fat than controls of normal weight [7]. The excessive weight of these athletes was due to hypertrophy of muscles rather than excessive adipose tissue [7]. Behnke's work rekindled an interest in studying the composition of the human body, an interest that had lain dormant for about 50 years.

THE COMPOSITION OF THE HUMAN ADULT BODY

As described by Friis-Hansen [8], the chemical composition of the human body was first described in 1859 in a book that dealt with the chemical composition of food.

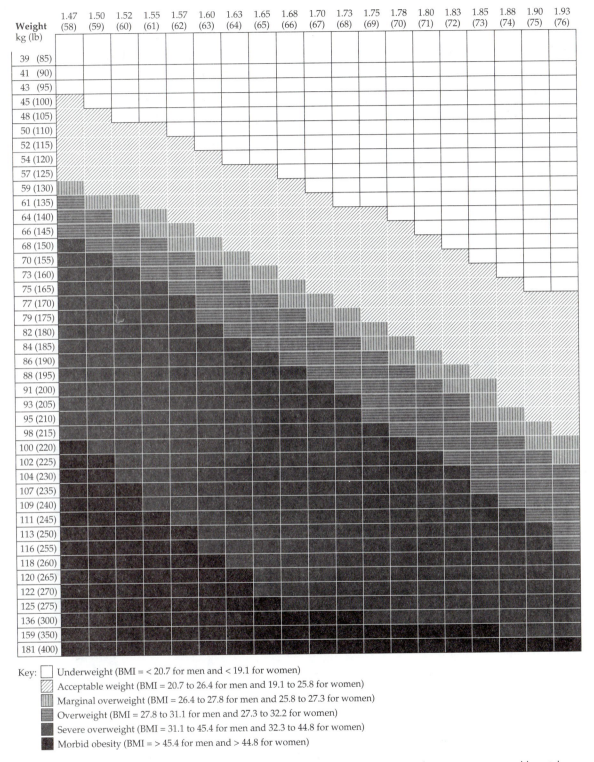

FIGURE 14.2 Acceptable weight for height based on body mass index (BMI). To determine your acceptable weight range, find your height in the top line. Look down the column below it and find the range represented by the shading. Look to the left column to see what weights are acceptable for you. *(Adapted from M. I. Rowland. A nomogram for computing body index. Dietetic Currents 16 (1989):8–9, used with permission from Ross Laboratories, Columbus, OH 43216. Copyright 1989 Ross Laboratories. Reprinted from Whitney EN, Rolfes SR. Understanding Nutrition, 6th ed. St Paul: West, 1993; inside cover.)*

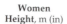

Women
Height, m (in)

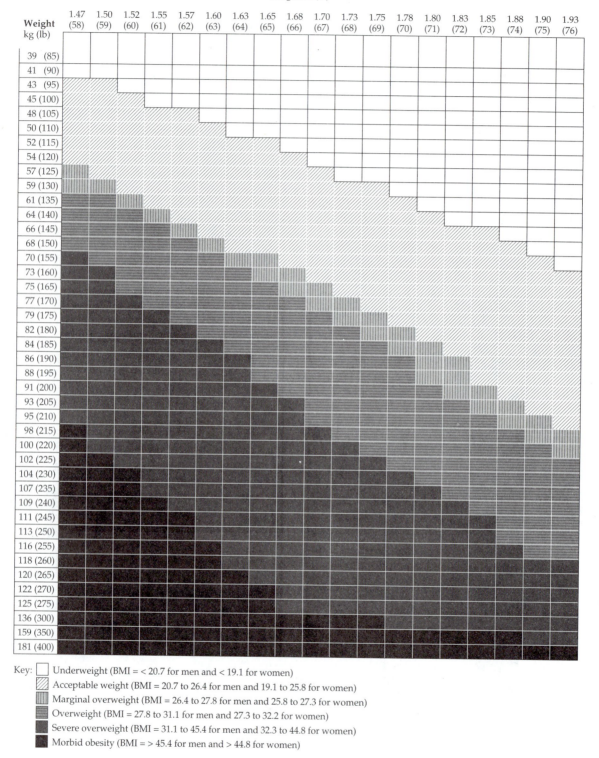

Key:
- ☐ Underweight (BMI = < 20.7 for men and < 19.1 for women)
- ▨ Acceptable weight (BMI = 20.7 to 26.4 for men and 19.1 to 25.8 for women)
- ⊞ Marginal overweight (BMI = 26.4 to 27.8 for men and 25.8 to 27.3 for women)
- ▦ Overweight (BMI = 27.8 to 31.1 for men and 27.3 to 32.2 for women)
- ▩ Severe overweight (BMI = 31.1 to 45.4 for men and 32.3 to 44.8 for women)
- ■ Morbid obesity (BMI = > 45.4 for men and > 44.8 for women)

FIGURE 14.3 Acceptable weight for height based on body mass index (BMI). To determine your acceptable weight range, find your height in the top line. Look down the column below it and find the range represented by the shading. Look to the left column to see what weights are acceptable for you. *(Adapted from M. I. Rowland. A nomogram for computing body index. Dietetic Currents 16 (1989):8–9, used with permission from Ross Laboratories, Columbus, OH 43216. Copyright 1989 Ross Laboratories. Reprinted from Whitney EN, Rolfes SR. Understanding Nutrition, 6th ed. St Paul: West, 1993; inside cover.)*

TABLE 14.5 Body Composition of Reference Man and Woman

Reference Man	Reference Woman
Age: 20–24 yr	Age: 20–24 yr
Height: 68.5 in	Height: 64.5 in
Weight: 154 lb	Weight: 125 lb
Total fat: 23.1 lb	Total fat: 33.8 lb
(15.0% body weight)	(27.0% body weight)
Storage fat: 18.5 lb	Storage fat: 18.8 lb
(12.0% body weight)	(15.0% body weight)
Essential fat: 4.6 lb	Essential fat: 15.0 lb
(3.0% body weight)	(12.0% body weight)
Muscle: 69 lb	Muscle: 45 lb
(44.8% body weight)	(36.0% body weight)
Bone: 23 lb	Bone: 15 lb
(14.9% body weight)	(12.0% body weight)
Remainder: 38.9 lb	Remainder: 31.2%
(25.3% body weight)	(25.0% body weight)
Average body density:	Average body density:
1.070 g/mL	1.040 g/mL

Source: McArdle WD, Katch FI, Katch VL. Exercise Physiology. Philadelphia: Lea & Febiger, 1981; p. 369. Adapted from Behnke AR, Wilmore JH. Evaluation and regulation of body build and composition. Englewood Cliffs, NJ: Prentice Hall, 1974.

Analytical chemistry was a rapidly growing science at the time, and figures describing chemical composition of the different tissues of the body were given in comparison with those for various foods.

Although additional chemical composition data from whole-body analysis of fetuses, children, and adults were collected during the next few decades, from around 1900 until about 1945 almost no similar work was carried out. With the advent of indirect measures or *in vivo* measurements of body composition such as hydrostatic weighing and isotope dilution, analysis of whole bodies again was carried out. Direct measurements of body composition were necessary to validate data obtained via indirect measurements [9–12].

The concept of the reference man and woman (Table 14.5) was developed by Behnke. These reference figures [13] are models based on average physical dimensions from measurements of thousands of subjects who participated in various anthropometric and nutrition surveys. The reference man and woman only provide a frame for comparisons.

As seen in Table 14.5, the reference man weighs 29 pounds more than the woman (nonpregnant) and is 4 inches taller. The man has 15% body fat versus the female with 27%. Of the 15% total body fat in the reference man only 3% is essential fat versus 12% essential fat in the reference woman's 27% total body fat. Essential fat is that fat associated with bone marrow, the cen-

tral nervous system (CNS), and viscera (internal organs). In females, essential fat also includes fat in mammary glands and the pelvic region. Note that in the reference man muscle accounts for 44.8% of body weight versus 36.0% of body weight in the female. The average body density of the reference man and woman are 1.070 and 1.040 g/mL respectively.

Table 14.6 provides information of the average values for body fat in U.S. men and women [14,15]. Based on data from physically active young adults and competitive athletes, a body fat content of about 15% (but not less than 8%) for men and between 15% and 25% for women has been recommended [15,16]. Female Olympic athletes (runners, jumpers, swimmers, divers, and gymnasts) had body fat levels of 11% to 16% [17].

METHODS FOR THE MEASUREMENT OF BODY COMPOSITION

Division of the body into components is used extensively for *in vivo* studies of body composition. In fact, densitometry, which is used to separate two components of the body, has become the standard against which most other indirect measurements of body composition have been evaluated [12].

The two-component model for body composition assessment divides the body into fat mass (which includes only the triacylglycerol quantity) and fat-free mass [8,18]. The terms *fat-free mass* and *lean body mass* are often used synonymously except that *lean body mass* includes essential fat. Several methods of body composition assessment are based on the two-component model.

Anthropometry

Anthropometry allows for estimation of body composition through measurement at various circumference and skin fold (fat) sites. Skin varies in thickness from 0.5 mm to 2 mm [19], thus fat beneath the skin typically represents the majority of the skin fold measurement. The assumption is that a direct relationship exists between total body fat and fat deposited in depots just beneath the skin (that is, subcutaneous fat).

Skin fold measurements can be used in two ways: (1) scores from the various measurements can be added and the sum used to indicate the relative degree of fatness among subjects or (2) scores can be plugged into various mathematical regression equations developed to predict

TABLE 14.6 Average Percentage of Body Fat for Women and Men from Selected Studies [15]

Study	Age Range	Stature (cm)	Mass (kg)	Fat (%)	68% Variation Limits[a]
Younger Women					
North Carolina, 1962	17–25	165.0 cm	55.5 kg	22.9%	17.5–28.5
New York, 1962	16–30	167.5	59.0	28.7	24.6–32.9
California, 1968	19–23	165.9	58.4	21.9	17.0–26.9
California, 1970	17–29	164.9	58.6	25.5	21.0–30.1
Air Force, 1972	17–22	164.1	55.8	28.7	22.3–35.3
New York, 1973	17–26	160.4	59.0	26.2	23.4–33.3
North Carolina, 1975		166.1	57.5	24.6	—
Massachusetts, 1993	17–30	165.3	57.7	21.8	16.7–27.2
Older Women					
Minnesota, 1953	31–45	163.3	60.7	28.9	25.1–32.8
Minnesota, 1953	43–68	160.0	60.9	34.2	28.0–40.5
New York, 1963	30–40	164.9	59.6	28.6	22.1–35.3
New York, 1963	40–50	163.1	56.4	34.4	29.5–39.5
North Carolina, 1975	33–50	—	—	29.7	23.1–36.5
Massachusetts, 1993	31–50	165.2	58.9	25.2	19.2–31.2
Younger Men					
Minnesota, 1951	17–26	177.8	69.1	11.8	5.9–11.8
Colorado, 1956	17–25	172.4	68.3	13.5	8.3–18.8
Indiana, 1966	18–23	180.1	75.5	12.6	8.7–16.5
California, 1968	16–31	175.7	74.1	15.2	6.3–24.2
New York, 1973	17–26	176.4	71.4	15.0	8.9–21.1
Texas, 1977	18–24	179.9	74.6	13.4	7.4–19.4
Massachusetts, 1993	17–30	178.2	76.3	12.9	7.8–18.1
Older Men					
Indiana, 1966	24–38	179.0	76.6	17.8	11.3–24.3
Indiana, 1966	40–48	177.0	80.5	22.3	16.3–28.3
North Carolina, 1976	27–50	—	—	23.7	17.9–30.1
Texas, 1977	27–59	180.0	85.3	27.1	23.7–30.5
Massachusetts, 1993	31–50	177.1	77.5	19.9	13.2–26.5

[a]Indicates the range of values for percentage of body fat that includes one standard deviation or about 68 out of every 100 people measured.
Source: Katch FI, McArdle WD. Introduction to nutrition, exercise, and health, 4th ed. Philadelphia: Lea and Febiger, 1993; p. 254.

body density or to calculate percentage of body fat [15,20]. Five sites commonly used for measuring skin fold thickness are shown in Figure 14.4. These sites are (A) the back of the upper arm (triceps) such that a vertical fold is measured at the midline of the upper arm halfway between the tip of the shoulder and the tip of the elbow; (B) subscapula—an oblique fat fold is measured just below the tip (interior angle) of the scapula; (C) suprailiac—a slightly oblique fold is measured just above the hip bone with the fold lifted to follow the natural diagonal line at this point; (D) abdomen—a vertical fold is measured 1 inch to the right of the umbilicus; and (E) thigh—a vertical fold is measured at midpoint of the thigh, between the knee cap to the hip (inguinal crease) [15,21]. Additional sites often include the pectoral (chest), midaxillary, and calf. The right side of the body is used for most measurements if comparisons are being made to standards derived from data from U.S. surveys that typically measured the right side of subjects. The handedness of the subject affects skin fold measurements taken on the arm such that measurements on the right exceed those on the left by 0.2 to 0.3 standard deviation units [22]. However, bias associated with the side of the measurement is less than error due to measurement [22]. All measurements should be repeated at least two to three times, and the average should be used as the skin fold value. The precision of skin fold thickness measurements depends on the skill of the anthropometrist; in general, a precision of within 5% can be obtained with a well-trained and experienced anthropometrist [23].

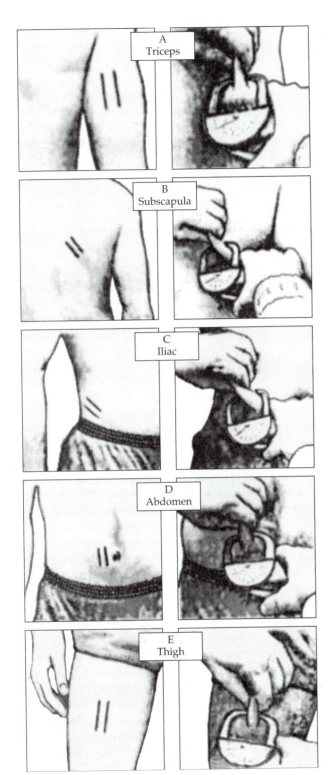

FIGURE 14.4 Anatomic location of the five fat fold sites: (A) triceps; (B) subscapular; (C) suprailiac; (D) abdomen; (E) thigh.

However, the use of anthropometry for predicting visceral fat content is of limited accuracy [24]. Nevertheless, the method is quite inexpensive, compared with the cost of other techniques.

Several different equations that are population specific have been developed for calculating total body fat from skin fold sites. Equations developed by Katch and McArdle [15] for predicting total body fat in young (aged 17 to 26 years) men and women from the triceps and subscapula skin folds are shown here:

Young women: % body fat = .55 (A) + .31 (B) + 6.13

Young men: % body fat = .43 (A) + .58 (B) + 1.47

where A = triceps fat fold measured in millimeters and B = subscapula fat fold measured in millimeters. Measurements from multiple (at least three) sites are deemed better for overall subcutaneous fat assessment than measurements from only one or two sites [15].

Circumference or girth measurements also may be used to assess body fat. Typical sites of measurement include the abdomen, buttocks, right thigh, and right upper arm. As with skin fold measurements, body fat prediction equations that are age and gender specific have been developed.

Circumference measurements of the waist (abdominal circumference) and hips (gluteal circumference) also provide an index of regional body fat distribution and have been shown to correlate with visceral fat [24]. A ratio of waist to hip circumference is calculated following measurement of both the subject's waist and hip. Waist measurements should be made below the rib cage and above the umbilicus in a horizontal plane at the most narrow site or site of least circumference. Hip circumference should be measured at the site with the greatest circumference around the hips or buttocks; soft tissue should not be compressed or indented during measurements. All measurements should be done with the subject standing. Reproducibility of circumference measurements is good at 2% [24]. Ratios greater than 0.8 in women and greater than 0.95 in men are thought to indicate increased health risk.

Densitometry

The principle of hydrostatic weighing on which densitometry is based can be traced to the Greek mathematician Archimedes. He discovered that the volume of an object submerged in water was equal to the volume of water displaced by the object. Specific gravity or density of an object can be calculated by dividing the object's weight (*wt*) in air by its loss of weight in water. For an individual who weighs 47 kg in air and 2 kg underwater, 45 kg represents the loss of body weight and the weight of the water displaced. Correction for residual air in the lungs and gas in the gastrointestinal tract (GI gas volume) must be made.

The calculation of body density is given as follows:

Body density =

$$\frac{\text{wt of body in air}}{\dfrac{(\text{wt of body in air} - \text{wt underwater})}{\text{density of water}} - \text{RLV} - \text{GI gas volume}}$$

Residual lung volume (RLV) is thought to be about 24% of vital lung capacity. The volume of gas in the gastrointestinal tract is estimated to range from 50 to 300 mL. This volume typically is either neglected or a value of 100 mL is used in calculations. The density of water or weight of water over a wide range of temperatures is also known and needs to be obtained for the calculation.

Calculating body density of the human body allows an estimation of body fat. At any known density, estimating percentage of body fat is made possible by an equation derived by Siri [25]:

$$\text{Percentage body fat} = \frac{495}{\text{body density}} - 450 \times 100$$

or by an equation derived by Brozek [16]:

$$\text{Percentage body fat} = \frac{457}{\text{body density}} - 414 \times 100$$

Calculations of body density are derived in part from the knowledge that the density of fat is 0.9 g/cm^3 and that of fat-free mass is 1.1 g/cm^3 (assuming fat-free mass is composed of 20.5% protein, 72.4% water, and 7.1% bone mineral). Once the percentage of body fat has been calculated, the weight of the fat and the weight of lean body mass can be estimated as follows [15]:

Body weight × percentage body fat = weight of body fat
Body weight − weight of body fat = lean body weight

Underwater weighing is considered a noninvasive and precise method for assessment of body fat. Standard error of estimate of body fat using densitometry has been estimated at 2.7% for adults and about 4.5% for children and adolescents [17]. Limitations of underwater weighing include its relatively high cost for the equipment, its impracticality for large numbers of subjects, and the extreme cooperation required from subjects who must be submerged and remain motionless for an extended time period. Thus the technique is not suit-

able for young children, older adults, and subjects in poor health.

Use of the two-component model of body composition was initially based on the assumption that fat weight of the body is variable and that lean body mass contains a relatively fixed amount of water and remains fairly constant once chemical maturity of the body had been reached [26]. Because of this assumption, measurement of total body water became a mechanism by which the fat content of the body could be estimated [6].

Total Body Water (TBW)

Quantification of total body water involves the use of isotopes, typically deuterium (D_2O), radioactive tritium (^3H_2O), or oxygen-18 (^{18}O). Water can be labeled with any one of the three isotopes. The water containing a specific amount (concentration) of the isotope is then ingested or injected intravenously. Following ingestion or injection, the isotope distributes itself throughout body water. Body water occupies about 73.2% of fat-free body mass. After a specified time period (usually two to six hours) for equilibration, samples of body fluids (usually blood and urine) are taken. Losses of the isotope in the urine must be determined. If ^{18}O is used, breath samples are collected for analysis. Concentrations of the isotope in the breath or body fluids are determined by scintillation counters or other instruments. The concentration (C_1) and volume (V_1) of the isotope given is equal to the final concentration of the isotope in the plasma (C_2) and the volume of total body water (V_2) and expressed as $C_1V_1 = C_2V_2$. Thus, total body water (V_2) = C_1V_1 divided by C_2. Once total body water has been determined, the percentage of lean body mass can be calculated. Fat-free mass equals total body water divided by 0.732. Body fat can be obtained by subtracting fat-free mass from body weight. A three-component model (consisting of total body water, body volume, and body weight) has been shown to measure changes in body fat as low as 1.54 kg in individuals [27].

Many studies, however, have shown that the degree of hydration varies considerably in lean body tissue of apparently healthy people. Therefore, implications about total body fat derived from the estimation of lean body mass via total body water may be misleading [6,15]. In addition, adipose tissue has been shown to contain as much as 15% water by weight [28]. Thus, measurement of extracellular fluid as well as total body water should be conducted and subtracted from total body water to get an indication of intracellular water and thus an indication of body cell mass. Because total body water involves radiation exposure if ^{3}H is used, the method is not suitable for use with some subjects (such as children or pregnant women). ^{18}O is in itself quite expensive and requires expensive mass spectrometry equipment for its analysis. Deuterated water (D_2O) is relatively inexpensive to purchase, but is expensive to measure [29].

Total Body Potassium (TBK)

Total body potassium is also used to assess fat-free mass; potassium is present within cells, but is not associated with stored fat. ^{40}K is a naturally occurring isotope that emits a characteristic gamma ray. About 0.012% of potassium occurs as ^{40}K. External counting of gamma rays emitted by ^{40}K provides the amount of total body potassium; however, getting accurate counts of ^{40}K may be difficult, because of external or background radiation. Alternately, ^{42}K may be administered to a subject orally or intravenously and the radioactivity measured. After measurement of potassium (^{40}K or ^{42}K) radiation from the body, calculation of total body potassium from the data is required. Fat-free mass can be estimated from the total body potassium based on any one of several conversion factors, which vary in men from 2.46 to 3.41 g potassium per kg fat-free mass, and in women from 2.28 to 3.16 g potassium per kg fat-free mass [28]. Total body fat can be calculated by subtracting fat-free mass from body weight. Overestimation of body fat in obese subjects has been reported with total body potassium [30]. The technique should not be used in people with potassium-wasting diseases.

Absorptiometry

Absorptiometry involves scanning the entire body or a portion of the body by a photon beam. Single-photon absorptiometry is used typically to investigate bone mineral content. Bone mineral is assumed to be directly proportional to the amount of photon energy absorbed by the bone being studied [23]. In dual-photon absorptiometry, the subject is scanned with photons at two different energy levels. Differential absorption is measured; the ratio of the two absorptions is linearly related to the percentage of body fat [28]. Reproducibility of abdominal fat mass by this method is about 12% [24]. Dual-photon absorptiometry can also be used to measure bone mass.

Limitations to the use of absorptiometry include the expense of the equipment and the exposure of subjects to radiation. Children, pregnant women, and subjects who are in poor health would not be suitable candidates for body composition assessment by absorptiometry.

Total Body Electrical Conductivity (TOBEC) and Bioelectrical Impedance (BEI) or Bioelectrical Impedance Analysis (BIA)

The TOBEC (total body electrical conductivity) technique is based on the change in electrical conductivity when a subject is placed in an electromagnetic field. Subjects lie face up on a bed, which is rolled into the TOBEC instrument. The instrument then induces an electrical current in the subject. Changes in conductivity are measured and are proportional to the body's electrolyte content. Since electrolytes in the body are found associated mostly with lean body mass, TOBEC allows for the estimation of lean body mass, and fat by difference. Hydration status, electrolyte imbalances, and variations in bone mass may however interfere with accuracy. In addition, while the procedure is fast and safe, the equipment is very expensive.

Bioelectrical impedance analysis (BIA) or bioelectrical impedance (BEI) is similar to TOBEC in that it also depends on changes in electrical conductivity. However in bioelectrical impedance analysis, measurement of electrical conductivity is made on the extremities and not on the whole body. Subjects lie face up on a bed with extremities away from the body. Electrodes are placed on the limbs in specific locations. An instrument generates a current that is passed through the body by means of the electrodes. Opposition to the current is called *impedance*. The body's resistance to the current is measured by the instrument. The lowest resistance value of an individual is used to calculate conductance and predict lean body mass. Tissues containing little water and electrolytes (such as fat) are poor conductors and have a high resistance to the passage of current [29].

Bioelectrical impedance is a safe, noninvasive, and rapid means to assess body composition. The equipment is portable, although it is also relatively expensive. Like TOBEC, bioelectrical impedance readings are affected by hydration and electrolyte imbalances. Thus, the technique is more useful for healthy subjects.

Computerized Tomography (CT)

Computerized or computed tomography (CT), involving an x-ray tube and detectors aligned at opposite poles of a circular gantry, allows the taking of visual images, and thus the determination of regional body composition such as visceral organ mass, regional muscle mass, subcutaneous, internal fat, and bone density. Subjects lie face up on a movable platform that passes through the instrument's circular gantry. Cross-sectional images of tissue are constructed by the scanner computer as the x-ray beam rotates around the person being assessed. Differences in x-ray attenuation are related to differences in the physical density of tissues [23]. Calculation of relative surface area or volume occupied by tissues, such as bone, adipose, and fat-free tissue, can be accomplished from the images produced by the instrument. Results are highly reproducible [24]. Excessively long exposure of subjects to ionizing radiation and the expense of the equipment are major drawbacks to the use of computerized tomography to assess body composition.

Magnetic Resonance Imaging (MRI)

Magnetic resonance imaging (MRI) is based on the principle that atomic nuclei behave like magnets when an external magnetic field is applied across the body. When the magnetic field is applied, the nuclei attempt to align with the field. The nuclei also absorb radio frequency waves directed into the body and in turn change their orientation in the magnetic field [23]. Abolishing the radio wave results in the emission of a radio signal by the activated nuclei. The emitted signal is used to develop a computerized image. Magnetic resonance imaging is used to measure body fat and fat distribution (subcutaneous, visceral, intra-abdominal). The technique is noninvasive and safe; however, the cost is quite high. Reproducibility of visceral fat area measured by magnetic resonance imaging is about 10 to 15% [24]. However, for assessment of adipose tissue distribution, magnetic resonance imaging provided the least variability when compared with skin fold, ^{40}K counting, bioelectrical impedance, total body water assessment with ^{18}O, and hydrostatic weighing [31].

Ultrasonography or Ultrasound

Ultrasound provides images of tissue configuration or depth readings of changes of tissue density [23]. Electrical energy is converted in a probe to high-frequency ultrasonic energy. The ultrasonic energy is transmitted through the skin and into the body in the form of short pulses or waves. The waves pass through adipose tissue until they reach lean body mass. At the interface between the adipose and lean tissues, part of the ultrasonic energy is reflected back to the receiver in the probe and is transformed to electrical energy. The echo is visualized. A transmission gel is used between the probe and skin and provides acoustic contact.

The equipment is portable, and the technique may provide information on the thickness of subcutaneous fat as well as muscle mass; however, the reproducibility is poor at 10 to 15%, and the validity of the method requires further research [24]. Anthropometry and computerized tomography appear to be superior in precision and accuracy to ultrasound [32]. Tissue interfaces are not as clearly delineated as with imaging techniques, and problems arise when the muscle–adipose tissue interface is irregular or there is fat layering [17,24].

Neutron Activation Analysis

Neutron activation analysis allows for an *in vivo* estimation of body composition including total body concentrations of nitrogen (TBN), calcium (TBCa), chloride (TBCl), sodium (TBNa), and phosphorus (TBP). A beam of neutrons is delivered to the individual being assessed. The body's atoms (nitrogen, calcium, chloride, sodium, and phosphorus) interact with the beam of neutrons to generate unstable radioactive elements, which emit energy as they revert back to their stable forms. The specific energy levels correspond with specific elements and the radiation's level of activity indicates the element's abundance [23]. The ability to measure nitrogen allows for lean body mass assessment. By subtracting lean body mass from total body water, total body fat can be calculated [33,34]. Two models for calculating total body fat have been used; the model used depends on the divisions identified as descriptors of components making up lean body mass. Division of lean body mass into body cell mass, extracellular water, and extracellular solids distinguishes better than the other model (protein + total body water + bone ash) between the actively metabolizing tissues and the relatively inactive tissues [33–35]. Tissues comprising body cell mass include muscle, viscera, brain, and reproductive system, while the extracellular solids are contributed primarily by the relatively inactive bone.

Table 14.7 [34] reports body composition information, derived from neutron activation, for males and females aged 20 to 79 years. Neutron activation analysis is noninvasive; however, the equipment is expensive and subjects are exposed to significant amounts of radiation.

Infrared Interactance

Infrared interactance is based on the principle that when material is exposed to infrared light, the light is absorbed, reflected, or transmitted, depending on the scattering and absorption properties of the material. For assessment of body composition, a probe that acts as an infrared transmitter and detector is placed on the skin. Infrared light of two wavelengths is transmitted by the probe. The signal penetrates the underlying tissue to a depth of 1 cm [23]. Infrared light also is reflected at the site from the skin and underlying subcutaneous tissues and detected by the probe. Estimates of body composi-

TABLE 14.7 Mean Body Composition Values for Healthy Males and Females[a]

Age (yr)	n	Body Weight (kg)	Protein (kg)	TBW (L)	Bone Ash (kg)	BCM (kg)	ECW (L)	ECS (kg)	TBF$_1$ (kg)	TBF$_2$ (kg)
Males										
20–29	12	80.1	13.1	44.9	3.53	35.7	19.8	6.77	18.6	16.8
30–39	12	73.7	11.2	42.3	3.44	32.5	19.0	6.61	16.8	15.6
40–49	12	84.6	12.4	47.2	3.59	35.1	19.8	6.88	21.4	23.0
50–59	12	82.0	12.1	45.0	3.43	33.3	19.3	6.58	21.5	20.7
60–69	10	78.5	11.8	42.1	3.33	30.7	19.9	6.39	21.3	21.5
70–79	10	80.5	11.1	40.4	3.17	27.6	20.3	6.08	25.8	26.5
Females										
20–29	17	64.6	9.0	33.3	2.78	23.1	16.1	5.33	19.4	20.0
30–39	10	69.3	9.3	33.6	2.69	22.9	16.5	5.17	23.7	24.7
40–49	11	65.2	8.7	31.4	2.60	21.3	15.9	4.99	22.5	22.9
50–59	9	73.6	8.4	31.7	2.40	20.5	15.9	4.61	29.1	22.6
60–69	13	61.7	7.8	28.6	2.26	18.0	15.4	4.34	23.0	23.9
70–79	9	58.3	7.3	27.6	2.03	17.6	14.5	3.89	21.4	22.3

[a]Protein = 6.25 × total body nitrogen; BCM (body cell mass) = 0.235 × total body potassium (g); ICW (intracellular water) = TBW (total body water) − ECW (extracellular water); BA (bone ash) = total body calcium (TBCa)/0.34; ECS (extracellular solids) = TBCa (total body calcium)/0.177; TBF (total body fat); TBF$_1$ = body weight − (protein + TBW + BA); TBF$_2$ = body weight − (BCM + ECW + ECS).

Source: Modified from Cohn SH, Vaswani AN, Yasumura S et al. Improved models for determination of body fat by in vivo neutron activation. Am J Clin Nutr 1984;40:255. © Am. J. Clin. Nutr., American Society for Clinical Nutrition. Reprinted with permission.

tion can be made by analyzing specific characteristics of the reflected light. The method is safe, noninvasive, and rapid; however, overestimates of body fat in lean (less than 8% body fat) subjects have been reported and underestimates of body fat in obese (greater than 30% body fat) subjects have been reported [30]. The accuracy of the technique requires further investigation.

To review the methods available to assess body composition, lean body mass or fat-free mass may be assessed by methods such as neutron activation analysis, total body potassium, intracellular water (total body water minus extracellular water), total body electrical conductivity, and bioelectrical impedance analysis. Body fat may be assessed by anthropometry, densitometry, dual-photon absorptiometry, and infrared interactance. Adipose tissue may be measured using computerized tomography, magnetic resonance imaging, and ultrasound. Table 14.8 [23,24,28,29,31] provides an overview of the methods discussed as well as a few additional methods.

PRIMARY INFLUENCES AND CHANGES IN BODY COMPOSITION WITH AGE

The effect of sex and age on lean body mass and its components including bone ash and extracellular solids can be observed in Table 14.7. However, additional sources of variation are race, heredity, and stature [36]. Although

stature accounts for only a small portion of the variance in lean body mass, its influence is sufficient to require that stature be taken into account in comparing body composition data among individuals or among groups of individuals. Taller children and adults have an advantage in lean body mass over their shorter peers [36].

Evidence suggests that bone density and fat-free weight are significantly affected by heredity. The effect of race is evidenced by the difference between North American whites and blacks. Blacks tend to have slightly larger lean body mass than whites, together with thicker and denser bones and hence a larger amount of total body calcium [35]. The influence of gender on body composition appears to exist from birth but becomes dramatically evident at puberty. The differences manifested at sexual maturation between males and females continue throughout life. Moreover, at menopause the female undergoes a further change in body composition as compared with the male. Accelerated loss of calcium from the bones, due in large part to the decline of estrogen production, causes a more rapid decrease in bone density of the elderly woman as compared to the elderly man.

The effect of maturation on body composition from infancy to adulthood is demonstrated in part in Table 14.9 [8], but data on the changes that occur during the time span from birth to adulthood are lacking. To help fill this gap, changes in body composition from birth to 10 years of age have been estimated through the use of

TABLE 14.8 Methods for Assessing Body Composition [20,21,25,26,29]

Method	Description of Method and Comments
Anthropometry	Skin fold thicknesses from a variety of locations, body weight, and limb circumferences can be used to calculate fat, fat-free mass, and muscle size. Measurements can be made in the field but require skilled technicians for accuracy. Skin folds can provide some information about regional subcutaneous fat as well as about total fat. Measurements may not be applicable to all population groups.
Densitometry	Measurement of total body density through determination of body volume by underwater weighing, helium displacement, or combination of water displacement by body and air displacement by head. Measurements can be used to determine body density, which in turn allows calculation of percentage of body fat and fat-free mass. Measurements are precise but must be conducted in laboratory; subject cooperation is necessary for underwater weighing. Method is unsuitable for young children and the elderly.
Total body water	Measured by dilution with deuterium (D_2O), tritium (^3H_2O), or oxygen-18 (^{18}O). TBW is used as index of human body composition based on findings that water is not present in stored triglycerides but occupies an approximate average of 73.2% of the fat-free mass. A specified quantity of the isotope is ingested or injected; then, following an equilibration period, a sampling is made of the concentration of the tracer in a selected biological fluid. TBW is calculated from equation $C_1V_1 = C_2V_2$, where V_2 represents TBW volume, C_1 is the amount of tracer given, and C_2 is the final concentration of tracer in the selected biological fluid. The ECF can be estimated by a variety of methods. Subtracting ECF from TBW allows calculation of fat-free mass. This is a difficult procedure with limited precision, and the cost can be great, particularly when ^{18}O is used as the tracer.
Total body potassium	^{40}K, a naturally occurring isotope, is found in a known amount (0.012%) in intracellular water and is not present in stored triglycerides. These facts allow fat-free mass to be estimated by the external counting of gamma rays emitted by ^{40}K. Instrument for counting ^{40}K is quite expensive and must be properly calibrated for precision. Method is limited to laboratories.
Urinary creatinine excretion	Creatinine is the product resulting from the nonenzymatic hydrolysis of free creatine, which is liberated during the dephosphorylation of creatine phosphate. The preponderance of creatine phosphate is located in the skeletal muscle; therefore urinary creatinine excretion can be related to muscle mass. Drawbacks to this method include large individual variability of creatinine excretion due to the renal processing of creatinine and the effect of diet. The creatine pool does not seem to be under strict metabolic control and is to some degree independent of body composition. Another technical difficulty is control of accurately timed 24-hour urine collections.
Total plasma creatinine	Because of the close relationship between total plasma creatinine and 24-hour urinary creatinine output, total plasma creatinine has been suggested as an index of total body skeletal mass. Calculated estimates supported by dissections of skeletal muscle in a few mature dogs indicate that each milligram of total plasma creatinine is equivalent to 0.88 kg skeletal muscle. A disadvantage is the range of error (0.5% to 10.8%) between predicted and observed mean mass values.
Endogenous 3-methyl-histidine excretion	3-methylhistidine has been suggested as a useful predictor of human body composition because this amino acid is located principally in the muscle and cannot be reused after its release from catabolized myofibrillar proteins (methylation of specific histidine residues occurs post-translationally on protein). Some concern exists over the use of 3-methylhistidine as a marker of muscle protein because of the potential influence of nonskeletal muscle protein (skin and gastrointestinal [GI] tract proteins) turnover on its excretory rate. Additional problems with this method are the need for consumption of a relatively controlled meat-free diet and complete and accurate urine collections.
Electrical conductance (a) Total body electrical conductivity	Method is based on the change in electrical conductivity when subject is placed in an electromagnetic field. The change is proportional to the electrolyte content of the body, and because fat-free mass contains virtually all the water and conducting electrolytes of the body, conductivity is far greater in the fat-free mass than in the fat mass. From measurement, LBM can be calculated and fat estimated by difference. A primary drawback to this method is the expense of the instrument required; this measurement is a laboratory procedure limited primarily to large clinical facilities.

TABLE 14.8 Methods for Assessing Body Composition [20,21,25,26,29] *(continued)*

Method	Description of Method and Comments
(b) Bioelectrical impedance analysis	This method is an adaptation of TOBEC; measurement of electrical conductivity is made on extremities rather than the whole body. Determinations of resistance and reactance are made, and the lowest resistance value for an individual is used to calculate conductance and to predict LBM. Equipment is portable and much less expensive than that required for TOBEC, yet precision is comparable.
Absorptiometry (a) Single-photon	Method is used in measurement of local or regional bone. The bone is scanned by a low-energy photon beam and the transmission monitored by a scintillation detector. Changes in transmission as the beam is moved across the bone are a function of bone mineral content (bone density) in that region. Disadvantages of this method are that the bone must be enclosed in a constant thickness of soft tissue, and measurements cannot be used to accurately predict total skeletal mass.
(b) Dual-photon	This method allows estimation of LBM as well as total bone mineral of the whole body. The body is scanned transversely in very small steps over its entire length by radiation from gadolinium-153 (^{153}Gd). This isotope emits two gamma rays of different energies; attenuation measurements at the two discrete photon energies allow quantitation of bone mineral and soft tissue. The equipment required for dual-photon absorptiometry is quite expensive, complicated calibration is required, and data collected requires complicated mathematical treatment. Use of this method is currently limited to research laboratories.
Computerized tomography	Method determines regional body composition. An image is generated by computerized processing of x-ray data. Fat, lean tissue, and bone can be identified by their characteristic density–frequency distribution. Information about regional fat distribution can be obtained; it has been used to determine the ratio of intra-abdominal to subcutaneous fat in humans. The size of the liver, spleen, and kidneys can be determined by computerized tomography (CT). Both cost of the equipment and technical difficulties are high. Method is a laboratory procedure presently limited primarily to large medical centers.
Ultrasound	Approach uses instrument in which electrical energy is converted in probe to high-frequency ultrasonic energy. Subsequent transmission of these sound waves through various tissues can be used to calculate tissue thickness. Method is used frequently to determine the thickness of subcutaneous fat layer. Large laboratory instruments and smaller portable equipment are available. Although data suggest a reasonable validity of method, its general use has been limited because the appropriate signal frequency of the probe has not been well defined and the needed constant pressure by the probe to the scan site is difficult to achieve. Changes in pressure by probe application can prejudice ultrasonic determination of adipose tissue thickness.
Infrared interactance	A relatively new method for measuring body fat. Measurement of body fat is made at various sites on the extremities through use of short wavelengths of infrared light. The amount of fat can be calculated from the absorption spectra and used through a prediction equation to estimate TBF. The method is considered to be in the developmental stage.
Magnetic resonance imaging	Approach is based on fact that atomic nuclei can behave like magnets. When external magnetic field is applied across a part of the body, each nucleus attempts to align with the external magnetic field. If these nuclei are simultaneously activated by a radio frequency wave, once the radio wave is turned off, the activated nuclei will emit the signal absorbed; this emitted signal is used to develop image by computer. Method has capability of generating images in response to intrinsic tissue variables and of representing such characteristics as level of hydration and fat content. This method appears to have much potential, but both the cost of equipment and technical difficulties are high.
Neutron activation analysis	This is the only technique currently available for measurement of multielemental composition of the human body. Low radiation doses produce isotopic atoms in tissues; the induced nuclides permit measurement of many elements, including nitrogen, calcium, phosphorus, magnesium, sodium, and chloride. Although precision of measurement is great, so are the technical difficulties and cost of equipment. Method of measuring body composition is limited to a very few laboratories in this country and abroad.

TABLE 14.9 Effect of Maturation on Body Composition

Chemical Components of Body (%)		Premature Infant	Term Infant	Adult Male
	Weight	1.5 kg	3.5 kg	70 kg
Protein (%)		11.3	12.5	18.0
Fat (%)		3.0	12.0	18.0
Water (%)		83.0	73.0	60.0
Ash (%)		2.7	3.2	5.2
Carbohydrate (%)		0.6	1.0	0.7

Source: Adapted from Friis-Hansen B. Body composition in growth. Pediatrics 1971;47:264.

"reference children" (Table 14.10) [37]. Table 14.11 [37] describes the composition of weight gain occurring during these years. Total body water decreases during the first year of life due primarily to a rapid increase in fat. The decrease in total body water during the first year of life is followed by a slight increase from age 12 months to about 6 or 7 years (Table 14.10) [37]. Although total body water gradually declines for the next three to four years, it still exceeds 60% of total body weight at age 10 years. Accompanying the changes in total body water is a change in the ratio of extracellular fluid (ECF) to intracellular fluid (ICF). ECF exceeds ICF volume in the fetus during gestation, but during infancy and childhood the ECF–ICF ratio progressively falls until ICF occupies the majority position [36]. The change in the ECF–ICF ratio occurs with the growth and maturation of the lean body mass. Cell hypertrophy and bone development encroach on the space occupied by ECF, while protein accrual results in an increased incorporation of ICF.

The rapid increase in lean body mass begun in the late fetal period continues for a while after birth and then decelerates. The deceleration is followed by a slower but fairly steady growth during the childhood years. The growth curve (body weight and lean body mass) for boys and girls is given in Figure 14.5 [36].

Despite the trend toward maturation of lean body mass during these childhood years, maturation appears to be incomplete until sometime during adolescence [36,38]. The percentage of water in lean body mass of reference children exceeds that considered average for the adult [38]. In addition, the value for minerals as a percentage of body weight is less than the adult average of 5.2% [8]. These differences in the components of lean body mass in children and adults decrease the density of lean body mass in children to below 1.10 g/mL, the average density for adults. Studies of children, both male and female, at various stages of maturation have confirmed the increased hydration of lean tissue and its lower density among people not yet having reached adulthood [38]. As a result of these studies, Lohman [39] has suggested that Siri's [25] equation for determining fatness (p. 450) be replaced by the following equation when body fat composition of prepubescent children is being estimated:

$$\text{Percentage fat} = \frac{5.30}{\text{body density}} - 4.89 \times 100$$

TABLE 14.10 Body Composition of Reference Children

Age	Weight		Fat		Protein		Water		Ash		Carbohydrate	
	Males	Females	Males	Females	Males	Females	Males	Females	Males	Females	Males	Females
Birth	3.545 kg	3.325 kg	13.7%	14.9%	12.9%	12.8%	69.6%	68.6%	3.2%	3.2%	0.5%	0.5%
4 mo	7.060	6.300	24.7	25.2	11.9	11.9	60.1	59.6	2.8	2.8	0.4	0.4
6 mo	8.030	7.250	25.4	26.4	12.0	12.0	59.4	58.4	2.8	2.7	0.4	0.4
12 mo	10.15	9.18	22.5	23.7	12.9	12.9	61.2	60.1	2.9	2.8	0.5	0.5
18 mo	11.47	10.78	20.8	21.8	13.5	13.5	62.2	61.3	3.1	3.0	0.5	0.5
24 mo	12.59	11.91	19.5	20.4	14.0	13.9	62.9	62.2	3.2	3.0	0.5	0.5
3 yr	14.675	14.10	17.5	18.5	14.7	14.4	63.9	63.5	3.4	3.1	0.5	0.5
4 yr	16.69	15.96	15.9	17.3	15.3	14.8	64.8	64.3	3.5	3.1	0.5	0.5
5 yr	18.67	17.66	14.6	16.7	15.8	15.0	65.4	64.6	3.7	3.1	0.5	0.5
6 yr	20.69	19.52	13.5	16.4	16.2	15.2	66.0	64.7	3.8	3.2	0.5	0.5
7 yr	22.85	21.84	12.8	16.8	16.5	15.2	66.2	64.4	3.9	3.1	0.5	0.5
8 yr	25.30	24.84	13.0	17.4	16.6	15.2	65.8	63.8	4.0	3.1	0.5	0.5
9 yr	28.13	28.46	13.2	18.3	16.8	15.1	65.4	63.0	4.1	3.1	0.5	0.5
10 yr	31.44	32.55	13.7	19.4	16.8	15.0	64.8	62.0	4.1	3.1	0.5	0.5

Source: Adapted from Foman SJ, Haschke F, Ziegler EE, Nelson SE. Body composition of reference children from birth to age 10 years. Am J Clin Nutr 1982;35:1171.

TABLE 14.11 Weight Increase and Its Components in Reference Children

Age	Weight Increase		Fat		Protein		Minerals	
	Males	Females	Males	Females	Males	Females	Males	Femals
0–1 mo	29.3 g/d	26.0 g/d	20.4%	21.4%	12.5%	12.5%	0.9%	0.8%
3–4 mo	20.8	18.6	39.6	39.3	10.9	11.3	0.5	0.4
5–6 mo	15.2	15.0	27.3	32.4	13.2	12.6	0.4	0.4
9–12 mo	10.7	10.0	9.0	11.9	17.0	16.7	0.4	0.3
12–18 mo	7.2	8.7	7.2	10.7	18.4	17.0	0.3	0.3
18–24 mo	6.1	6.2	6.6	7.8	18.7	17.5	0.3	0.2
2–3 yr	5.7	6.0	5.8	7.9	19.1	17.6	0.2	0.2
3–4 yr	5.5	5.1	4.0	8.1	19.7	17.5	0.3	0.2
4–5 yr	5.4	4.7	3.2	11.3	19.9	17.0	0.3	0.2
5–6 yr	5.5	5.1	3.7	13.9	19.8	16.6	0.3	0.2
6–7 yr	5.9	6.4	6.3	19.6	19.5	15.6	0.3	0.2
7–8 yr	6.7	8.2	14.8	21.9	17.9	15.2	0.3	0.2
8–9 yr	7.8	9.9	15.2	24.5	17.9	14.8	0.4	0.3
9–10 yr	9.1	11.2	18.0	27.2	17.5	14.3	0.4	0.3

Source: Adapted from Foman SJ, Haschke F, Ziegler EE, Nelson SE. Body composition of reference children from birth to age 10 years. Am J Clin Nutr 1982;35:1174. © Am. J. Clin. Nutr., American Society for Clinical Nutrition. Reprinted with permission.

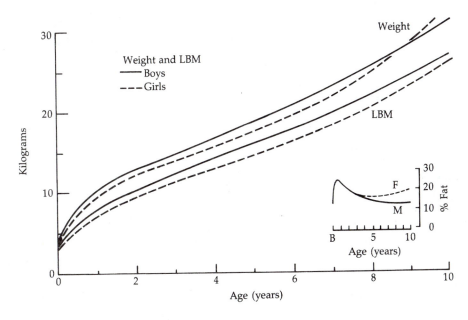

FIGURE 14.5 Graph of average body weight and lean body mass (LBM) for boys and girls from birth to 10 years. *(Forbes GB. Human body composition. New York: Springer-Verlag, 1987:154.)*

Although some gender differences are evidenced in the body composition of prepubescent children (Tables 14.10, 14.11, and Fig. 14.5), these are not of great magnitude. The significant gender differences occur during adolescence and, once established, persist throughout adulthood. Lean body mass is the body component most significantly affected by gender. In both sexes serum testosterone levels rise during adolescence, but the rise is much greater in boys, with their testosterone values approaching ten times those found in girls. As a result of high testosterone production, boys increase their lean body mass by approximately 33 to 35 kg between the age of 10 and 20 years. The increment in girls, however, is only about half as much, approximately 16 to 18 kg [36,40–42]. The female achieves her maximum lean body mass by about 18 years, whereas the male continues accretion of lean body mass until about 20 years or so [33,38]. By age 15 years the male-to-female ratio of lean body mass is 1.23:1, and by 20 years the ratio has increased to 1.45:1. This male-to-female ratio for lean body mass (1.45:1) is well above that for body weight (1.25:1) and stature (1.08:1). The pronounced gender difference in lean body mass is the primary reason for the gender difference in nutrition requirements [36].

TABLE 14.12 Body Composition in Young and Elderly Males and Females

Parameters	Males		Females	
	Young (n = 10) (18–23 yr)	Elderly (n = 20) (61–89 yr)	Young (n = 10) (18–23 yr)	Elderly (n = 20) (60–89 yr)
Body weight (kg)	72.60 ± 10.34	61.60 ± 10.40	54.90 ± 2.71	56.10 ± 9.21
TBW (mL/kg)	586.1 ± 64.3	579.9 ± 54.4	531.0 ± 89.9	442.3 ± 57.3
Intracellular volume (mL/kg)	378.2 ± 42.3	375.7 ± 41.8	328.9 ± 64.7	248.3 ± 26.3
LBM (g/kg)	800.7 ± 87.9	790.3 ± 78.1	725.4 ± 112.9	603.6 ± 77.8
TBF (g/kg)	199.3 ± 87.9	212.7 ± 66.2	274.6 ± 112.9	396.4 ± 77.8
Extracellular water volume (mL/kg)	207.9 ± 30.8	204.2 ± 37.0	192.1 ± 31.0	192.6 ± 19.4
Interstitial volume (mL/kg)	167.7 ± 20.8	157.2 ± 19.7	172.5 ± 41.5	148.9 ± 21.2
Plasma volume (mL/kg)	43.2 ± 7.6	47.03 ± 6.2	29.6 ± 5.2	45.1 ± 10.1

Source: Adapted from Fulop T, Worum I, Csongor J, Foris G, Leovey A. Body composition in elderly people. Gerontology 1985;31:6. Karger, Basel.

The sharp increase in lean body mass that occurs in boys during the adolescent growth spurt is accompanied by a decrease in the percentage of body fat. The average percentage of body fat in boys aged 6 to 8 years is about 13–15%; this percentage decreases to 10–12% for boys aged 14–16 years [16]. Although the adolescent female also increases her lean body mass during the growth spurt, a higher percentage of the weight gain is due to accretion of essential sex-specific fat. Girls aged 6 to 8 years have about 16–18% body fat and by age 14 to 16 years percentage of body fat ranges from 21–23% [16].

After 25 years of age weight gain is usually due to body fat accretion [34]. Although the percentage of body weight due to fat remains lower in males than females, a slow sustained rise in fat in both sexes occurs throughout adulthood and later years [8,43]. The onset of menarche seems to affect the amount of fat accrued by the female through the early adulthood years [44]. Earlier sexual maturity in women appears to result in a greater amount of storage fat and a greater risk for obesity. In addition to increased body fat with age, a redistribution of body fat also occurs [7,45,46]. Subcutaneous fat decreases with age, but internal or visceral fat increases [29]. The significance of this change in distribution is thought to lie with its difference in functional behavior [47].

Table 14.12 [48] illustrates the differences between the young and the elderly in the various body components. More marked changes were seen in aging females than in males. However, with aging in both males and females, a decrease in lean body mass (due primarily to a decrease in body cell mass) occurs [43,48]. Skeletal muscle loss may be due in part to decreased physical activity and alterations in protein metabolism that may be affected by diminished anabolic hormone concentrations [29]. Decreased lean body mass causes a decrease in total body water. The decrease in total body water is much greater in the female than the male. Further examination of the body water shows that extracellular fluid volume remains virtually unchanged. However, a redistribution occurs such that interstitial fluid decreases, but plasma volume increases [48]. Loss of bone mass and atrophy of organs also occurs with aging.

SUMMARY

Although differences in weight for height among individuals have been used traditionally for estimating body fatness, height–weight tables provide limited information about true body composition. Obtaining information on body composition is very complex because it entails study of the body as a whole. *In vivo* (or indirect) determinations of body components must be noninvasive; therefore, the *in vivo* measurements require validation against direct analyses of whole bodies (cadavers). The complexity of making *in vivo* determinations of body components is evidenced by the lack of agreement among researchers concerning descriptors to be used for the components. For instance, should the body component that makes up the percentage of fatness be described as fat, adipose tissue, or storage fat, or should it be divided between a desirable percentage of fat and obesity tissue? Also, what is the most appropriate nomenclature for the nonfat tissue? Should it be described as *lean body mass* or *fat-free body mass*?

Because the components of fat-free tissue vary among individuals even within the same population group for age and sex, no really valid constants exist for estimation of components. For this reason, the two-component model of body composition does not give a complete profile of the individual. To obtain a true composite, measurements of all components of the body must be made. Equipment for making such measurements is presently available in a few medical centers, but the measurements are very expensive and available only to a small segment of the population. Trying to find simplified measurements that are still valid is an area of much current research.

Presently, estimations of body composition for the general public are derived from anthropometric measurements. With an accurate measure of height, weight, and skin folds from selected areas of the body, the percentage of body fat can be determined. Then by difference, lean body mass can be estimated. Certain skin fold or circumference measurements can even provide some information about distribution of body fat, a factor that may be as important, or even more important, to health than the percentage of total body fat.

Despite the differences in the various body components that have been noted in individuals and population groups, it is probably undeniable that the component showing the greatest variability is the one over which we have the most control—total body fat!

References Cited

1. Weigley ES. Average? Ideal? Desirable? A brief review of height–weight tables in the United States. J Am Diet Assoc 1984;84:417–423.
2. Schulz LO. Obese, overweight, desirable, ideal: Where to draw the line in 1986? J Am Diet Assoc 1986;86:1702–1704.
3. Build Study 1979. Chicago: Society of Actuaries and Association of Life Insurance Medical Directors of America, 1980.
4. Callaway CW. Weight standards: Their clinical significance. Ann Intern Med 1984;100:296–298.
5. Andres R. Mortality and obesity: The rationale for age-specific height–weight tables. In: Andres R, Bierman EL, Hazzard WR, eds. Principles of geriatric medicine. New York: McGraw-Hill, 1985:311–318.
6. Micozzi MS, Albanese D, Jones DY, Chumlea WC. Correlations of body mass indices with weight, stature, and body composition in men and women in NHANES I and II. Am J Clin Nutr 1986;44:725–731.
7. Behnke AR, Feen BG, Welham WC. The specific gravity of healthy men. JAMA 1942;118:495–498.
8. Friis-Hansen B. Body composition in growth. Pediatrics 1971;47:264–274.
9. Mitchell HH, Hamilton TS, Steggerda FR, Bean HW. The chemical composition of the adult human body and its bearing on the biochemistry of growth. J Biol Chem 1945;158:625–637.
10. Widdowson EM, McCance RA, Spray CM. The chemical composition of the human body. Clin Sci 1951;10:113–125.
11. Forbes RM, Cooper AR, Mitchell HH. The composition of the human body as determined by chemical analysis. J Biol Chem 1953;203:359–366.
12. Clarys JP, Martin AD, Drinkwater DT. Gross tissue weights in the human body by cadaver dissection. Hum Biol 1984;56:459–473.
13. Behnke AR, Wilmore JH. Evaluation and regulation of body build and composition. Englewood Cliffs, NJ: Prentice Hall, 1974.
14. McArdle WD, Katch FI, Katch VL. Exercise physiology, 3rd ed. Philadelphia: Lea and Febiger, 1991.
15. Katch FI, McArdle WD. Introduction to nutrition, exercise, and health, 4th ed. Philadelphia: Lea and Febiger, 1993;223–258.
16. Nieman DC. Fitness and Sports Medicine: An introduction. Palo Alto: Bull, 1990.
17. Barr SI, McCargar LJ, Crawford SM. Practical use of body composition analysis in sport. Sports Med 1994;17:277–282.
18. Brozek J, Grande F, Anderson JT, Keys A. Densitometric analysis of body composition: Revision of some quantitative assumptions. Ann NY Acad Sci 1963;110:113–140.
19. Clarys JP, Martin AD, Drinkwater DT, Marfell-Jones MJ. The skinfold: Myth and reality. J Sports Sci 1987;5:3–33.
20. Sinning WE, Dolny DG, Little KD, et al. Validity of "generalized" equations for body composition analysis in male athletes. Med Sci Sports Exerc 1985;17:124–130.
21. Harrison GG, Buskirk ER, Carter JEL, Johnston FE, et al. Skinfold thicknesses and measurement technique. In: Lohman TG, Roche AF, Martorell R. Anthropometric standardization reference manual. Champaign, IL: Human Kinetics Books, 1988;55–80.
22. Martorell R, Mendoza F, Mueller WH, Pawson IG. Which side to measure: Right or left. In: Lohman TG, Roche AF, Martorell R. Anthropometric standardization reference manual. Champaign, IL: Human Kinetics Books, 1988;87–91.
23. Lukaski HC. Methods for the assessment of human body composition: Traditional and new. Am J Clin Nutr 1987;46:537–556.
24. van der Kooy K, Seidell JC. Techniques for the measurement of visceral fat: A practical guide. Internl J Obesity 1993;17:187–196.
25. Siri WE. Gross composition of the body. In: Lawrence, JH, Tobias CA, eds. Advances in biological and medical physics. New York: Academic Press, 1956:239–280.
26. Pace N, Rathbun EN. Studies on body composition: III. The body water and chemically combined nitrogen content in relation to fat content. J Biol Chem 1945;158:685–691.
27. Jebb AS, Murgatroyd PR, Goldberg GR, Prentice AM, Coward WA. In vivo measurement of changes in body composition: Description of methods and their validation against 12-d continuous whole-body calorimetry. Am J Clin Nutr 1993;58:455–462.

28. Jensen MD. Research techniques for body composition assessment. J Am Diet Assoc 1992;92:454–460.
29. Heymsfield SB, Matthews D. Body composition: Research and clinical advances. JPEN 1994;18:91–103.
30. Garrow JS. New approaches to body composition. Am J Clin Nutr 1992;35:1152–1158.
31. Fuller MF, Fowler PA, McNeill G, Foster MA. Imaging techniques for the assessment of body composition. J Nutr 1994;124:1546S–1550S.
32. Orphanidou C, McCargar L, Birmingham CL, Mathieson J, Goldner E. Accuracy of subcutaneous fat measurement: Comparison of skinfold calipers, ultrasound, and computed tomography. J Am Diet Assoc 1994;94:855–858.
33. Cohn SH, Vartsky D, Yasumura S, Vaswani AN, Ellis KJ. Indexes of body cell mass: Nitrogen versus potassium. Am J Physiol 1983;244:E305–310.
34. Cohn SH, Vaswani AN, Yasumura S, Yuen K, Ellis KJ. Improved models for determination of body fat by in vivo neutron activation. Am J Clin Nutr 1984;40:255–259.
35. Moore FD, Olesen KH, McMurrey JD, et al. The body cell mass and its supporting environment: Body composition in health and disease. Philadelphia: Saunders, 1963.
36. Forbes GB. Human body composition—growth, aging, nutrition and activity. New York: Springer-Verlag, 1987.
37. Foman SJ, Haschke F, Ziegler EE, Nelson SE. Body composition of reference children from birth to age 10 years. Am J Clin Nutr 1982;35:1169–1175.
38. Boileau RA, Lohman TG, Slaughter MH, et al. Hydration of the fat-free body in children during maturation. Hum Biol 1984;56:651–666.
39. Lohman TG. Research relating to assessment of skeletal status. In: Body composition assessment in youth and adults. Report of the Sixth Ross Conference on Medical Research. Columbus, OH: Ross Laboratories, 1985:38–41.
40. Nutr MD. Body composition changes during adolescence. 1986;12:2.
41. Tepperman J, Tepperman HM. Metabolic and endocrine physiology, 5th ed. Chicago: Year Book Medical, 1987.
42. Baker ER. Body weight and the initiation of puberty. Clin Obstet Gynecol 1985;28:573–579.
43. Forbes GB, Reina JC. Adult lean body mass declines with age: Some longitudinal observations. Metabolism 1970;19:653–663.
44. Garn SM, LaVelle M, Rosenberg KR, Hawthorne VM. Maturational timing as a factor in female fatness and obesity. Am J Clin Nutr 1986;43:879–883.
45. Borken GA, Hults DE, Gerzof SG, et al. Comparison of body composition in middle-aged and elderly males using computed tomography. Am J Phys Anthropol 1985;66:289–295.
46. Komiya S. Aging, total body water and fat mass in males between ages 9 and 77 years. Ann Physiol Anthropol 1984;3:149–151.
47. Bray GA. General discussion of adipose tissue. In: Body-composition assessments of youth and adults. Report of the Sixth Ross Conference on Medical Research. Columbus, OH: Ross Laboratories, 1985:20–21.
48. Fulop T, Worum I, Csougor J, Foris G, Leovey A. Body composition in elderly people. Gerontology 1985;31:6–14.

Suggested Reading

van der Kooy K, Seidell JC. Techniques for the measurement of visceral fat: A practical guide. Internl J Obesity 1993;17:187–196.

Heymsfield SB, Matthews D. Body composition: Research and clinical advances. JPEN 1994;18:91–103.

Jensen MD. Research techniques for body composition assessment. J Am Diet Assoc 1992;92:454–460.

Lukaski HC. Methods for the assessment of human body composition: Traditional and new. Am J Clin Nutr 1987;46:537–556.

These four articles provide a complete compilation and description of various methods used in assessing body composition. The precision and cost of each method along with any associated technical difficulties are identified.

Friis-Handen B. Body composition in growth. Pediatrics 1971;47:264–174.

This is an excellent, concise discussion of body composition in general with emphasis on the influence of maturation.

Body-composition assessment in youth and adults. Report of the Sixth Ross Conference on Medical Research. Columbus, OH: Ross Laboratories 1985.

This compilation of papers was presented at the Ross Conference on Body Composition. The report brings together the research of many outstanding scientists engaged in studying body composition.

Fulop T, Worum I, Csougar J, Foris G, Leovey A. Body composition in elderly people. Gerontology 1985;31:6–14.

This is an excellent discussion of changes in body composition of the elderly. Sex-related variations are delineated.

Forbes GB. Human body composition—growth, aging, nutrition and activity. New York: Springer-Verlag, 1987.

This comprehensive 350-page book on body composition was written by a recognized expert in the field. Information is presented in an easy-to-read, understandable fashion.

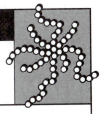

PERSPECTIVE

Maintenance of Desirable Skeletal Status

Skeletal tissue, although a relatively inactive component of the lean body tissue or fat-free mass, is not static. The fact that its composition changes with aging is quite evident in Table 14.7 [1]. Of particular importance to public health is the difference between bone ash in elderly women as compared with young women. From measurement by neutron activation analysis, bone ash for women between 70 and 79 years was, on the average, approximately 73% of that in women 20 to 29 years of age. Many estimates place percentage of bone diminution throughout life even higher than the 27% shown in Table 14.7.

Excessive demineralization or diminution of bone, termed *osteoporosis* or *osteopenia*, develops asymptomatically and often goes undiagnosed until the condition is far advanced. Diagnosis quite often may be made only as a result of a fracture or a complaint of severe, chronic, back pain. X rays are unable to pick up a decrease in bone mass until 30 to 50% of bone mineral has been lost [2,3].

Osteoporosis affects an estimated 20 to 25 million people in the United States, over the age of 45 years [4]. Over twice as many women as men are affected, with the highest prevalence found in postmenopausal women [2,3]. Between the age of 20 and 70 years, bone density decreases from 1.064 to 1.036 g/mL in males and from 1.034 to 1.013 g/mL in females [5].

Both types of bone in the body—the trabecular or honeycomb-like bone (found in the vertebrae of the spine, pelvis, and ends of long bones) and the cortical or compact bone (found in the shaft of long bones of the limbs)—are demineralized with aging. Mineral loss from the trabecular bone begins earlier, at about 20 years of age than cortical bone, and proceeds in a linear fashion. The rate of demineralization is approximately 1% per year in women and about one half that in men [3,6]. Cortical bone, in contrast, continues to increase in density until the middle of the second decade and probably into the third, at which time density plateaus. But by about age 50 years, a persistent, gradual demineralization of cortical bone occurs. This cortical bone loss is greater in women than in men.

Type I osteoporosis is characterized by demineralization of the vertebrae (especially the lumbar region) and the distal radius. Type I osteoporosis occurs mostly in postmenopausal women aged 51 to 65 years, or about 10 to 15 years after menopause [7]. Some cortical bone loss occurs, but to a lesser extent than tra-

becular bone loss. Type I osteoporosis, also called *postmenopausal osteoporosis*, is linked with menopause and reduced estrogen production. The influence of estrogen on bone mineralization is discussed further in the next section, "Levels of Endogenous Estrogen."

Type II osteoporosis is characterized by demineralization of the vertebrae, hip, pelvis, humerus, and tibia. It occurs in both men and women over 75 years of age [7]. In Type II osteoporosis, trabecular and cortical bone are affected due to age-induced decreased bone cell activity, especially osteoblast activity. In addition, decreased synthesis of vitamin D (caused by decreased 1-hydroxylase activity in the kidney) and decreased intestinal calcium transport occur with aging and contribute to Type II osteoporosis. When these events are coupled with a low calcium intake, parathyroid hormone concentrations increase. High blood parathyroid hormone concentrations stimulate bone resorption and promote bone demineralization.

Loss of trabecular and cortical bone in women is shown in Figures 1 and 2, respectively. Generally, more trabecular bone is lost than cortical bone in women over a lifetime [4]. Osteoporosis is associated with kyphosis (hunchback-type curvature of the spine),

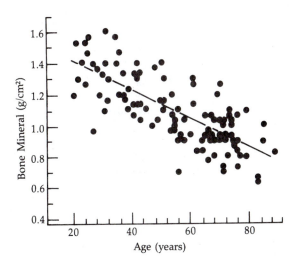

FIGURE 1 Regression of lumbar spine density in normal women as determined by dual-photon absorptiometry. *(Reproduced, with permission, from the Annual Review of Nutrition, Volume 4, © 1984 by Annual Reviews, Inc.)*

PERSPECTIVE (continued)

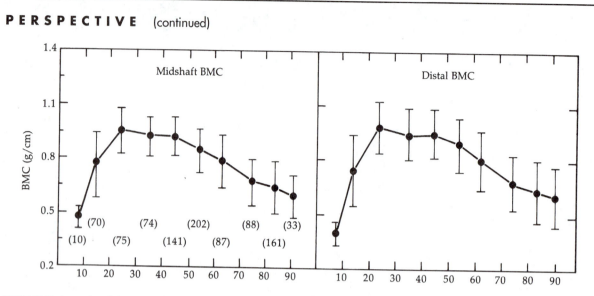

FIGURE 2 Age-related changes in bone mass content (BMC) of radius in white women measured by single-photon absorptiometry. *(Reproduced, with permission, from the Annual Review of Nutrition, Volume 4, © 1984 by Annual Reviews, Inc.)*

chronic pain, bed rest-induced pressure sores, and decreased mobility [4]. A decrease in the alveolar bone (the bone comprising the bony processes of the maxilla, mandible, and surrounding and containing the teeth) also has been attributed to osteoporosis by some researchers [8]. Thus, osteoporosis may contribute to adult tooth loss and to ill-fitting dentures as the alveolar bone decreases in density [8].

The high prevalence of osteoporosis among women makes this condition a public health problem. Although the effects of aging and genetic factors cannot be eliminated, perhaps other factors promoting bone demineralization in women can be altered so as to allow attainment or maintenance of a more desirable skeletal status. Some of the alterable factors that impinge on bone loss and that will be addressed include [4,6] level of endogenous estrogen, physical activity, smoking, calcium nutriture, and other miscellaneous dietary constituents.

Level of Endogenous Estrogen

Estrogen has a positive effect on the bone mineralization, and its influence is evidenced at puberty. Although epiphyseal closure and cessation of longitudinal bone growth signal maturity of the skeletal tissue, remodeling of bone continues. The average density of the skeleton can increase perhaps as late as age 35 years [9]. The rate of resorption (loss) of existing bone and deposition of new bone to replace that lost is affected by circulating estrogen levels. If levels of estrogen become low, bone responsiveness to parathyroid hormone appears to increase and contributes to bone

resorption [4]. Low estrogen levels occur with menopause, but also in many women athletes and women with the eating disorder anorexia nervosa. Young women, often teenagers, are thus at increased risk for bone loss unless estrogen levels can be maintained. How estrogen protects bone is not fully understood, but evidence supports a role for estrogen in bone mineralization via the osteoblasts. Estrogen receptors have been isolated on osteoblasts [10,11], suggesting that estrogen may affect the bone-forming (osteoblast) cells directly.

Because of the protective effect of estrogen on bone, many gynecologists believe that estrogen replacement should be recommended on an individual basis especially to women who are immediately postmenopausal or who are going through menopause. After the age of 65 years, the therapeutic benefit of estrogen replacement becomes somewhat doubtful [6]. Estrogen replacement therapy (ERT) appears to be helpful in preventing many cortical bone fractures associated with osteoporosis, but ERT protects little against the spinal "dowager's hump." Bone loss from the spine begins quite early (Fig. 1) and is likely due to factors other than (or at least in addition to) decreased estrogen levels [3].

Physical Activity

The negative influence of weightlessness on mineral balance has long been recognized. It follows, therefore, that weight bearing by the bone will influence positively mineral balance. This supposition has proved to be true. Weight-bearing exercises on a regular basis

PERSPECTIVE (continued)

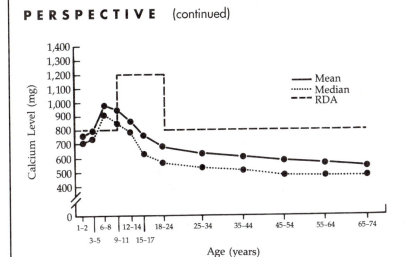

FIGURE 3 Daily calcium intake (mg) for a U.S. female population, 1976–1980.

have a protective effect on bone and decreases the age-related demineralization of bone [2,5,6,12].

An interesting longitudinal study of elderly men and women [12] has demonstrated the effect of body weight on the density of the heel bone of the right foot. From the first measurement at age 75 years, the degree of demineralization was related to the weight borne on the heel bone. Elderly people who regularly carried around more weight had less bone loss.

Extremes in physical activity, however, when associated with amenorrhea (lack of menstruation) are counterproductive to maintaining bone mass. Low blood estrogen concentrations are found with amenorrhea. Bone mineral density (especially in the vertebrae) of amenorrheic women is typically much lower than that of control eumenorrheic women.

Smoking

Smoking is associated with lower bone density, earlier menopause in women, and increased postmenopausal bone loss [13]. Smoking decreases circulating estrogen concentrations and thereby contributes to bone loss [13].

Calcium Nutriture

Although calcium intake remains important during life's later years, the crucial period for calcium intake is during the years when positive calcium balance is possible (when bone density can increase). Sufficient calcium should be available so that attainment of the full genetic expression of peak skeletal mass is possible. Attainment of peak bone density probably does not occur before age 25 years and may be as late as 35 years of age, several years after linear growth has been completed [9]. For this reason, the 1,200 mg calcium rec-

ommended for adolescents has been extended through age 24 years in the tenth edition of the RDA [14]. New recommendations for calcium intakes have been suggested by a 1994 U.S. National Institutes of Health Concensus Panel [15]. Calcium intakes for children aged 1–10 years are 800–1,200 mg (1989 RDA 800 mg), for adolescents and young adults 1,200–1,500 mg (RDA 1,200 mg), for women aged 25–50 years 1,000 mg (RDA 800 mg) and for pregnant and lactating women 1,400 mg (RDA 1,200 mg) [15]. Intakes of 1,500 mg/day for postmenopausal women who are not receiving estrogen therapy also have been recommended [15]. The calcium intake of females throughout their lives is given in Figure 3; it can be seen that the average calcium intake (about 600 mg) is below the recommended dietary allowance (RDA) except during a part of the childhood years [8].

Attainment of dense bones during the early years offers the best prevention of weakened bones in later years. Calcium supplements of 2,000 mg per day were unable to decrease trabecular bone loss and had only a minor positive effect on cortical bone in postmenopausal women [16]. In contrast to these findings, calcium supplements (1,000 mg daily for two years) reduced by 43% total body bone density loss in postmenopausal (at least 3 years) women [17]. The rate of bone mineral density loss in the legs was 35% and loss was eliminated in the trunk [17]. Thus, calcium supplements benefit both appendicular cortical and axial bone mass in postmenopausal women.

One danger of inadequate calcium intake is the effect of low blood calcium levels on secretion of parathyroid hormone. The primary secretagogue for parathyroid hormone is a decreased pool of circulating ionized calcium [3]. A more generous intake of calcium may not correct the problem of decreased circulating calcium, but it more than likely will raise the plasma calcium level somewhat. Perhaps in this indirect way, an adequate calcium intake can prevent excessive parathyroid hormone production, thereby slowing calcium release from bone for maintenance of plasma calcium.

Other Miscellaneous Dietary Constituents

Several other dietary or diet-related substances have been implicated as impinging on bone mineralization. These substances include fluoride, phosphorus, protein, vitamin D, alcohol, and caffeine. There has been much controversy about the benefits of fluoride. Although it has been shown that fluoride used as a drug stimulates bone formation (osteoblast activity) and increases trabecular bone mass [6], research has suggested that highly fluoridated water does not protect against bone loss [18]. In fact, the more highly fluoridated water appeared to have a detrimental effect on bone density unless calcium intake was at an acceptable level. Combining a calcium supplement (400 mg) with a slow-release fluoride tablet (25 mg) appears to hold promise in the treatment of patients with spinal osteoporosis. Patients treated with this fluoride–calcium combination are showing a 3 to 6% increase per year in spinal mass and incidence of spinal fractures is decreasing [19]. At present, fluoride therapy in the United States is still in the experimental stages.

In contrast to earlier studies suggesting that a high intake of phosphorus decreased bone mineralization, recent studies have shown a beneficial effect of dietary phosphorus on calcium use [2]. Phosphorus, by stimulating parathyroid hormone secretion, increases indirectly the reabsorption of calcium by the renal tubules so that less calcium is lost in the urine. Thus, although phosphorus causes loss of calcium by increasing calcium secretion into the gastrointestinal tract, its overriding effect is to conserve calcium. Potassium also reduces urinary calcium excretion [20]. However, high phosphorus intake coupled with inadequate calcium intake can produce elevated blood parathyroid hormone concentrations in young adult women [21]. High parathyroid hormone concentrations stimulate bone resorption with possible long-term detrimental effects on bone mineral content [21,22].

Proteins and a variety of amino acids (especially sulfur-containing amino acids—methionine and cysteine) have been shown to increase excretion of calcium in the urine. Dietary protein directly influences calcium [23]; doubling of protein intake without changing intake of other nutrients results in about a 50% increase in urinary calcium [23,24]. These pro-

teins and amino acids, however, are usually combined in natural foods with substances that counteract their effect on calcium excretion. A high intake of protein from natural food sources appears to have no deleterious effect on calcium balance [2].

Sodium has also been shown to be detrimental to body calcium. A sodium load of 100 mmol (2.3 g) per day increased urinary calcium excretion by 1 mmol (40 mg) per day [25,26]. Sodium is excreted in the urine with calcium.

Many elderly people may benefit from vitamin D supplementation because of marginal intake of the vitamin, little exposure to sunlight, and decreased efficiency of transformation of the vitamin into its active metabolite, 1,25-dihydroxy cholecalciferol due to decreased renal 1-hydroxylase activity [6]. Furthermore, the amount of vitamin D_3 produced in aging skin during exposure to the ultraviolet rays of the sun may be decreased to one-half of that produced in young skin [27].

Chronic alcoholism can lead to excessive bone loss. People consuming excessive alcohol generally have lower bone mass and reduced osteoblast activity. Factors affecting bone and its loss include insufficient intake of nutrients (especially calcium, protein, and/or vitamin D) coupled with poor absorption of nutrients [2]. Malabsorption often occurs and may be secondary to pancreatic insufficiency associated with alcoholism [2].

Caffeine has also been considered by some as a detriment to calcium balance [28,29]. Caffeine is thought to reduce the renal reabsorption of calcium, which leads to increased urinary calcium losses [29]. It has been estimated that one cup of coffee can contain enough caffeine to cause an extra loss of 6 mg calcium in the urine per day [28]. Caffeine (300 to 400 mg) increased urinary calcium (0.25 mmol or 10 mg/day) and increased secretion of calcium into the gut [7,29].

Maintenance of desirable skeletal status in women appears to be multifactorial. Nevertheless, achievement of potential peak bone mass during early adulthood is probably the most important factor in its later maintenance. Achievable bone mass appears to be programmed by genetic factors and mechanical loading (weight-bearing exercises) of the skeleton, but the potential is influenced by the endocrine and nutritional environment [30]. Most important in this environment are the hormone estrogen and the nutrient calcium. One's genetic makeup cannot be changed nor can the physiological changes accompanying aging be reversed. The individual usually does have the option, however, of choosing a lifestyle in which weight-bearing exercise and good nutrition are practiced regularly. Exercise and an adequate calcium intake throughout life appear to foster the maintenance of a healthy skeleton in the later years.

PERSPECTIVE (continued)

References Cited

1. Cohn SH, Vaswani AN, Yasumura S, Yuen K, Ellis KJ. Improved models for determination of body fat by in vivo neutron activation. Am J Clin Nutr 1984;40:255–259.
2. Spencer H, Kramer LB. Nutrition and other factors influencing skeletal state. In: Body-composition assessments in youth and adults. Report of the Sixth Ross Conference on Medical Research. Columbus, OH: Ross Laboratories 1985;33–37.
3. Avioli LV. Calcium and osteoporosis. Ann Rev Nutr 1984;4:471–491.
4. Wardlaw GM. Putting osteoporosis in perspective. J Am Diet Assoc 1993;93:1000–1006.
5. Lohman TG. Research relating to assessment of skeletal status. In: Body-composition assessments in youth and adults. Report of the Sixth Ross Conference on Medical Research. Columbus, OH: Ross Laboratories 1985;38–41.
6. Marcus R. Calcium, skeletal aging and osteoporosis. Nutr. MD 1985;11(3):1.
7. Harward MP. Nutritive therapies for osteoporosis: The role of calcium. Med Clin N Am 1993;77:889–898.
8. The role of calcium in health. Dairy Council Dig 1984;55:1–8.
9. Heaney RP. Calcium, bone health, and osteoporosis. In: Peck WA, ed. Bone and mineral research. New York: Elsevier Science 1986;4:255–301.
10. Komm BS, Terpening CM, Benz DJ, et al. Estrogen binding, receptor mRNA, and biologic response in osteoblast-like osteosarcoma cells. Science 1988;241:81–84.
11. Eriksen EF, Colvard DS, Berg NJ, et al. Evidence of estrogen receptors in normal human osteoblast-like cells. Science 1988;241:84–86.
12. Recker RR. The role of calcium in bone health. Nutr News 1984;47:5–6.
13. Jensen J, Christiansen C, Rodbro P. Cigarette smoking, serum estrogens, and bone loss during hormone-replacement therapy early after menopause. N Eng J Med 1985;313:973–977.
14. National Research Council. Recommended dietary allowances, 10th ed. Washington, DC: National Academy Press, 1989.
15. Rowe PM. New US recommendations on calcium intake. Lancet 1994;343:1559–1560.
16. Riis B, Thomsen K, Christiansen C. Does calcium supplementation prevent postmenopausal bone loss? N Engl J Med 1987;316:173–177.
17. Reid IR, Ames RW, Evans MC, Gamble GD, Sharpe SJ. Effect of calcium supplementation on bone loss in postmenopausal women. N Engl J Med 1993;328:460–464.
18. Sowers MR, Wallace RB, Lemke JH. The relationship of bone mass and fracture history to fluoride and calcium intake: A study of three communities. Am J Clin Nutr 1986;44:889–898.
19. Fackelmann KA. Fluoride-calcium combo builds better bones. Sci News 1989;135:36.
20. Lemann J, Pleuss JA, Gray RW. Potassium causes calcium retention in healthy adults. J Nutr 1993;123:1623–1626.
21. Calvo MS, Kumar R, Heath H. Persistently elevated parathyroid hormone secretion and action in young women after four weeks of ingesting high phosphorus, low calcium diets. J Clin Endocrinol Metab 1990;70:1334–1340.
22. Anderson JJB. The role of nutrition in the functioning of skeletal tissue. Nutr Rev 1992;50:388–394.
23. Allen LH, Wood RJ. Calcium and phosphorus. In: Shils ME, Olson JA, Shike M. Modern nutrition in health and disease, 8th ed. Philadelphia: Lea and Febiger, 1994;144–163.
24. Heaney RP. Protein intake and the calcium economy. J Am Diet Assoc 1993;93:1259–1260.
25. Massey LK. Dietary factors influencing calcium and bone metabolism: Introduction. J Nutr 1993;123:1609–1610.
26. Nordin BEC, Need AG, Morris HA, Horowitz M. The nature and significance of the relationship between urinary sodium and urinary calcium in women. J Nutr 1993;123:1615–1622.
27. MacLauglin J, Holick MF. Aging decreases the capacity of human skin to produce vitamin D_3. J Clin Invest 1985;76:1536–1538.
28. Heaney RP, Recker RR. Effects of nitrogen, phosphorus and caffeine on calcium balance in women. J Lab Clin Med 1982;99:46–55.
29. Massey LK, Whiting SJ. Caffeine, urinary calcium, calcium metabolism and bone. J Nutr 1993;123:1611–1614.
30. Seeman E, Hopper JL, Bach LA, et al. Reduced bone mass in daughters of women with osteoporosis. N Engl J Med 1989;320:554–558.

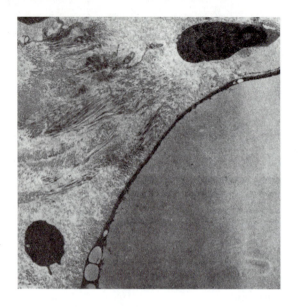

ENERGY BALANCE AND WEIGHT CONTROL

Photo: A portion of an adipocyte engorged with lipid, showing the compressed cytoplasm as a thin strand. Smaller cells are leukocytes.

Whether body weight is being maintained, increased, or decreased depends primarily on the extent to which the energy requirements of the body (i.e., total energy expenditure) have been met by energy intake. Thus, the first step in the study of an individual's energy balance or weight control is the determination of the person's energy expenditure.

COMPONENTS OF ENERGY EXPENDITURE

Total energy expenditure [1–3] is composed primarily of

- Basal metabolic rate (BMR), resting energy expenditure (REE), or resting metabolic rate (RMR)

- Diet-induced thermogenesis (DIT)—also called *specific dynamic action (SDA), specific effect of food (SEF),* or *thermic effect of food (TEF)*

- Effect of physical activity or exercise

A fourth component, adaptive thermogenesis, is sometimes included. The average division of energy expenditure among the components is given in Figure 15.1.

Basal Metabolic Rate, Resting Energy Expenditure, and Resting Metabolic Rate

Although the terms *basal* and *resting* are often used interchangeably, differences exists. The word *basal*, as in BMR, is more precisely defined than is *resting*, as in REE. Measurement of oxygen consumed and carbon dioxide produced, used for the calculation of energy expenditure necessary to support life (i.e., BMR), is made under closely controlled and standardized conditions. An individual's BMR is determined when he or she is in a postabsorptive state (i.e., no food intake for at least 12 hours), is lying

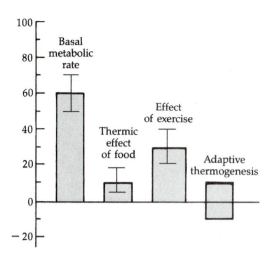

FIGURE 15.1 Components of energy expenditure and their approximate percentage contribution.

down, and is completely relaxed, preferably very shortly after awakening from sleep in the morning. In addition, the temperature of the room in which the measurement occurs is made as comfortable as possible for the individual. Any factors that could influence the internal work of the individual are minimized as much as possible.

In contrast to BMR, REE is not usually measured under basal conditions [3]. REE is measured when the individual is at rest in a comfortable environment; however, he or she need not have fasted for 12 hours. Usually the fast for REE is about two to four hours. REE is usually slightly higher than BMR [4] due to its less stringent conditions of measurement; however, typically, BMR and REE differ by about 10% [3]. REE is thought to account for about 65 to 75% of daily total energy expenditure [4]. BMR accounts for about 50 to 70% of daily total energy expenditure [5].

Basal metabolism is a result of energy exchanges occurring in all cells of the body. The rate of oxygen consumption, however, is most closely related to the actively metabolizing cells or that component of the body called *lean body mass* or *body cell mass* [6]. The BMR per unit body weight is affected not only by the ratio of body cell mass to the less active body components such as fat, but also by changes in proportions of tissues that make up the active cell mass. In aging, fat increases at the expense of body cell mass, and BMR decreases. With maturation, the proportion of supporting structures (i.e., bone and muscle) increases more rapidly than does total body weight. Bone and muscle, although components of body cell mass, have a much lower metabolic ac-

tivity than organ tissues, but much greater than adipose tissue. This difference in rate of weight accretion between the less active and more active components of cell mass means a decrease in the overall metabolic activity of cell mass and a concurrent decrease in BMR per unit body weight [6]. These changes that occur in maturation explain the lower REE of children as compared with very young infants.

A look at the metabolic activity among the different components of the cell mass in an adult male illustrates its variability in metabolic activity. Under normal circumstances, approximately 5% of total body weight can be attributed to weight of the brain, liver, heart, and kidney, while about 40% of body weight is due to muscle mass [6]. At the same time, the metabolic activity of the organ tissues accounts for approximately 60% of basal oxygen consumption, while the muscle mass accounts for only about 25% [6]. Thus, change in BMR can occur whenever the proportions of body tissues change in relation to each other [6]. Because of the many variations among individuals as well as the changes that can occur within individuals themselves, estimating energy expenditures may result in significant errors [1]. Accurate energy expenditures are much more likely to be obtained from actual measurements of these expenditures.

Diet-Induced Thermogenesis, Specific Dynamic Action, Specific Effect of Food, or Thermic Effect of Food

A second component of energy expenditure is the metabolic response to food, also referred to as *diet-induced thermogenesis, specific dynamic action,* or the *thermic* or *specific effect of food.* Diet-induced thermogenesis represents the body's processing of food. This includes the work associated with the digestion, absorption, transport, metabolism, and storage of energy from ingested food. The percentage increase in energy expenditure over BMR due to diet-induced thermogenesis has been estimated to range from about 5 to 15% [7,8]. The value most commonly used for the metabolic effect of food is 10% of the caloric value of a mixed diet consumed within 24 hours [1,5]. However, diet-induced thermogenesis is not a fixed percentage of calories ingested; diet-induced thermogenesis varies with the composition of the diet and the antecedent dietary practices of the individuals in whom measurements are being made [1,8]. A mixed diet increases diet-induced thermogenesis more positively when the ratio of carbohydrate to fat is high [4]. The rise in metabolism following food consumption appears to reach a maximum

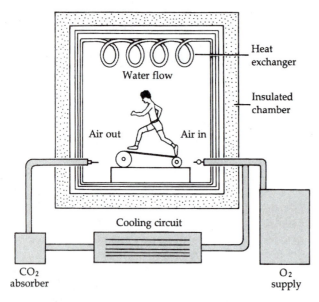

FIGURE 15.2 A simplified version of the human calorimeter used to measure direct body heat loss, that is, energy expenditure.

approximately one hour after eating and is absent four hours postprandial (after eating) [3].

Physical Activity

The effect of physical activity or exercise is the most variable of the components; it is also the only component that is easily altered. Although on an average physical activity accounts for about 20 to 40% of the total energy expenditure, it can be considerably less in a truly sedentary person or much more in a very physically active person [1,5]. Factors impinging on energy expenditure during exercise beside the actual activity itself include the intensity, duration, and frequency with which the activity is performed, the body mass of the person, his or her efficiency at performing the activity, and also any extraneous movements that may accompany the activity.

Other Components of Energy Expenditure

An additional component of energy expenditure that is of some importance is adaptive thermogenesis, also called *nonshivering*, *facultative*, or *regulatory thermogenesis*. The term *adaptive thermogenesis* refers to the alteration in metabolism that occurs due to environmental, psychological, or other influences. Some of the possible factors affecting adaptive thermogenesis are unconscious or spontaneous movements or activities, hormone levels, responses to changes in nutrient and caloric intake, adaptations to changes in ambient temperature and

to emotional stress, and activation or suppression of futile metabolic cycles.

MEASUREMENT OF ENERGY EXPENDITURE

Measurement of the total energy expenditure can be determined by direct calorimetry, which measures the dissipation of heat from the body [9]. Heat dissipation is measured via an isothermal principle, a gradient-layer system, or a water-cooled garment [9,10]. A very simplified version of calorimetry for humans based on the isothermal principle is given in Figure 15.2. Total heat loss consists of sensible heat loss and heat of water vaporization. In the isothermal calorimeter (Fig. 15.2), sensible heat loss is determined by the difference in the water temperature and in the amount of water flowing in and out of the pipes situated within the walls of the chamber where the subject has been placed. Heat removed by vaporization of water is calculated from the moisture of air leaving the calorimeter and being absorbed in sulfuric acid. Although the concept of direct calorimetry is relatively simple, direct measurement of body heat loss is expensive, cumbersome, and usually rather unpleasant for the subject or subjects involved [1].

Basal metabolic rate is usually measured indirectly. Indirect calorimetry measures the consumption of oxygen and the expiration of carbon dioxide. In other words, indirect calorimetry measures the heat produced by oxidative processes [9], although urinary nitrogen excretion should also be measured, since for every 1 g of nitrogen excreted approximately 6 L of oxygen are consumed and 4.8 L carbon dioxide are produced [11].

The amount of heat being produced can be calculated from the ratio of the carbon dioxide expired to the oxygen inhaled. This ratio is known as the *respiratory quotient (RQ)*.

Examination of respiratory quotients provides meaningful information with respect to overall substrate oxidation; however, no information about substrate oxidation in individual organs and tissues is gained [9]. An RQ equal to 1.0 suggests carbohydrate is being oxidized, because the amount of oxygen required in the combustion of glucose equals the amount of carbon dioxide produced, as shown here:

$$C_6H_{12}O_6 + 6O_2 \longrightarrow 6CO_2 + 6H_2O;$$
$$RQ = 6CO_2/6O_2 = 1.0$$

The RQ for a fat is less than 1.0 because it is a much less oxidized fuel source. For example, a fat such as tristearin, as shown in the following equation, requires 163

TABLE 15.1 Thermal Equivalent of O_2 and CO_2 for Nonprotein RQ

Nonprotein RQ	Caloric Value of 1 L O_2	Caloric Value of 1 L CO_2	Source of Calories	
			Carbohydrate (%)	Fat (%)
0.707	4.686	6.629	0	100
0.71	4.690	6.606	1.10	98.9
0.72	4.702	6.531	4.76	95.2
0.73	4.714	6.458	8.40	91.6
0.74	4.727	6.388	12.0	88.0
0.75	4.739	6.319	15.6	84.4
0.76	4.751	6.253	19.2	80.8
0.77	4.764	6.187	22.8	77.2
0.78	4.776	6.123	26.3	73.7
0.79	4.788	6.062	29.9	70.1
0.80	4.801	6.001	33.4	66.6
0.81	4.813	5.942	36.9	63.1
0.82	4.825	5.884	40.3	59.7
0.83	4.838	5.829	43.8	56.2
0.84	4.850	5.774	47.2	52.8
0.85	4.862	5.721	50.7	49.3
0.86	4.875	5.669	54.1	45.9
0.87	4.887	5.617	57.5	42.5
0.88	4.899	5.568	60.8	39.2
0.89	4.911	5.519	64.2	35.8
0.90	4.924	5.471	67.5	32.5
0.91	4.936	5.424	70.8	29.2
0.92	4.948	5.378	74.1	25.9
0.93	4.961	5.333	77.4	22.6
0.94	4.973	5.290	80.7	19.3
0.95	4.985	5.247	84.0	16.0
0.96	4.998	5.205	87.2	12.8
0.97	5.010	5.165	90.4	9.58
0.98	5.022	5.124	93.6	6.37
0.99	5.035	5.085	96.8	3.18
100	5.047	5.047	100	0

Source: This table was adapted from McArdle W, Katch F, Katch V. Exercise physiology, 2nd ed. Philadelphia: Lea and Febiger 1986;127. The original source is Weber. Die bedeutung de verschiedenen nährstoffe als erzeuger der muskelkraft. Pflügers Archiv zür Physiologie, 1901:83(1):557–571.

mol of oxygen for the production of 114 mol of carbon dioxide:

$$2C_{57}H_{110}O_6 + 163O_2 \longrightarrow 114CO_2 + 110H_2O;$$
$$RQ = 114CO_2/163O_2 = 0.70$$

Calculating the RQ for protein oxidation is more complicated because metabolic oxidation of amino acids requires removing the nitrogen and some oxygen and carbon as urea, a urinary excretory compound. Urea nitrogen represents a net loss of energy to the body; only the remaining carbon chain of the amino acid can be oxidized in the body. The following equation illustrates the oxidation of a small protein molecule into carbon dioxide, water, sulfur trioxide, and urea:

$$C_{72}H_{112}N_{18}O_{22}S + 77O_2 \longrightarrow$$
$$63CO_2 + 38H_2O + SO_3 + 9CO(NH_2)_2$$

The RQ of this small protein molecule is equal to 0.818.

The average figures of 1.0, 0.7, and 0.8 are accepted as the representative RQs for carbohydrate, fat, and protein, respectively. The RQ for an ordinary mixed diet consisting of the three energy-producing nutrients is usually considered to be about 0.85. An RQ of 0.82 represents the metabolism of a mixture of 40% carbohydrate and 60% fat [12]. RQs that are actually computed from gaseous exchange and that come closer to 1.0 or nearer to 0.7 would indicate that more carbohydrate or fat, respectively, was being used for fuel. In clinical practice, an RQ < 0.8 suggests that a patient may be underfed, an RQ < 0.7 suggests starvation or ingestion of a low-carbohydrate or high-alcohol diet, while an RQ > 1.0 suggests lipogenesis is occurring [9].

Once the RQ has been computed from gaseous exchange, the calculation of heat production is rather simple. Table 15.1 (p. 469) gives the caloric value for 1 L of oxygen and for 1 L of carbon dioxide. When the amount of oxygen and/or carbon dioxide in the exchange has been determined, the total caloric value represented by the exchange may be calculated. It is also possible to determine the amount of carbohydrate and fat being oxidized in production of these calories.

For example, if under standard conditions for the determination of BMR a person consumed 15.7 L oxygen/hr and expired 12.0 L carbon dioxide, the RQ = 12.0/15.7, or 0.7643. From Table 15.1, the caloric equivalent for an RQ of 0.76 is 4.751 for 1 L oxygen or 6.253 for 1 L carbon dioxide. Based on the caloric equivalent for oxygen, calories produced/hr are $15.7 \times 4.751 = 74.59$. Based on caloric equivalent for carbon dioxide, calories produced/hr are $12.0 \times 6.253 = 75.04$. If we then use 75 kcal/hr as the caloric expenditure, then under basal conditions, the BMR for the day would approximate 1,800 kcal (75 kcal/hr $\times$ 24 hr). At this RQ of 0.76, fat is supplying almost 81% of energy expended.

Because under ordinary circumstances the contribution of protein to energy metabolism is so small, the oxidation of protein is ignored in the determination of the so-called nonprotein RQ. If a truly accurate RQ is required, a correction, although minimal, can be made by measuring the amount of urinary nitrogen in a specified time period. As mentioned earlier, for every 1 g of nitrogen excreted, approximately 6 L of oxygen are consumed and 4.8 L carbon dioxide are produced. The amount of oxygen and carbon dioxide exchanged in the release of energy from protein can then be subtracted from the total amount of measured gaseous exchange.

Measurement of energy expended in various activities has also been made primarily through indirect calorimetry. The method for measuring gas exchange, however, differs from that used for determining BMR. The subject performing the activity for which energy expenditure is being determined inhales ambient air, which has a constant composition of 20.93% oxygen, 0.03% carbon dioxide, and 78.04% nitrogen. Air exhaled by the subject is collected in a spirometer (used to measure respiratory gases) and is analyzed to determine how much less oxygen and more carbon dioxide it contains as compared to ambient air. The difference in the composition of the inhaled air and exhaled air reflects the energy release from the body [12]. A lightweight portable spirometer (Fig. 15.3) can be worn during performance of almost any sort of activity, and freedom of movement outside the laboratory is possible. In the laboratory the Douglas Bag is used routinely to collect expired air [12].

Tables are available that list for a wide variety of activities the kilocalories expended per kilogram body weight per minute or hour. Table 15.2, an example of such a table, indicates various activities grouped together according to their average level of energy expenditure.

ESTIMATING TOTAL ENERGY EXPENDITURE

Estimating basal metabolic rate or resting energy expenditure rather than measuring it has been the practice among clinicians since about 1925. Many different methods for estimating energy needs have been used over the years. Estimations have been based on body surface area, body weight, and/or calculations from equations that take into account the person's gender, age, weight, and height. One of the best estimates of BMR for all mammals, including humans, is based on body weight raised to the power of three-fourths, or 0.75 [6,13]. The equation

$$BMR \text{ (kcal/day)} = 70 \times W^{0.75}$$

uses weight (W) measured in kg and raised to the power of 0.75 multiplied by 70 for estimating BMR. Table 15.3 lists body weights ranging from 1 to 100 kg that have been raised to the power of 0.75. Because of the relatively narrow range in human body size, calculations from the preceding equation give an estimate that is reasonably close to the BMR value obtained from the formula of 1 kcal/kg/hr for men and 0.9 kcal/kg/hr for women. Estimation of the BMR of a 70-kg man using these two methods illustrates their comparable results:

1. BMR (kcal/day) = $70 \times 70^{0.75}$ which, using Table 15.3, = $70 \times 24.2 = 1,694$ kcal/day
2. BMR = 1 kcal $\times$ 70 kg $\times$ 24 hr = 1,680 kcal/day

The equations probably most often used [7] to estimate BMR in the clinical setting are those derived by Harris and Benedict in 1919 [14], and only slightly modified. Using the Harris Benedict equation, BMR (kcal/day) is predicted in separate equations for men and women based on W (weight in kilograms), H (height in centimeters), and A (age in years):

Men:
BMR = $66.5 + (13.7 \times W) + (5.0 \times H) - (6.8 \times A)$
Women:
BMR = $655.1 + (9.56 \times W) + (1.85 \times H) - (4.7 \times A)$

Another equation, by Mifflin and St. Jeor [15], predicts REE (kcal/day) for men and women as

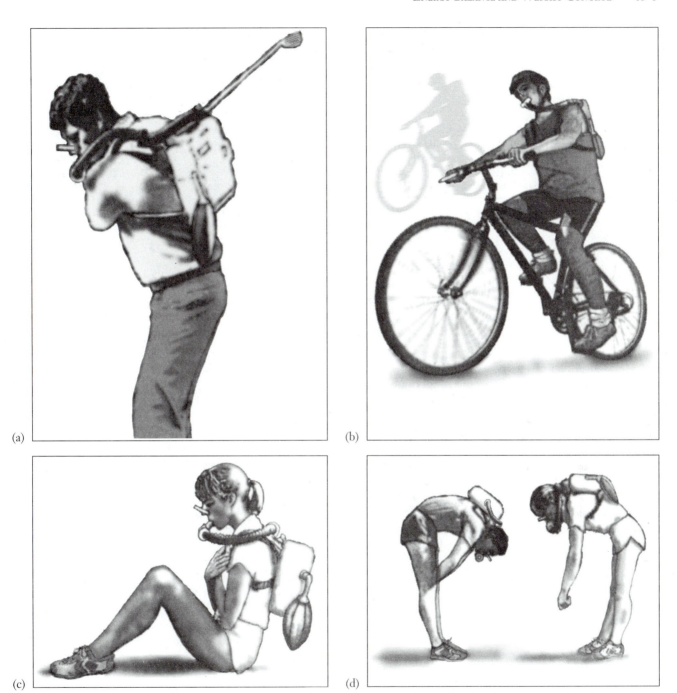

FIGURE 15.3 Measurement of oxygen consumption by portable spirometer during (a) golf; (b) cycling; (c) sit-ups; (d) calisthenics.

Men: REE = (10 × W) + (6.25 × H) − (5 × A) + 5
Women:
REE = (10 × W) + (6.25 × H) − (5 × A) − 161

W refers to weight in kilograms, *H* refers to height in centimeters, and *A* is for age in years.

Using the two equations, a female who is 35 years old, weighs 125 lb (56.82 kg), and is 5 ft, 5 in tall (165.1 cm) would have a BMR of 1,339 kcal (Harris Benedict equation) and an REE of 1,264 kcal (Mifflin St. Jeor equation).

The various equations, along with the calculated energy values, are re-evaluated regularly in scientific literature. Recent re-evaluations have shown that predicted values for BMR are often higher than the actual expenditure and may not be applicable to all individuals, such

TABLE 15.2 The Energy Cost Associated with Different Activities

Energy Level	Type of Activity	Energy (kcal/kg/min[a])	
		Woman	Man
a	Sleep or lying still, relaxed[b]	0.000	0.000
b	Sitting or standing still (such as sewing, writing, eating)	0.001–0.007	0.003–0.012
c	Very light activity (driving a car, walking slowly on level ground)	0.009–0.016	0.014–0.022
d	Light exercise (sweeping, eating, walking normally, carrying books)	0.018–0.035	0.023–0.040
e	Moderate exercise (fast walking, dancing, bicycling, cleaning vigorously, moving furniture)	0.036–0.053	0.042–0.060
f	Heavy exercise (fast dancing, fast uphill walking, hitting tennis ball, swimming, gymnastics)	0.055	0.062

[a]Measured in kcalories per kilogram per minute above basal energy. Where ranges are given, pick the midpoint within the range, unless you have reason to believe you are unusually relaxed or energetic when performing the activity. For example, for "sitting," a man should normally pick 0.007; if he is sitting very relaxed, 0.003; if very tense, 0.012.
[b]For purposes of this exercise, these are assumed to be at the basal level of activity.
(*Modified from:* Whitney E, Cataldo C. Understanding normal and clinical nutrition. St. Paul, MN: West, 1983.)

as those who are obese [7,8,16]. Thus, dietitians must be alert to literature for recent findings and recognize the limitations and implications of the use of these various equations.

Once basal or resting energy needs have been determined, energy needs for diet-induced thermogenesis and for physical activity must be added to the basal or resting energy needs to estimate total daily energy needs. Energy for diet-induced thermogenesis typically represents an additional 10% (range 5 to 15%) of basal energy needs. Depending on the type, duration, intensity, and frequency of physical activity, energy needs for physical activity may vary from 20 to 70% or more of basal metabolism. A rough estimate of an individual's total energy expenditure for one day (basal metabolic rate + diet-induced thermogenesis + physical activity) can be made through use of Table 15.2 and Forms 1, 2, and 3, found in Appendix C.

ENERGY INTAKE AND ITS REGULATION

Food consumption is influenced by many more factors than energy expenditure. Although appetite appears to be a voluntary act influenced by external cues, it is also regulated internally. Weingarten [17] suggests that newborns may be the only true depletion-driven eaters; that is, the only individuals whose feeding behavior is regulated totally by internal control. After the neonatal period, people have increased experiences with food, with feeding, and with the rituals associated with eating. These experiences cause development of the incentive-based hunger system. As a result, for the rest of a person's life, the incentive-based hunger system will

interact with the physiologic depletion signals to control both hunger and eating [17].

Appetite is thought initially to be increased by the smell and sight of food, which provide afferent signals. Along with the taste and texture of food in the mouth, sensory cues about the quality of food provide positive feedback signals to continue food ingestion [18]. The presence of food or chyme in the stomach and small intestine is detected by mechanoreceptors and chemoreceptors that monitor distention and other physiological activities in these organs. Information detected by these receptors is then sent to the brain. The brain receives sensory input by the vagus nerve. Information sent to the brain is thought to pertain to the amount of food ingested, its nutrient composition, and the rate of nutrient digestion [19,20].

Gastrointestinal or regulatory peptides released from the gastrointestinal tract also provide signals to the brain to affect appetite. Examples of some of these peptides include somatostatin, cholecystokinin, and bombesin. Somatostatin and cholecystokinin act from the periphery, providing satiety signals that are relayed by sensory nerve fibers to the brain [19]. Bombesin acts both peripherally and directly on the brain to induce satiety (i.e., inhibit hunger or inhibit further eating). In addition, it appears that some of the gastrointestinal peptides work synergistically. Bombesin stimulates the release of cholecystokinin, which, in the presence of glucagon, has an even greater effect on satiety [19].

In addition to the gastrointestinal peptides, many neurotransmitters also regulate food intake. Opioids (beta-endorphin) and neuropeptide Y are thought to be principal stimulants of food intake [18,19,21]. Galanin also stimulates food intake while serotonin and corticotropin-releasing factor (CRF) diminish appetite. A

TABLE 15.3 Body Weights in Kilograms Raised to Power of .75

Weight (kg)	Weight.75 (kg)	Weight (kg)	Weight.75 (kg)
1	1.0	51	19.1
2	1.68	52	19.4
3	2.28	53	19.6
4	2.83	54	19.9
5	3.34	55	20.2
6	3.83	56	20.5
7	4.30	57	20.8
8	4.75	58	21.0
9	5.19	59	21.3
10	5.62	60	21.6
11	6.04	61	21.8
12	6.44	62	22.1
13	6.84	63	22.4
14	7.24	64	22.6
15	7.62	65	22.9
16	8.00	66	23.2
17	8.38	67	23.4
18	8.75	68	23.7
19	9.10	69	23.9
20	9.46	70	24.2
21	9.8	71	24.4
22	10.2	72	24.7
23	10.5	73	25.0
24	10.8	74	25.2
25	11.2	75	25.5
26	11.5	76	25.8
27	11.8	77	26.0
28	12.2	78	26.2
29	12.5	79	26.5
30	12.8	80	26.7
31	13.1	81	27.0
32	13.5	82	27.2
33	13.8	83	27.5
34	14.1	84	27.7
35	14.4	85	28.0
36	14.7	86	28.2
37	15.0	87	28.5
38	15.3	88	28.7
39	15.6	89	29.0
40	15.9	90	29.2
41	16.2	91	29.4
42	16.5	92	29.7
43	16.8	93	29.9
44	17.1	94	30.2
45	17.4	95	30.4
46	17.7	96	30.7
47	18.0	97	30.9
48	18.2	98	31.1
49	18.5	99	31.4
50	18.8	100	31.6

Source: Adapted from Pike R, Brown M. Nutrition: An integrated approach, 3rd ed. New York: Macmillan (formerly Wiley) 1984:749.

reciprocal or inverse relationship exists between the effect of some neurotransmitters on food intake and the effect of the neurotransmitter on sympathetic nervous system activity [22].

Nutrients and products of their metabolism also influence appetite. Following absorption of nutrients through the enterocytes (intestinal cells), nutrients enter the blood for circulation to tissues, especially the liver. Uptake of glucose by glucose-sensitive liver cells has been shown to change the frequency of impulses reaching areas of the brain via vagal sensory nerve fibers [19,23]. Liver cells appear to monitor the oxidation of fatty acids as well as glucose [24,25]. With high oxidative metabolism of nutrients such as glucose, satiety occurs; inhibition of fatty acid oxidation may stimulate feeding [21,23]. In addition, products of lipid metabolism, such as 3-hydroxybutyrate, can cross the blood–brain barrier and bind to specific chemoreceptors, influence neurotransmitter synthesis, or alter some aspect of neuronal metabolism to affect appetite [20].

Hormones such as glucagon and insulin also affect appetite. Insulin, a hormone released from the pancreas during ingestion of food, rises in the blood, cerebrospinal fluid, and finally the brain. Although high plasma insulin concentrations stimulate hunger, the binding of insulin to receptors in the brain is thought to stimulate satiety [19,26]. High plasma insulin concentrations also enable the amino acid tryptophan to more readily cross the blood–brain barrrier (see Chapter 16). Within the brain, tryptophan may be converted into serotonin. Serotonin stimulates satiety and is thought to suppress the actions of norepinephrine and opioids, both of which stimulate food intake [19].

Mechanisms by which body composition modulates appetite also have been proposed. Specifically, an unidentified signal(s) regarding body composition is thought to be sent from adipocytes and/or other tissues to the central nervous system [27]. The size of the fat depot in individuals may be one of many determinants affecting long-term control of food intake [13].

Individual balances of the macronutrients (carbohydrate, fat, and protein) in the body also appear to affect energy balance. Satiation coincides with carbohydrate intake [28]. Ingestion of a meal high in carbohydrates stimulates carbohydrate oxidation; however, this does not occur with lipid ingestion [11,29]. In other words, ingestion of a high-fat diet does not stimulate fat oxidation, and diets high in fat and low in carbohydrate decrease carbohydrate oxidation by diminishing the postprandial insulin response [28]. To increase fat oxidation, an increase in body fat mass is needed [11,28]. Thus, energy balance is thought to be equivalent to fat balance [29].

The high-fat diet ingested by many U.S. citizens may be one of many possible causes of obesity. Several other hypotheses have been generated with respect to energy balance and causes of several types of obesity. Although the latter is beyond the scope of this book, reviews of the subject are available; see reference 22, by George Bray.

CREATING AN ENERGY BALANCE

Energy balance and weight control require energy intake and energy expenditure to be equal; simple in theory but often difficult in practice. How the control of body weight impacts on the individual depends on the person's weight in relation to his or her ideal body weight (IBW). Estimation of a desirable weight for height can provide a guide for an appropriate energy intake and expenditure.

Many formulas and tables for determining IBW have been devised. Some of the methods more commonly used include the Quetelet body mass index (BMI) [13,30] and the Devine [31] formulas, used initially in pharmacokinetics [31,32]. For women and men aged 19 to 34 years, a BMI between 19 and 25 kg/m² is considered acceptable, and for men and women over 35 years, a BMI between 21 and 27 kg/m² is considered acceptable [33]. A BMI of 25 or 27 to 30 kg/m² is considered overweight and if > 30 kg/m² is considered obese [33].

The formulas suggested by Devine [31,32] to calculate ideal body weight (IBW) are as follows:

IBW for men = 50 kg + 2.3 kg/in > 5 ft
IBW for women = 45 kg + 2.3 kg/in > 5 ft

These formulas have been modified somewhat and converted into the following familiar empirical formulas:

IBW for men = 110 lb + 5 lb/in > 5 ft
IBW for women = 100 lb. + 5 lb/in > 5 ft

A slightly modified formula for men is also used:

IBW for men = 106 lb + 6 lb/in > 5 ft

A 10% range minus and plus the calculated ideal weight allowing for the differences in weight due to a small or large frame size, respectively, is usually included in the Devine formula.

Using the formulas, a man who is 5ft, 11in tall with a medium frame should weigh either 165 lb [110 + (5 × 11) = 165 lb] or 172 lb [106 + (6 × 11) = 172 lb] depending on which formula was used. If the man had a small frame, ideal body would be 10% less than that calculated for a medium frame size (i.e., 165 lb − 16.5 lb = 148.5 lb or 172 lb − 17.2 lb = 154.8 lb, respectively). A

female who is 5 ft, 6 in, and has a large frame has an ideal body weight of 143 lb [that is, 100 + (5 × 6) = 130 lb + 13 lb (accounting for the 10% addition for the large frame size) = 143 lb].

Regression equations purported to be more nearly accurate in estimating IBW have been based on the 1959 Metropolitan Life Insurance Company height–weight tables and the IBW tables used by Grant [34] in nutrition assessment. These equations are rather complicated, but they account for gender and frame size without sacrificing accuracy. The equation based on the 1959 Metropolitan Life Insurance Company tables (with indoor clothing and shoes) is as follows [35]:

y (or IBW in lb) =
  $-139.17 + 3.86(\text{height}) + 9.52(\text{frame}) + 5.01(\text{sex})$

Based on Grant's tables, corrected for nude height and weight, the equation becomes

$y = -133.99 + 3.86(\text{height}) + 9.52(\text{frame}) + 3.08(\text{sex})$

In these two equations, height is in inches. Figures used for frame size are 1 for small, 2 for medium, and 3 for large. Figures for sex are +1 for male and −1 for female.

Another equation for determining an ideal or desirable body weight is based on body composition and requires measurement of body fat [12].

$$\text{Desirable body weight} = \frac{\text{lean body weight}}{1 - \%\ \text{fat desired}}$$

Calculations would be as follows for a woman who weighs 130 lb, with a measured 30% of this weight due to fat:

130 lb × 0.30 = 39 lb (fat weight)
130 lb − 39 lb = 91 lb (lean body weight)

Since a desirable amount of fat in males is 15% or less, and in females is 25% or less [36,37], a figure of 25% (0.25) is figured in the following equation for the sample woman:

Desirable body weight =
  91/(1 − 0.25) = (91/0.75) = 121 lb

Once IBW has been estimated, a decision can be made concerning the individual's energy balance and weight control. If actual body weight is the same as desirable body weight, little may need to be done with respect to modifying energy intake and expenditure. Should actual body weight deviate from ideal body weight, changes in energy intake and energy expenditure may be needed.

Aberrations in body weight include conditions of overweight and obesity, along with eating disorders, especially anorexia nervosa. Although the etiologies of

TABLE 15.4 The Balance Between Adipose Tissue and Muscle Functions in Central Energy Metabolism in Upper- and Lower-Body Obesity

	Adipose Tissue	Consequences	Muscle	Consequences	Net Results In Muscle	In Glucose Homeostasis
Upper-body obesity	Abdominal adipose tissues enlarged; elevated FFA mobilization	Excess FFA[a] turnover	Few slow-twitch fibers; many fast-twitch fibers	Slow oxidative capacity	Decreased glucose transport; insulin resistance	Insulin resistance; decreased glucose tolerance; diabetes mellitus
Lower-body obesity	Femoral-gluteal adipose tissues enlarged; low FFA mobilization	Normal FFA turnover	Many slow-twitch fibers; few fast-twitch fibers	High oxidative capacity	Normal glucose transport; insulin sensitivity	Normal glucose tolerance

[a]FFA = free fatty acids.

Source: Björntorp P. Classification of obese patients and complications related to distribution of surplus fat. Am J Clin Nutr 1987;45 (suppl.):1124. © Am. J. Clin. Nutr., American Society for Clinical Nutrition. Reprinted with permission.

these disorders are multifactorial and beyond the scope of this book, this chapter briefly addresses some approaches to weight loss and gain. The "Perspective" section at the end of this chapter addresses eating disorders.

Creating a Negative Energy Balance

According to the National Center for Health Statistics [38], 28.4% of adults 25 to 74 years of age examined between 1976 and 1980 were overweight (or exceeded normal weight by at least 20%). Individuals weighing greater than 150 kg (330 lb) represent close to 0.1% of the population [33]. The prevalence of excessive body weight is increasing. Of particular concern is the increased incidence of obesity, which appears to be occurring in children [39]. The limitations associated with anthropometric measurements taken in the various national surveys, however, have impaired the ability to accurately describe trends in obesity for children and adolescents in the United States [40].

Defining overweight and/or obesity has been difficult because of the differences in criteria used. One common method for classifying obesity is based on percentage of overweight, whereby those people 28 to 40% over IBW are deemed to be mildly overweight, those 41 to 100% over IBW are moderately overweight, and those people greater than 100% over IBW are severely obese. One problem in using percentage overweight as the basis for obesity classification is the difficulty of identifying individual IBW. Another classification of obesity is based on the BMI (W/H^2). Classifications of BMI for assessment of obesity and health risks associated with obesity are as follows [33].

Class	BMI (kg/m²)	Risk of Health Problems
O	20–25	None
I	25–30	Low health risk from obesity
II	30–35	Moderate health risk from obesity
III	35–40	High health risk from obesity
IV	>40	Very high health risk from obesity

Although health risks associated with class I obesity may be low, mild obesity cannot be ignored totally because it may be a transition from a mild state into a class with more serious health consequences.

Obesity can be classified not only according to its degree of severity, but also according to body distribution. Table 15.4 and Figure 15.4 show the differences between upper-body or abdominal obesity and lower-body obesity. Also shown in Table 15.4 are the increased health risks associated with upper-body obesity. Upper-body obesity is associated with an increased risk for heart disease, stroke, noninsulin-dependent diabetes mellitus, and some types of cancers [41,42]. Adipocytes making up abdominal fat tissue differ from those found in the gluteal fat. Abdominal fat has a preponderance of beta receptors, whereas alpha receptors predominate in the gluteal fat [43–45]. Alpha receptors promote accumulation of lipids within the cells, whereas the beta receptors favor mobilization of fat stores (higher rate of lipolysis) [43–45]. In addition, abdominal or upper-body obesity is associated with decreased peripheral glucose metabolism and increased hepatic synthesis and release of triglycerides and very low density lipoproteins into the blood.

Because of the prevalence of excessive body weight and the health risks associated with serious obesity, the

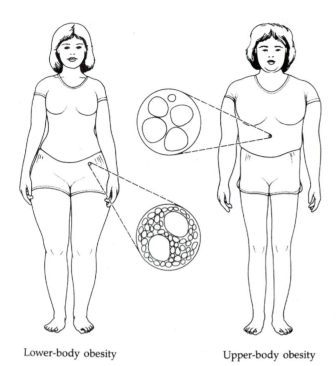

Lower-body obesity   Upper-body obesity

FIGURE 15.4 Lower- and upper-body obesity and adipocyte differences in these two obesity types.

rest of the chapter reviews some strategies, tools, and techniques used in the control of body weight. It needs to be noted, however, that effective treatment for one obese person may be inappropriate for another. Moreover, while each overweight person attempting to lose weight should be matched to an individually appropriate treatment, guidelines for such matching are not available.

Negative energy balance (weight loss) is accomplished when energy expenditure exceeds energy intake:

$$\text{Energy expenditure} > \text{energy intake} = \\ - \text{energy balance}$$

Two routes exist for creating a negative relationship between energy expenditure and energy intake: food (energy intake) can be decreased and/or physical activity (energy expenditure) can be increased.

Before weight loss is attempted, current body weight, desirable body weight, and the difference between the two should be calculated. With this information and knowledge of energy intake needed to equal energy expenditure at the body's present weight, one can undertake a systematic approach to weight loss.

For example, a 25-year-old woman of small frame stands 5 ft, 5 in, tall, weighs 140 lb, and has a current maintenance caloric intake of 2,000 kcal. First, her de-

sirable weight is calculated by the modified Devine formula [IBW = (100 lb + 5 lb/in > 5 ft) − 10% due to small frame] such that IBW = (100 + 25) − 12.5 = 112.5 or 113 lb. The young woman presently weighs 140 lb and wants to reach her IBW of 113 lb; the weight loss needed is 27 lb. Because her actual body weight exceeds her IBW by approximately 25% (27/113 × 100), this young woman would be considered mildly obese. Weight reduction in mildly obese or overweight people can be accomplished by diet, physical exercise, and behavior modification, whereas weight reduction for the moderately or severely obese often requires additional medical intervention and/or supervision [46].

The caloric equivalent of 1 pound of weight is estimated to be approximately 3,500 kcal. Therefore, theoretically 1 lb of tissue should be lost whenever maintenance energy intake is reduced by 3,500 kcal. All the weight lost, however, is not from adipose tissue, a fact addressed in the following section. If all the weight lost were fat, 1 lb would equal 4,086 kcal [454 grams (which equals 1 lb) × 9 kcal/g = 4,086 kcal].

Because the young woman in the preceding example is maintaining her current weight of 140 lb with an energy intake of 2,000 kcal per day, the next calculation will be to determine by how much she can reduce her energy intake and still maintain nutritional adequacy. To ensure adequate nutrition, a caloric intake of no less than 10 kcal/lb current weight is advised for women [46], thus 10 kcal/lb × 140 lb = 1,400 kcal, which represents the minimum daily energy intake. Energy intake at which weight was maintained (2,000 kcal) minus minimum energy intake (1,400 kcal) equals an energy deficit of −600 kcal. Thus, if every pound of weight loss is equivalent to 3,500 kcal, then with a daily caloric deficit of 600 kcal, this young woman should expect to lose in one week approximately 1.2 lb (600 kcal/day × 7 days = 4,200 kcal/3,500 kcal/lb). If, in addition, physical activity were increased so as to create an even greater deficit during the week (e.g., − 1,000 kcal), then weight loss might be expected to approximate 1.5 lb/week.

Composition and Rate of Weight Loss Weight loss does not proceed in quite such a uniform manner as just outlined. The composition of weight loss, and, consequently, its caloric equivalency vary with the duration of caloric restriction. With continued caloric restriction, the rate of weight loss decreases, while the caloric equivalency increases. The quality of weight loss is said to improve (i.e., increase loss of body fat) as its quantity decreases! The changes in composition of weight loss in young men during caloric restriction and enforced physical activity are shown in Figure 15.5. During the first few

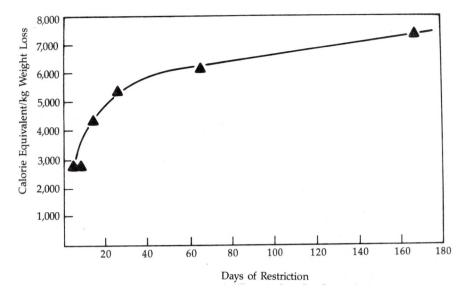

FIGURE 15.5 Caloric equivalent of weight loss in relation to the duration of caloric restriction. Results of six experimental periods of caloric restriction are plotted; duration of caloric restriction ranged from 4 days to 168 days. The caloric equivalent of weight loss after 168 days of restriction more than doubled that for a restriction lasting only 4 to 5 days. (Adapted from Grande, F. Nutrition and energy balance in body composition studies. In: Techniques for measuring body composition. Washington, DC: National Academy of Sciences-National Research Council, 1961.)

Experiment	No. of Subjects	Duration (Days)	Average Weight Loss (kg)	Total Calorie Deficit	Caloric Equivalent
1	1	4	2.85	8,107	2,845
2	6	5	5.50	15,590	2,835
3	6	12	5.90	25,368	4,300
4	13	24	7.60	40,480	5,326
5	12	63	14.10	87,000	6,170
6	32	168	16.82	126,420	7,516

days, weight loss was rapid. Water comprised about 70% of the weight loss, with an additional 25% coming from fat and 5% from protein. After about three weeks, weight loss was slower, but 85% of the weight loss was now fat and 15% protein. The caloric equivalency of 1 lb of weight loss increased from 1,180 kcal during the first three days of energy deficit to 3,955 during days 22 and 24.

Weight loss, regardless of the duration of caloric restriction, entails a loss of lean body mass as well as fat because obesity tissue contains substantial amounts of cell residue. An estimate of fat-free mass accrued in weight gain amounts to 22 to 25% [6,48]; therefore, during weight loss no more than 22 to 25% of the loss should be of fat-free origin. The initial water loss associated with caloric restriction is not due entirely to a shift in body fluids. Some of the water loss comes from fat-free mass and the small amount of available glycogen catabolized to provide energy [6].

Caloric restriction results in a drop in BMR. For each kilogram of weight lost due to a hypocaloric diet, energy expenditure is estimated to be reduced by approximately 20 kcal [35]. Reduction in weight decreases the energy cost of physical activities, and spontaneous activity lessens when calories are restricted [6]. The energy conservation caused by a hypocaloric diet therefore slows down the rate of weight loss. Nevertheless, individuals show considerable differences in their rate of weight loss; consequently, predicting the amount and rate of weight loss that can be expected by any one person is very difficult. No real constants exist in weight control!

The fact remains that energy conservation in response to a hypocaloric diet is operative at some level in all humans. Repeated caloric restrictions, therefore, may result in the body's becoming increasingly efficient in its use of food. As a result, each time weight reduction is attempted, weight comes off more slowly, and when refeeding occurs, weight is gained more rapidly [45]. Figure 15.6 exemplifies this so-called yo-yo effect. The many various fad diets to which much of the public subscribes cannot be the answer to weight control because the maintenance of weight loss assumes as much or more importance than does weight loss itself. Effective weight control demands a treatment and manipulation of energy balance that can be employed for the rest of one's life [49].

Components of Weight Loss or Weight Control Programs The young woman in the just-mentioned example who is attempting to lose weight would be well

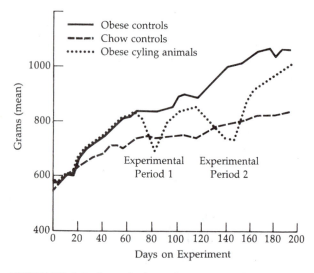

FIGURE 15.6 Body weight changes in experimental animals subjected to cyclic dieting. The "yo-yo" effect of cyclic caloric restriction is illustrated by the difference in rate of weight change during experimental periods 1 and 2. Weight loss was slower and weight gain more rapid during experimental period 2. *(Brownell K. Nutrition Today 1987;22(3):7. © by Williams & Wilkins, 1987.)*

advised to include physical activity and make behavior modifications part of her weight control program. Most successful weight loss programs for the mildly obese include dietary management, increased physical activity, and behavior modification. The latter fosters the development of new patterns into true habits. More drastic treatment—that is, with drugs, very low calorie diets, or even surgery—may be necessary for severe obesity.

Dietary Management Deciding on the appropriate caloric intake is only the first step in the dietary management component of a weight control program. In addition to providing the designated energy level, the diet should meet the following criteria [50]:

- Satisfy all nutrition needs except calories.
- Be acceptable to tastes and habits of the individual.
- Minimize hunger and fatigue.
- Be readily available and socially acceptable.
- Favor establishment of lasting pattern of eating.
- Be conducive to improvement of overall health.

Nutrition education is a very important aspect of dietary management. Most individuals need to learn more about the importance of the various nutrients and the food sources of these nutrients. An excellent tool for teaching nutrient and energy contributions from foods is the Exchange Lists for Meal Planning compiled by the American Diabetes Association and the American Dietetic Association. The exchange lists are found in Appendix D. Informed use of these exchange lists allows the development of eating patterns that meet all the criteria just listed.

Choosing foods based solely on their caloric content is a very dangerous practice nutritionally. Diet composition may be just as important as the caloric content in the reduction of body weight [51]. Decreasing dietary fat intake is consistent with caloric restriction because of the high energy value of fat (9 kcal/g or perhaps as high as 11 kcal/g) [52] as compared with carbohydrate or protein (4 kcal/g). In addition, dietary fat does not generate as strong a gastrointestinal peptide and neurotransmitter response to induce satiety as does carbohydrate [20]. Moreover, diets high in fat and low in carbohydrate decrease carbohydrate oxidation by diminishing the postprandial insulin response [28]. Efficacy in weight control also may be improved with a high-carbohydrate, low-fat diet, because dietary fat is stored more efficiently in body fat than is dietary carbohydrate when energy intake is consumed in excess of energy needs. Dietary fat can be converted into triglycerides of adipose tissue at a metabolic cost of only 3% of ingested calories, while the cost of storing dietary carbohydrate in fat requires an expenditure of 23% of energy ingested [4].

According to the current evidence about the relationship between the macronutrients and improvement of overall health, probably the best division of a hypocaloric diet is 55 to 60% of total energy from carbohydrate with emphasis on complex carbohydrates, 25% of total energy from fat, and 15 to 20% of total energy from protein. This division would be appropriate for the 1,400-kcal diet being followed by the young woman in the example given earlier. Protein supplied at this level would ensure an intake of at least 0.8 g/kg body weight. At her present weight of 140 lb (or 63.6 kg), this young woman should receive approximately 51 g protein/day. If 15% of the 1,400 kcal comprising her reduction diet comes from protein, her intake of protein will be 52 g.

Once the number of grams of carbohydrate, protein, and fat to be included in each day's food intake has been determined, the diet prescription can be converted into meal patterns for the day through use of the exchange lists. Inclusion each day of foods from all groups of foods (exchange lists) and variety in the choice of foods from each list will allow nutrition needs to be satisfied provided the caloric intake remains as high as 1,200 to 1,500 kcal. A diet as calorically restricted as this permits very few empty calories. Most of the foods selected for inclusion in the diet must be of high nutrient density (i.e., the ratio of nutrient content to energy value must be high).

Increased Physical Activity Physical activity as part of a weight control program may need to be divided into two categories: (1) programmed episodes of concentrated exercise and (2) general activity forming part of lifestyle. Simple lifestyle changes in activity could include parking one's car some distance from the destination and then walking to the destination. Also, walking up and down stairs rather than using escalators and elevators can be a helpful change [50]. Lifestyle changes of this sort may have only a minimal effect on weight loss per se, but they can improve overall fitness and should be used as an adjunct to the programmed physical activities that are of a more strenuous nature. Realistically, these simple lifestyle changes may be the only physical activity that the obese can be expected to undertake initially. For the very sedentary, these changes make an excellent beginning!

Exercise should occur in programmed episodes with specified intensity, duration, and frequency. Each episode of exercise needs to create an uncompensated deficit of kcal and should be performed no less than three times per week. Expenditure of approximately 300 kcal, for example, can be accomplished by 20 to 30 minutes of running, swimming, or bicycling. Walking briskly for 40 to 60 minutes will cause a similar energy expenditure. There is some evidence to suggest that the timing of the exercise can affect the amount of energy expended. Specifically, physical exercise occurring shortly after meals may cause a greater than normal expenditure of energy [49]. If the young woman in the example wants to increase her energy deficit by another 1,000 kcal per week through exercise, she will need to exercise three times per week using at least 300 kcal during each episode of exercise.

Regular exercise has several benefits. Particularly important is the sparing effect of exercise on the fat-free mass of the body [53]. Caloric restriction alone can cause substantial losses of lean body mass, but when exercise is incorporated into a weight control program, these losses are decreased [12,49,50]. Exercise also may partially offset the decline in BMR that is induced by calorically restricted diets [53]. A long-term potential benefit of regular exercise is its role in the maintenance of the weight loss that has been achieved. The modest deficit in calories made possible by regular exercise allows the maintenance diet to be a bit more liberal. Being able to find more enjoyment in eating while still maintaining a desirable weight could be a strong motivation for continued interest in weight control. Furthermore, modest amounts of regular exercise may have the benefit of suppressing appetite among sedentary individuals [50,54].

Behavior Modification Two behaviors that need modifying in overweight individuals to promote weight loss and/or weight maintenance are those already discussed: eating and exercise. Old habits must be "unlearned" and a new lifestyle developed. Seven elements that may be included in conservative treatments for obesity [54] or behavior modification [45,50,54] are (1) self-monitoring or keeping records of behavior to be changed (Fig. 15.7); (2) control of the stimuli that precede eating (Table 15.5); (3) development of techniques to control the act of eating (e.g., putting fork down between mouthfuls, chewing thoroughly before swallowing, leaving some food on the plate); (4) reinforcement of prescribed behavior through systemized rewards; (5) cognitive restructuring; (6) nutrition education; and (7) increasing physical activity. Cognitive restructuring is a particularly important component of behavior modification because it focuses on an improved mental attitude of the dieters toward themselves and toward weight reduction. It is designed to overcome the self-defeating attitudes that commonly plague those attempting weight loss and to help them maintain their motivation toward weight reduction. Support from family and close friends can be particularly helpful.

An interesting behavioral approach to weight loss is the comprehensive program developed by Brownell [45] in which nutrition, physical exercise, and behavioral modification have been incorporated under the acronym LEARN:

L = lifestyle, which refers to changes in eating behavior or "behavior modification."

E = exercise.

A = attitudes and encompasses the cognitive restructuring already mentioned. People are encouraged to adopt flexible goals and are instructed in developing positive attitudes toward occasional failures in diet compliance.

R = relationships emphasizing the importance of support from family, friends, neighbors, co-workers, and the like.

N = nutrition and the importance of an adequate diet provided through attractive low-calorie meals.

Behavior modification, a complex subject, is addressed only in a cursory manner in this chapter. Concise reviews of the subject are provided by Brownell [45], Blundell [49], and Stunkard [55]. An important point made by Blundell [49] is that behavior modification appears to be particularly appropriate for the treatment of mild obesity because treatment effectiveness lasts for

Day of Week_____   Name_____

Time	Minutes Spent Eating	M/S	H	Body Position	Activity While Eating	Location of Eating	Food Type and Quantity	Eating with Whom	Feeling While Eating
6:00 A.M.									
11:00 A.M.									
4:00 P.M.									
9:00 P.M.									

Abbreviations:
M/S; meal or snack; H: degree of hunger (0 = none, 3 = maximum)
body position: 1 = walking; 2 = standing, 3 = sitting, 4 = lying down

FIGURE 15.7 Illustration of a food diary particularly appropriate for the person embarking on a behavioral weight reduction program. *(Stunkard AJ. Food diary for first week of a behavioral weight-reduction program. Am J Clin Nutr 1987;45:1152. © Am J Clin Nutr, American Society for Clinical Nutrition. Reproduced with permission.)*

about 25 weeks, with a weight loss of approximately 1 lb per week being the norm.

Creating a Positive Energy Balance

Although a positive energy balance is necessary for the growing child, the need to gain weight is not a major problem among the healthy adult population of the United States. Nevertheless, the problem does affect some individuals and can be quite troublesome to those affected.

Creating a positive energy balance requires an intake of calories that more than offsets energy expenditure; that is, energy intake > energy expenditure = + energy balance or weight gain.

As discussed earlier in the chapter, the greatest variable in energy expenditure is physical activity; therefore, physical activity should be maintained at a modest level among adults attempting a weight gain. Some physical activity is desirable for everyone because of its fitness factor, but for the person needing to gain weight a modest caloric expenditure in exercise is appropriate.

TABLE 15.5 Stimulus Control

A. Shopping
  1. Shop for food after eating.
  2. Shop from a list.
  3. Avoid ready-to-eat foods.
  4. Don't carry more cash than you need for shopping.
B. Plans
  1. Plan to limit intake.
  2. Substitute exercise for snacking.
  3. Eat meals and snacks at scheduled times.
  4. Don't accept foods offered by others.
C. Activities
  1. Store food out of sight.
  2. Keep all food out of sight.
  3. Remove food from inappropriate storage areas in house.
  4. Keep serving dishes off the table.
  5. Use smaller dishes.
  6. Avoid being the food server.
D. Holidays and parties
  1. Plan eating habits before parties.
  2. Eat a low-calorie snack before parties.
  3. Practice polite ways to decline food.

Source: Adapted from Stunkard, AJ. Conservative treatents for obesity. Am J Clin Nutr 1987;45:1142–1154. © Am J Clin Nutr., American Society for Clinical Nutrition. Reprinted with permission.

A positive energy balance of approximately 3,500 kcal is needed for a 1-lb gain in body weight [5]. About one-fourth of this energy is required for the synthesis of the protein and fat components of the gain; therefore, the caloric equivalency of a 1-lb gain in body weight is only 2,700 kcal. Approximately 30% of the weight gain is water, 5.6% is protein, and 64% is fat [5]. Based on the assumption that fat-free mass is 72.7% water and 25.7% protein, the percentage of fat-free mass in weight gain can be estimated to approximate 22% [5,48].

Because approximately 3,500 kcal are needed for every pound of weight gain, increasing the intake of energy-rich foods becomes of prime importance for the person attempting weight gain. Research on sensory-specific satiety has shown that the greater variety of foods presented in a meal, the better the appetite of people consuming the meal [35]. To increase the food intake of people needing to gain weight, emphasis needs to be placed on food variety in each meal. Foods with different colors, smells, tastes, and textures should comprise the meal. Sufficient time should be allowed for meal enjoyment, and eating should occur in a pleasant, relaxed atmosphere.

Calories in addition to those ingested at meals can be obtained through high-energy snacks eaten shortly after completion of meals. Snacks consumed approximately one hour after meals probably will have no effect on the appetite for the next meal if there is as much as a five-hour interval between meals. A high-calorie snack at bedtime is a particularly good idea.

SUMMARY

Weight control is an individual matter. Although changes in energy balance produce weight changes, the extent of these changes varies from person to person. Trying to devise a formula that will accurately predict a specific amount of weight loss or weight gain for any population group is a hopeless task. One of the greatest problems in making predictions centers around estimation of energy expenditure. Energy expenditure has three defined components: basal metabolic rate, diet-induced thermogenesis, and the effect of exercise or physical activity, none of which is constant. To make energy metabolism even more complex, there is the possibility that adaptive thermogenesis can increase or decrease energy expenditure.

Losing excess weight may appear to be a formidable task, but actually it is easier than the maintenance of weight loss. A sufficiently negative energy balance, regardless of the manner in which it is obtained, will allow weight loss. Maintenance of this weight loss, however, requires a continual struggle. New eating and exercise habits have to be incorporated into a continuing lifestyle. Behavior modification assumes much importance in any successful weight control program.

References Cited

1. Horton ES. Introduction: An overview of the assessment and regulation of energy balance in humans. Am J Clin Nutr 1983;38:972–977.
2. Devlin JT, Horton ES. Energy requirements. In: Brown ML, ed. Present knowledge in nutrition, 6th ed. Washington, DC: International Life Sciences Institute Nutrition Foundation, 1990:1–6.
3. Food and Nutrition Board, Commission on Life Sciences, National Research Council. Recommended Dietary Allowances, 10th ed. Washington, DC: National Academy Press, 1989;24–38.
4. Danforth E. Diet and obesity. Am J Clin Nutr 1985;41:1132–1145.
5. Ravussin E, Bogardus C. A brief overview of human energy metabolism and its relationship to essential obesity. Am J Clin Nutr 1992;55:242S–245S.
6. Grande F. Body weight, composition and energy balance. In: Olson RE, Broquist HP, Chichester CO, Darby WJ, Kolbye AC Jr, Stalvey RM, eds. Nutrition Reviews' pre-

sent knowledge in nutrition, 5th ed. New York: The Nutrition Foundation, 1984:7–18.

7. Daly JM, Heymsfield SB, Head CA, Harvey LP, Nixon DW, Katzeff H, Grossman GD. Human energy requirements: Overestimation by widely used prediction equation. Am J Clin Nutr 1985;42:1170–1174.

8. Owen OE, Kavle E, Owen RS, Polansky M, Caprio S, Mozzoli MA, Kendrick ZV, Bushman MC, Boden G. A reappraisal of caloric requirements in healthy women. Am J Clin Nutr 1986;44:1–19.

9. Jequier E, Acheson K, Schutz Y. Assessment of energy expenditure and fuel utilization in man. Ann Rev Nutr 1987;7:187–208.

10. Webb P. Human calorimeters. New York: Praeger, 1985.

11. Westerterp KR. Food quotient, respiratory quotient, and energy balance. Am J Clin Nutr 1993;57:759S–765S.

12. McArdle WD, Katch FI, Katch VL. Exercise physiology, 2nd ed. Philadelphia: Lea and Febiger, 1986.

13. Garrow JS. Energy balance in man—an overview. Am J Clin Nutr 1987;45:1114–1119.

14. Harris J, Benedict F. A biometric study of basal metabolism in man. Publication 279. Washington, DC: Carnegie Institution, 1919.

15. Mifflin MD, St Jeor ST, Hill LA, Scott BJ, Daugherty SA, Koh YO. A new predictive equiation for resting energy expenditure in healthy individuals. Am J Clin Nutr 1990;51:241–247.

16. Heshka S, Feld K, Yang M-U, Allison DB, Heymsfield SB. Resting energy expenditure in the obese: A cross-validation and comparison of prediction equations. J Am Diet Assoc 1993;93:1031–1036.

17. Weingarten HP. Stimulus control of eating: Implications for a two-factor theory of hunger. Appetite 1985;6:387–401.

18. Bray GA. Treatment of obesity: A nutrient balance/nutrient partition approach. Nutr Rev 1991;49:33–45.

19. Norton P, Falciglia G, Gist D. Physiologic control of food intake by neural and chemical mechanisms. J Am Diet Assoc 1993;93:450–454,457.

20. Blundell JE, Lawton CL, Hill AJ. Mechanisms of appetite control and their abnormalities in obese patients. Horm Res 1993;39(suppl.3):72–76.

21. Blundell JE. Appetite disturbance and the problems of overweight. Drugs 1990;39(suppl. 3):1–19.

22. Bray GA. Obesity, a disorder of nutrient partitioning: The MONA LISA hypothesis. J Nutr 1991;121:1146–1162.

23. Martin RJ, White BD, Hulsey MG. The regulation of body weight. Am Sci 1991;79:528–541.

24. Friedman MI, Ramirez I. Relationship of fat metabolism to food intake. Am J Clin Nutr 1985;42:1093–1098.

25. Novin D, Robinson K, Culbreth LA, Tordoff MG. Is there a role for the liver in the control of food intake? Am J Clin Nutr 1985;42:1050–1062.

26. Woods SC, Porte D, Bobbioni E, Ionescu E, Sauter JF, Rohner-Jeanrenaud F, Jeanrenaud B. Insulin: Its relationship to the central nervous system and to the control of food intake and body weight. Am J Clin Nutr 1985;42:1063–1071.

27. Weigle DS. Appetite and the regulation of body composition. FASEB J 1994;8:302–310.

28. Astrup A, Raben A. Obesity: An inherited metabolic deficiency in the control of macronutrient balance. Eur J Clin Nutr 1992;46:611–620.

29. Ravussin E, Swinburn BA. Pathophysiology of obesity. Lancet 1992;340:404–408.

30. Stavig GR, Leonard AR, Igra A, Felten P. Indices of relative body weight and ideal weight charts. J Chron Dis 1984;37:255–262.

31. Devine BJ. Gentamicin therapy. Drug Intell Clin Pharm 1974;8:650–655.

32. Robinson JD, Lupklewica SM, Palenik L, Lopez LM, Ariet M. Determination of ideal body weight for drug dosage calculations. Am J Hosp Pharm 1983;40:1016–1019.

33. Bray GA. Pathophysiology of obesity. Am J Clin Nutr 1992;55:488S–494S.

34. Grant A, DeHoog S. Anthropometry. In: Nutritional assessment and support, 3rd ed. Seattle: Grant, 1985;11.

35. Giannini VS, Giudici RA, Nerrukk DL. Determination of ideal body weight. Am J Hosp Pharm 1984;41:883–887.

36. Katch FI, McArdle WD. Introduction to nutrition, exercise, and health, 4th ed. Philadelphia: Lea and Febiger, 1993;223–258.

37. Nieman DC. Fitness and sports medicine: An introduction. Palo Alto: Bull Publishing, 1990;107–139.

38. National Center for Health Statistics. Health, United States, 1986. U.S. Dept. of Health and Human Services publication no. (PHS) 87–1232. Public Health Service. Washington, DC: U.S. Government Printing Office, 1986.

39. Gortmaker SL. Increasing pediatric obesity in the United States. Am J Dis Child 1987;141:535–540.

40. Kuczmarski RJ. Trends in body composition for infants and children in the U.S. Crit Rev Food Sci Nutr 1993;33:375–387.

41. Jequier E. Energy, obesity and body weight standards. Am J Clin Nutr 1987;45(suppl.):1035–1036.

42. Björntorp P. Classification of obese patients and complications related to distribution of surplus fat. Am J Clin Nutr 1987;45(suppl.):1120–1125.

43. Kolata G. Why do people get fat? Science 1985;227:1327–1328.

44. Leibel RL, Hirsch J. Metabolic characterization of obesity. Ann Int Med 1985;103:1000–1002.

45. Brownell KD. Obesity and weight control: The good and bad of dieting. Nutr Today 1987;22(3):4–9.

46. Stunkard AJ. The current status of treatment for obesity in adults. In: Stunkard AJ, Steller E, eds. Eating and disorders. New York: Raven Press, 1984:157–173.

47. The American Dietetic Association's nutrition recommendations for women. J Am Diet Assoc 1986;86:1663–1664.

48. Webster JD, Hesp R, Garrow JS. The composition of excess body weight in obese women estimated by body den-

sity, total body water and total potassium. Hum Nutr: Clin Nutr 1984;38C:299–306.

49. Blundell JE. Behavior modification and exercise in the treatment of obesity. Postgrad Med J 1984;60(suppl. 3):37–49.

50. Weinsier RL, Wadden TA, Ritenbaugh C, Harrison GG, Johnson FS, Wilmore JH. Recommended guidelines for professional weight control programs. Am J Clin Nutr 1984;40:865–872.

51. Miller WC. Diet composition, energy intake, and nutritional status in relation to obesity in men and women. Med Sci Sport Exercise 1991;23:280–284.

52. Donato K, Hegsted DM. Efficiency of utilization of various sources of energy for growth. Proc Natl Acad Sci USA 1985;82:4866–4870.

53. Hill JO, Sparling PB, Shields TW, Heller PA. Effects of exercise and food restriction on body composition and metabolic rate in obese women. Am J Clin Nutr 1987;46:622–630.

54. Pi-Sunyer FX, Woo R. Effect of exercise on food intake in human subjects. Am J Clin Nutr 1985;42:983–990.

55. Stunkard AJ. Conservative treatments for obesity. Am J Clin Nutr 1987;45(suppl.):1142–1154.

Suggested Reading

Forbes GB. Body composition as affected by physical activity and nutrition. Fed Proc 1985;44:343–347.

Foreyt JP, Goodnick GK. Living without dieting. Houston: Harrison, 1992.

Roberts SB. Energy expenditure and the development of early obesity. Ann NY Acad Sci 1993;699:18–25.

Wood PD. Impact of experimental manipulation of energy intake and expenditure on body composition. Crit Rev Food Sci Nutr 1993;33:369–373.

American Journal of Clinical Nutrition 1992; 55(2) whole issue.

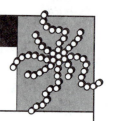

PERSPECTIVE

Eating Disorders

Despite its increasing prevalence in our society, obesity is still considered unacceptable. Few things can create such a sensation in the media as a new weight reduction diet guaranteed to remove that unwanted fat. The authors of the sensational new diet are interviewed on television talk shows; newspapers give publicity to the new diet (and their authors); and the book promoting the "new and revolutionary" diet joins its companions on the shelves of all bookstores. The fact that the new diet book has so many companions in the bookstores attests to the fact that none of these "new and revolutionary" diets is successful in reducing weight and keeping it off. Nevertheless, following some sort of weight reduction diet appears to be a way of life among many Americans, particularly women.

The desire by girls and women to be thin has foundation: the ideal female body image is dictated to a large extent by fashion magazines, *Playboy* centerfolds, and beauty pageant contestants. Children as young as 9 years of age have been found curtailing their food intake to avoid becoming fat [1]. In addition to wanting to conform for aesthetic reasons to the ideal body image, there are advantages of being thin, or at least of normal weight, for educational and professional reasons [2]. Obese girls are less likely to be admitted to college and/or programs of professional training. Furthermore, obese women (as compared with thin women or those of normal weight) have less likelihood of being hired for desirable jobs and/or of being promoted.

Concerns with excessive restriction of body weight include possible stunted growth and delayed sexual maturity of children, but also possible development of eating disorders such as anorexia nervosa and bulimia. Eating disorders are particularly prevalent among young females; in fact, 90 to 95% of the people affected by anorexia nervosa and bulimia are young, white females from middle-class and upper-middle-class families [3]. Some male athletes also appear to be affected. The prevalence of eating disorders among U.S. adolescent girls and young women is estimated between 1 and 4% [4,5].

Anorexia nervosa, described over 100 years ago as "loss of appetite due to a morbid mental state," is actually misnamed because its victims do not have a loss of appetite unless they have reached a moribund state. Anorectics remain thin through self-inflicted starvation and excessive amounts of strenuous exercise. Diagnos-

tic criteria for anorexia nervosa (Table 1) include refusal to maintain at least 85% of normal weight for height, denial of a low current body weight, fear of gaining weight, and amenorrhea (absence of at least three consecutive menstrual cycles) [6]. In addition, preoccupation with food and abnormal food consumption patterns are typical of anorexia nervosa.

Eating patterns of individuals with anorexia nervosa mostly fall into one of two categories [4,7]: the restricting type or the binge eating–purging type. Anorectics with restricting-type eating will eat to a limited extent without regularly inducing vomiting or misusing laxatives or diuretics. Individuals with binge eating- and purging-type anorexia nervosa alternate between restricting food intake and bouts of binge eating or purge behavior with laxative and/or diuretic misuse or self-induced vomiting [4,8].

TABLE 1 Diagnostic Criteria for 307.1 Anorexia Nervosa

A. Refusal to maintain body weight at or above a minimally normal weight for age and height (e.g., weight loss leading to maintenance of body weight less than 85% of that expected; or failure to make expected weight gain during period of growth, leading to body weight less than 85% of that expected).

B. Intense fear of gaining weight or becoming fat, even though underweight.

C. Disturbance in the way in which one's body weight or shape is experienced, undue influence of body weight or shape on self-evaluation, or denial of the seriousness of the current low body weight.

D. In postmenarcheal females, amenorrhea, i.e., the absence of at least three consecutive menstrual cycles. (A woman is considered to have amenorrhea if her periods occur only following hormone, e.g., estrogen, administration.)

Specify type:

Restricting Type: during the current episode of Anorexia Nervosa, the person has not regularly engaged in binge-eating or purging behavior (i.e., self-induced vomiting or the misuse of laxatives, diuretics, or enemas)

Binge-Eating/Purging Type: during the current episode of Anorexia Nervosa, the person has regularly engaged in binge-eating or purging behavior (i.e., self-induced vomiting or the misuse of laxatives, diuretics, or enemas)

Source: Diagnostic and statistical manual of mental disorders, 4th ed. Washington, DC: American Psychiatric Association, 1994:544–545.

PERSPECTIVE (continued)

TABLE 2 Some Potential Physical Consequences of Anorexia Nervosa and Bulimia

System Affected	Manifestation	
	Anorexia Nervosa	Bulimia
Endocrine/metabolic	Amenorrhea Osteoporosis ↓ Norepinephrine secretion ↑Growth hormone Abnormal temperature regulation	Menstrual irregularities
Cardiovascular	Bradycardia Hypotension Arrhythmias	Cardiac failure (vomiting induced—often via Ipecac)
Renal	↑ Blood urea nitrogen (BUN) ↓ Glomerular filtration rate Edema	Hypokalemia (diuretic induced)
Gastrointestinal	↓ Gastric emptying Constipation	Acute gastric dilation Parotid enlargement Tooth enamel erosion Esophagitis Esophageal tears
Hematologic	Anemia Leukopenia	Hypokalemia (vomiting and laxative induced)
Pulmonary		Aspiration pneumonia

Source: Herzog D, Copeland P. Eating disorders. N Engl J Med 1985;313:295. Reprinted by permission.

The cause(s) of anorexia nervosa is/are unknown, but it seems to be a multifactorial disease. At least two sets of issues and behaviors are entangled. Issues include those concerning food and body weight, and those involving relationships with oneself and with others [9]. Conflict regarding maturation and problems with separation, sexuality, self-esteem, and compulsivity often are associated with the development of anorexia nervosa [10].

The initial weight loss of the anorectic may not always be a result of a deliberate decision to diet; weight loss may occur unintentionally, for example, as the result of the flu or a gastrointestinal disorder [4]. However, following the initial weight loss, whatever its cause, additional diet restriction often coupled with excessive exercise to induce further weight loss is deliberate. Weight loss or control of body weight becomes the overriding goal in life, especially during stressful periods [4,5]. Because the anorectic has such a disturbed body image and such an intense fear of becoming fat, she may continue starving herself to emaciation and even death, should intervention be delayed too long.

The effects of anorexia nervosa on the body are similar to the effects of starvation. Growth and development slow. Adipose tissue, lean body mass, and bone mass are lost. Organ mass may be lost, and/or organ function may become impaired. Hormone and nutrient levels in the blood become altered. Skin typically becomes dry, hair loss occurs, and body temperature drops. Table 2 describes some additional potential physical consequences of anorexia nervosa and of bulimia nervosa.

Bulimia nervosa, another eating disorder, is a condition in which there is recurring binge eating coupled with self-induced vomiting and misuse of laxatives, diuretics, or other medications to prevent weight gain. Binge eating is characterized by a sense of lack of control over eating during the binge episode [6]. A binge is defined as eating an amount of food that is larger than most people would eat during a similar time period and under similar circumstances [6]. Bulimia denotes a ravenous appetite (or "ox hunger") associated with powerlessness to control eating [4]. The incidence of bulimia nervosa is thought to exceed that of anorexia nervosa [7]; however, depending on diagnostic criteria used in the prevalence studies, the prevalence estimates of bulimia vary widely [11]. Criteria [6] for the diagnosis of bulimia nervosa are shown in Table 3.

Bulimia occurs primarily in young women, especially college-aged women who are normal weight or

PERSPECTIVE (continued)

TABLE 3 Diagnostic Criteria for 307.51 Bulimia Nervosa

A. Recurrent episodes of binge eating. An episode of binge eating is characterized by both of the following:
   (1) eating, in a discrete period of time (e.g., within any 2-hour period), an amount of food that is definitely larger than most people would eat during a similar period of time and under similar circumstances
   (2) a sense of lack of control over eating during the episode (e.g., a feeling that one cannot stop eating or control what or how much one is eating)
B. Recurrent inappropriate compensatory behavior in order to prevent weight gain, such as self-induced vomiting; misuse of laxatives, diuretics, enemas, or other medications; fasting; or excessive exercise.
C. The binge eating and inappropriate compensatory behaviors both occur, on average, at least twice a week for 3 months.
D. Self-evaluation is unduly influenced by body shape and weight.
E. The disturbance does not occur exclusively during episodes of Anorexia Nervosa.
Specify type:
   Purging Type: during the current episode of Bulimia Nervosa, the person has regularly engaged in self-induced vomiting or the misuse of laxatives, diuretics, or enemas
   Nonpurging Type: during the current episode of Bulimia Nervosa, the person has used other inappropriate compensatory behaviors, such as fasting or excessive exercise, but has not regularly engaged in self-induced vomiting or the misuse of laxatives, diuretics, or enemas

Source: Diagnostic and statistical manual of mental disorders, 4th ed. Washington, DC: American Psychiatric Association, 1994:549–550.

slightly overweight. The typical bulimic, rather than being overly concerned with losing weight and being very thin like the individual with anorexia nervosa, seeks to be able to eat without gaining weight [4]. Bulimia starts with dieting attempts in which hunger feelings get out of control. These dieting attempts, usually based on food abstinence, lead to binge eating. Once binge eaters discover they can undo the consequences of their overeating by vomiting out the ingested food, they no longer binge only when they are hungry, but also when they are experiencing any distressing emotion [4]. Most binge eating is done privately in the afternoon or evening, with an intake of about 3,500 kcal [12,13]. Favorite foods for binging usually are dessert and snack foods, very high in carbohydrate. Embarrassment usually prevents the bulimic from revealing his or her food-related behavior even to those closest to him or her [3].

Although bulimia may begin around 17 to 18 years of age, diagnosis may not occur until the bulimic is in her (or his) thirties or forties [3]. Diagnosis is usually dependent on self-reported symptoms or treatment for related problems or conditions. Conditions that may develop as the result of repeating vomiting include skin lesions on the dorsal side of the hands especially over the joints, severe dental erosion, swollen enlarged neck glands, reddened eyes, headache, and fluid and electrolyte imbalances. Laxative misuse may exacerbate fluid and electrolyte losses, and when coupled with vomiting, may lead to heart failure. Other potential consequences of bulimia are shown in Table 2.

Eating disorders (Table 4) [6] not meeting the diagnostic criteria of anorexia nervosa or bulimia nervosa also are present with the U.S. population. Characteristics of disordered eating include fear of fatness, restrained eating, binge eating, purge behavior, and distorted body image [14]. Further research is needed to determine if these unspecified eating disorders lead to the development of anorexia nervosa or bulimia nervosa.

Early identification and treatment of eating disorders are crucial if serious complications are to be avoided. Rehabilitation requires a multidisciplinary treatment approach [9]. Yet, even with rehabilitation, many former anorectics and bulimics are unable to totally overcome psychological and/or physical impairment and may return to their dietary practices [3,4]. Clearly, being too thin or engaging in bizarre behaviors to keep from becoming overweight carries health risks just as great or greater than being obese [9]. Combatting these eating disorders is difficult because not only must the victims be treated, but it still appears that the images and values of society must be rehabilitated [15].

References Cited

1. Pugliese MT, Lifshitz F, Grad G, Fort P, Marks-Katz M. Fear of obesity. N Engl J Med 1983;309: 513–518.
2. Love S, Johnson CL. Etiological factors in the development of bulimia. Nutr News 1985;48:5–7.

PERSPECTIVE   (continued)

TABLE 4 307.50 Eating Disorder Not Otherwise Specified

The Eating Disorder Not Otherwise Specified category is for disorders of eating that do not meet the criteria for any specific Eating Disorder. Examples include

1. For females, all of the criteria for Anorexia Nervosa are met except that the individual has regular menses.
2. All of the criteria for Anorexia Nervosa are met except that, despite significant weight loss, the individual's current weight is in the normal range.
3. All of the criteria for Bulimia Nervosa are met except that the binge eating and inappropriate compensatory mechanisms occur at a frequency of less than twice a week or for a duration of less than 3 months.
4. The regular use of inappropriate compensatory behavior by an individual of normal body weight after eating small amounts of food (e.g., self-induced vomiting after the consumption of two cookies).
5. Repeatedly chewing and spitting out, but not swallowing, large amounts of food.
6. Binge-eating disorder: recurrent episodes of binge eating in the absence of the regular use of inappropriate compensatory behaviors characteristic of Bulimia Nervosa.

Source: Diagnostic and statistical manual of mental disorders, 4th ed. Washington, DC: American Psychiatric Association, 1994:550.

3. Herzog DB, Copeland PM. Eating disorders. N Engl J Med 1985;313:295–303.
4. Casper RC. The pathophysiology of anorexia nervosa and bulimia nervosa. Ann Rev Nutr 1986;6:299–316.
5. Revised diagnostic subgroupings for anorexia nervosa. Nutr Rev 1994;52:213–215.
6. Diagnostic and statistical manual of mental disorders, 4th ed. Washington, DC: American Psychiatric Association, 1994.
7. Edwards KI. Obesity, anorexia, and bulimia. Med Clin N Am 1993;77:899–909.
8. Emerson E, Stein D. Anorexia nervosa: Emperical basis for the restricting and bulimic subtypes. J Nutr Ed 1993;25:329–336.
9. Reiff DW, Reiff KKL. Position of the American Dietetic Association: Nutrition intervention in the treatment of anorexia nervosa, bulimia nervosa, and binge eating. J Am Diet Assoc 1994;94:902–907.
10. Practice guidelines for eating disorders. Am J Psychiatry 1993;150:212–218.
11. Stein DM. The prevalence of bulimia: A review of the empirical research. J Nutr Ed 1991;23:205–213.
12. Muuss RE. Adolescent eating disorder: Bulimia. Adolescence 1986;21:257–267.
13. Mitchell JE, Pyle RL, Eckert ED. Frequency and duration of binge-eating episodes in patients with bulimia. Am J Psychiatry 1981;138:835–836.
14. Mellin LM, Irwin CE, Scully S. Prevalence of disordered eating in girls: A survey of middle-class children. J Am Diet Assoc 1992;92:851–853.
15. Bulimia among college students. Nutr Rev 1987;45:10–11.

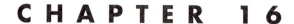
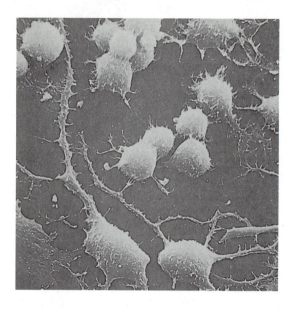

NUTRITION AND THE CENTRAL NERVOUS SYSTEM

Nutrient Precursors of Neurotransmitters
Tryptophan
Tyrosine
Choline and Lecithin

Sugar

Caffeine

Glutamic Acid and Monosodium Glutamate

Aspartame

Perspective: **Hyperactivity in Children**

Photo: Neurons

Energy metabolism in the brain and other parts of the central nervous system (CNS) is very similar to that in other organs and tissues in the body. However, it is the brain's neurological function that is its distinguishing characteristic, and our emotions, behavior, mood, and memory are squarely the responsibility of this organ. A nutritional quest that has generated a great deal of interest is to determine if, and to what extent, the foods we eat affect our neurological characteristics.

Studies designed to explore a correlation between diet and manifestations such as anxiety or sedation, sleepiness or alertness, or even memory capacity span many years. Although such a correlation has not yet been firmly established by scientific investigation, the popular belief throughout the population that it does exist is unrelenting. Consequently, the subject has been fertile ground for scientific inquiry.

The behavioral consequences of malnutrition are well established. Protein calorie malnutrition and vitamin deficiencies interfere in various ways with the normal development of the brain and other tissues of the central nervous system (CNS). Adequate intake of the trace minerals is also necessary for normal brain development, and certain mineral deficiencies, such as those of zinc and iodine, have been implicated in a variety of behavioral alterations such as deficits in long- and short-term memory, apathy, irritability, and depression. It has been reported that lower levels of essential fatty acids were found in the serum of hyperactive youths compared to age- and sex-matched controls [1]. Also, the effect of dietary intervention with essential fatty acids on behavior and learning ability in rats and mice has been extensively researched [2]. The effects of nutritional deficiencies on central nervous system development and behavior are not discussed further in this chapter. However, the subject has been extensively reviewed for the interested reader [3,4].

The focus of this chapter is (1) to discuss nutrient precursors that are required for the synthesis of selected neurotransmitters, and the effect on behavior of their dietary manipulation, and (2) to examine the impact on behavior of several selected food additives and other dietary components that have "rightly or wrongly" been implicated in behavior alteration.

NUTRIENT PRECURSORS OF NEUROTRANSMITTERS

Examples of compounds that are constituents of a normal diet, and that have a neurological association due to their biochemical conversion to neurotransmitters, are tryptophan, tyrosine, and choline. Tryptophan and tyrosine, which are commonly occurring amino acids, are provided by dietary protein. The major source of choline is lecithin. The fact that these substances can be converted into neurotransmitters raised the interesting speculation that foods might produce changes in behavior by altering the levels of brain neurotransmitters that are linked to various psychologic functions. Not all neurotransmitters are influenced by the availability of their dietary precursors, however. It has been proposed that several conditions must be met in order for precursor control of neurotransmitter synthesis and release to occur [5]. These conditions are as follows:

- Plasma levels of the precursor substance must vary in parallel with that of the dietary intake. In other words, there cannot be a control mechanism that regulates the plasma concentration within narrow limits regardless of intake.
- The precursor must be able to cross the blood–brain barrier so that synaptic synthesis of the transmitter can take place.
- The transport mechanism by which the nutrient precursor is carried from the blood into the cells of the brain must not be saturated, allowing it to accommodate more precursor as plasma levels of the precursor rise.
- The enzyme(s) catalyzing the conversion of precursor to transmitter must be of low affinity (high K_m; see p. 19). Under such a condition, the amount of precursor available becomes the rate-limiting factor in neurotransmitter synthesis.
- There cannot be feedback inhibition of the catalytic enzyme(s) as the level of product (neurotransmitter) rises.

All five of these conditions are met for the neurotransmitter serotonin, produced in the brain from the amino acid tryptophan, and for acetylcholine, formed from choline or lecithin. Although less dramatically demonstrated, control of the synthesis of the neurotransmitters norepinephrine (NE) and dopamine (DA) from their precursor tyrosine has also been observed. Before beginning a discussion of the biosynthesis and physiology of these neurotransmitters, a brief review of the process of synaptic transmission may be appropriate.

The cellular units that make up the brain and peripheral CNS are called *neurons*, which are estimated to number nearly 100 billion in the brain alone. Each neuron transmits and receives electrical signals through filamentous appendages called *axons* and *dendrites*. Signals pass through the axon of a transmitting neuron and impinge on the dendrite of a receiving neuron. The transmission of the impulse from an axon to the receiving cell takes place across a narrow gap referred to as the *synapse* and is mediated by chemical substances known as *neurotransmitters*. An average neuron possesses several thousand synaptic junctions, and these can be situated between intercellular axon and axon, dendrite and dendrite, and axon and cell body as well as between axon and dendrite.

Nutrient precursors of the neurotransmitters must be transported from the brain capillaries into the neurons where the synthesis of the transmitters takes place. The junctions between the capillary endothelial cells in the brain are too tight to allow passage by diffusion of tryptophan, tyrosine, or choline, and therefore these precursors must be transported through the capillary wall (cross the blood–brain barrier) by carrier molecules. The capillary receptor sites at which the precursors are picked up by the carrier molecule are not absolutely specific, and a competition among structurally similar compounds for a given receptor may take place. This is exemplified by the competition for a common carrier of large, neutral amino acids (LNAAs), included among which are tryptophan and tyrosine. This explains why neuronal serotonin synthesis is stimulated by dietary carbohydrate even though the neurotransmitter is derived from the amino acid tryptophan. This is discussed in more detail in the following section on tryptophan. The enzymatic conversion of choline, tryptophan, and tyrosine into their respective neurotransmitters, acetylcholine, serotonin, and norepinephrine, takes place in the presynaptic terminal of the neuron, where they are stored.

When a signal entering the brain or traveling from one brain cell to another arrives at the synapse, it causes the neurotransmitters to be released into the synaptic gap. The compounds complete the synaptic transmission of the signal by interacting with specific receptors on the postsynaptic terminal of the cell. Following completion

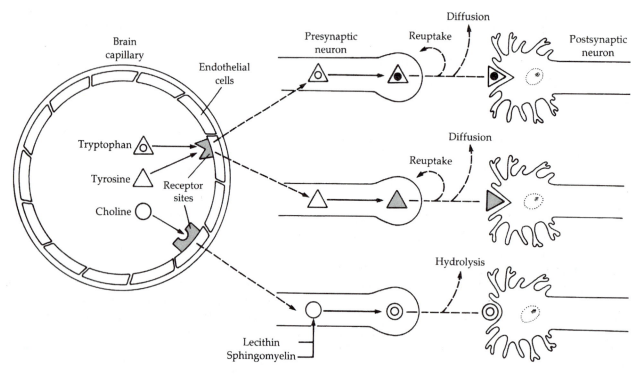

FIGURE 16.1 The conversion of the nutrient precursors tryptophan, tyrosine, and choline into their respective neurotransmitters, serotonin (△), norepinephrine (▲), and acetylcholine (◎). Migration of the transmitters across the synaptic junction and interaction with postsynaptic receptors complete a nerve signal. Also indicated is the competition between tryptophan and tyrosine (as well as other LNAAs) for common receptor sites on the capillary endothelium.

of the transmission of the signal, the neurotransmitters must be inactivated to prevent protracted "firing" of the synapse. In the case of acetylcholine, the molecule is hydrolyzed by acetylcholinesterase into the products acetic acid and choline. The choline may then be taken up by the presynaptic terminal or returned to the blood stream, from which it can once again re-enter the brain cells by carrier-mediated transport, as described previously. Inactivation of the catecholamine neurotransmitters norepinephrine and dopamine is primarily by their reuptake at the presynaptic terminal. However, the portion escaping reuptake can be enzymatically inactivated by monoamine oxidase (MAO) and catechol-O-methyl transferase (COMT). MAO is also involved in the enzymatic inactivation of serotonin. Figure 16.1 summarizes the transport of blood-borne nutrient precursors into the neuron, their conversion into neurotransmitters, and the release and reuptake of the neurotransmitters in bringing about a transynaptic signal.

Tryptophan

Conversion to Serotonin The behavioral effects of tryptophan, an amino acid present in nearly all dietary

sources of protein, is due to its biochemical conversion to serotonin in the neuron (see 16A).

Behavioral Effects Numerous studies correlating dietary tryptophan consumption with psychologic manifestations such as activity and aggression, sensory responses, sleep, mood, and performance have not produced clearly definitive conclusions. It is generally conceded, however, with substantial experimental backing, that tryptophan does exert a calming effect, inducing drowsiness and alleviating aggressive behavior. It may do this either by elevating brain serotonin levels or by reducing the amount of tyrosine entering the neurons because of competition for a common carrier across the capillary endothelium. As discussed later, tyrosine can elevate mood in certain cases of depression, and its deficiency can result in lethargy.

Tryptophan, being an essential amino acid, cannot be synthesized by humans or other mammals. Since the body's nutritional supply of tryptophan is acquired through dietary protein, it is logical to assume that a meal rich in protein should elevate tryptophan and therefore serotonin, resulting in a calming, drowsy effect. In actu-

(16A)

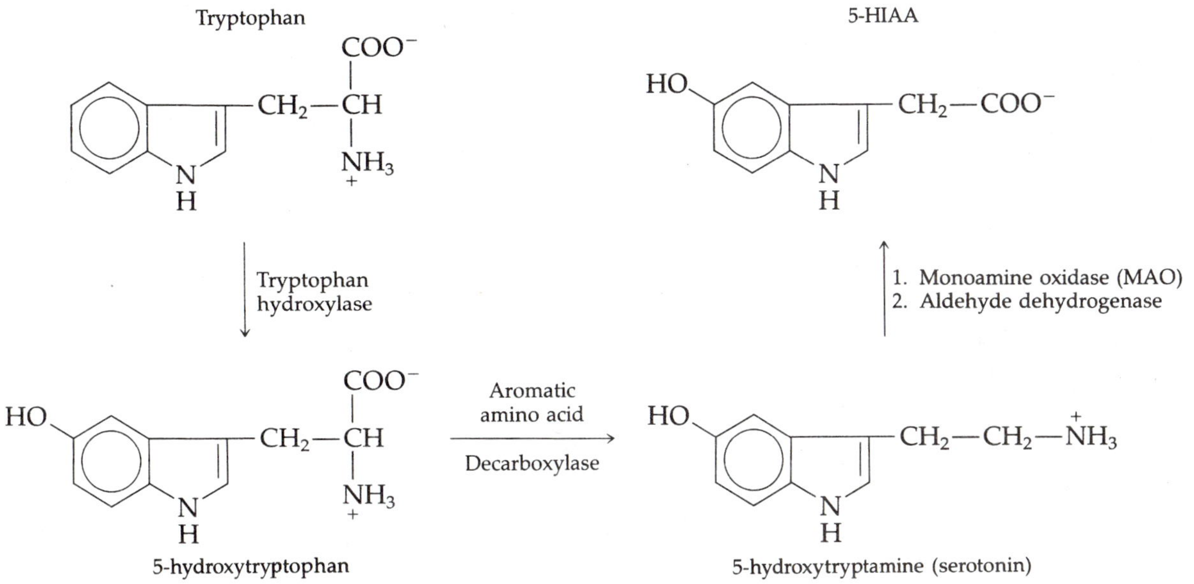

Tryptophan

5-HIAA

Tryptophan hydroxylase

1. Monoamine oxidase (MAO)
2. Aldehyde dehydrogenase

5-hydroxytryptophan

Aromatic amino acid Decarboxylase

5-hydroxytryptamine (serotonin)

ality, the opposite occurs. Following a protein-rich meal, brain levels of tryptophan and serotonin decline. This is because most dietary protein contains considerably more LNAAs, such as valine, leucine, tyrosine, and phenylalanine, than tryptophan; and since all the LNAAs compete for a common carrier molecule for transport into the neurons, the brain influx of tryptophan declines relative to its competitors. Tyrosine uptake would therefore take preference over tryptophan uptake, and the mood affectation would predictably be more stimulatory than sedating. Paradoxically, it is the meal low in protein but rich in carbohydrate that increases brain tryptophan and serotonin even though the food may lack tryptophan completely. This is because a protein-poor, carbohydrate-rich meal increases the ratio of plasma tryptophan to the other LNAAs, a fact attributed to the carbohydrate-induced release of insulin that stimulates the uptake into muscle cells of most of the LNAAs other than tryptophan. It has been shown that among subjects who have fasted overnight, insulin secretion triggered by carbohydrate intake causes a 40 to 60% decline in plasma valine, leucine, and isoleucine and a 15 to 30% decrease in tyrosine. Plasma tryptophan levels, in contrast, do not decline, an observation thought to be due to its binding to albumin molecules at sites previously occupied by free fatty acids that were released by the action of the hormone. As a result, less receptor competition from other LNAAs causes an increased brain influx of tryptophan, resulting in ele-

vated neuronal serotonin. The effectiveness of the "milk and cookies before bedtime" regimen to help induce sleepiness and sedation is not, as once believed, due to the tryptophan in the casein but rather to the high carbohydrate content of that favorite combination. Figure 16.2 illustrates the relationship between brain tryptophan levels and the ingestion of meals having varying proportions of protein and carbohydrate [6].

The sedating effect of serotonin (and therefore carbohydrate intake) and how it relates to certain emotional disorders is exemplified by the fact that patients afflicted with either seasonal affective disorder (SAD), carbohydrate-craving obesity (CCO), or premenstrual syndrome (PMS) appear to share a tendency to crave carbohydrate snacks [7]. Among SAD patients, the seasonal effect on eating disorders is evidenced in Figure 16.3, which shows that carbohydrate snacking constitutes a significantly higher percentage of total carbohydrate intake during the fall of the year compared to springtime.

Further corroboration of the relationship between serotonin levels and carbohydrate craving is found in the effect of drugs that prolong the neuronal effect of serotonin. d-Fenfluramine, which releases serotonin into brain synapses and prolongs its action by blocking its reuptake, selectively suppresses carbohydrate snacking in CCO patients and simultaneously eases symptoms of depression [8]. There is recent evidence that it may be similarly effective in the treatment of PMS [7].

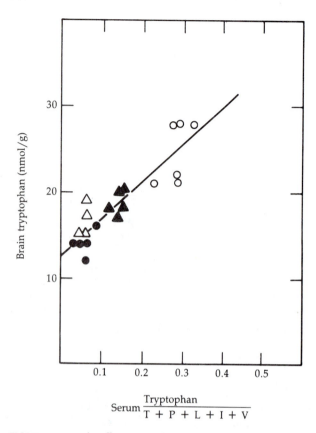

$$\text{Serum} \frac{\text{Tryptophan}}{\text{T + P + L + I + V}}$$

FIGURE 16.2 The effect in rats of variations in the ratio of dietary protein to carbohydrate on the relationship between serum tryptophan and the brain uptake of tryptophan. (○), animals ingesting no protein (high carbohydrate); (▲), rats consuming 18% protein; (△), rats consuming 40% protein; (●), fasting controls. Capital letters denote the other LNAAs: T (tyrosine), P (phenylalanine), L (leucine), I (isoleucine), V (valine). *(Fernstrom JD, Faller DV. Neutral amino acids in the brain: Changes in response to food ingestion. J Neurochem 1978;30:1531–1538.)*

Tyrosine

Conversion to Dopamine, Norepinephrine, and Epinephrine Dopamine, norepinephrine, and epinephrine are compounds referred to as *catecholamines* because they are derivatives of catechol (see 16B).

It would be appropriate to regard the essential amino acid phenylalanine as a precursor of these catecholamine transmitters also, since it is readily converted to tyrosine by the action of phenylalanine hydroxylase (p. 175). However, it has been estimated that nearly 90% of the brain catecholamines are synthesized directly from naturally occurring tyrosine. The biosynthetic pathway of the catecholamines is shown in 16C.

Certain neurons contain the enzymes tyrosine hydroxylase (TOH) and aromatic amino acid decarboxylase (AAAD) but lack dopamine-β-hydroxylase

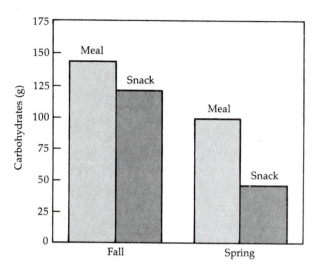

FIGURE 16.3 The seasonal effect of carbohydrate craving in SAD patients. In the fall of the year, carbohydrate snacks account for nearly 50% of the total carbohydrate intake whereas they represent less than 30% in the spring. *(Wurtman RS, Wurtman JJ. Carbohydrates and depression. Sci Am 1989;260:68–75. Copyright © 1989 by Scientific American, Inc. All rights reserved.)*

(16B)

Catechol

(DBH). Dopamine therefore becomes the final product in these neurons. In contrast, noradrenergic neurons have DBH activity in addition to TOH and AAAD, and therefore the dopamine produced in these cells is rapidly β-hydroxylated to norepinephrine. Neurons generally have little phenylethanolamine-N-methyl transferase (PNMT) activity and consequently synthesize only small amounts of epinephrine. Most of this hormone is produced in the adrenal medulla, where a considerably higher activity of PNMT exists. Although it is a potent stimulator of glycogenolysis (p. 82) and elevates blood pressure by interaction with blood vessel β-receptors, epinephrine's role as a brain neurotransmitter is of little importance and will not be discussed further in this connection.

Behavioral Effects There exist two popularly held explanations for the primary form of depression—that which is brought on by a neurochemical imbalance. One

(16C)

Phenylalanine → Tyrosine →(TOH)→ Dihydroxyphenylalanine (DOPA) →(AAAD)→ Dopamine →(DBH)→ Norepinephrine →(PNMT)→ Epinephrine

explanation attributes the condition to a deficiency of serotonin; the other, to inadequate norepinephrine. Evidence that there may be some validity to these theories is that primary depression can be treated with drugs such as MAO inhibitors, which maintain higher brain levels of these neurotransmitters. It is therefore not unreasonable to assume that similar results may be achieved by increasing the level of these neurotransmitters through an increased dietary intake of their precursors. But although the concentration of brain cell norepinephrine and dopamine do rise, concomitant with increased precursor (tyrosine) intake, the effect of tyrosine loading on behavior alteration remains controversial. One reason for the lack of a clear-cut relationship between tyrosine administration and behavior modification may be that the effect on a given neuron of an increased supply of the nutrient depends on the firing rate of that neuron [9]. This is evidenced by the observation that tyrosine administration does not ordinarily increase the release of dopamine from dopamine-releasing neurons, even though brain concentrations of tyrosine increase. Yet under conditions in which the firing frequency of the neurons is markedly increased, such as would occur with dopamine-depleting lesions, dopamine receptor blockade by drugs, or Parkinson's disease, tyrosine does enhance the release of the neurotransmitter.

Choline and Lecithin

Nearly all the choline consumed in a normal diet is in the form of choline phosphatides such as lecithin and sphingomyelin, since free choline is present in only small amounts in foods. The richest food sources of

lecithin are natural; for example, eggs, liver, soybeans, wheat germ, and peanuts.

The free choline pool from which the neurotransmitter acetylcholine (discussed next) is synthesized is maintained through several mechanisms, one of which is the enzymatic hydrolysis of lecithin and sphingomyelin. The phospholipases that are responsible for this hydrolytic breakdown are quite active in brain cells, thereby releasing choline directly into the cholinergic neurons where acetylation then occurs. Free choline can also enter cerebral cells from the plasma by a choline-specific transport system across the blood–brain barrier. In the maintenance of neuronal concentrations of free choline, however, the outward flux of choline from the cells into the plasma exceeds the cellular uptake. Nevertheless, the specific transport system is believed to play a key role in the use of choline for acetylcholine synthesis. The richest source of precursor choline, however, is the reuse of endogenous choline formed from the hydrolysis of acetylcholine by acetylcholinesterase following synaptic transmission.

Taken in large amounts, dietary lecithin increases the plasma concentration of choline and therefore its intracellular brain levels. Unlike free choline, the glycerophosphatide is believed not to cross the blood–brain barrier to a significant degree, because of its tenacious binding to plasma albumin. These facts, taken together, therefore suggest that the higher plasma concentrations of choline arise from an accelerated peripheral hydrolysis of the additional lecithin. It appears that the relationships among blood and brain choline, dietary choline and choline-containing lipids, and brain acetylcholine are quite complex. The possibility exists that any behavioral effects (discussed later) of feeding large quantities of choline or lecithin may be indirect and may arise through mechanisms that are not as yet clearly understood.

Conversion to Acetylcholine   In the presynaptic terminal of the neuron, acetylcholine is formed by a reversible reaction between choline and acetyl CoA. The reaction is catalyzed by choline acetyltransferase (CAT):

$$\text{Choline + acetyl CoA} \xrightarrow{\text{choline acetyltransferase (CAT)}} \text{acetylcholine + CoA}$$

Experiments have demonstrated that the level of choline in cholinergic neurons is well below the K_m of CAT. Therefore the enzyme is not normally saturated, a condition that, it will be recalled, must be in effect if nutrient precursor concentrations are to have a bearing on the rate of transmitter formation.

Although the source of acetyl CoA for the synthesis of acetylcholine continues to be investigated, it is generally accepted that acetyl CoA is formed indirectly from glucose by neuronal glycolysis and directly through the action of the pyruvate dehydrogenase complex of enzymes (p. 92). The source of the free choline has already been discussed.

Behavioral Effects   There is evidence for a linking of the central cholinergic system to learning and memory in both experimental animals and humans. The most convincing findings supporting this connection have been pharmacologic. In normal people, cholinergic antagonists such as scopolamine, which block the interaction of acetylcholine with its postsynaptic receptors, produce memory deficits. Such deficits resemble those observed among elderly people. The disturbance can be reversed by physostigmine, a cholinesterase inhibitor that prevents the degradation of acetylcholine by acetylcholinesterase within the synapse. It is not surprising therefore that since the intake of large amounts of acetylcholine precursors increases the neuronal concentration and release of the neurotransmitter, there is a great deal of interest in the possible enhancement of cognitive ability and memory through dietary precursor loading.

The beneficial effect of dietary choline in bringing about an improvement in memory remains controversial, due in part to the fact that an age factor appears to be involved. Choline has been found to produce an improvement in memory among normal young subjects. In contrast, when tested on elderly people for whom memory disturbance may represent a significant clinical problem, acetylcholine precursor feeding has yielded disappointing results. It has been proposed that a combination of lecithin loading together with physostigmine administration may alleviate memory deficits in the elderly.

It is believed that among the neurologic disturbances of Alzheimer's disease is a cholinergic deficiency attributable to a reduction in the activity of choline acetyltransferase. Predictably, any measures that would tend to increase neuronal acetylcholine may therefore help to allay the deficiency in recall memory associated with this disease. Temporary improvement has been observed following physostigmine treatment, but dietary loading with neurotransmitter precursors has had marginal benefit. A study in which lecithin was fed to Alzheimer's patients in the early stages of the disease indicated that an improvement in learning ability occurred in some of the patients and that the improvement reversed after discontinuation of the lecithin loading [10]. Only a small number of subjects was used in the study, however, and it is clear that more research is required to establish any efficacy of lecithin or choline feeding in the treatment of this disease. Lecithin is generally preferred to choline in such studies because of the foul odor of trimethylamine, produced by the enzymatic breakdown of free choline in the digestive tract.

The most convincing clinical evidence for a link between nutrient precursor loading and neurotransmitter function concerns patients afflicted with tardive dyskinesia, a condition characterized by uncontrollable movements of the face and upper body. In most patients it is caused by the prolonged administration of certain antipsychotic drugs and is considered to be the major side effect limiting the use of those drugs [9]. Following studies that showed physostigmine to be effective in calming the abnormal movements, it was subsequently demonstrated also that increasing brain acetylcholine by feeding choline had a similar effect. The results of these particular investigations are considered reliable in view of the large number of subjects involved and the fact that a double-blind, placebo-controlled protocol was used. For the reason mentioned earlier, lecithin has largely replaced choline as a dietary test precursor.

The behavioral effects of the nutrients tryptophan, tyrosine, and choline and lecithin have been reviewed in depth by Spring [5]. The review also includes an informative discussion of the methods by which mood and/or behavioral effects of nutrients are assessed; it is recommended as supplemental reading.

Clearly, the nutrients discussed to this point, those that serve as precursors for the neurotransmitters, are of vital importance, because neurotransmitters are essential for normal neurologic function. Furthermore, the importance of the nutrients dictates that they be readily available through a normal diet. Proteins and choline-containing lipids furnish these precursors for the neurotransmitters discussed. However, other food components that can be categorized as nutritive or non-nutritive additives are commonly included in a typical diet, and affect, or allegedly affect, behavior and CNS function. In the following sections, several representative compounds of current interest are discussed.

SUGAR

No dietary substance has received more bad press than sugar in its alleged negative effect on behavior. Fostering this belief are the sensational reports linking sugar consumption to a multiplicity of behavioral disturbances such as hyperactivity, depression, mental confusion, and antisocial behavior. An example of society's negative view of sugar is revealed in the celebrated case of a fatal shooting in 1979 of the San Francisco mayor and another city official. Lawyers for the perpetrator in the case argued that their client had acted irrationally, and suffered "diminished mental capacity" as a result of his over-consumption of sugar-containing junk foods. The argument has come to be called the "Twinkie defense." It was successful in reducing the charge against the perpetrator from first-degree murder to manslaughter, an outcome that still makes some forensic experts cringe.

The hypothesized connection between antisocial behavior and sugar consumption exists in two parts: (1) the belief that the intake of simple sugars causes reactive hypoglycemia due to an insulin response to the elevated blood sugar, and (b) reports, such as that of Virkkunen [11], that reactive hypoglycemia may correlate with the habitual violent behavior displayed by some criminals and delinquents. Such conclusions must be viewed with caution, however, considering that simple sugars do not necessarily increase blood sugar levels any more than do foods containing complex carbohydrates. Secondly, low blood glucose levels do not necessarily correlate with the clinical symptoms of hypoglycemia, which include (1) low circulating blood glucose levels (<50 mg/dL); (2) symptoms including sweating, palpitations, anxiety, headaches, weakness, and hunger; and (3) alleviation of these symptoms when plasma glucose levels are restored to normal following food ingestion. Low blood glucose levels can occur in the absence of any symptoms of the condition, and conversely, symptoms of reactive hypoglycemia may manifest in the absence of low blood glucose levels [12].

Studies linking sugar intake to antisocial behavior have also been complicated by a weakness in their experimental design. The independent variable, sugar intake, is difficult to quantify and control, and the dependent variable, changes in antisocial behavior, is also very difficult to measure objectively. Despite the experimental shortcomings of the investigations, the public's view persists that sugar can contribute to antisocial behavior and also to hyperactivity (the subject of this chapter's "Perspective" section). Convincing arguments in support of the alleged sugar–behavior connection have not yet been forthcoming, but it is a premise that is important enough to warrant further, well-designed studies.

CAFFEINE

Caffeine belongs to a group of compounds referred to as the *methylxanthines*. Its chemical name is 1,3,7-trimethylxanthine, and it is one of the most widely consumed, pharmacologically active dietary substances. It occurs naturally in several plant components such as coffee bean, tea leaf, kola nut, and cacao seed, most of it being consumed in the form of beverages containing extracts of these plant sources. Among the major caffeine-containing beverages are coffee (50 to 150 mg/cup), tea (approximately 50 mg/cup), and cola drinks (about 35 mg/12 oz). Table 16.1 lists average daily consumption of caffeine by consumer age, according to a survey by the Market Research Corporation of America. A detailed and comprehensive review of the human consumption of caffeine, based on extensive market research surveys, has been published [13].

Caffeine is also present in various over-the-counter medications, including analgesics, appetite suppressants, and CNS stimulants (see 16D). Chocolate contains some caffeine but contains a much larger amount of another methylxanthine, theobromine (3,7-dimethylxanthine), which exerts pharmacologic effects similar to those of caffeine. Although it is not a food or food component, the methylxanthine theophylline (1,3-dimethylxanthine) warrants mention at this point. It is a synthetic drug used in the treatment of pulmonary disorders such as emphysema and asthma, and predictably, its side affects are pharmacologically caffeine-like.

The brain seems to be the organ most sensitive to caffeine. Wakefulness or sleep latency is probably the most common manifestation of caffeine consumption, the period of sleep latency nearly doubling in some subjects by a single serving of 1 to 2 mg/kg body weight (equivalent to about two cups of coffee). The "alerting" effects of caffeine, those that allow an individual to func-

Table 16.1 Mean Daily Consumption of Caffeine (mg/kg Body Weight) by Age According to the Market Research Corporation of America Survey

Age (years)	Source				
	All Sources	Coffee	Tea	Soft Drinks	Chocolate
Under 1	0.18	0.009	0.13	0.02	0.02
1–5	1.20	0.11	0.57	0.34	0.16
6–11	0.85	0.10	0.41	0.21	0.13
12–17	0.74	0.16	0.34	0.16	0.08
18 and over	2.60	2.1	0.41	0.10	0.03

Source: Barone JJ, Roberts H. Human consumption of caffeine. In: Dews PB, ed. Caffeine: Perspectives from human research. Berlin: Springer-Verlag, 1984:66.

(16D)

Caffeine

tion in the face of fatigue, can be experienced in regular caffeine consumers after a single dose of 2 to 3 mg/kg body weight. In fact, regular users experience improved visual reaction times and auditory alertness at much lower doses (0.5 mg/kg) [14]. Interestingly, doses of this magnitude can cause irritability and nervousness among nonconsumers of caffeine, and even among regular consumers who have abstained from the substance for a period of time.

Although the excitatory effect of the methylxanthines on the CNS is obvious, their mechanism of action is not fully understood. Earlier proposed mechanisms focused on the ability of these agents to inhibit the action of phosphodiesterase, an enzyme that hydrolyzes cyclic adenosine monophosphate (cAMP). This would tend to maintain elevated levels of cAMP, resulting in neural excitation, since cAMP is considered to be a second messenger for neurotransmitter–receptor systems. The results of much research in this area, however, indicate that such a mechanism cannot be wholly responsible for the stimulatory action of the methylxanthines. Probably the most significant revelation in this regard is that the concentration of methylxanthines required to inhibit phosphodiesterase *in vivo* is generally higher than that at which CNS stimulation occurs.

A second proposed mechanism of action of caffeine derives from its ability to inhibit the passage of chloride ions across neuronal membranes at sites referred to as *chloride channels.* The chloride channel is closely associated with neuronal inhibition. As the chloride flux increases, the membrane conductance to chloride ion increases in parallel, resulting in suppression of neuronal activity. By antagonizing this effect, caffeine reduces chloride conductance and therefore stimulates neuronal activity.

Perhaps the single, most convincing explanation for the effect of caffeine on the CNS relates to its action as an antagonist to the naturally occurring substance adenosine. Adenosine can inhibit neuronal activity and behavior both through direct action at postsynaptic sites on neurons as well as by an indirect effect involving presynaptic inhibition of neurotransmitter release. The structural similarity of caffeine and adenosine allows the successful competition of caffeine for adenosine receptors, thereby countering the inhibitory effect of adenosine on the neuron. It appears, however, that chronic caffeine intake may lead to an increase in the number of adenosine receptor sites. As a consequence, the effect of endogenous adenosine would be magnified, and larger amounts of exogenous caffeine would therefore be necessary to restore the adenosine–caffeine balance. If this balance should suddenly be shifted by decreasing or abruptly stopping caffeine intake, the excess adenosine receptors would no longer be blocked by caffeine, thereby intensifying the adenosine effect. It has been suggested that the exaggerated response to adenosine that would follow contributes to caffeine withdrawal symptoms [15].

Stimulant drugs are the medication of choice in the treatment of attention deficit disorder associated with hyperactivity in children. Consequently, an interest in caffeine developed in this regard, particularly since early

(16E)

$$CH_2—COOH$$
$$|$$
$$CH_2$$
$$|$$
$$\overset{+}{H_3N}—CH—COOH$$
Glutamic acid

$$CH_2—COOH$$
$$|$$
$$CH_2$$
$$|$$
$$\overset{+}{H_3N}—CH—COO^-Na^+$$
Monosodium glutamate (MSG)

(16F)

$$COO^-$$
$$|$$
$$CH_2$$
$$|$$
$$CH_2$$
$$|$$
$$\overset{+}{H_3N}—CH—COO^-$$
Glutamate

$$\xrightarrow[\text{CO}_2]{\text{Glutamate}\atop\text{decarboxylase}}$$

$$COO^-$$
$$|$$
$$CH_2$$
$$|$$
$$CH_2$$
$$|$$
$$\overset{+}{H_3N}—CH_2$$
γ-aminobutyrate

reports claimed it to be as beneficial as methylphenidate hydrochloride (Ritalin), a frequently prescribed stimulant [16]. A much more recent study [17] also showed that high doses of caffeine (600 mg/d) significantly eased hyperactive behavior. The untoward side effects of such high intake levels of caffeine (nausea, insomnia) argue against the use of the substance clinically. Furthermore, there is a consensus that, based on the majority of experimental results, caffeine offers little therapeutic value compared to prescription drugs [18].

GLUTAMIC ACID AND MONOSODIUM GLUTAMATE

Glutamic acid is one of several amino acids known to be active as neurotransmitters (see 16E). It is one of the most active neuroexcitatory substances present in the CNS of vertebrates. Other amino acids having neurotransmitter activity are aspartic acid and γ-amino butyric acid (GABA). In the brain, glutamate functions as the precursor for GABA, a very important inhibitory transmitter. The conversion involves the removal of the γ-carboxyl group of glutamate by the enzyme glutamate decarboxylase, which is therefore instrumental in maintaining an excitatory–inhibitory steady state (see 16F).

Interest in glutamate and particularly its monosodium salt arose from the observation that it can cause anatomic lesions in the hypothalamus of certain animal species that had received large quantities of the substance. In addition, the incidence of discomforts that may occur among consumers of monosodium glutamate (MSG) as a dietary additive invited a great deal of research and speculation as to the etiology of the symptoms. It should be emphasized that there is no evidence linking these physiologic effects of MSG to the transmitter role of glutamate. Furthermore, behavior alteration *per se* is not among the effects reported as a result of ingesting the substance. The justification for devoting a small portion of this chapter to a discussion of gluta-

mate is the interesting paradox that it can be toxic to the body in spite of the fact that it is a natural, ubiquitous amino acid present in most dietary proteins.

It is known from studies dating back to 1969 [19] that MSG, if administered in large quantities by either gavage or parenterally to infant mice, has neurotoxic effects. Specifically it results in a selective lesion of the hypothalamus, marked by the destruction of neurons in the nucleus arcuatus of that portion of the brain. It became known as the nucleus arcuatus of the hypothalamus (NAH) lesion, and it was subsequently shown to be inducible in other animal species. Reports on behavior modification by MSG are sketchy at best, however, even when the compound is administered in NAH-inducing amounts. Some such reports allude to a deficiency of discriminatory learning in certain laboratory animals. It is important to note that there is a clear-cut difference in the neurotoxicity of MSG when administered parenterally or by gavage, on the one hand, and by dietary administration, on the other. No threshold dose of dietary MSG causing neurotoxicity has been detected in any animal species. This is explained by the fact that even at high doses, MSG consumed as part of the diet never induces the elevated plasma levels obtained with much lower doses administered by gavage or subcutaneously.

MSG is widely used as a taste and flavor enhancer, or as a salt substitute, in western and particularly Asian countries. As mentioned previously, its ingestion by some individuals can cause physiologic distress referred to as the "Chinese restaurant syndrome," which is most commonly marked by headache, lightheadedness, and a tightening feeling in the face. The syndrome is particularly interesting in view of the normal abundance of cellular glutamate in mainstream metabolism. Again, the relationship of the symptoms to the neuroexcitatory function of glutamate has not been established, and the cause for the idiosyncratic distress remains obscure. The possibility that the symptoms are related to an allergic reaction has not been ruled out.

(16G)

$$\underset{\text{Aspartame}}{\overset{+}{H_3N}-\overset{\overset{\displaystyle COO^-}{|}}{\underset{|}{CH_2}}-\overset{\overset{\displaystyle CH_2}{|}}{\underset{|}{CH}}-\overset{\overset{\displaystyle O}{||}}{C}-NH-\overset{\overset{\displaystyle CH_2}{|}}{\underset{|}{CH}}-\overset{\overset{\displaystyle O}{||}}{C}-O-CH_3}$$

ASPARTAME

The popularity of the artificial sweetener aspartame within our weight-conscious population stems from the fact that although it has the same number of calories per gram as sucrose, it delivers 180 to 200 times the sweetening power of the sugar.

Chemically, aspartame, commonly known by its trade name Nutrasweet, is a methyl ester of a dipeptide (L-aspartyl-L-phenylalanine methyl ester, see 16G).

Aspartame is possibly the most thoroughly studied food additive ever approved by the U.S. Food and Drug Administration (FDA) in terms of the total number of studies conducted prior to approval. This is because the widespread use of the sweetener provoked reports of various reactions attributed to a sensitivity to the substance. The Centers for Disease Control (CDC) investigated 517 consumer complaints and found that 67% involved neurologic or behavioral symptoms, primarily headaches. The results of this study are recorded in Table 16.2 [20]. Whether or not neurotoxic effects are indeed experienced by some aspartame consumers is still being debated. Among the investigators who subscribe to the relationship, some have proposed mechanisms for the neurotoxicity of aspartame based on the manner in which it is metabolized in the body.

Ingested aspartame is absorbed and metabolized in one of two ways. It may be hydrolyzed in the intestinal lumen to aspartate, phenylalanine, and methanol by hydrolytic enzymes. These components are absorbed from the lumen and reach the portal blood in a manner similar to that of amino acids and methanol arising from dietary protein or polysaccharides. Alternatively, aspartame may be demethylated in the intestinal lumen to yield the dipeptide aspartyl-phenylalanine and methanol. The dipeptide is then absorbed directly into mucosal cells by peptide transport mechanisms, with subsequent hydrolysis to aspartate and phenylalanine within the en-

Table 16.2 CDC Evaluation of Consumer Complaints Related to Aspartame Use

System	Complaint
CNS	Mood changes
	Insomnia
	Seizures
Gastrointestinal	Abdominal pain
	Nausea
	Diarrhea
Gynecologic	Irregular
	menses

Source: Morbidity and mortality weekly report. Atlanta: Centers for Disease Control 1984(33)43:605.

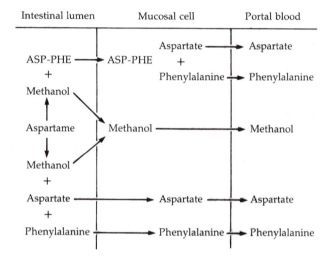

FIGURE 16.4 The hydrolysis of aspartame in the intestinal lumen and the mucosal cell. The hydrolytic products aspartate, phenylalanine, and methanol are delivered to the portal circulation as shown. (Stegink CD. The aspartame story. A model for the clinical testing of a food additive. Am J Clin Nutr 1987;46:204–215. © Am J Clin Nutr American Society for Clinical Nutrition.)

terocytes. In either case the ingestion of large doses of aspartame releases aspartate, phenylalanine, and methanol into the portal blood, and these must be metabolized and/or excreted. Aspartame metabolism is summarized in Figure 16.4.

Proposed mechanisms for aspartame neurotoxicity have focused on the resulting increase in plasma phenylalanine. This is not surprising in view of the frank brain damage manifested by the high plasma/brain cell concentrations of phenylalanine and its metabolites in the disease phenylketonuria (PKU) (p. 175). To put doses and toxicities in their proper perspective, however, it should be pointed out that although the toxic plasma threshold is estimated to be nearly 100 μmol/dL for normal adults, a loading dose of 34 mg aspartame/kg body weight increases plasma phenylalanine levels from 6 μmol/dL to only 11 μmol/dL. This is still well within the normal range. A loading dose of 200 mg/kg, equivalent to consuming 24 L of aspartame-sweetened beverage, increases the plasma phenylalanine value to approximately 49 μmol/dL, still well below the toxicity threshold. Nevertheless, the impaired metabolism of phenylalanine in the PKU patient would of course result in correspondingly higher plasma concentrations, and it is for this reason that all aspartame-containing products are mandated by the FDA to display the warning label "Phenylketonurics: Contains Phenylalanine." Another concern, even among normal people, is the possibility that phenylalanine neurotoxicity may be linear rather than threshold. The threshold concept implies that no toxicity results until a certain threshold plasma concentration is attained. The threshold level of nearly 100 μmol/dL cited earlier is based on the observation that while mental retardation is evident in PKU children having plasma concentrations of 120 to 600 μmol/dL, it is not discernible among patients having levels up to 50 μmol/dL. If the relationship between hyperphenylalaninemia and brain effects is a linear function, however, then increases in plasma phenylalanine up to 100 μmol/dL may have subtle but definite effects on the brain that may not be observed clinically.

Phenylalanine may have neurologic effects at a blood and brain concentration well below the neurotoxic levels associated with PKU. The basis for this premise is that elevated phenylalanine concentrations may reduce normal neurotransmitter (serotonin) levels and consequently affect behavior and mood and even induce seizures. Prompting the proposal was the report that a few, otherwise healthy adults had suffered seizures after ingesting very high doses of aspartame. The suggested mechanism for this relates to the competition of phenylalanine, tryptophan, and other LNAAs for a common carrier across the blood–brain barrier (p. 491). Compared to dietary protein that would release various amounts of all the LNAAs, aspartame dosing creates a phenylalanine imbalance when its blood level is selectively raised relative to the other LNAAs. The imbalance becomes even more pronounced if the aspartame "meal" also includes carbohydrate. This is because of the effect of insulin in causing primarily the branched-chain amino acids to leave the bloodstream and to be taken up by skeletal muscle (p. 177). Plasma tryptophan, the precursor of brain serotonin, must then compete for a common carrier with the disproportionately high concentration of

phenylalanine. Not only would phenylalanine have the competitive edge from the standpoint of concentration, but it also has a lower K_m for the carrier than tryptophan (that is, it is bound more tightly by the carrier). Therefore, consumption of aspartame, particularly along with carbohydrate, could cause a reduction in brain serotonin, with associated neurologic symptoms.

Although the speculation that aspartame may influence neurotransmitter levels, and the mechanism by which it may do so is of academic interest, the results of several studies have failed to establish a link between dietary aspartame/carbohydrate and brain tryptophan levels. In addition, recent investigations involving aspartame effects on behavior alteration showed no significant correlation, and showed that it did not differ in this respect from other sweeteners such as sucrose [21].

Based on the data it has reviewed, the FDA has concluded that while aspartame increases blood and brain phenylalanine concentrations, there is insufficient evidence that aspartame alone or in conjunction with carbohydrate alters behavior or functional neurotransmitter activity.

The methanol and aspartate moieties of the aspartame dipeptide have also been studied from the standpoint of their possible effects on behavior and/or neurotoxicity [22]. The toxicity of methanol is, of course, well known. Its ingestion in large quantities leads to a variety of adverse effects, including metabolic acidosis and blindness. The toxicity reflects the accumulation of the methanol metabolite formate, rather than the methanol itself. It has been of interest, therefore, to study the plasma level of formate as a function of aspartame ingestion. The results of such studies showed that no significant rise in plasma formate occurred even when abuse doses of aspartame as high as 200 mg/kg were fed to humans.

Aspartate is also toxic in very large quantities and has been reported to induce brain lesions in experimental animals. Like the methanol moiety, however, plasma levels of the amino acid were not markedly elevated by aspartame loading because of its rapid clearance from the plasma.

In summary, if high-dose aspartame administration does have an effect on the brain, the effect is likely to be mediated via phenylalanine and not by way of the intact dipeptide or the aspartate or methanol moieties. The effect on the brain of aspartame-derived phenylalanine is also subject to question. If such a consequence does exist, however, it will occur only when the intake of the sweetener is sufficiently high so as to cause a substantial imbalance in the concentration of plasma phenylalanine relative to the other LNAAs. To date, measurable neurologic disturbances have not been convincingly demonstrated as a result of abuse dosing with the sweetener.

SUMMARY

The normal diet includes compounds that can affect mood or behavior. The effect may be direct, without structural alteration of the compounds, or it may be exerted following their metabolic conversion to active products such as neurotransmitters. Examples of nutrient precursors, along with their corresponding neurotransmitters, are listed here:

Nutrient	Neurotransmitter
Tryptophan	Serotonin
Tyrosine	Epinephrine
	Norepinephrine
	Dopamine
Choline (as lecithin)	Acetylcholine
Glutamic acid	Gamma-aminobutyric acid (GABA)

To function as a neurotransmitter, the nutrient must enter the neurons from the bloodstream (cross the blood–brain barrier). The process requires the nutrient's binding to receptors on the capillary endothelial cells followed by carrier-mediated transport through the cells. The nutrient–carrier interaction is not absolutely specific, however, resulting in a competition among large, neutral amino acids (LNAAs), including tryptophan and tyrosine, for common receptor sites. The calming effect of tryptophan, via conversion to serotonin, is therefore enhanced by a diet that minimizes the competition from the other LNAAs, allowing a larger portion of circulating tryptophan to cross the blood–brain barrier. Although this effect can be achieved by a reduction in the dietary intake of competing LNAAs, it is more dramatically expressed by a high-carbohydrate diet, which, through the release of insulin, diverts competing LNAAs into muscle. This action proportionately increases the amount of tryptophan available for brain uptake.

Because tyrosine is a progenitor of the stimulatory neurotransmitters norepinephrine, dopamine, and epinephrine, it is tempting to speculate that alterations in the dietary intake of the amino acid may affect mood by parallel changes in brain levels of the transmitters. The relationship has not been firmly established, however.

Choline, the dietary source of which is principally lecithin, is convertible to the neurotransmitter acetylcholine, a depletion of which has been linked to deficits in learning and memory. The therapeutic benefit of dietary loading of the nutrient to alleviate these symptoms has been investigated, but the results of the studies remain controversial.

Among the most widely consumed psychoactive dietary substances is caffeine, a CNS stimulant well known for its induction of wakefulness and "alerting" effects. The effectiveness of the stimulant prescription drug Ritalin, used in treating attention-deficit disorders associated with hyperactivity in children, fostered interest in caffeine as a possible alternative stimulant. The high doses required to achieve positive effects, however, preclude its therapeutic use.

Glutamic acid is rather unique among the neuroactive nutrients in that its activity can be stimulatory or inhibitory depending on its metabolic route. Structurally unaltered, glutamic acid is a potent neuroexcitatory transmitter; however, it can be decarboxylated in the brain to form the inhibitory transmitter GABA. The ubiquitousness of glutamic acid, and its high concentration throughout the body tissues, including the brain, hamper studies on the effect of its dietary intake on neuroactivity. A link between the physiologic distress reported by some people following the eating of glutamate as its monosodium salt MSG and the neuroactive effects of glutamate or GABA has not been established.

Another commonly ingested substance that reportedly can be identified with neurologic symptoms is the artificial sweetener aspartame. At very high dietary levels of the dipeptide, such symptoms may be accounted for by the resulting increased concentration of plasma phenylalanine, which may impede neuronal uptake of tryptophan. This effect is potentiated if carbohydrate is consumed along with the sweetener.

References Cited

1. Mitchell EA, Aman MG, Turbott SH, Manku M. Clinical characteristics and serum essential fatty acids in hyperactive children. Clinical Pediatrics 1987;26:406–411.

2. Wainwright PE. Lipids and behavior: The evidence from animal models. In: Lipids, learning, and the brain: Fats in infant formulas. Report of the 103rd Ross Conference on Pediatric Research. Columbus OH: Ross Laboratories, 1993:69–88.

3. Kanarek RB, Marks-Kaufman R. Nutrition and behavior: New perspectives. New York: Van Nostrand Reinhold, 1991.

4. Robinson J, Ferguson A. Food sensitivity and the nervous system: Hyperactivity, addiction, and criminal behavior. In: Nutr Res Rev 1992;5:203–223.

5. Spring B. Effects of foods and nutrients on the behavior of normal individuals. In: Wurtman RJ, Wurtman JJ, eds.

Nutrition and the brain. New York: Raven Press, 1986;7:1–47.

6. Fernstrom JD, Faller DV. Neutral amino acids in the brain: Changes in response to food ingestion. J Neurochem 1978;30:1531–1538.

7. Wurtman RJ, Wurtman JJ. Carbohydrates and depression. Sci Am 1989;260:68–75.

8. Wurtman J, Wurtman R, Mark S, et al. d-Fenfluramine selectively suppresses carbohydrate snacking by obese subjects. J Eat Dis 1985;4(1):89–99.

9. Wurtman RJ. Nutrients that modify brain function. Sci Am 1982;246:50–59.

10. Etienne P, Gauthier S, Dastoor D, et al. Alzheimer's disease: Clinical effect of lecithin treatment. In: Barbeau A, Growdon JH, Wurtman RJ, eds. Nutrition and the brain. New York: Raven Press, 1979;5:389–396.

11. Virkkunen M. Reactive hypoglycemic tendency among habitually violent offenders. Nutr Rev 1986;44(Suppl.): 94–103.

12. Ferguson HB, Stoddart C, Simeon JG. Double blind challenge studies of behavioral and cognitive effects of sucrose-aspartame ingestion in normal children. Nutr Rev 1986;44(Suppl.):144–150.

13. Barone JJ, Roberts H. Human consumption of caffeine. In: Dews PB, ed. Caffeine: Perspectives from recent research. Berlin: Springer-Verlag, 1984:59–73.

14. Zwyghuizen-Doorenbos A, Roehrs TA, et al. Effects of caffeine on alertness. Psychopharmacology 1990;100: 36–39.

15. Griffiths RR, Woodson PP. Caffeine physical dependence: A review of human and laboratory animal studies. Psychopharmacology 1988;94:437–451.

16. Schnackenberg RC. Caffeine as a substitute for schedule II stimulants in hyperactive children. Am J Psychiatry 1973;130:796–798.

17. Schecter MD, Timmons GD. Objectively measured hyperactivity II. Caffeine and amphetamine effects. J Clin Pharmacol 1985;25:276–280.

18. Rumsey JM, Rapoport JL. Assessing behavioral and cognitive effects of diet in pediatric populations. In: Wurtman RJ, Wurtman JJ, eds. Nutrition and the brain. New York: Raven Press, 1983;6:101–161.

19. Olney JW. Brain lesions, obesity, and other disturbances in mice treated with monosodium glutamate. Science 1969;164:719–721.

20. Morbidity and mortality weekly report. Atlanta: Centers for Disease Control 1984;43(33):605.

21. Kruesi MJP, Rapoport JL. Diet and human behavior: How much do they affect each other? Ann Rev Nutr 1986;6:113–130.

22. Stegink LD. The aspartame story: A model for the clinical testing of a food additive. Am J Clin Nutr 1987; 46:204–215.

Suggested Reading

Kruesi MJP, Rapoport JL. Diet and human behavior: How much do they affect each other? Ann Rev Nutr 1986;6: 113–130.
Included is a review of pertinent research evaluation along with the behavioral effects of specific dietary constituents.

Spring B. Effects of foods and nutrients on the behavior of normal individuals. In: Wurtman RJ, Wurtman JJ, eds. Nutrition and the brain, New York: Raven Press, 1986;7:1–47.
In-depth coverage is provided of the methodologic issues involved in researching nutrient versus behavior correlations as well as selected nutrient effects in both human and animal studies.

Diet and behavior: A multidisciplinary evaluation. Proceedings of a symposium, Arlington, VA. Nutr Rev 1986;44 (Suppl. May):1–252.
This article provides a broad, multitopic treatment of the effects of nutrients on both brain function and patterns of behavior. The inclusion of a section on the strategies for improving pertinent research adds to the strength of this review.

Praag HM, Lemus C. Monoamine precursors in the treatment of psychiatric disorders. In: Wurtman RJ, Wurtman JJ, eds. Nutrition and the brain. New York: Raven Press, 1986;7:89–138.
This is a thorough, data-and-statistics approach relating to the rationale for and the results of the administration of nutrient monoamine precursors in treating psychiatric disorders.

Hyperactivity in Children

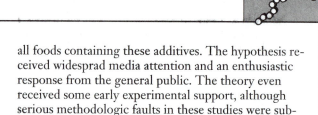

There has been a long-standing public belief that diet affects behavior. Scientific evidence for the relationship was the revelation that brain levels of neurotransmitters can be affected by the dietary intake of their precursors. Research on diet and behavior consists of two general types: correlational and experimental. The experimental design, because of its ability to establish cause-and-effect relationships, is the more widely used. It involves manipulation of the variables (for example, a dietary constituent such as tyrosine) to examine their effect on dependent measures such as behavior and/or cognitive factors. Cognitive assessment is quantitative and readily measurable. Examples of cognitive measures are continuous performance test (CPT) results or the ability to recall information as a result of diet manipulation. Behavioral assessment, in contrast, is difficult to quantitate, and consequently, conclusions are often subjective and anecdotal. Regardless of whether it is cognition or behavior that is the dependent variable, research employing experimental designs is capable of establishing causal relationships.

Correlational designs examine behavioral characteristics of individual subjects in relation to their eating habits. The correlational approach requires a large number of subjects, and its chief weakness is its inability to distinguish cause from effect.

Following this brief review of research terminology, the possible effect of certain food substances on hyperactivity in children will be considered. This condition has received considerable publicity in recent years largely because of the debatable overuse of the stimulant drug Ritalin, used to allay the symptoms. Hyperactivity is a syndrome characterized by restlessness and hyperkinesis as well as a compromised attention span and an inability to concentrate. Since the syndrome is a distortion of normal behavior, it is not surprising that a dietary link to this condition gradually surfaced. Historically, artificial food additives such as colors (dyes) and flavors and, more recently, sweeteners, particularly sucrose, have been implicated in promoting the symptoms of hyperactivity.

In 1975 Feingold offered the hypothesis that the ingestion of artificial food additives (colors and flavors) and naturally occurring salicylates in foods results in hyperactivity and learning disabilities in children. On the basis of this conclusion it was suggested that treatment be implemented through the Feingold Kaiser-Permanente (K-P) diet, which is designed to eliminate all foods containing these additives. The hypothesis received widesprad media attention and an enthusiastic response from the general public. The theory even received some early experimental support, although serious methodologic faults in these studies were subsequently reported.

The National Advisory Committee on Hyperkinesis and Food Additives was formed to study the Feingold theory. It concluded that more data were needed to substantiate the hypothesis unequivocally. Finally, in 1983 a meta-analysis [1] of the controlled studies completed by that time provided a generally negative relationship between food additives and hyperactivity. It was concluded from the study that the Feingold K-P diet afforded only a marginal, limited benefit compared with control diets. The findings did not preclude rare, individual exceptions.

There has also been considerable public concern that refined sugar, chiefly sucrose, may be linked to hyperactivity. This speculation received support from the results of a study showing positive correlations between dietary carbohydrate–protein ratios and directly observed restless and aggressive behavior in a sample of hyperactive children. As a correlational study, however, it could not establish causality. For example, a tendency toward hyperactivity may have encouraged the children to consume more carbohydrate because of its calming effect (p. 491). Alternatively, there is the possibility that both the hyperactivity and the heightened carbohydrate intake result from a third variable, a higher metabolic rate.

A number of double-blind, placebo-controlled experimental design studies have been conducted examining the effect of sugar on children's behavior and cognition. A variety of "effect" parameters have been used in these studies, such as playroom or classroom observation, wrist and ankle actometers (designed to measure physical activity) and CPT. CPT is a cognitive measure, generally used to assess sustained attention and impulsiveness. Regardless of the assessment method used, there is lack of evidence that sugar challenge has any effect on the behavior or cognition of hyperactive boys [2]. Although a few of the studies did indicate an increased level of activity and a decreased attention span as a result of sugar challenge, others curiously showed precisely the opposite effect. The majority of the investigations revealed no correlation between sugar loading and behavior or cognition.

PERSPECTIVE (continued)

Studies have also been conducted on normal and supposedly "sugar sensitive" children, in which the effects on behavior and cognition of different sweetener diets, sucrose, aspartame, and saccharin (as placebo), were measured. It was concluded that even if intake exceeds typical dietary levels, neither sucrose nor aspartame affects children's behavior or cognitive ability [3].

In summary, artificial food additives and sucrose, the two major alleged dietary culprits in the cause or exacerbation of hyperactivity, cannot be proven guilty, based on the results of extensive research employing the use of double-blind studies. Whether or not the symptoms of hyperactivity are completely independent of dietary factors awaits further study. Meanwhile, the cause of the condition remains a mystery.

References Cited

1. Kavale KA, Forness SR. Hyperactivity and diet treatment: A meta-analysis of the Feingold hypothesis. J Learn Disabil 1983;16:324–330.
2. Woolraich M, Milich R, Stumbo P, et al. The effects of sucrose ingestion on the behavior of hyperactive boys. J Pediatr 1985;106:575–582.
3. Wolraich ML, Lindgren SD, Stumbo PJ, et al. Effects of diets high in sucrose or aspartame on the behavior and cognitive performance of children. N Engl J Med 1994;330:301–307.

NUTRITION KNOWLEDGE BASE

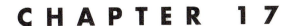

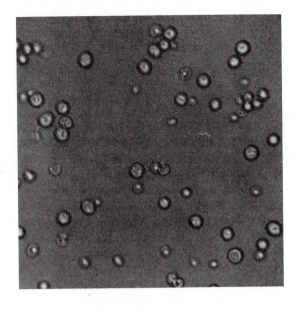

EXPERIMENTAL DESIGN AND CRITICAL INTERPRETATION OF RESEARCH

Photo: Budding yeast cells (Saccharomyces)

Research can be defined as a process that uses a scientific method to solve puzzling problems and to resolve previously unanswered questions [1]. As such, research owes its beginning to Antoine Lavoisier, who, in the late eighteenth century, introduced the scientific approach (or research process) to problem solving [2–4]. Up until that time, inquiry into problems had been only a philosophic exercise.

Lavoisier initiated the experimental method of research with its primary components: (1) formulation of hypothesis (or hypotheses), (2) experimentation under controlled conditions, (3) interpretation of results, and (4) formulation of theory. His approach to problem solving is illustrated by the following steps [2,3]:

- Using Priestley's earlier discovery that oxygen is involved in burning, Lavoisier formulated the *hypothesis* that respiration in animals was a form of combustion.

- Lavoisier carried out *experimentation under controlled conditions* on animals (guinea pigs). Oxygen consumption, heat production, and production of carbon dioxide by animals confined in airtight chambers were carefully measured.

- With the measurements (data) collected, Lavoisier *interpreted the results:* A pattern could be identified between oxygen consumption, carbon dioxide production, and heat emanating from the animal body.

- Based on his interpretation of the data, Lavoisier *formulated the theory* that consumption of oxygen is related to the amount of carbon burned or heat produced in the animal body. Then, to validate his theory, he performed similar controlled experiments on other animals, including humans.

Research design, particularly that which lends itself to the physical and biological sciences, must include the components just discussed. To be considered a fact, the theory formulated must be verified by other investigators who carry out the re-

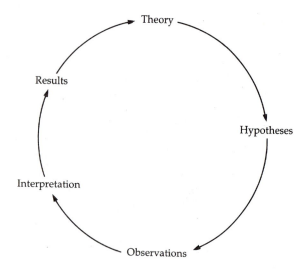

FIGURE 17.1 Relationship of theory to research. *(Reprinted by permission from Research Methods in Human Ecology/Home Economics by J. Touliatos and N. H. Compton © 1988 by Iowa State University Press, Ames, IA.)*

search under the same controlled conditions used in the original research. If the theory is verified, it becomes accepted as fact until advances in research can disprove it.

INTERRELATIONSHIP OF KNOWLEDGE BASE, TECHNOLOGY, THEORY, AND RESEARCH

The components of research, described in the preceding section, can be thought of as occupying a cyclic relationship to each other. This is illustrated in Figure 17.1, which shows the inseparable linkage between research and theory. The hypotheses comprising theory are constantly being tested by research. Research both tests and stimulates theory, contributes to the refinement of methods and procedures, and leads to the development of new or modified theory [5].

Nutrition research, the mechanism for expanding the nutrition knowledge base, which began with Lavoisier's revelations about energy metabolism (around 1789)[3] moved at a rather slow pace until the beginning of the twentieth century. At this time, many important discoveries and technologic advances allowed a rapid expansion of the nutrition knowledge base. Throughout the twentieth century, nutrition research, along with technologic advances, has continued to progress.

The cyclic nature of research makes clear that one prerequisite of productive research is an investigator

who is familiar with what is already known about the subject under study, and how others have investigated the subject [5]. This prerequisite is provided admirably in the studies of Rose [6] and Young [7], who investigated the dietary essentiality of amino acids. Their studies are described briefly here to provide an example of well-planned research and to emphasize the cyclic nature of the investigative process.

Protein composition and metabolism has been a particularly fertile field in nutrition and biochemical research. Scientific inquiry has been directed toward identification of the indispensable amino acids followed by quantitative determination of human requirements for these amino acids and for total protein. Rose [6], after comparing the work of previous investigators (Osbourne and Mendel, Fischer and others) on the amino acid composition of proteins with that from his own laboratory, undertook the identification of those amino acids that are indispensable to animals and/or humans. He began his investigations with weanling rats and then extended experimentation to humans (graduate students!). The data obtained from rats were used as the starting point for the more difficult and costly studies on human beings. Keeping one amino acid as the single independent variable in the diet and using maximum weight gain as the criterion (dependent variable), Rose found through a series of experiments that only 10 of the 19 to 20 amino acids ordinarily found in proteins are required by the rat: arginine, histidine, isoleucine, leucine, lysine, methionine, phenylalanine, threonine, tryptophan, and valine.

In his follow-up study on humans, Rose [6] used nitrogen equilibrium as the criterion (dependent variable) for determining indispensability; but one amino acid remained the single independent variable in the test diet. Rose's 13-year study on the indispensable amino acids and their requirements in the adult male (1942 to 1955) resulted in identification of the amino acids indispensable (essential) to human beings, along with the range of requirements, a tentatively proposed minimal requirement, and a definitely safe intake (Table 17.1). One troubling aspect of the study was the increased caloric intake required by the subjects to maintain nitrogen equilibrium when they were fed amino acids rather than protein as their nitrogen source. In the discussion of his studies, Rose cites their limitations, noting particularly the small number of subjects, the artificiality of using diets containing mixtures of amino acids rather than proteins, and the attendant need for increased caloric intake on the part of the subjects. Rose concludes his studies thus [6, p. 644]: "By reference to Table 3 [Table 17.1 in this text], it should be possible to predict with reasonable accuracy how much of a given protein or diet, if its content of

TABLE 17.1 The Daily Amino Acid Requirements of Young Men

Amino Acid	Quantitative Experiments (no.)	Range of Requirements Recorded (g)	Minimum Proposed Tentatively (g)	Definitely Safe Intake (g)	Subjects in N Balance on Safe Intake or Less (no.)
L-tryptophan	3[a]	0.15–0.25	0.25	0.50	42
L-phenylalanine	6	0.80–1.10[b]	1.10	2.20	32
L-lysine	6	0.40–0.80	0.80	1.60	37[c]
L-threonine	3[d]	0.30–0.50	0.50	1.00	29
L-methionine	6	0.80–1.10[e]	1.10	2.20	23
L-leucine	5	0.50–1.10	1.10	2.20	18
L-isoleucine	4	0.65–0.70	0.70	1.40	17
L-valine	5	0.40–0.80	0.80	1.60	33

All values were determined with diets containing the eight essential amino acids and sufficient extra nitrogen to permit the synthesis of the nonessential amino acids.
[a]Fifteen other young men were maintained in nitrogen balance on a daily intake of 0.20 g, though their exact minimum needs were not established. Of the 42 subjects maintained on the *safe* intake or less, 33 had 0.30 g daily or less.
[b]These values were obtained with diets devoid of tyrosine. In two experiments, the presence of tyrosine was found to spare the phenylalanine requirement to the extent of 70 and 75%.
[c]Ten of these subjects had an intake of 0.80 g or less.
[d]In addition to these 3 subjects, 4 young men had diets containing 0.60 g L-threonine daily and 16 others had 0.80 g daily. No attempt was made to determine the exact minimum requirements of these 20 subjects, but all were in positive balance on the amounts shown.
[e]These values were obtained with diets devoid of cystine. In three experiments, the presence of cystine was found to spare the methionine requirement to the extent of 80 to 89%.
Source: Rose WC, Wixom RL, Lockhart HB, et al. The amino acid requirements of man, XV. The valine requirement: Summary and observations, J. Biol. Chem. 1955;217:992. Reprinted with permission.

amino acids is known, would be required to maintain nitrogen equilibrium, provided the moderate quantity of extra nitrogen needed by the body for synthesis is already present or is added to the food. Such calculations must take account of the availability of the amino acids in the materials under investigation, since the processing and preservation of foods and their preparation for consumption may modify the nutritional usefulness of the component proteins."

Up to the present, these studies by Rose, published in 1957, have been used to a large degree as the basis for the estimation of adults' needs for the indispensable amino acids. They also have provided a basis for development of an amino acid pattern against which the biological value or "completeness" of a protein is measured.

The hypotheses comprising Rose's theory began to be tested by Young [7] in the late 1960s, and continues today. Young's research has contributed to the refinement of methods and procedures in assessing the amino acid needs of humans and probably is leading to a new, increased estimate of adults' amino acid requirements. This modification of the amino acid requirements in adult humans that may result from Young's research does not negate in any way the usefulness of Rose's theory. According to Turner [8], when a theory is rejected, science has advanced because the theories that do survive offer, at least for the time being, the most nearly accurate picture of the world.

During the last 30 years, the time in which Young has been conducting research on amino acid metabolism, many weaknesses in the use of nitrogen balance as the dependent variable for studying protein metabolism have been identified [7]: (1) nitrogen equilibrium gives no specifics about protein metabolism in individual tissues or organs; (2) results using the nitrogen balance technique often overestimated need because losses of nitrogen through the skin seldom are measured, and various other sources of error are also possible; (3) nitrogen balance is significantly affected by energy intake; and (4) nitrogen balance can be greatly influenced by the length of the experimental period, making interpretation of a specific nitrogen balance difficult. As he became aware of the limitations of nitrogen balance as a criterion for amino acid adequacy, and having available (through technologic advances) some alternative methods for assessment of protein status, Young [7] began a new series of studies on amino acid requirements in adults. An alternative, dependent variable that he used extensively during the late 1960s and early 1970s was the plasma amino acid response curve [9–12]. Subsequently, following the advent of stable isotopes, the tracing of amino acid distribution and use within the body became possible. As a consequence, distribution and use of an amino acid replaced the amino acid response curve as the dependent variable. Concurrently, by combining the isotope tracer technique with the measurement of nitrogen balance, Young collected some convincing evidence to support his hypothesis that adults need more of the indispensable amino acids than had been indicated through the measurement of nitrogen balance alone.

These examples of research efforts illustrate the effect on outcome by (1) a broadening of the knowledge base and (2) advancing technology. Young had available to him the knowledge of the positive effect of increased caloric intake on nitrogen balance, along with other disadvantages associated with nitrogen balance studies, which Rose did not. In addition, Young gained advantage from the advent of isotope tracer techniques and other technological advances.

According to Leedy [1], a barrier imposed by limitations of knowledge and technology separate data from the realm of ultimate truth. This barrier allows only a portion of the light of truth to shine through. No research conclusions can be stated in absolute terms!

RESEARCH METHODOLOGIES

Many different types, or classifications, of research exist. One of the broadest classifications of research is according to *application:* is the research basic or applied? Basic research seeks to expand existing knowledge by discovering new knowledge. Applied research, in contrast, seeks to solve problems primarily in a field setting. Other classifications of research can be according to *strategy* (historical, survey), *degree of experimental control* (experimental versus non-experimental), *time dimension* (cross-sectional versus longitudinal), *setting* (laboratory, field), *character of data collected* (qualitative, quantitative), or *purpose* (descriptive or analytic).

Despite the diversity of research classifications, the methods by which research can be carried out are more concisely categorized. It has been proposed that regardless of which classification of research is undertaken, the research effort can follow any one of four discrete methodologies. These are historical methods, descriptive survey methods, analytical survey methods, and experimental methods, each of which will be described briefly.

Historical Method

Historical research seeks to explain the cause of past events and to interpret current happenings on the basis of these findings. Sources of information for the historical researcher are primarily documentary, existing in the form of written records and accounts of past events, as well as literary productions and critical writings. The researcher relies, if possible, only on primary data, a term that implies that the data are "first hand" and therefore minimally distorted by the channels of communication. Generally, information gathered by historical research does not need to be analyzed by any form of statistical treatment or data analysis.

Descriptive Survey Method

One word that distinguishes the descriptive survey method from other research methods is *observation.* The investigator observes, across a defined population group, whatever variable is under study. The variable may be physical (size, shape, color, strength, and so on) or cognitive (achievement, beliefs, attitudes, intelligence). The researcher (1) observes very closely the population bounded by the parameters that were set for the study, and then (2) carefully records what was observed, for future interpretation. It is important to note that observation does not involve only visual perception, but is very likely conducted through tests, questionnaires, attitude scales, inventories, and other evaluative measures. In fact, most descriptive surveys use well-designed questionnaires as the instrument of observation.

Data gathered by the descriptive survey method are analyzed by appropriate statistical treatment, including ranges, frequencies, modes, cross-tabulation, and so on.

Analytical Survey Method

The analytical survey method is best described by contrasting it with the descriptive survey method just discussed. Although the descriptive survey method involves observations that can be described in words and concluded from those words, the analytical survey uses a different language, a language not of words but of *numbers.* Because values obtained from an analytical survey are numerical, the data are said to be *quantitative.* The verbal data obtained from historical or descriptive studies, are, by contrast, qualitative data.

The quantitative data of an analytical survey are analyzed by statistical tools from which conclusions can be inferred. Statistical analysis may be directed at frequency distribution (mean, median, mode), measures of dispersion (standard deviation, coefficient of variation), measures of correlation (correlation coefficient, chi square), or regression analyses.

Experimental Method

The hallmark of the experimental method is control. So basic is control to this method that this means of searching for truth is frequently referred to as the *control group–experimental group design*. Such a study uses two or more population groups with the subjects of each group matched, characteristic by characteristic, as closely as possible to the subjects of the other group(s). One of the groups serves as a control, and as such is not exposed to some extraneous change. The experimental group is exposed to the alteration under study, and whatever change is noted, relative to the subjects of the control group, is presumed to be caused by the extraneous variables. The experimental method can also use just one group, a method sometimes called a pretest–posttest approach. In short, the experimental method is based on *cause and effect*. Many traditional descriptive and inferential statistical tools can be used to analyze the data.

To illustrate some of the research methodologies described, several examples of actual research, taken from the nutrition literature, are presented next. For the purpose of the discussion, the methodological approaches used in these examples are broadly classified as descriptive studies or analytical studies. These classifications include certain sub-classifications that exemplify one of the types of methodologies discussed. The research examples will be identified by the corresponding methodology.

DESCRIPTIVE STUDIES

Descriptive studies help to establish associations among different factors. However, they do not measure cause-and-effect relationships. The descriptive studies cited here include qualitative research, case reports or case studies, and survey research [13]. Each of these types of studies exemplifies the descriptive survey approach to research.

Qualitative Research

Qualitative research is exploratory and allows the investigator to watch for clues, and to gain insight into a situation or phenomenon [14]. Data collected for qualitative research is gained through interviews, questionnaires, or observations. Such studies often precede the use of other types of research design. Qualitative research may be particularly important when the subject of interest is new or is an old one in which little has been done.

Goldberger's work on pellagra illustrates the use of qualitative research. Goldberger [14] described qualitatively the population and environment at two orphanages in Mississippi in 1914 as a preliminary study in his research on pellagra. By careful, systematic observation, he noted (1) the incidence or absence of pellagra among both the orphan residents and staff, (2) age groups affected by disease or free of the disease, (3) opportunity for close contact among groups, (4) sanitary conditions, and (5) foods eaten by the different groups of residents and staff. In this preliminary inquiry he found that the disease pellagra was confined almost exclusively to a group of 6- to 12-year-old children. The different diet given to the 6- to 12-year-old groups was the only factor he observed at this point to explain a possible cause of the disease. The finding led him to test his hypothesis in later experimental dietary studies. The prevalent theory at the time of Goldberger's work was that pellagra was an infectious disease spread by unsanitary conditions. Goldberger's ability as a researcher is exemplified by his refusal to be constrained by these prevailing beliefs.

Case Report or Case Series

A case report is a report of observations on one subject, whereas a case series involves observations on more than one subject. Generally the subjects being observed have a condition or disease in common. This form of research design is useful in an attempt to identify variables or generate hypotheses that may be important in the etiology, care, or outcome of patients with a particular disease or condition.

An example of a case report is the investigation by Sedlet and Ireton-Jones [16]. These researchers studied energy expenditure in a patient who, on initial evaluation at an eating disorder clinic, presented with a semifast–binge eating pattern. Findings of the investigation were documented as a case report study, preliminary to further research. Energy expenditure in the subject was assessed prior to and following nutrition intervention. Basal energy expenditure (BEE) was estimated by use of the Harris Benedict equation (p. 470). Actual measured energy expenditure (MEE) was determined by indirect calorimetry. The investigators found that the patient's BEE was 53% higher than her MEE when, on initial evaluation, she was in the semifast–binge eating pattern. Modification of her eating pattern to three meals a day, providing a total of approximately 1,200 kcal/day, was accomplished over a four- to six-week period. After the modification, her MEE increased

TABLE 17.2 Energy Intake Versus Expenditure of JK (a bulimic patient)

Treatment Period	Intake (kcal/day range)	BEE (kcal/day)	MEE (kcal/day)	BEE/MEE (% difference)
Pretreatment semifast–binge	600–3,800	1,266	829	53
Nutrition counseling follow-up				
2 months	1,000–1,200	1,257	1,203	4
6 months	1,000–1,200	1,252	1,193	5
7 months	1,000–1,200	1,252	1,202	4

Source: Sedlet KL, Ireton-Jones CS. Energy expenditures and the abnormal eating pattern of a bulimic: A case report. J Am Diet Assoc 1989;89:16.

and was essentially the same as her BEE (Table 17.2), while her activity level remained the same throughout treatment. The subject seemed more willing to continue the modified eating pattern (3 meals/day) when she was able to eat each day and not gain weight.

Findings from this case report helped to generate an ongoing research project to determine whether data presented can be substantiated in a study involving a group of patients with bulimia. There is limited information about actual versus estimated energy expenditure in bulimia, and also about ways acceptable to patients to modify their food intake pattern.

Data for case series studies are often collected from existing records and are considered retrospective studies, meaning "looking back." A disadvantage of the retrospective study is that observations of the different variables of interest may not have been recorded in a standardized way and thus may not be comparable. Alternately, data for case series may be collected concurrently, providing an opportunity to standardize procedures. An advantage of case series studies is that they are relatively easy to perform and are inexpensive. They may provide data to justify the need for future analytic study, especially when concerned with a condition or disease about which information is limited.

Bulimia (p. 485), a disease requiring nutrition intervention but about which little is known, has been studied by observation. Pyle et al. [15] reported a case series study of 34 subjects with bulimia. Findings regarding frequency of binge eating, fasting, self-induced vomiting, and use of laxatives were among the characteristics described. An eating pattern of binge eating combined with periods of fasting was common.

Survey Research

Survey research provides information through data collected from the observation of a specific population [13]. Data obtained are not numerical (quantitative), and the research therefore follows the descriptive sur-

vey mode. The Ten State Survey [17] and the National Health and Nutrition Examination Survey (NHANES I and II) [18] are examples of large surveys. These surveys can also be classified as "cross-sectional" studies; that is, all subjects across the population are studied at approximately the same time, and each is studied once, not continuously.

The Ten State Survey was designed to oversample among low-income populations in selected states in the United States. Thus, application of findings (external validity) was limited and could not be applied to the U.S. population in general. Findings from the Ten State Survey provided some evidence for the need to expand food programs in low-income populations. The NHANES data were collected from a statistically elected sample to represent the 194 million noninstitutionalized civilians aged 1 to 74 years in the United States. Data were collected systematically and by standardized methods of measurement from the sample population. Data from the NHANES are considered baseline information for the U.S. population at the time of the survey.

One example of use of data from NHANES was the development of new standards of anthropometric reference values such as weight and skinfold measurements by age, sex, and height for adults [19]. Figures 17.2 and 17.3 illustrate the anthropometric changes identified between the first health examination survey (HES) and its follow-up, which included nutrition (NHANES I).

ANALYTICAL STUDIES

Analytical research is designed to test hypotheses. Unlike descriptive studies, causal relationships can be detected through this type of research. Examples of analytical research that will be presented here include observational research designs (analytical survey method) and experimental research designs (experimental method). Each of these designs will be discussed.

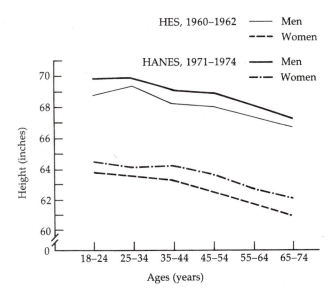

FIGURE 17.2 Mean height of adults in 1960–1962 and 1971–1974 by age and sex.

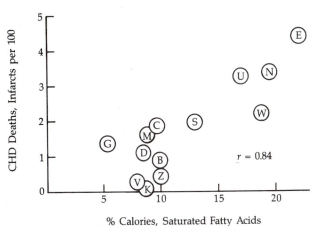

FIGURE 17.4 Diet–heart associations. (B, Belgrade faculty; C, Crevalcore; D, Dalmatia; E, East Finland; G, Corfu; K, Crete; N, Zutphen; M, Montegiorgio; S, Slavonia; U, U.S. railroad; V, Velika Krsna; W, West Finland; Z, Zrenjanin) *(Inter-society commission for Heart Disease Resources, Atherosclerosis group. Keys A, ed. Coronary heart disease in seven countries. Circulation 1970(1)41:211. Reprinted with permission.)*

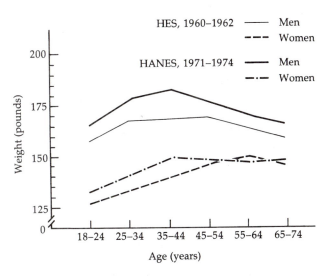

FIGURE 17.3 Mean weight of adults in 1960–1962 and 1971–1974 by age and sex.

Observational Research Designs

The use of the word *observational* in describing this type of research may at first seem confusing since observation is also the hallmark of descriptive surveys, as discussed earlier. Remember, however, that the observational research designs discussed here are examples of an analytical study, and as such, produce numerical, quantitative data, interpretable by the application of statistics. Descriptive surveys, although based on observation, rely on written data, and are not quantitative. Observational de-

signs, such as epidemiological or cohort studies, do not involve experiment-induced changes in variables. Epidemiology has been defined by Burr [20] as "the study of the distribution of a disease or condition in the population and the factors that influence the distribution" [20, p. 259]. A cohort is a group of subjects entered into a study at the same time and followed up at intervals over a period of time. A cohort study is also called a *prospective* study, meaning "looking ahead."

Two examples of observational nutrition-related studies are the Seven Countries Studies reported by Keyes [21], and the Framingham Study [22]. In the Seven Countries Studies, the outcome of interest was coronary heart disease (CHD). Possible associated major factors under consideration were dietary total calories, total fat, animal fat, saturated fat, total protein, animal protein, and sucrose. Data regarding CHD and the dietary factors were collected from population groups in each country by systematic, standardized methods of measurement by trained teams. Data were statistically analyzed for possible association of any of the studied dietary factors. Figure 17.4 shows the relationship of one dietary factor, saturated fat, to the incidence of CHD.

The Framingham Study, a cohort study, is a long-term, longitudinal study, initiated in the town of Framingham, Massachusetts, in 1948. A longitudinal study is one conducted on the subjects of a study group over a certain period of time. It was designed to study the dis-

Risk of heart attack increases
as blood cholesterol goes up

Heart attack rate per 1,000 men per 10 years

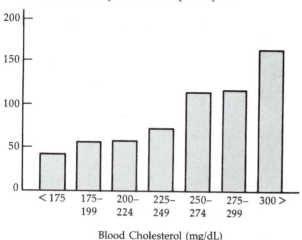

Blood Cholesterol (mg/dL)

FIGURE 17.5 Risk of heart attack as related to blood cholesterol level. (*Inter-society Commission for Heart Disease Resources, Atherosclerosis Group. Primary prevention of the atherosclerotic disease. Circulation Dec 1977 42:A55–95. Reprinted with permission.*)

TABLE 17.3 Major Characteristics of Diets

	Atherogenic	Low Fat	Corn Oil
Protein	16	19	15
Carbohydrate	43	77	45
Fat	41	4	40
Cholesterol	1.2	0	0

Values for protein, carbohydrate, and fat are percentages of total calories; cholesterol values are percentages by weight.
Source: Armstrong ML, Warner ED, Connor WE. Regression of coronary atheromatosis in rhesus monkeys. Circ Res 1970;27:60. Reprinted with permission of the American Heart Association, Inc.

tribution of CHD in the sample population and possible causal factors associated with the disease. The study began with a cohort of 2,336 men and 2,873 women aged 29 to 62 years, randomly selected from the population. Data regarding the cardiovascular condition and the possible causal factors of CHD were systematically collected from subjects at specified time intervals, using standardized methods of measurement. Data from the Framingham Study showed that hypercholesterolemia, hypertension, and cigarette smoking are three major risk factors in CHD. Information from that study was used also to show comparative risk at different levels of blood cholesterol (Fig. 17.5).

Experimental Research Designs

Experimental research designs allow the investigator to control or manipulate one or more variables in an effort to examine the relationship between the variables. Variables typically are designated as dependent and independent. The *independent variable* is that which is controlled or manipulated by the investigator. The *dependent variable* occurs as the result of the influence of the independent variable. In other words, the dependent variable reflects the effects of the independent variable.

Numerous examples can be given to illustrate use of the experimental method in nutrition research. This

methodology is the one most frequently employed in biological studies [1].

Armstrong et al. [23] using the experimental research design, tested the hypothesis that diet-induced atheromas may regress in primates by use of appropriate diet (the independent diet). The investigators conducted their study with 40 adult, male, rhesus monkeys. To serve as *controls*, 10 of the monkeys were fed a low-fat, cholesterol-free diet throughout the study. The other 30 were fed the same low-fat, cholesterol-free diet for a control period of six weeks, and then were given a high-fat, high-cholesterol diet (atherogenic diet) for 17 months. Composition of the diets is given in Table 17.3. The 30 monkeys were then divided into three groups matched for body weight and hyperlipidemia. Group 1 was autopsied for determination of baseline atherosclerosis. Group 2 was fed a low-fat, cholesterol-free diet, and group 3 a linoleate-rich diet for a 40-month period. All diets throughout the study included supplements to make them complete in all essential nutrients. Control and study animals were autopsied at the end of the study to determine the degree of atheromatosis (the dependent variable). Autopsies showed that the cross-sectional area of the lumen of five major coronary arteries was significantly greater in monkeys fed the regression diets (group 2, low-fat diet; group 3, linoleate-enriched diet) than in the monkeys with baseline atherosclerosis (group 1). Comparison of the groups is given in Table 17.4. The investigators were able to show for the first time regression of atheromatosis in nonhuman primates by modification of diet.

It may be appropriate at this point to remind the reader that examples of the invaluable role of animals in experimental method research are almost innumerable. However, the use of animals in research is threatened by efforts of organized animal rights activists. Recent advances in the care and protection of animals in research need to be carefully preserved and made known to these

TABLE 17.4 Luminal Narrowing (%)

	Main coronary				
Group	Left	Right	LAD	L c'flex	R dist
1	60 ± 8	56 ± 7	53 ± 18	57 ± 9	65 ± 10
2	17 ± 4	14 ± 3	21 ± 4	22 ± 6	16 ± 5
3	25 ± 5	26 ± 3	30 ± 5	23 ± 6	18 ± 5

Abbreviations of branch arteries: LAD, left anterior descending;
L c'flex, left circumflex; R dist, distal continuation of right main coronary artery.
Values are means ± SE (standard error).
Source: Armstrong ML, Warner ED, Connor WE. Regression of coronary atheromatosis in rhesus monkeys. Circ Res 1970;27:61. Reprinted with permission of the American Heart Association, Inc.

activists. Currently each institution in which animals are used in research is required to have a committee to oversee animal care and treatment, and to review all research plans in which animals are used [5].

The randomized clinical trial, an experimental research design, is frequently used in medical research studies in humans. Clinical trials are usually conducted after preliminary trials have been done in experimental animals, and typically test the benefits of one or more treatments.

Subjects in clinical trials are those who have the condition to be treated and should be representative of the population to which results are to be applied. Subjects are assigned randomly to a treatment group. In some instances only one treatment is available, and a placebo is used for the control group. Subjects who enroll in the study must be informed that they have an equal chance of being assigned either to the treatment or to the control group. Ideally, to avoid bias, a clinical trial should be "double blind," with neither the subject nor the investigator knowing which group is which.

An example of a clinical trial is The Lipid Research Clinics Coronary Primary Prevention Trial (LRC-CPPT) [24]. This research project, sponsored by the National Heart, Lung, and Blood Institute of the National Institutes of Health (NIH), illustrates a number of important points that must be considered in the design of a randomized clinical trial.

The LRC-CPPT was undertaken to determine if reducing blood cholesterol levels lowers the risk of CHD in humans. Earlier studies had shown that elevated blood cholesterol levels were a major risk factor in CHD. Numerous studies had shown also that blood cholesterol levels could be reduced by diet and drugs in animals and in humans. Previous clinical trials had not been considered conclusive because of a number of problems in research design. These previous clinical trials, however, along with findings from earlier studies, such as epidemiologic studies, clinical investigations, and animal studies, were extremely useful in designing the LRC-CPPT. A particularly helpful aspect of the earlier clinical trials was the identification of pitfalls in experimental design: absence of double-blind testing, too-small sample size, treatment groups that were not identical, and questionable statistical procedures. Typical problems and pitfalls in research are considered later in the chapter.

In the LRC-CPPT, the study population consisted of people known to be at high risk of CHD. Those under consideration for the study, therefore, were men aged 35 to 59 years of age, asymptomatic for CHD but exhibiting primary hypercholesterolemia (a plasma cholesterol of 265 mg/dL or greater). Subjects were 3,810 men, screened from approximately 48,000 age-eligible men. Informed consent was received from each subject entered into the trial.

Subjects were randomly selected to receive either the drug cholestyramine (a resin previously tested for safety and effectiveness in reducing total cholesterol and low-density lipoprotein cholesterol), or a placebo. Both subjects and investigators were unaware of the treatment assignment (that is, it was double blind). A moderate cholesterol-lowering diet, designed to lower cholesterol levels 3 to 5%, was prescribed to all subjects. Maintaining all the subjects on the same diet throughout the study minimized the opportunity for confounding the study results because of different dietary intakes.

Twelve Lipid Research Clinics (LRCs) participated in the trial. To ensure comparability of data over the entire study period, a common protocol documenting all procedures in detail was adhered to by clinic personnel trained and certified in standardized procedures. All aspects of the study were carefully monitored by the Central Patient Registry and Coordinating Center and by the Program Office.

Table 17.5 illustrates the close similarity of the drug and placebo groups before and during treatment for selected variables that include the major, known risk factors for CHD. If there had been a change in risk factors other than cholesterol levels during the treatment period, this could have posed an alternative explanation for the observed treatment benefit.

The results of the trial showed that the cholestyramine group experienced a 19% reduction in the risk of the primary end point (that is, definite CHD death and/or definite nonfatal myocardial infarction). The data also showed that a 1% reduction in blood cholesterol level yields approximately a 2% reduction in CHD rates.

TABLE 17.5 Selected Variables Before and During Treatment

Variable	Placebo			Cholestyramine Resin		
	Pre-entry	First Year	Seventh Year	Pre-entry	First Year	Seventh Year
Mean systolic blood pressure, mm Hg	121	120	122	121	120	122
Mean diastolic blood pressure, mm Hg	80	79	78	80	78	78
Mean Quetelet index, g/cm²	2.6	2.6	2.7	2.6	2.6	2.7
Mean weight, kg	81	81	83	80	80	82
% current smokers	37	35	26	38	36	27
Mean cigarettes/d for current smokers	25	24	25	26	25	26
% regular exercisers	30	a	27	31	a	28
Median alcohol consumption, g/wk	61	58	51	64	57	53

aNo assessment of exercise was done in the first year.

Source: Lipid Research Clinics Program: The Lipid Research Clinics Primary Prevention Trial Results. I. Reduction in incidence of coronary heart disease to cholesterol lowering. JAMA 1984;251:357.

Subjects were followed for a minimum of 7 years and for as long as 10 years, the average follow-up being 7.4 years. Subjects attended clinics every two months during the follow-up. At clinic visits, subjects received the drug or placebo, dietary and drug counseling to encourage adherence, and standardized examinations and evaluations according to the detailed protocol. All subjects who entered the study were followed to the completion of the trial irrespective of their levels of adherence or frequency of visits. At the completion of the trial, contact was made with all men who discontinued visits during the trial. Thus, it was possible to know the vital status of every subject.

Experience in the LRC-CPPT met design goals in several features of the study, as shown in Table 17.6. Twenty-seven percent of subjects did not adhere (nonadherers) to taking cholestyramine for seven years. This percentage was less than the expected goal of 35%. However, a nonadherer was defined as a subject taking less than one-half packet medication daily. The prescribed dose was six packets of medication per day. Thus, many subjects, although considered to be adherers, were not taking the total prescribed dose. As a consequence, the goal of 28% reduction in cholesterol levels of men assigned to cholestryamine treatment was not met. Actual reduction in cholesterol levels amounted to 13.9%. In addition, although the 19% reduction in the primary end point (incidence of CHD death) was well below the goal of 36%, the reduction in CHD deaths has been judged to be clinically significant.

Investigators in the LRC-CPPT expressed caution that the results of the study could not be extrapolated to predict results from use of drugs that are not bile acid sequestrants like cholestyramine. In addition, the study was not designed to show whether cholesterol lowering

TABLE 17.6 Comparison of LRC-CPPTa Design Goals and Actual Experience

Design Feature	Goal	Experience
Sample size	3,550	3,808b
Duration of follow-up, year	7	7–10
Lost to follow-up	0	0
Reduction of plasma total cholesterol levels in placebo group	4%	4.8%
Nonadherersc at year 7	35%	27%
Reduction of plasma total cholesterol levels in men adheringd to cholestyramine resin treatment	28%	13.9%d
Seven-year incidence of primary end point in placebo group	8.7%	8.6%
Reduction in primary end point	36%	19%

aLRC-CPPT indicates Lipid Research Clinics Coronary Primary Prevention Trial.
bAfter removal of four type III participants.
cA nonadherer is someone averaging less than half a packet of cholestyramine resin per day.
dComputed for seventh year.

Source: Lipid Research Clinics Program: The Lipid Research Clinics Primary Prevention Trial Results. I. Reduction in incidence of coronary heart disease to cholesterol lowering. JAMA 1984;251:360.

by diet decreased CHD deaths. It is known, however, that cholesterol levels can be reduced by dietary modification [23], and findings from the LRC-CPPT support the view that cholesterol lowering by diet would be beneficial. That view was later strongly supported by the Consensus Conference on lowering blood cholesterol to prevent heart disease [25]. The LRC-CPPT was a long, complex, expensive clinical trial. Nevertheless, the experimental design method involving randomized clinical trials, can be used for much less expensive studies.

TERMS THAT DESCRIBE RESEARCH QUALITY

Descriptive terms that reflect the effectiveness or quality of a research effort include *validity, accuracy, precision,* and *reliability.*

The "truth" of research lies within the *validity* of its collected data. Validity represents the extent to which the process or technique that is being used is measuring what it is supposed to be measuring. Validity is concerned with the *effectiveness of the measuring instrument* [1]. The term *instrument*, as it applies in research, is broadly defined, ranging from survey questionnaires to pieces of scientific equipment.

There are several types of validity. *Face validity* relies on the subjective judgment of the researcher, and involves asking the questions (1) Is the instrument measuring what it is supposed to be measuring? (2) Does the sample being measured adequately represent the behavior or trait being measured? *Criterion validity* uses as an essential component a reliable and valid criterion; that is, a standard against which to measure the results of the instrument that is doing the measuring. Validity can also be expressed as *internal* or *external*, both of which are very important in research. The term *internal validity* refers to causal relationships; that is, did an experimental treatment make (cause) a difference? The term *external validity* refers to the generalizability of the results of the research to a population group that was not studied.

The terms *reliability* and *accuracy* are related because they are both concerned with how close to the "truth" a measurement is. The term *reliability* refers to how accurate is the instrument used to make the measurement, while *accuracy* is a quantitative measure of the instrument's reliability. Accuracy is expressed as the difference between the measured values of an instrument and the true values [13]. The more accurate a measurement, the closer is the result to the true value. This concept can be illustrated by the use of a sundial as an instrument for telling time. It is a reliable timepiece if one is only concerned with whether the time of day is early afternoon or late afternoon. However, the sundial has poor reliability for more precise timing such as informing the observer as to when to turn on the television to see a favorite show, or when to leave to catch a bus. In both of these cases, the sundial's accuracy—that is, the quantitatively expressed nearness of the measured time to the true time—is poor.

The term *precision* is a very useful expression of the consistency or repeatability of multiple analyses performed on the same sample or subject. Procedures used in research should generate the same data from the same sample with repetition. For example, multiple assays of serum glucose performed on the same serum sample provide an indication of the precision of the instrument used. It is important to understand the difference between precision and accuracy. A method may be highly precise—that is, replicate values may be very close to one another—yet it may not be accurate. In contrast, widely disparate replicate values—that is, poor precision—might yield an accurate *average* value. However, imprecise measurements are not a property of quality research.

INITIATION OF RESEARCH

The only prerequisite for initiation of research is an inquiring mind. The novice is likely to be intimidated by reports of sophisticated research that has required expensive equipment, extensive personnel, and a generous budget. Not all research needs to be conducted at this level; it can be simple and inexpensive while still serving the purpose of broadening the knowledge base.

Initiation of research requires familiarity with the characteristics of research. These characteristics are shown in Table 17.7. The first characteristic suggests that research begins with a question—that is, why does something occur, or what causes something? Second, research demands that the problem be identified and stated clearly. Research requires a plan. It seeks direction through hypotheses. Research deals with data and their meaning. And research is circular, as shown previously in Figure 17.1.

To be certain that all these characteristics are included in a research project, the following four steps should be followed [5].

1. Select the research topic or problem to be solved. Selection of a topic or problem narrow enough to be manageable often can be difficult. A review of published literature in relation to the selected research topic is necessary to have a basis on which to build present research, and to help to precisely define the research.

2. State clearly the question to be researched. Components of the question include *who (which)*, that is, the subjects or units being assessed are identified; *what*, that is, the factor of interest is stated specifically; *how assessed*, that is, the outcome to be assessed is stated specifically [5,20].

3. Prepare a research plan/proposal. The proposal should include

    a. A statement of the research question (from step 2)
    b. A review of literature (from step 1)
    c. The significance of the research

d. A description of research design, which should specify the specifics of the investigation (that is, methods, data analysis, and the appropriate statistical analysis).

Putting the plan in writing forces the researcher to think through all aspects of the investigation and can serve as a clearly defined guide for carrying out the project. The plan becomes a working document that can be converted into the research report [5].

Depending on the level of the research, the plan may range from a simple outline to a complicated, detailed request for funding from a foundation or government agency. Regardless of the level of investigation, whenever live subjects are used, established guidelines must be followed. Review of proposed research projects by committees on ethical standards ensures that procedures are acceptable. These committees exist in academic institutions at the departmental and university level. Funding agencies and organizations are very careful about considering only those proposals that strictly adhere to these guidelines.

4. Plan for the collection and preparation of data. Once the method for data collection has been selected (or designed), a pilot study can point out any adjustments that need to be made in the data collection method. The pilot study may also provide a good indication of the value of the data being collected. Improvements in research design often result from a pilot study.

Once the research procedures have been refined, the planning stage is finished, and the research study can be conducted. Carrying out the research involves the collection of data, followed by the crucial step of interpreting the data, and reporting the results. The problem that initiated the research finally is addressed, and results of the investigation are interpreted in the framework of existing theory and past research, if such is attainable. The problem is either solved, or the process must begin again [1,5].

Many valuable outcomes are possible from even the simplest research projects if they are well planned. An interest in problem solving coupled with a diligence in planning an orderly, stepwise progression in problem solution provides the essentials for scientific inquiry.

EVALUATION OF RESEARCH AND SCIENTIFIC LITERATURE

Evaluation, like initiation, of research also requires familiarity with the characteristics of research (Table 17.7). The library research paper cannot be considered research because it is not gathering "new" data or using existing data for a "new" purpose. The research paper, however, does involve the selection and transfer of existing information, and therefore, requires careful evaluation of scientific literature. Table 17.8 lists some questions that may be helpful in identifying published research reports (articles) that possess the characteristics described in Table 17.7. The type of publication in which the research article is published is also important. Publication in a "peer reviewed" or refereed journal in-

---

TABLE 17.7 Characteristics of Research

1. *Research begins with a question* in the mind of the researcher—Why?, What is the cause of that?, or similar questions are the point at which research begins.
2. *Research demands identification of a problem,* stated in clear, unambiguous terms. At the very beginning of research, a statement sets forth exactly what the ultimate goal of the research is.
3. *Research requires a plan.* The whole research effort must be governed by a purposeful design.
4. *Research deals with the main problem through appropriate subproblems.* The researcher needs to recognize the integral components within the larger problem and then to divide the main problem into its subproblems. Resolution of all the subproblems results in the solution of the primary research problem.
5. *Research seeks direction through appropriate hypotheses and is based on obvious assumptions.* Hypotheses are conjectural suppositions or reasonable guesses generated from background information. The data gathered and their interpretation will determine whether or not the suppositions are valid or invalid. Assumptions are conditions that are taken for granted and without which the research effort would be impossible.
6. *Research deals with data and their meaning.* Data must be collected and organized into meaningful aggregates so that they can be analyzed and interpreted. The significance of the data depends upon the way they are interpreted. Research begins when the investigator interprets the accumulated data so that it has meaning for the problem that initiated the research in the first place. The data to be gathered determine the research method that is chosen, and legitimate interpretation of the data often requires expert statistical design.
7. *Research is circular.* The problem that initiated the research finally is addressed with the interpretation of the gathered data. The problem is either solved, or the process must begin over again. Even though the initial problem may be resolved, its resolution always gives rise to further unexplored questions.

Source: Adapted from Leedy PD. Practical research: Planning and design, 2nd ed. New York: Macmillan, 1980:4–7.

dicates that the article has been reviewed by some of the researcher's peers to determine its worth for publication. Peer review helps enhance the quality of a research publication. However, it is not a guarantee of a high-quality study.

Although most quality research articles appear in refereed journals, many excellent invited reviews from prestigious investigators may appear in other journal publications, such as *Nutrition Today*, *Nutrition in Clinical Practice*, or *Contemporary Nutrition*. These reviews are not original research but are summaries of research in a particular area (subject) and are based on information formerly published in refereed journals. The information in review articles is secondhand, and thus may have become somewhat distorted because of the imperfections inherent to communication [1]. Review articles, however, can be extremely helpful in providing an overview of some particular topic. When specifics are important, the original report should always be consulted.

PROBLEMS AND PITFALLS IN RESEARCH

In general, a clear understanding of the steps or components of the research process provides a good checklist against which to evaluate research presented in publications or to plan one's own research study. Attention to these components also provides a guide against problems and pitfalls that can plague research.

The logical progression of components in the research process has been discussed earlier in the chapter under "Initiation of Research" and has been reproduced in checklist form in Table 17.8. A complete plan for this logical progression of the elements of the research process, including the question, research design, and exact statistical analysis, should be in place before any research activity begins. If this is done, then the research study will in fact be following a predetermined protocol, in a manner similar to a National Aeronautics and Space Administration (NASA) launch.

Despite the best-laid plans, there are some problems that can occur during a research study. As summarized in an editorial by Vaisrub [26], problems that can be considered as either "soluble" or "insoluble" may arise in the course of a research study. Examples of such problems are given in Table 17.9.

One of the more difficult and error-prone areas of research is the application of statistics in the analysis of data. In view of the magnitude of the subject, data analysis is not addressed in this chapter. However, excellent pertinent references are available to the interested reader [27–29].

SUMMARY

This chapter has identified characteristics of research, noted the process for evaluating scientific literature, and identified problems that can plague a research study. It also has described methodologies used in research, giving examples of nutrition-related research in which various methodologies were used.

Certainly one chapter cannot provide sufficient depth of information for performing outstanding research. Study and course work in the various elements of the research process, as well as apprenticeship to a more experienced investigator, are normally required. It is

TABLE 17.8 Checklist for the Evaluation of Research

1. Is the central problem for research (and its subproblems) clearly stated?
2. Does the research evidence plan and organization?
3. Has the researcher stated his or her hypotheses?
4. Are the hypotheses related to the principal problem or the subproblems of the research?
5. Are the assumptions stated? Are these assumptions realistic for the research undertaken?
6. Is the research methodology that has been employed clearly stated?
7. If the research is of experimental design, was it *in vivo* or *in vitro* work? If *in vivo*, were humans or animals used? Was there a control group? What was the sex, number, and age of experimental (and control) subjects? What was the length of the experiment? Was there sufficient number of subjects and/or sufficient time allowed to warrant meaningful conclusions?
8. Is the statistical treatment of data clearly defined and statistics presented in a straightforward manner?
9. Are the conclusions that the researcher presents justified by the facts presented?
10. Is there any indication whether the hypotheses are supported or rejected?
11. Are limitations of the study identified?
12. Is there any reference to or discussion of related literature or studies by other investigators?
13. Are specific areas for further research suggested?
14. By whom was the research sponsored? Could results be influenced in any way by the source of funding?

TABLE 17.9 Commonly Encountered Problems in Research

Insoluble problems in studies
  Lack of representative sampling
  Vague target population definition with poor selection of subjects
  Lack of random allocation of treatments
  Lack of proper handling of confounding (nuisance) variables
  Lack of appropriate controls
  Lack of blinded subjects and evaluators
  Lack of objective measurement or assessment of outcome
Possibly soluble problems in studies
  Inadequate assurance of group comparability
  Inappropriate choice of sample units
  Use of calculated normal limits for skewed distributions; multiple significance testing
  Incorrect denominators for rates, risks, or probabilities
  Misuse and incorrect presentation of age data
  Improper handling of problems arising from incomplete follow-up in longitudinal studies
  Spurious associations between diseases or between a disease and apparent risk factors
  Ambiguity concerning descriptive statistics used
  Improper handling of nonnormal data
  Unnecessary categorization of continuous variable values
  Incorrect use of the terms *incidence* and *prevalence*
  Inadequate information on reliability checks
  Absence of confidence intervals for percentage data
  No assurance regarding choice of sample sizes
  Finally, trivial differences judged statistically significant based on large sample sizes, with no evaluation of clinical significance

hoped, however, that the material offered in the chapter, together with the supplemental references, have at least armed the reader with new insight as to proper research protocol, and imparted a higher level of confidence to become a more critical reviewer of the literature.

Expansion of the nutrition knowledge base depends on ongoing nutrition research at every level. Knowledge about the total human depends on research at the molecular, cellular, organ or tissue, and system levels. Examples of research at different levels have been given in this chapter and throughout the book.

References Cited

1. Leedy PD. Practical research: Planning and design, 2nd ed. New York: Macmillan, 1980.
2. Lusk G. The basics of nutrition. New Haven, CT: Yale University Press, 1923.
3. McCollum EV. A history of nutrition. Boston: Houghton Mifflin, 1957.
4. Taylor CM, Pye OF. Foundations of nutrition, 6th ed. New York: Macmillan, 1966.
5. Touliatos J, Compton N. Research methods in human ecology and home economics. Ames: Iowa State University Press, 1988.
6. Rose WC. The amino acid requirements of adult man. Nutr Abst Rev 1957;27:631–647.
7. Young VR. 1987 McCollum Award lecture. Kinetics of human amino acid metabolism: Nutritional implications and some lessons. Am J Clin Nutr 1987;46:709–725.
8. Turner, JH. The structure of sociological theory, 4th ed. Homewood, IL: Dorsey, 1986.
9. Young VR, Scrimshaw NS. Endogenous nitrogen metabolism and plasma free amino acids in young adults given a "protein free" diet. Br J Nutr 1968;22:9–20.
10. Young VR, Hussein MA, Murray E, et al. Plasma tryptophan response curve and its relation to tryptophan requirements in young adult men. J Nutr 1971;101:45–60.
11. Ozalp I, Young VR, Nagchaudhuri J, et al. Plasma amino acid response in young men given diets devoid of single essential amino acids. J Nutr 1972;102:1147–1158.
12. Young VR, Toutisrin K, Ozalp I, et al. Plasma amino acid response and amino acid requirements in young men: Valine and lysine. J Nutr 1972;102:1159–1170.
13. Monsen ER, Cheney CL. Research methods in nutrition and dietetics: Design, data analysis, and presentation. J Am Diet Assoc 1988;88:1047–1065.
14. Terris M, ed. Goldberger on pellagra. Baton Rouge: Louisiana State University Press, 1964.
15. Pyle RL, Mitchell JE, Eckart ED. Bulimia: A report of 34 cases. J Clin Psychiatry 1981;42:60–64.
16. Sedlet KL, Ireton-Jones CS. Energy expenditure and the abnormal eating pattern of a bulimic: A case report. J Am Diet Assoc 1989;89:74–77.
17. U.S. Department of Health, Education and Welfare. Ten-state nutrition survey, 1968–1970. Washington, DC: U.S. Government Printing Office, 1972.
18. National Center for Health Statistics. Plan and operation of the health and nutrition examination survey. Rockville, MD: U.S. Department of Health and Human Services, 1975.

19. Frisancho RA. New standards of weight and body composition by frame size and height for assessment of nutritional status of adults and the elderly. Am J Clin Nutr 1984;40:808–809.

20. Burr ML. Epidemiology for nutritionists. 1. Some general principles. Hum Nutr Appl Nutr 1983;34A:259–264.

21. Keys A, ed. Coronary heart disease in seven countries. Circulation 1970;41(suppl. 1):1–211.

22. Gordon T, Kannel WB. Premature mortality from coronary heart disease. The Framingham Study. JAMA 1971;215:1617–1625.

23. Armstrong ML, Warner ED, Connor WE. Regression of coronary atheromatosis in rhesus monkeys. Circ Res 1970;27:59–67.

24. Lipid Research Clinics Program: The Lipid Research Clinics Coronary Primary Prevention Trial Results. I. Reduction in incidence of coronary heart disease to cholesterol lowering, and II. The relationship of reduction in incidence of coronary heart disease to cholesterol lowering. JAMA 1984;251:351–364,365–374.

25. Lowering blood cholesterol to prevent heart disease. Consensus Conference. JAMA, 1985;253:2080–2086.

26. Vaisrub N. Manuscript review from a statistician's perspective (editorial). JAMA 1985;253:3145–3147.

27. Daniel WW. Biostatistics: A foundation for analysis in the health sciences, 4th ed. New York: Wiley, 1987.

28. Remington RD, Schork MA, Johnson RA, Wichern DW, eds. Statistics and applications to the biological and health sciences, 2nd ed. Englewood Cliffs, NJ: Prentice Hall, 1985.

29. Altman DG, Gore SM, Gardner MJ. Statistical guidelines for contributors to medical journals. Br Med J 1983;286:1489–1493.

Suggested Reading

Touliatos J, Compton NH. Research methods in human ecology/home economics. Ames, IA: Iowa State University Press, 1988.
This is an excellent up-to-date book on the "how-tos" of applied research.

Monsen ER, Cheney CL. Research methods in nutrition and dietetics: Design, data analysis and presentation. J Am Diet Assoc 1988;88:1047–1065.
This extremely useful article can serve as a guide for students who are learning the mechanics of research as well as for practitioners in the field of nutrition. Practical examples of research that could be conducted inexpensively in the work setting are given.

The Surgeon General's Report on Nutrition and Health. DHHS (PHS) publication no. 88-50210. Washington, DC: U.S. Government Printing Office, 1988.
This 725-page report includes extensive evidence for the relationship between nutrition and several chronic diseases. Results of research reported to support evidence of relationship are based on a wide array of studies: dietary studies, experiments with laboratory animals, genetic and metabolic research, and epidemiologic studies. Issues of special priority for continuing research are listed after discussion of each disease.

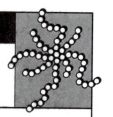

Fatty Acids and CHD: A Story Unfolds

As indicated in this chapter, research is considered to develop as a circular process. However, it may more realistically be considered a helix than a circle [1]. The helix concept of research pictures the process as a spiral, continuing progressively onward as the solution to one research problem gives rise to other unanswered questions [1]. Research dealing with the relationship of dietary fatty acids to the development of CHD (coronary heart disease) is a fitting example of the helical concept of research.

Research conducted by international epidemiologists during the years following World War II consistently revealed relationships among diet, serum cholesterol level, and CHD [2,3]. A connection between high plasma cholesterol levels and the incidence of CHD was well documented during that time, and research then began to focus on the influence of various dietary lipids on plasma cholesterol levels. Two researchers who vigorously investigated the relationship between habitual fat intake and serum cholesterol were Keys and his associates [4] and Hegsted and his associates [5]. They studied this relationship by comparing a series of different fats for their effect on total plasma cholesterol concentrations. In their analysis of the results, they attempted to quantify the relative effects of saturated fatty acids, polyunsaturated fatty acids (linoleic acid), and oleic acid on the plasma cholesterol level [6]. Although working separately, they both came to approximately the same conclusion, which was expressed in the following equation, designated as the Keys equation [7]:

$$\Delta C = 2.7\Delta S - 1.35\Delta P + 1.5Z^{1/2}$$

where ΔC is the change in plasma cholesterol; ΔS and ΔP are the changes in the percentages of dietary calories provided by saturated and polyunsaturated fatty acids, respectively; and Z is the mg of dietary cholesterol/1,000 kcal. The monounsaturates (oleic acid) were assigned a neutral role; that is, they had no effect and were used as a baseline by which to compare other fatty acids. Relative to oleic acid, the saturated fatty acids raised cholesterol while the polyunsaturated fatty acids lowered it, but the saturated acids raised total cholesterol about twice as much as linoleic acid lowered it. These relationships among these three classes of fatty acids in their effect on plasma cholesterol were accepted from the time of this research (late 1950s and early 1960s) until quite recently. People suffering from hypercholesterolemia have been advised to restrict cholesterol intake while adjusting fat intake so that the ratio of polyunsaturated fatty acids to saturated acids is at least 1:1. However, the knowledge on which certain assumptions were based in the earlier studies has since been proven shallow, as the research spiral continues. For example, polyunsaturated fatty acid effects had been equated primarily to the effects of linoleic acid feeding, and the saturated fatty acids (C12:0 through C18:0) were considered to be quite similar in their cholesterol-elevating effect. The similarity is implied in the Keys equation, which makes no distinction among the various saturated fatty acids regarding their effect on cholesterol levels.

New information from a variety of sources has caused a re-examination of this classic view of the relation of various fatty acids to CHD:

- Research was carried out to discover why CHD was absent in Greenland Eskimos despite their high intake of fat, very little of which is polyunsaturated [8]. This research revealed that the principal polyunsaturated fatty acids in the Eskimo diet were omega-3 fatty acids—eicosapentaenoic acid (EPA) and docosahexaenoic acid (DHA)—and that they were metabolized differently from the omega-6 fatty acids (linoleic and arachidonic). No longer could all polyunsaturates be considered equal. (α-Linolenic acid, also an omega-3 fatty acid, is found in small amounts of certain plant products and can be converted slowly in the body to EPA and DHA.)

  How omega-3 fatty acids provide protection against CHD is unclear, but their inhibition of platelet aggregation and their anti-inflammatory effect are considered important reasons for their protective action [9,10]. Their protective effect probably is not related to their influence on plasma cholesterol, because that influence is variable [3].

- The discovery that the low-density lipoprotein (LDL) fraction is the atherogenic fraction while high-density lipoproteins (HDL) are antiatherogenic has made it necessary to re-examine the effects of the various fats on serum cholesterol. It became apparent that research needed to focus more on the distribution of cholesterol between these fractions rather than on total cholesterol. During the course of stud-

PERSPECTIVE   (continued)

ies on the effect of polyunsaturated fatty acids (primarily linoleic acid) on the cholesterol fractions, it was discovered that not only was the LDL cholesterol lowered but, to some extent, so was the HDL cholesterol. Therefore, the beneficial effect (lower LDL) of the polyunsaturates was partially offset by their HDL-lowering property. The HDL-lowering effect of polyunsaturates was particularly noticeable when these fatty acids were administered in large amounts [6]. It has been reported that polyunsaturated fats may reduce the HDL fraction by inhibiting the synthesis of apolipoprotein A-I, the major protein of that fraction [11].

- Interest in the cholesterolemic effects of the mono-unsaturated fats began to develop, probably spurred by the negative (HDL-lowering) aspects of certain polyunsaturates. Early indications as to the favorable effects of the monounsaturates arose through observations made in the Seven Countries Study [2] showing that Cretan men were virtually free of CHD although they habitually consumed a diet in which 40% of the calories was provided by fat. Usually a diet this high in fat is accompanied by a high incidence of CHD. One striking feature of the Cretan diet was its high content of the monounsaturate oleic acid, due to generous intakes of olive oil [6,12]. Studies into the effect of oleic acid on the total plasma cholesterol and its fractions have revealed that when oleic acid replaces saturated fat, it lowers total plasma cholesterol and LDL cholesterol while having little effect on the level of HDL cholesterol. Rather than being neutral in its effect, oleic acid therefore appears to rival the polyunsaturates in its cholesterol-lowering effect when it is substituted for saturated fatty acids in the diet [6,12]. Although the mechanism by which the polyunsaturates and oleic acid lower plasma cholesterol is unclear, it is believed that in their replacing the saturated fatty acids, the polyunsaturates and monounsaturates inhibit the suppressing effect of the saturates on LDL receptor activity.

- Additional findings that challenge the classic view of the relationship between fatty acids and CHD involve the varied effects of different saturated fatty acids on plasma cholesterol. Recent studies clearly show that the C12:0 through C18-0 fatty acids are not equivalent in this property. Since cocoa butter, which is high in stearic acid (C18:0), had been shown to not increase plasma cholesterol as much as other saturated fatty acids (lauric, C12:0; myristic, C14:0; or palmitic, C16:0), Bonanome and Grundy [13] studied the metabolic effects of stearic acid on

plasma lipoprotein levels in 11 human subjects. Rather than raising total plasma cholesterol and LDL cholesterol, stearic acid actually caused a decrease in their levels. These investigators concluded that stearic acid was comparable to oleic acid in its plasma cholesterol-lowering effect when it replaced palmitic acid in the diet. Because the oleic acid content of plasma triacylglycerols and cholesteryl esters increased significantly during the period of high stearic acid intake, the investigators suggested that stearic acid was being converted rapidly to oleic acid, which, in turn, exerted its cholesterol-lowering effect. This positive impact of stearate has been reinforced by other recent reports [14] that it more favorably affects plasma lipids and factor VII coagulant activity, compared to the C12:0–C16:0 saturates. Reaction to reports on the possible cholesterol-lowering effect of stearic acid has been quick. Much more research on stearic acid metabolism is being urged before it is assumed that this saturated fatty acid acts like oleic acid or the polyunsaturates in the body [15]. There is concern that new foods containing generous amounts of stearic acid will be engineered and promoted on their cholesterol-lowering action.

Research on the cholesterolemic effects of the shorter chain saturates—lauric (C12:0), myristic (C14:0), and palmitic (C16:0) acids—has become very active. In comparison to stearic acid [13] and lauric acid [16], palmitate appeared to reduce cholesterol values less effectively than either of the other two. This negative impact of palmitate is compounded by the fact that it is the most heavily consumed saturated fatty acid in a typical diet. In other studies, however, palmitate appears to be less villainous than an ingested combination of laurate and myristate. In a double-blind, cross-over study, it was found that palmitic acid lowered plasma cholesterol in normocholesterolemic males to a greater extent than an equal caloric intake of laurate and myristate consumed in combination [17].

And so the spiral continues!

As truth is discovered, we all reap the benefits. The particular studies presented in this "Perspective" section illustrate this. These investigations, together with others that will assuredly follow, may ultimately reveal to us a diet's ideal lipid component, one that minimizes our risk for cardiovascular disease, and improves our chance for a longer and healthier life.

References Cited

1. Leedy PD. Practical research: Planning and design, 2nd ed. New York: Macmillan, 1980.

PERSPECTIVE (continued)

2. Keys A, ed. Coronary heart disease in seven countries. Circulation 1970;41(suppl. 1):1–211.
3. Kris-Etherton PM, Krummel D, Dreon D, et al. The effect of diet on plasma lipids, lipoproteins, and coronary heart disease. J Am Diet Assoc 1988;88: 1373–1400.
4. Keys A, Anderson JT, Grande F. Prediction of serum cholesterol responses of man to changes in fats in the diet. Lancet 1957;2:959–966.
5. Hegsted DM, McGandy RB, Myers ML, et al. Quantitative effects of dietary fat on serum cholesterol in man. Am J Clin Nutr 1965;17:281–295.
6. Grundy SM. Monounsaturated fatty acids, plasma cholesterol, and coronary heart disease. Am J Clin Nutr 1987;45:1168–1175.
7. Keys A, Anderson JT, Grande F. Serum cholesterol response to changes in the diet IV. Particular saturated fatty acides in the diet. Metabolism 1965; 14:776–87.
8. Bang HO, Dyerberg J, Nielsen AB. Plasma lipid and lipoprotein pattern in Greenlandic West Coast Eskimos. Lancet 1971;1:1143–1145.
9. Mehta J, Lopez LM, Wargovich, T. Eicosapentaenoic acid: Its relevance in atherosclerosis and coronary artery disease. Am J Cardiol 1987;59:155.
10. Leaf A, Weber PC. Cardiovascular effects of n-3 fatty acids. N Engl J Med 1988;318:549–557.
11. Shepherd J, Packard CJ, Patsch JR, Gotto AM Jr., Taunton OD. Effect of dietary polyunsaturated and saturated fat on the properties of high density lipoproteins and the metabolism of apolipoprotein A-1. J Clin Invest 1978;60:1582–92.
12. Mattson FH. A changing role for dietary monounsaturated fatty acids. J Am Diet Assoc 1989;89:387–391.
13. Bonanome A, Grundy SM. Effect of dietary stearic acid on plasma cholesterol and lipoprotein levels. N Engl J Med 1988;318:1244–1248.
14. Tholstrup T, Marckmann P, Jespersen J, Sandstrom B. Fat high in stearic acid favorably affects blood lipids and factor VII coagulant activity in comparison with fats high in palmitic or high in myristic and lauric acids. Am J Clin Nutr 1994;59:371–377.
15. Green MH. A perspective on dietary fats, plasma cholesterol and atherosclerosis. Nutr Today 1989; 24:6–8.
16. Denke MA, Grundy SM. Comparison of effects of lauric acid and palmitic acid on plasma lipids and lipoproteins. Am J Clin Nutr 1992;56:895–898.
17. Sundram K, Hayes KC, Siru OH. Dietary palmitic acid results in lower serum cholesterol than does a lauric-myristic acid combination in normolipemic humans. Am J Clin Nutr 1994;59:841–846.

RECOMMENDED DIETARY ALLOWANCES 1989

Food and Nutrition Board, National Academy of Sciences—National Research Council Recommended Dietary Allowances,[a] Revised 1989

Category	Age (years) or Condition	Weight[b] (kg)	Weight[b] (lb)	Height[b] (cm)	Height[b] (in)	Protein (g)	Fat-Soluble Vitamins Vitamin A (µg RE)[c]	Vitamin D (µg)[d]	Vitamin E (mg α-TE)[e]	Vitamin K (µg)
Infants	0.0–0.5	6	13	60	24	13	375	7.5	3	5
	0.5–1.0	9	20	71	28	14	375	10	4	10
Children	1–3	13	29	90	35	16	400	10	6	15
	4–6	20	44	112	44	24	500	10	7	20
	7–10	28	62	132	52	28	700	10	7	30
Males	11–14	45	99	157	62	45	1,000	10	10	45
	15–18	66	145	176	69	59	1,000	10	10	65
	19–24	72	160	177	70	58	1,000	10	10	70
	25–50	79	174	176	70	63	1,000	5	10	80
	51+	77	170	173	68	63	1,000	5	10	80
Females	11–14	46	101	157	62	46	800	10	8	45
	15–18	55	120	163	64	44	800	10	8	55
	19–24	58	128	164	65	46	800	10	8	60
	25–50	63	138	163	64	50	800	5	8	65
	51+	65	143	160	63	50	800	5	8	65
Pregnant						60	800	10	10	65
Lactating	1st 6 months					65	1,300	10	12	65
	2nd 6 months					62	1,200	10	11	65

[a]The allowances, expressed as average daily intakes over time, are intended to provide for individual variations among most normal people as they live in the United States under usual environmental stresses. Diets should be based on a variety of common foods in order to provide other nutrients for which human requirements have been less well defined.

[b]Weights and heights of reference adults are actual medians for the U.S. population of the designated age, as reported by FHANES II. The median weights and heights of those under 19 years of age were taken from Hamill et al. (1979). The use of these figures does not imply that the height-to-weight ratios are ideal.

[c]Retinol equivalents. 1 retinol equivalent = 1 µg retinol or 6 µg β-carotene. See text for calculation of vitamin A activity of diets as retinol equivalents.

[d]As cholecalciferol. 10 µg cholecalciferol = 400 IU of vitamin D.

[e]α-tocopherol equivalents. 1 mg d-α tocopherol = 1 α-TE. See text for variation in allowances and calculation of vitamin E activity of the diet as α-tocopherol equivalents.

Sources: Recommended dietary allowances 10th ed., © 1989 by the National Academy of Sciences, National Academy Press, Washington, DC. Also Hamill PVV, Drizd TA, Johnson CL, Reed RB, Roche AF, Moore WM. Physical growth: National Center for Health Statistics percentiles. Am J Clin Nutr 1979;32:607–629.

Recommended Dietary Allowances (continued)

Age (years) or Condition	Water-Soluble Vitamins							Minerals						
	Vitamin C (mg)	Thiamin (mg)	Riboflavin (mg)	Niacin (mg NE)f	Vitamin B6 (mg)	Folate (µg)	Vitamin B12 (µg)	Calcium (mg)	Phosphorus (mg)	Magnesium (mg)	Iron (mg)	Zinc (mg)	Iodine (µg)	Selenium (µg)
0.0–0.5	30	0.3	0.4	5	0.3	25	0.3	400	300	40	6	5	40	10
0.5–1.0	35	0.4	0.5	6	0.6	35	0.5	600	500	60	10	5	50	15
1–3	40	0.7	0.8	9	1.0	50	0.7	800	800	80	10	10	70	20
4–6	45	0.9	1.1	12	1.1	75	1.0	800	800	120	10	10	90	20
7–10	45	1.0	1.2	13	1.4	100	1.4	800	800	170	10	10	120	30
11–14g	50	1.3	1.5	17	1.7	150	2.0	1,200	1,200	270	12	15	150	40
15–18g	60	1.5	1.8	20	2.0	200	2.0	1,200	1,200	400	12	15	150	50
19–24g	60	1.5	1.7	19	2.0	200	2.0	1,200	1,200	350	10	15	150	70
25–50g	60	1.5	1.7	19	2.0	200	2.0	800	800	350	10	15	150	70
51+ g	60	1.2	1.4	15	2.0	200	2.0	800	800	350	10	15	150	70
11–14h	50	1.1	1.3	15	1.4	150	2.0	1,200	1,200	280	15	12	150	45
15–18h	60	1.1	1.3	15	1.5	180	2.0	1,200	1,200	300	15	12	150	50
19–24h	60	1.1	1.3	15	1.6	180	2.0	1,200	1,200	280	15	12	150	55
25–50h	60	1.1	1.3	15	1.6	180	2.0	800	800	280	15	12	150	55
51+h	60	1.0	1.2	13	1.6	180	2.0	800	800	280	10	12	150	55
Pregnant	70	1.5	1.6	17	2.2	400	2.2	1,200	1,200	320	30	15	175	65
Lactatingi	95	1.6	1.8	20	2.1	280	2.6	1,200	1,200	355	15	19	200	75
Lactatingj	90	1.6	1.7	20	2.1	260	2.6	1,200	1,200	340	15	16	200	75

fNE (niacin equivalent) is equal to 1 mg of niacin or 60 mg of dietary tryptophan.

gA male in that age group.

hA female in that age group.

i1st 6 months.

j2nd 6 months.

Estimated Safe and Adequate Daily Dietary Intakes of Selected Vitamins and Minerals[a]

Category	Age (years)	Vitamins Biotin (μg)	Pantothenic Acid (mg)
Infants	0–0.5	10	2
	0.5–1	15	3
Children and adolescents	1–3	20	3
	4–6	25	3–4
	7–10	30	4–5
	11+	30–100	4–7
Adults		30–100	4–7

Category	Age (years)	Trace Elements[b] Copper (mg)	Manganese (mg)	Fluoride (mg)	Chromium (μg)	Molybdenum (μg)
Infants	0–0.5	0.4–0.6	0.3–0.6	0.1–0.5	10–40	15–30
	0.5–1	0.6–0.7	0.6–1.0	0.2–1.0	20–60	20–40
Children and adolescents	1–3	0.7–1.0	1.0–1.5	0.5–1.5	20–80	25–50
	4–6	1.0–1.5	1.5–2.0	1.0–2.5	30–120	30–75
	7–10	1.0–2.0	2.0–3.0	1.5–2.5	50–200	50–150
	11+	1.5–2.5	2.0–5.0	1.5–2.5	50–200	75–250
Adults		1.5–3.0	2.0–5.0	1.5–4.0	50–200	75–250

[a]Because there is less information on which to base allowances, these figures are not given in the main table of RDA and are provided here in the form of ranges of recommended intakes.

[b]Since the toxic levels for many trace elements may be only several times usual intakes, the upper levels for the trace elements given in this table should not be habitually exceeded.

CALCULATION OF AVAILABLE DIETARY IRON

Three factors are involved in the calculation of the amount of iron absorbed from a meal:

1. The amount of iron that is heme iron and the amount that is nonheme

2. The amount of vitamin C consumed in the meal

3. The amount of meat, fish, or poultry (MFP) consumed in the meals

Based on these three factors, meals may be classed as high availability, medium availability, or low availability, as shown here:

A *high-availability meal* would be one containing

- 90 g lean raw MFP (about 69 g cooked)
- or 75 mg of ascorbic acid
- or 30 g MFP *plus* 25 mg ascorbic acid

Absorption of nonheme iron from a high-availability meal would be 8% for the individual with iron stores of 500 mg.

A *medium-availability meal* would be one containing either

- 30 to 60 g lean raw MFP (about 23 to 46 g cooked)
- or 25 to 75 mg of ascorbic acid

Absorption of nonheme iron from a medium-availability meal would be 5% for the individual with iron stores of 500 mg.

A *low-availability meal* would be one containing

- less than 30 g lean raw MFP (about 23 g cooked)
- or less than 25 mg of ascorbic acid

Absorption of nonheme iron from a low-availability meal would be 3% for the individual with iron stores of 500 mg.

Heme iron is found only in meat, fish, and poultry, but only 40% of the iron in these foods is *heme*; the other 60% is nonheme. Absorption of heme iron is not variable like nonheme iron but can be calculated at 23% of available heme iron. For example, 3 oz sirloin steak supplies 3.3 mg iron, 40% of which (1.3 mg) is heme iron and the rest of which is nonheme (2.0 mg). Therefore the heme iron absorbed would be 1.3 mg × 23% or 0.3 mg. The amount of the total nonheme iron in the meal that is absorbed is dependent on how the meal is classified. As indicated, in a high-availability meal nonheme iron has an average absorbability of 8%, whereas in one of low availability only 3% of the nonheme iron is absorbed.

Table B.1 demonstrates the calculation of available iron from a typical day's intake.

TABLE B.1 Calculation of Available Iron from a Typical Day's Intake

Time of	(1) Food/beverage (in meal/snack groupings)	(2) Weight (g)	(3) MFP[a] Iron (mg)	(4) Other[b] Iron (mg)	(5) Ascorbic Acid (as served) (mg)	(6) MFP (g)	(7) Availability of Meal Iron H M L	(6) Available MFP Iron (mg)	(9) Available Other Iron (mg)	(10) Total Available Iron (mg)
7:30 A.M.	Oatmeal, 1 cup	240	—	1.4	—	—				
	Brown sugar, 1 T	9	—	0.3	—	—				
	Milk, 1 cup	245	—	0.1	2	—				
	Orange juice, 6 oz	187	—	0.2	90	—				
	Wheat toast, 1 slice	21	—	0.8	—	—				
	Honey, 1 T	21	—	0.1	—	—				
	Subtotals		0	2.9	92	0	✓	0	0.23	0.23
10:30 A.M.	Coffee, 1 cup	180	—	0.2	—	—				
	Subtotals		0	0.2	0	0	✓	0	0.01	0.01
1:00 P.M.	Tuna sandwich									
	Tuna, 1½ oz	45	0.9	—	—	45				
	Wheat bread, 2 slices	50	—	1.6	—	—				
	Carrot sticks	50	—	0.3	4	—				
	Radishes	50	—	0.5	12	—				
	Banana	200	—	1.0	14	—				
	Subtotals		0.9	3.4	30	45	✓	0.13	0.27	0.40
4:00 P.M.	Coffee	180	—	0.2	—	—				
	Peanuts	10	—	0.2	—	—				
	Subtotals		0	0.4	0	0	✓	0	0.01	0.01
6:45 P.M.	Pork loin chop, lean with fat, 3 oz	85	3.0	—	—	85				
	Baked potato, 1	202	—	1.1	31	—				
	Green peas, ½ cup	80	—	1.5	10	—				
	Tossed salad	80	—	1.6	6	—				
	Applesauce, ⅔ cup	170	—	0.9	2	—				
	Gingersnaps, 3	21	—	0.5	—	—				
	Subtotals		3.0	5.6	49	85	✓	0.42	0.45	0.87
10:00 P.M.	Hot cocoa, 1 cup	250	—	1.0	0.3	—				
	Subtotals		0	1.0	0.3	0	✓	0	0.03	0.03
	Total available iron									1.55

Total available iron = 1.6 mg

[a]MFP: Meat, fish, or poultry.
[b]Other iron: All food iron except MFP iron.

Source: Monsen, ER. Simplified method for calculating available dietary iron. Food & Nutr. News 1980;51. © Food & Nutr. News, Natl. Live Stock and Meat Bd.

FORMS FOR ESTIMATING TOTAL ENERGY EXPENDITURE

TABLE 1 Minutes Spent at Each Energy Level

Clock Time	Total Minutes	Activity	Energy Level[a]							
			a	b	c	d	e	f	g	h
7:00–7:45	45	Dressing			23	22				
7:45–8:15	30	Eating		26	4					
8:15–9:00	45	Bike to school			4	25	16			
Total										

[a]See Table 15.2, p. 472, for explanation of energy level.

Source: Whitney E, Cataldo C. Understanding normal and clinical nutrition. St. Paul: West, 1983;255.

TABLE 2 Energy Cost for Activities (exclusive of basal metabolism and the effect of food)

Energy Level	Total Minutes Spent	Energy Cost per Minute (kcal/kg/min)					Total Energy Cost per kg (kcal/kg)
			(women)		(men)		
a		×	0.000		0.000	=	0.000
b		×	0.001 −0.007	or	0.003 −0.012	=	
c		×	0.009 −0.016	or	0.014 −0.022	=	
d		×	0.018 −0.035	or	0.023 −0.040	=	
e		×	0.036 −0.053	or	0.042 −0.060	=	
f		×	0.055	or	0.062		

Subtotal 1,440
Extra energy spent on stairs:

Flights down		+	0.012		=	
Flights up		+	0.036		=	

Total kcal/kg/24 hours
Now multiply by body weight (kg)
to arrive at   × _____

Total energy spent on activities for the day: = [   ]
                                                                                                                      kcal/day

Source: Whitney E, Cataldo C. Understanding normal and clinical nutrition. St. Paul: West, 1983;257.

TABLE 3 Estimation of Total Energy Expenditure

A. Calculate energy spent on basal metabolism using the factor
   1 kcal/kg/hour (for men) or 0.9[a] kcal/kg/hour (for women).

   _____ kcal/kg/hour × _____ kg × 24 hours   =   A. _____ kcal (round off to whole number)

B. Transfer from Table 2 the total kilocalories you spent on muscular
   activities in 24 hours exclusive of basal metabolism.   B. _____ kcal (round off to whole number)
C. To approximate thermic effect of food (TEF), add A + B and take 10% of the total:

   (A _____ kcal + B _____ kcal) × 0.10   C. _____ kcal (round off to whole number)

Total energy expenditure for 24 hours = A + B + C   =   _____ kcal
This is your personalized "RDA" for energy.

[a]0.9 kcal is used for women rather than the 1 kcal/kg body weight used for men because of the higher percentage of body fat in women.
Source: Whitney E, Cataldo C. Understanding normal and clinical nutrition. St. Paul: West, 1983;258.

FOOD EXCHANGE LISTS

STARCH AND BREAD LIST

Each item in this list contains approximately 15 g of carbohydrate, 3 g of protein, a trace of fat, and 80 calories. Whole-grain products average about 2 g of fiber per serving. Some foods are higher in fiber. Those foods that contain 3 g or more of fiber per serving are identified with the symbol *.

You can choose your starch exchanges from any of the items on this list. If you want to eat a starch food that is not on this list, the general rule is that

- ½ cup of cereal, grain, or pasta is one serving
- 1 oz of a bread product is one serving

Your dietitian can help you be more exact.

Cereals/Grains/Pasta

Bran cereals, concentrated*	⅓ cup
Bran cereals, flaked* (such as Bran Buds,® All Bran®)	½ cup
Bulgur (cooked)	½ cup
Cooked cereals	½ cup
Cornmeal (dry)	2½ T
Grapenuts	3 T
Grits (cooked)	½ cup
Other ready-to-eat unsweetened cereals	¾ cup
Pasta (cooked)	½ cup
Puffed cereal	1½ cup
Rice, white or brown (cooked)	⅓ cup
Shredded wheat	½ cup
Wheat germ*	3 T

Dried Beans/Peas/Lentils

Beans and peas* (cooked) (such as kidney, white, split, blackeye)	⅓ cup
Lentils (cooked)*	⅓ cup
Baked beans*	¼ cup

Starchy Vegetables

Corn*	½ cup
Corn on cob, 6 in. long*	1
Lima beans*	½ cup
Peas, green* (canned or frozen)	½ cup
Plantain*	½ cup
Potato, baked	1 small (3 oz)
Potato, mashed	½ cup
Squash, winter (acorn, butternut)	¾ cup
Yam, sweet potato, plain	⅓ cup

*3 grams or more of fiber per serving

The Exchange Lists are the basis of a meal planning system designed by a committee of the American Diabetes Association and The American Dietetic Association. While designed primarily for people with diabetes and others who must follow special diets, the Exchange Lists are based on principles of good nutrition that apply to everyone. © 1986 American Diabetes Association, Inc., American Dietetic Association.

Bread

Bagel	½ (1 oz)
Bread sticks, crisp, 4 in. long × ½ in.	2 (⅔ oz)
Croutons, low fat	1 cup
English muffin	½
Frankfurter or hamburger bun	½ (1 oz)
Pita, 6 in. across	½
Plain roll, small	1 (1 oz)
Raisin, unfrosted	1 slice (1 oz)
Rye, pumpernickel*	1 slice (1 oz)
Tortilla, 6 in across	1
White (including French, Italian)	1 slice (1 oz)
Whole wheat	1 slice (1 oz)

Crackers/Snacks

Animal crackers	8
Graham crackers, 2½ in square	3
Matzo	¾ oz
Melba toast	5 slices
Oyster crackers	24
Popcorn (popped, no fat added)	3 cups
Pretzels	¾ oz
Rye crisp, 2 in × 3½ in	4
Saltine-type crackers	6
Whole-wheat crackers, no fat added (crisp breads, such as Finn®, Kavli®, Wasa®	2–4 slices (¾ oz)

Starch Foods Prepared with Fat

(Count as 1 starch/bread serving, plus 1 fat serving.)

Biscuit, 2½ in across	1
Chow mein noodles	½ cup
Corn bread, 2-in cube	1 (2 oz)
Cracker, round butter type	6
French-fried potatoes, 2 in to 3½ in long	10 (1½ oz)
Muffin, plain, small	1
Pancake, 4 in across	2
Stuffing, bread (prepared)	¼ cup
Taco shell, 6 in across	2
Waffle, 4 ½-in square	1
Whole-wheat crackers, fat added (such as Triscuits®)	4-6 (1 oz)

MEAT LIST

Each serving of meat and substitutes on this list contains about 7 g of protein. The amount of fat and number of calories varies, depending on what kind of meat or substitute you choose. The list is divided into three parts based on the amount of fat and calories: lean meat, medium-fat meat, and high-fat meat. One ounce (one meat exchange) of each of these includes:

	Carbohydrate (g)	Protein (g)	Fat (g)	Calories
Lean	0	7	3	55
Medium-fat	0	7	5	75
High-fat	0	7	8	100

You are encouraged to use more lean and medium-fat meat, poultry, and fish in your meal plan. This will help decrease your fat intake, which may help decrease your risk for heart disease. The items from the high-fat group are high in saturated fat, cholesterol, and calories. You should limit your choices from the high-fat group to three (3) times per week. Meat and substitutes do not contribute any fiber to your meal plan.

Tips

1. Bake, roast, broil, grill, or boil these foods rather than frying them with added fat.

2. Use a nonstick pan spray or a nonstick pan to brown or fry these foods.

3. Trim off visible fat before and after cooking.

4. Do not add flour, bread crumbs, coating mixes or fat to these foods when preparing them.

5. Weigh meat after removing bones and fat, and after cooking. Three ounces of cooked meat is about equal to 4 ounces of raw meat. Some examples of meat portions are:

2 oz meat (2 meat exchanges) =
  1 small chicken leg or thigh
  ½ cup cottage cheese or tuna

3 oz meat (3 meat exchanges) =
1 medium pork chop
1 small hamburger
½ of a whole chicken breast
1 unbreaded fish fillet
cooked meat, about the size of a deck of cards

6. Restaurants usually serve prime cuts of meat, which are high in fat and calories.

Lean Meat and Substitutes

(One exchange is equal to any one of the following items.)

Beef:	USDA Good or Choice grades of lean beef, such as round, sirloin, and flank steak; tenderloin; and chipped beef†	1 oz
Pork:	Lean pork, such as fresh ham; canned, cured or boiled ham; canadian bacon†, tenderloin	1 oz
Veal:	All cuts are lean except for veal cutlets (ground or cubed). Examples of lean veal are chops and roasts	1 oz
Poultry:	Chicken, turkey, cornish hen (without skin)	1 oz
Fish:	All fresh and frozen fish	1 oz
	Crab, lobster, scallops, shrimp, clams (fresh or canned in water†)	2 oz
	Oysters	6 medium
	Tuna† (canned in water)	¼ cup
	Herring (uncreamed or smoked)	1 oz
	Sardines (canned)	2 medium
Wild game:	Venison, rabbit, squirrel	1 oz
	Pheasant, duck, goose (without skin)	1 oz
Cheese:	Any cottage cheese	¼ cup
	Grated parmesan	2 T
	Diet cheeses† (with less than 55 calories/oz)	1 oz
Other:	95% fat-free luncheon meat	1 oz
	Egg whites	3 whites

†All foods that have 400 mg or more of sodium per exchange are indicated with this symbol.

	Egg substitutes with less than 55 calories/¼ cup	¼ cup

Medium-Fat Meat and Substitutes

(One exchange is equal to any one of the following items.)

Beef:	Most beef products fall into this category. Examples are all ground beef, roast (rib, chuck, rump), steak (cubed, porterhouse, T-bone), and meatloaf	1 oz
Pork:	Most pork products fall into this category. Examples are chops, loin roast, Boston butt, cutlets.	1 oz
Lamb:	Most lamb products fall into this category. Examples are chops, leg, and roast.	1 oz
Veal:	Cutlet (ground or cubed, unbreaded)	1 oz
Poultry:	Chicken (with skin), domestic duck or goose (well drained of fat), ground turkey	1 oz
Fish:	Tuna† (canned in oil and drained)	¼ cup
	Salmon† (canned)	¼ cup
Cheese:	Skim or part-skim milk cheeses, such as	
	Ricotta	¼ cup
	Mozzarella	1 oz
	Diet cheeses† (with 56–80 calories/oz)	1 oz
Other:	86% fat-free luncheon meat†	1 oz
	Egg (high in cholesterol, limit to 3/week)	1
	Egg substitutes with 56–80 calories/¼ cup	¼ cup
	Tofu (2½ in × 2¾ in × 1 in)	4 oz
	Liver, heart, kidney, sweetbreads (high in cholesterol)	1 oz

High-Fat Meat and Substitutes

Remember, these items are high in saturated fat, cholesterol, and calories and should be used only three (3) times per week. (One exchange is equal to any one of the following items.)

Beef:	Most USDA Prime cuts of beef, such as ribs, corned beef†	1 oz
Pork:	Spareribs, ground pork, pork sausage† (patty or link)	1 oz

Lamb:	Patties (ground lamb)	1 oz
Fish:	Any fried fish product	1 oz
Cheese:	All regular cheeses[†], such as American, blue, cheddar, Monterey, Swiss	1 oz
Other:	Luncheon meat[†], such as bologna, salami, pimento loaf	1 oz
	Sausage[†], such as Polish, Italian	1 oz
	Knockwurst, smoked	1 oz
	Bratwurst[†]	1 oz

| Frankfurter[†] (turkey or chicken) | 1 frank (10/lb) |
| Peanut butter (contains unsaturated fat) | 1 T |

Count as one high-fat meat plus one fat exchange:

| Frankfurter[†] (beef, pork, or combination) | 1 frank (10/lb) |

VEGETABLE LIST

Each vegetable serving on this list contains about 5 g of carbohydrate, 2 g of protein, and 25 calories. Vegetables contain 2 to 3 g of dietary fiber. Vegetables that contain 400 mg of sodium per serving are identified with a [†] symbol.

Vegetables are a good source of vitamins and minerals. Fresh and frozen vegetables have more vitamins and less added salt. Rinsing canned vegetables will remove much of the salt.

Unless otherwise noted, the serving size for vegetables (one vegetable exchange) is

• ½ cup of cooked vegetables or vegetable juice

• 1 cup of raw vegetables

Artichoke (½ medium)

Asparagus

Beans (green, wax, italian)

Bean sprouts

Beets

Broccoli

Brussels sprouts

Cabbage, cooked

Carrots

Cauliflower

Eggplant

Greens (collard, mustard, turnip)

Kohlrabi

Leeks

Mushrooms, cooked

Okra

Onions

Pea pods

Peppers (green)

Rutabaga

Sauerkraut[†]

Spinach, cooked

Summer squash (crookneck)

Tomato (one large)

Tomato/vegetable juice[†]

Turnips

Water chestnuts

Zucchini, cooked

Starchy vegetables such as corn, peas, and potatoes are found on the Starch/Bread List.

For free vegetables, see Free Food List on page 000.

FRUIT LIST

Each item on this list contains about 15 g of carbohydrate and 60 calories. Fresh, frozen, and dried fruits have about 2 g of fiber per serving. Fruits that have 3 g or more of fiber per serving have a * symbol. Fruit juices contain very little dietary fiber.

The carbohydrate and calorie content for a fruit serving are based on the usual serving of the most commonly eaten fruits. Use fresh fruits or fruits frozen or canned without sugar added. Whole fruit is more filling than fruit juice and may be a better choice for those who are trying to lose weight. Unless otherwise noted, the serving size for one fruit serving is

- ½ cup of fresh fruit or fruit juice
- ¼ cup of dried fruit

Fresh, Frozen, and Unsweetened Canned Fruit

Apple (raw, 2 in across)	1 apple
Applesauce (unsweetened)	½ cup
Apricots (medium, raw) or	4 apricots
Apricots (canned)	½ cup, or 4 halves
Banana (9 in long)	½ banana
Blackberries (raw)*	¾ cup
Blueberries (raw)*	¾ cup
Cantaloupe (5 in across) (cubes)	⅓ melon 1 cup
Cherries (large, raw)	12 cherries
Cherries (canned)	½ cup
Figs (raw, 2 in across)	2 figs
Fruit cocktail (canned)	½ cup
Grapefruit (medium)	½ grapefruit
Grapefruit (segments)	¾ cup
Grapes (small)	15 grapes
Honeydew melon (medium) (cubes)	⅛ melon 1 cup
Kiwi (large)	1 kiwi
Mandarin oranges	¾ cup
Mango (small)	½ mango
Nectarine (1½ in across)*	1 nectarine

Orange (2½ in across)	1 orange
Papaya	1 cup
Peach (2¾ in across)	1 peach, or ¾ cup
Peaches (canned)	½ cup, or 2 halves
Pear	½ large, or 1 small
Pears (canned)	½ cup or 2 halves
Persimmon (medium, native)	2 persimmons
Pineapple (raw)	¾ cup
Pineapple (canned)	⅓ cup
Plum (raw, 2 in across)	2 plums
Pomegranate*	½ pomegranate
Raspberries (raw)*	1 cup
Strawberries (raw, whole)*	1¼ cup
Tangerine (2½ in across)	2 tangerines
Watermelon (cubes)	1¼ cup

Dried Fruit

Apples*	4 rings
Apricots*	7 halves
Dates	2½ medium
Figs*	1½
Prunes*	3 medium
Raisins	2 T

Fruit Juice

Apple juice/cider	½ cup
Cranberry juice cocktail	⅓ cup
Grapefruit juice	½ cup
Grape juice	⅓ cup
Orange juice	½ cup
Pineapple juice	½ cup
Prune juice	⅓ cup

MILK LIST

Each serving of milk or milk products on this list contains about 12 g of carbohydrate and 8 g of protein. The amount of fat in milk is measured in percent (%) of butterfat. The calories vary, depending on what kind of milk you choose. The list is divided into three parts based on the amount of fat and calories: skim/very low fat milk, low-fat milk, and whole milk. One serving (one milk exchange) of each of these includes

	Carbohydrate (g)	Protein (g)	Fat (g)	Calories
Skim/very low fat	12	8	Trace	90
Low-fat	12	8	5	120
Whole	12	8	8	150

Milk is the body's main source of calcium, the mineral needed for growth and repair of bones. Yogurt is also a good source of calcium. Yogurt and many dry or powdered milk products have different amounts of fat. If you have questions about a particular item, read the label to find out the fat and calorie content.

Milk is good to drink, but it can also be added to cereal and to other foods. Add life to plain yogurt by adding one of your fruit servings to it.

Skim and Very Low Fat Milk

Skim milk	1 cup
½% milk	1 cup
1% milk	1 cup
Low-fat buttermilk	1 cup

Evaporated skim milk	½ cup
Dry nonfat milk	⅓ cup
Plain nonfat yogurt	8 oz

Low Fat Milk

2% milk	1 cup fluid
Plain low-fat yogurt (with added nonfat milk solids)	8 oz

Whole Milk

The whole-milk group has much more fat per serving than the skim and low-fat groups. Whole milk has more than 3¼% butterfat. Try to limit your choices from the whole-milk group as much as possible.

Whole milk	1 cup
Evaporated whole milk	½ cup
Whole plain yogurt	8 oz

FAT LIST

Each serving on the fat list contains about 5 g of fat and 45 calories.

The foods on the fat list contain mostly fat, although some items may also contain a small amount of protein. All fats are high in calories and should be carefully measured. Everyone should modify fat intake by eating unsaturated fats instead of saturated fats. The sodium content of these foods varies widely. Check the label for sodium information.

Unsaturated Fats

Avocado	⅛ medium
Margarine	1 t
Margarine, diet‡	1 T
Mayonnaise	1 t
Mayonnaise, reduced-calorie‡	1 T
Nuts and seeds	
Almonds, dry roasted	6 whole

Cashews, dry roasted	1 T
Pecans	2 whole
Peanuts	20 small or 10 large
Walnuts	2 whole
Other nuts	1 T
Seeds, pine nuts, sunflower (without shells)	1 T
Pumpkin seeds	2 t
Oil (corn, cottonseed, safflower, soybean, sunflower, olive, peanut	1 t
Olives‡	10 small or 5 large
Salad dressing, mayonnaise type	2 t
Salad dressing, mayonnaise type, reduced calorie	1 T
Salad dressing (all varieties)‡	1 T
Salad dressing, reduced calorie†	2 T

(Two tablespoons of low-calorie salad dressing is a free food.)

‡If more than one or two servings are eaten, these foods have 400 mg or more of sodium.

Saturated Fats

Butter	1 t
Bacon‡	1 slice
Chitterlings	½ oz
Coconut, shredded	2 T
Coffee whitener, liquid	2 T
Coffee whitener, powder	4 t
Cream (light, coffee, table)	2 T
Cream, sour	2 T
Cream (heavy, whipping)	1 T
Cream cheese	1 T
Salt pork‡	¼ oz

FREE FOODS

A *free food* is any food or drink that contains less than 20 calories per serving. You can eat as much as you want of those items that have no serving size specified. You may eat two or three servings per day of those items that have a specific serving size. Be sure to spread them out through the day.

Drinks:

Bouillon† or broth without fat
Bouillon, low sodium
Carbonated drinks, sugar free
Carbonated water
Club soda
Cocoa powder, unsweetened (1 T)
Coffee/tea
Drink mixes, sugar free
Tonic water, sugar free

Nonstick pan spray

Fruit:

Cranberries, unsweetened (½ cup)
Rhubarb, unsweetened (½ cup)

Vegetables:
(raw, 1 cup)

Cabbage
Celery
Chinese cabbage*
Cucumber
Green onion
Hot peppers
Mushrooms
Radishes
Zucchini*

Salad greens:

Endive
Escarole
Lettuce
Romaine
Spinach

Sweet substitutes:

Candy, hard, sugar free
Gelatin, sugar free
Gum, sugar free
Jam/Jelly, sugar free (2 t)
Pancake syrup, sugar free (1–2 T)
Sugar substitutes (saccharin, aspartame)
Whipped topping (2 T)

Condiments:

Catsup (1 T)
Horseradish
Mustard
Pickles†, dill, unsweetened
Salad dressing, low calorie (2 T)
Taco sauce (1 T)
Vinegar

Seasonings can be very helpful in making food taste better. Be careful of how much sodium you use. Read the label, and choose those seasonings that do not contain sodium or salt.

Basil (fresh)
Celery seeds
Cinnamon
Chili powder
Chives
Curry
Dill

Flavoring extracts (vanilla, almond, walnut, peppermint, butter, lemon, etc)

Garlic

Garlic powder

Herbs

Hot pepper sauce

Lemon

Lemon juice

Lemon pepper

Lime

Lime juice

Mint

Onion powder

Oregano

Paprika

Pepper

Pimento

Spices

Soy sauce[†]

Soy sauce, low sodium ("lite")

Wine, used in cooking (¼ cup)

Worcestershire sauce

GLOSSARY

(ACAT) *acyl coenzyme A: cholesterol acyl transferase* An enzyme forming a cholesterol ester from free cholesterol by attachment of a CoA-activated fatty acid.

(ACP) *acyl carrier protein* A pantothenic acid, protein, thioethanolamine structure upon which fatty acid biosynthesis occurs.

(ADH) *antidiuretic hormone* Conserves body water by increasing water permeability of the distal tubule and collecting duct. Also referred to as vasopressin.

(ADP) *adenosine diphosphate* A dephosphorylated form of adenosine triphosphate, serving as phosphate group acceptor in the adenosine triphosphate energy cycle.

(AMP) *adenosine monophosphate* A dephosphorylated form of adenosine diphosphate sometimes acting as a modulator in metabolic regulation.

(ATP) *adenosine triphosphate* The principal form of stored energy in the body, contained within the phosphate anhydride bonds of the molecule. ATP serves as phosphate donor in the energy cycle of the cell.

(BCAAs) *branched chain amino acids* The amino acids valine, leucine, and isoleucine. A metabolic disorder associated with an inability to catabolize these compounds normally is called maple syrup urine disease.

(BEE) *basal energy expenditure* Equivalent to basal metabolic rate (BMR)

(BMI) *body mass index* A term used in the estimation of ideal body structure, calculated as the body weight divided by the square of the height (W/H^2).

(BMR) *basal metabolic rate* The rate of oxygen consumption of a body at complete rest, long after a meal.

(cAMP) *cyclic 3′, 5′-adenosine monophosphate* An activator of protein kinases in serving as a second messenger in the hormonal stimulation of a cell.

(CCK) *cholecystokinin* A hormone released from the duodenal mucosa, causing contraction of the gall bladder.

(CHD) *coronary heart disease* Impairment of circulation in the vasculature of the heart due primarily to the deposition of arterial fatty plaque. Also referred to as coronary artery disease (CAD).

(CoA) *coenzyme A* A pantothenic acid-containing activator of acyl compounds.

(CoQ) *coenzyme Q* Also called ubiquinone, a carrier of hydrogens and electrons in the mitochondrial electron transport chain.

(CRBP) *cellular retinol-binding protein* A protein capable of binding retinol (vitamin A), located in the absorptive cells of the small intestine.

(DHAP) *dihydroxyacetone phosphate* A phosphorylated triose occurring as an intermediate in the glycolytic pathway. It serves as a precursor for the synthesis of the glycerol portion of triacylglycerols, therefore functioning as an important link between carbohydrate and fat metabolism.

(DNA) *deoxyribonucleic acid* The nuclear polynucleotide ultimately responsible for protein synthesis and the transmittance of genetic information.

($E_0′$) *standard reduction potential* A measure of the relative capacity of a reducing agent to release electrons.

(ECF) *extra cellular fluid* Fluids external to cellular compartments.

(ER) *endoplasmic reticulum* A subcellular particle involved in communication between a cell's nucleus and its exterior.

(FAD) *flavin adenine dinucleotide* A riboflavin-containing coenzyme serving as a hydrogen and electron carrier in certain dehydrogenase reactions.

541

(FADH$_2$) *flavin adenine dinucleotide reduced form*   Flavin adenine dinucleotide (FAD) reduced by its aquisition of hydrogen atoms and electrons.

(FCR) *fractional catabolic rate*   The rate of catabolism of a substance, most commonly pertaining to that of the lipoprotein fractions.

(FIGLU) *formiminoglutamic acid*   An intermediate in the conversion of histidine to glutamic acid. The formation of FIGLU is folate dependent.

(FMN) *flavin mononucleotide*   A nucleotide coenzyme containing riboflavin, functioning as a component of the mitochondrial electron transport chain.

(G) *Gibb's free energy*   An expression of energy, which, upon its release, is capable of doing work.

(GABA) *gamma aminobutyric acid*   A neurotransmitter formed from the decarboxylation of glutamic acid.

(GDP) *guanosine diphosphate*   A dephosphorylated form of GTP, important in the activation of substances participating in the biosynthesis of proteins.

(GIP) *gastric inhibitory peptide*   A peptide hormone inhibiting gastric motility and acid secretion.

(GI tract) *gastrointestinal tract*   The system of the body responsible for the intake, digestion, and absorption of nutrients.

(GLUT) *glucose transporter protein*   These proteins transport glucose across the membranes of certain cell types.

(GRP) *gastrin-releasing peptide*   A neuroactive peptide originating in nerves of the gut, and stimulating the release of gastrin from gastrin cells.

(GSH) *glutathione (reduced)*   See GSSG for description of function.

(GSSG) *glutathione (oxidized)*   A tripeptide containing glutamic acid, cysteine, and glycine. Its sulfhydryl group can undergo reversible oxidation and reduction, allowing the molecule to serve as a sulfhydryl buffer. An important function is to act as a reductant of toxic peroxides through the action of glutathione peroxidase. It is designated GSH in its reduced form.

(GTF) *glucose tolerance factor*   A potentiator of insulin action, comprised of niacin, glutathione, and trivalent chromium.

(GTP) *guanosine triphosphate*   A high energy phosphate-containing compound sometimes used in the activation of other compounds, particularly in protein synthesis processes.

(HANES) *Health and Nutrition Examination Survey*   A survey designed to investigate the nutritional status of the population.

(HDL) *high density lipoprotein*   A plasma lipid/protein complex rich in phospholipid and cholesterol. Considered to be of benefit in reducing the risk of cardiovascular disease.

(HMG CoA) *3-hydroxy 3-methylglutaryl coenzyme A*   An intermediate in the pathway of cholesterol biosynthesis.

(IBW) *ideal body weight*   A parameter useful in determining recommended changes in energy intake and energy expenditure balance.

(ICF) *intracellular fluid*   Fluid within cellular compartments.

(IDDM) *insulin-dependent diabetes mellitus*   A juvenile onset form of diabetes due to pancreatic islet cell injury. Also referred to as type I diabetes.

(IF) *intrinsic factor*   A glycoprotein secreted by the parietal cells of the gastric mucosa, responsible for the absorption of vitamin B$_{12}$.

(IP$_3$) *inositol 1,4,5-triphosphate*   Released from phosphatidyl inositol by hydrolysis, it acts as a second messenger in the release and activation of cellular calcium.

(ISF) *interstitial fluid*   Fluid surrounding extravascular cells, providing a medium for passage of nutrients from the bloodstream to the cells.

(K$_a$) *acid dissociation constant*   Reflects in a direct relationship the strength, ie the proton-releasing tendency, of an acid.

(K$_{eq}$) *equilibrium constant*   Relates the specific concentrations of reactants and products in a chemical reaction at equilibrium.

(K$_m$) *Michaelis constant*   The substrate concentration at which an enzyme shows one half of its maximum velocity.

(LCAT) *lecithin-cholesterol acyltransferase*   An enzyme forming a cholesterol ester from free cholesterol by the transfer of a fatty acid from lecithin.

(LBM) *lean body mass*   The mass of living tissue devoid of all storage fat, allowing for the relatively small amount of essential fat.

(LDL) *low density lipoproteins*   A lipid/protein complex circulating in the plasma, transporting most of the blood cholesterol. This lipoprotein fraction is implicated in the risk of cardiovascular disease.

(LES) *lower esophageal sphincter*   A region of increased tonic pressure just above the juncture of the esophagus and stomach, functioning to prevent gastric reflux.

(LHA) *lateral hypothalmic area*   The hunger center of the hypothalamus.

(LNAAs) *large, neutral amino acids* The branched chain and aromatic amino acids, all of which compete for a common carrier across the blood brain barrier.

(MAO) *monoamine oxidase* An enzyme which reduces neural transmission by inactivating amine neurotransmitters such as serotonin and the catecholamines.

(MEE) *measured energy expenditure* A quantification of expended energy by calorimetry.

(MMC) *migrating motility complex* A series of contractions having several phases moving distally along the stomach and intestinal tract.

(mRNA) *messenger ribonucleic acid* The template for the synthesis of proteins from amino acids. Having nucleotide sequences complementary to DNA nucleotide sequences, it is responsible for carrying the genetic message from the nucleus to the ribosome.

(MSG) *monosodium glutamate* Occasionally used as a flavor-enhancing additive to foods. Alleged to elicit various neurological symptoms in some individuals—the so-called Chinese restaurant syndrome.

(MUFAs) *monounsaturated fatty acids* Fatty acids possessing a single double bond.

(NAD) *nicotinamide adenine dinucleotide* A coenzyme, or cosubstrate, formed from niacin, functioning as carrier of hydrogen atoms and electrons in certain dehydrogenase reactions.

(NADH) *nicotinamide adenine dinucleotide (reduced form)* Nicotinamide adenine dinucleotide (NAD) reduced by the aquisition of a hydrogen atom and electrons from a substrate undergoing oxidation.

(NADP) *nicotinamide adenine dinucleotide phosphate* A coenzyme/cosubstrate functionally like NAD but possessing an additional phosphate group, and having a different enzyme specificity.

(NADPH) *nicotinamide adenine dinucleotide phosphate (reduced form)* Nicotinamide adenine dinucleotide phosphate (NADP) reduced by the acquisition of a hydrogen atom in a dehydrogenase-catalyzed reaction.

(NIDDM) *non-insulin dependent diabetes mellitus* A maturity onset form of diabetes associated with obesity. Referred to as type II diabetes.

(NDpCal%) *net dietary protein calories percent* The percentage of dietary calories contributed by protein.

(NPU) *net protein use* A measure of protein digestibility together with essential amino acid content.

(NSP) *non-starch polysaccharides* Indigestible polysaccharides originating primarily in plant cell walls, and serving as an important component of dietary fiber.

(PEP) *phosphoenolpyruvic acid* A very high energy phosphate-containing compound occurring as an intermediate in carbohydrate metabolism. Its phosphate group can be transferred to ADP, producing ATP, in the process of substrate level phosphorylation of ADP.

(PGI$_2$) *prostaglandin I$_2$* A potent platelet antiaggregative factor formed from arachidonate by cyclo-oxygenase. It is thought to be a factor in the antithrombotic properties of the n-3 polyunsaturated fatty acids. Also referred to as prostacyclin.

(PKU) *phenylketonuria* A metabolic disease caused by a deficiency of the enzyme phenylalanine hydroxylase, resulting in an inability to form tyrosine from phenylalanine.

(PLP) *pyridoxal phosphate* A coenzyme derived from vitamin B$_6$, required in transamination reactions and amino acid decarboxylations.

(PRPP) *5-phosphoribosyl 1-pyrophosphate* An activated form of ribose used in the synthesis of ribose nucleotides.

(PTH) *parathyroid hormone* A hormone intimately involved in calcium homeostasis, acting to conserve the metal and increase its concentration in extracellular fluids.

(PUFAs) *polyunsaturated fatty acids* Fatty acids possessing more than one double bond.

(PVN) *paraventricular nucleus (hypothalamic)* A regulator of the release of pituitary hormones affecting food intake.

(RBC) *red blood cell* Non-nucleated, hemoglobin-enriched blood cells responsible for the transport of oxygen from lungs to tissues.

(RBP) *retinol-binding protein* A protein synthesized in the liver, and, as a complex with a second protein, transthyretin (TTR), is responsible for the plasma transport of retinol.

(RBW) *relative body weight* A body weight index obtained by dividing a person's weight by the midpoint of the weight range for his or her estimated frame size.

(RDA) *recommended dietary allowances* The Food and Nutrition Board's recommendation for daily dietary intake of nutrients.

(RE) *retinol equivalent* A measure of vitamin A activity used in statements of dietary standards. One RE equals 1 µg of retinol or 6 µg of β-carotene.

(REE) *resting energy expenditure* The measurement of metabolic rate while the subject is at rest.

(RER) *rough endoplasmic reticulum* That portion of the endoplasmic reticulum of a cell which is granular due to studding with ribosomes.

(RIA) *radioimmunoassay* A sensitive analytical technique for determining levels of a substance in body fluids, based on specific immunological reactions and the use of a radiolabelled form of the substance being determined.

(RNA) *ribonucleic acid* A polynucleotide, the synthesis of which is directed by DNA. Important in protein synthesis and as a ribosomal structural component.

(RQ) *respiratory quotient* The ratio of the volume of expired CO_2 in a subject to the volume of the consumed O_2.

(SAM) *S-adenosyl methionine* One of the principal methyl group donors in the transfer of single carbon units among metabolic intermediates.

(SER) *smooth endoplasmic reticulum* That portion of the cellular endoplasmic reticulum serving as the site of synthesis of various lipids, and the detoxification of drugs.

(SFA) *saturated fatty acids* Fatty acids possessing no double bonds.

(SOD) *superoxide dismutase* An enzyme protecting against damage from accumulating superoxide radicals by reducing the radicals to hydrogen peroxide and oxygen.

(T₃) *triiodothyronine* A thyroid hormone which, like thyroxin (T_4), is involved in the regulation of metabolic rate. Although occurring at a lower concentration than T_4, its molar activity is more potent.

(T₄) *thyroxin* The major hormone of the thyroid gland, important in the regulation of metabolic rate.

(TBF) *total body fat* A parameter of body composition, related to overall body fitness.

(TBG) *thyroxin-binding globulin* The major protein participating in the plasma transport of thyroxin and triiodothyronine.

(TBW) *total body water* A parameter of body composition sometimes used to estimate lean body mass.

(TDP) *thiamin diphosphate* Commonly called thiamin pyrophosphate (TPP), a coenzyme required in the decarboxylation of certain alpha ketoacids.

(TEE) *thermal effect of exercise* The exercise component of energy expenditure.

(TEF) *thermic effect of food* A component of energy expenditure, estimated to account for 6% to 15% of energy expenditure over the basal metabolic rate.

(TGN) *trans Golgi network* A segment of the Golgi apparatus of the cell.

(THFA) *tetrahydrofolic acid* The reduced form of folic acid, the form in which the compound is capable of acquiring and transferring single carbon units.

(TPN) *total parenteral nutrition* A method of meeting all nutrient requirements by intravenous administration.

(TPP) *thiamin pyrophosphate* An alternative term for thiamin diphosphate (see TDP).

(TSH) *thyroid stimulating hormone* A product of the anterior pituitary gland, stimulating the formation and release of thyroid hormones from the thyroid gland.

(tRNA) *transfer ribonucleic acid* Forms of ribonucleic acid, each specific for the various amino acids with which they attach and then bring to specific ribosomal sites for protein synthesis.

(TTR) *transthyretin* Formerly called prealbumin, this protein binds thyroid hormones and retinol binding protein.

(TXA₂) *thromboxane A₂* Like prostacyclin (PGI₂), an eicosanoid formed from arachidonate by the cyclo-oxygenase pathway, but antagonistic to prostacyclin in being a potent platelet aggregative factor.

(UDP) *uridine diphosphate* A dephosphorylated form of uridine triphosphate (UTP). Involved in activation of intermediates in carbohydrate synthesis.

(UTP) *uridine triphosphate* A high energy phosphate-containing compound used in the activation of certain intermediates in carbohydrate synthesis.

(VIP) *vasoactive intestinal peptide* A neuropeptide (neuro-crine) originating in the nerves of the gut.

(VLDL) *very low density lipoprotein* A triacylglycerol-rich endogenous complex of lipid and protein. Compared to the LDL and HDL fractions, it circulates at a relatively low concentration in the plasma.

(VMN) *ventromedial nucleus* Believed to be the satiety center of the hypothalamus.

(VO₂ₘₐₓ) *maximum oxygen consumption* An exertional workload which places the highest possible demand on a working muscle.

INDEX

Page numbers in italic indicate figures; t following a page number indicates tabular information.

0-314-04467-1

9 780314 044679

90000